Lifelong Motor Development

CARL P. GABBARD, EdD
Texas A&M University

Seventh Edition

Wolters Kluwer

Philadelphia • Baltimore • New York • London
Buenos Aires • Hong Kong • Sydney • Tokyo

Acquisitions Editor: Michael Nobel
Product Development Editor: John Larkin
Editorial Assistant: Tish Rogers
Marketing Manager: Shauna Kelley
Production Project Manager: David Orzechowski
Design Coordinator: Steve Druding
Manufacturing Coordinator: Margie Orzech
Prepress Vendor: Absolute Service, Inc.

Seventh edition

9 8 7 6 5 4 3 2 1
Printed in China

Library of Congress Cataloging-in-Publication Data

Names: Gabbard, Carl, 1948- author.
Title: Lifelong motor development / Carl P. Gabbard.
Description: Seventh edition. | Philadelphia : Wolters Kluwer Health, [2018]
| Includes bibliographical references and index.
Identifiers: LCCN 2016022858 | ISBN 9781496346797
Subjects: | MESH: Human Development | Motor Activity—physiology
Classification: LCC QP301 | NLM WE 103 | DDC 612/.04—dc23 LC record available at https://lccn.loc.gov/2016022858

LWW.com

RRS1607

To the Student

Once again, I want to address you in this special section because I realize not all students are overwhelmed at the notion of reading the preface of a college text. The seventh edition of *Lifelong Motor Development* is a study in one of the most fascinating and relevant subjects you will encounter. What could be more interesting than understanding how we develop and change across the life span—a look back and, perhaps more intriguing, a glance at days to come? This text is a window into the dynamics of one of our most natural, joyful, and important behaviors—movement! You are about to begin a fascinating journey through the study of motor behavior and the marvelous machine that controls it from its prenatal beginnings to older adulthood. Let the journey of a lifetime begin!

Carl Gabbard

P.S. Hints for success—read, know the objectives and key terms, work with a study group, and use the Website resources, especially *thePoint*. That is all there is to it!

Preface

The seventh edition of *Lifelong Motor Development* is the most comprehensive research-based text of its kind. The ***developmental systems perspective*** provides a unique framework for the ***study of change*** in growth and motor behavior across the life span. *Lifelong Motor Development* is the study of coordinated movement and the processes that underscore perception and action. With this approach, students are provided information from multiple perspectives from which a broader and more in-depth understanding of development may be acquired. The developmental systems perspective advocates that development is the product of dynamic interacting processes between the various biological systems and environmental contexts. This approach incorporates, for example, Gibson's ecological theory, dynamic systems theory, the constraints model, and the latest environmental perspectives. All of which are being visualized into one of the most promising "fields" of development study—*Developmental Cognitive Neuroscience*. Furthermore, this edition is deeply rooted in the applied aspects of motor development and how it applies to your chosen career field (e.g., physical/occupational therapy, teaching, coaching, medical professions).

We also wish to note that in addition to information stated as important for future professional school attendees (i.e., medically related), chapter objectives conform to the published *Undergraduate Motor Development Competencies* by the Society for Health and Physical Educators (SHAPE).

WHAT'S NEW TO THIS EDITION?

Students will benefit from a variety of new content and features in the seventh edition, including:

- The text has been streamlined to present information in a more concise manner. This is especially evident in regard to the scientific approaches and theories that explain developmental *change* in physical growth and the processes driving perception to action.
- Expanded *Think About It* questions (margin boxes) that address science and applied aspects of content, many from the contemporary "constraints" model perspective.
- *Focus on Change* notations (boxes) are also found in the margin. These complement the central theme of studying *change* in human motor development by highlighting significant change effects.
- **NEW!** *WebLink* in the margins adjacent to associated discussion. These provide expanded information and video illustrations. In addition, *WebLink* provides access to information as it changes.

  New with this feature are videos of motor behavior across the life span, including access to fundamental motor skills for observation and analysis training.

- **NEW!** Information on special populations and its application to the text has been expanded to a new chapter—*Atypical Motor Behavior*. This section includes commonly observed atypical behavior frequently noted with special populations.
- **NEW!** Updated and new motor assessment instruments, including *TGMD-3* and *BMAT* for older populations.
- **NEW!** Latest information on physical activity patterns, obesity, and physical fitness statistics. *WebLink* provides for updates as new reports are created.
- Expanded *Focus on Application* features highlighting real-world issues and practical observations of relevance to the future professional (e.g., concussions, obesity, hormones, new research discoveries).
- **NEW!** One of the primary objectives with this edition was to expand the number of *Learning Activities* with relevance to likely career avenues, namely, teaching, physical and occupational therapy, coaching, and medicine. *Learning Activities* are found at the end of each chapter and *Supplemental Learning Activities* at *thePoint* Website.
- Accompanying this edition of *Lifelong Motor Development* is access to *thePoint*, http://thepoint.lww.com/gateway. This feature, one of the best in the industry, provides Instructor's Resources that includes updated guidelines for course development, a course outline, chapter objectives and key terms section, *Think About It* questions, *Focus on Change* section, and sample test questions and answer key. Also available is a general PowerPoint presentation offering comprehensive chapter outlines with key points and visuals from the text.

BASIC ORGANIZATION

Lifelong Motor Development presents a topical and chronological approach to the study of human motor development. Although good arguments exist for using either approach entirely, the intent is to provide the student with a multidimensional perspective of *change*. The topical sections offer a rich feel for the interrelatedness of the lifelong developmental process. On the other hand, conceptualizing life-span development within a framework for study and placement of significant events necessitates a "general" time-related continuum; this text provides such a developmental framework.

The basic organization of the text is not different from the previous edition. For first-time users (in brief), *Lifelong Motor Development* is divided into six parts. Part One consists of a single chapter that presents a multidisciplinary overview of lifelong human development with emphasis on basic developmental principles, terms, issues, and theoretical approaches. Also provided is a conceptual model of the phases of motor behavior used as the framework for the material presented in Part Four, "Motor Behavior Across the Life Span." Part Two is devoted to topical discussions on the body of information related to lifelong biological growth and development. Chapters 2, 3, and 4 provide information on the various hereditary, neurological, and physical characteristics that, together with experience, form the bases for motor behavior across the life span. Chapter 5 deals with factors and conditions that may affect the course of biological growth and development.

Chapters 6 and 7 (Part Three) present comprehensive, topical discussions of lifelong perceptual development, and information-processing characteristics, including the latest theories on perception to action. The chapters in Part Four (8 through 11) provide a chronological (phase model) description of motor behavior characteristics across the life span. Coverage begins with early movement behavior (Chapter 8). It extends through early childhood (Chapter 9); later childhood and adolescence (Chapter 10); motor behavior during the adult years characterized by peak performance and, with older age, regression (Chapter 11); and finally, Chapter 12 (new) describes atypical motor behaviors associated with special populations.

Part Five (Chapter 13) offers a broad perspective on the diversity of motor assessment techniques and discusses the considerations for selecting and implementing a wide variety of assessment instruments. Part Six (Chapter 14) presents a discussion of the influence and importance of sociocultural factors on motor development from a lifelong perspective.

PEDAGOGICAL FEATURES

An important goal in creating this text was to make it a teachable resource with an *effective learning system*. Each of the six parts of the text begins with an overview of its content. Included in the introduction of each chapter are *chapter objectives* and *key terms*. The objectives reflect the conceptual framework used by identifying the important facts, topics, and concepts to be covered. Marginal notations are provided to aid the reader in identifying text material related to chapter objectives. Consistent feedback from users suggests that these characteristics are quite useful in developing (customizing) course materials. For example, in some instances, instructors may wish to designate selected (rather than all) chapter objectives for course coverage. This can be especially useful for advanced studies of motor development. **Key terms** appear in boldfaced type in the text and pinpoint the words of greatest importance to understanding the broader concepts of each chapter; these and other significant terms are highlighted (italicized) throughout.

Think About It questions are found in the margins of each chapter with the intent of stimulating critical thinking and active involvement with the subject matter. Like the objectives, they can be used for a variety of instructional purposes.

Focus on Change notations, also found in the margins, are intended to highlight significant characteristics of lifelong change effects.

WebLinks found in the margins and adjacent to the associated discussion. These, too, help clarify and expand on information. They may also be used to assist with assigned learning activities and projects.

Focus on Application features, which highlight real-world issues and practical observations, are found in selected chapters.

A chapter *Summary*, list of *Think About It* questions, *Learning Activities*, and *Suggested Readings* are presented at the end of each chapter. The *Learning Activities* are provided to stimulate interest and expand on chapter content. Additional learning activities are found at *thePoint* student and instructor resource.

Supplements available with the seventh edition of *Lifelong Motor Development* include a Student Quiz Bank, an Instructor's Manual, a PowerPoint presentation with lecture outlines, key figures and tables from the text, Test Generator and Image Bank.

And finally, a much-desired outcome of the seventh edition of *Lifelong Motor Development* is that the reader will feel the excitement associated with studying and understanding human motor development from a life-span perspective.

ACKNOWLEDGMENTS

The seventh edition of *Lifelong Motor Development* is the outcome of much more than my efforts. I am most grateful for the continuous and diligent efforts of the scientific community in providing the knowledge base. Much of the inspiration for creating the seventh edition came from comments of current users, colleagues, and students. Many thanks to the following reviewers: Mike Bamman, Huntington College; Alberty Cordova, University of Texas; Jennifer J. Gorecki, Kent State University; Adam King, Truman State University; Yuhua Li, University of Memphis; Gerard Lyons, Idaho State University; Timothy A. Mirtz, Bethune-Cookman University; Timothy Sawicki, Canisius College; and Sara Winges, Louisiana State University.

With this edition, I also owe a special debt of gratitude to the staff at Wolters Kluwer, specifically Michael Nobel, John Larkin, and Shauna Kelley, for their support and dedication in making this edition the very best text in *Lifelong Motor Development*.

Finally, this edition is dedicated to all the students from the past and present who continue to fuel my desire to contribute to this exciting field of study.

Brief Contents

Contents

part one

An Overview of Lifelong Human Development

Chapter 1: Introduction to the Developmental Perspective

part one presents an overview of lifelong human and motor development, which involves the study of *change* in growth and motor behavior as influenced by biology and the environment. Much of this section focuses on its fundamentals. Basic developmental principles, terms, and theoretical approaches and issues are provided to aid the reader in forming a developmental systems perspective of human development and motor behavior across the life span.

Along with the basic framework of developmental systems, Chapter 1 provides the initial introduction to the ways in which motor development parallels other human experience across the life span. Highlighting this section is a conceptual model of the developmental continuum of life-span motor behavior. This model provides a basis (conceptual framework) for describing and integrating much of the material presented in subsequent chapters.

To complement the continuum, the reader is provided information that addresses one of the most important issues in contemporary motor development: What factors underlie *change* across the life span? In addition to examining change in physical growth, we will explore change in the ability to acquire and maintain coordinated movement, the study of

Perception → Action

Chapter 1

Introduction to the Developmental Perspective

OBJECTIVES

Upon completion of this chapter, you should be able to

1.1 Explain the *developmental systems perspective* and describe its relationship to motor development.

1.2 Define the term *motor development* and describe its association with the life-span perspective.

1.3 Discuss the multidisciplinary approach to studying motor development.

1.4 Briefly describe the five major goals of the developmental specialist.

1.5 Describe the primary determinants of motor development and behavior.

1.6 Define the general terms associated with motor development.

1.7 Discuss and support the major observations (assumptions) associated with human development.

1.8 Outline the periods of life-span development.

1.9 Illustrate and briefly describe the developmental continuum for life-span motor behavior.

1.10 Discuss the purpose of and identify the primary strategies used in conducting research in the scientific study of life-span development.

1.11 Name and describe the major theoretical views and approaches to study human development.

1.12 Identify careers associated with the field of motor development.

KEY TERMS

developmental systems perspective
epigenesis
quantitative change
qualitative change
motor development
life-span perspective
multidisciplinary approach
environmental contexts
affordances
developmentally appropriate
aging
stages
phase
individual differences
critical period
sensitive period
heredity
growth
development
maturation
motor behavior
cephalocaudal development
proximodistal development
plasticity
periods of life-span development
developmental continuum
bioecological systems theory
Gibson's ecological perspective
information-processing view
developmental biodynamics
constraints model

focus on change

The study of human and motor development involves the *changing person* (biology) and his or her *changing environmental context*.

Objective 1.1

As a general philosophy for the study of lifelong human and motor development, this text supports and is firmly grounded in the **developmental systems perspective**. This approach advocates the notion that human development is *the product of changing relations between the developing person and his or her changing multilevel environmental contexts*. A person is a dynamic, self-organizing unit consisting of several systems (e.g., neurological, muscular, skeletal, and cognitive) with multiple levels within each system. Examples of environmental contexts, known as *ecological systems*, include the home, school, culture, and social influences within (e.g., family, peers, and coaches). The interpretation of human development emphasizes the reciprocal interactions between all our biological characteristics and the environment. Closely associated with this line of thought (the developmental systems perspective) is **epigenesis**. This idea is that development is the result of an ongoing, bidirectional interchange between one's biological characteristics (including heredity) and the environment. This view suggests a strong interdependence of heredity and the environment in one's resulting phenotype (observable traits). Prominent theories that complement the systems approach and add to our understanding of lifelong motor development are the focus in this and subsequent chapters. Although the *developmental systems* perspective was introduced over a decade ago (Lerner, 2002), its basic tenets are seen in more contemporary writings (Lerner, 2012), including those that study motor behavior (e.g., Adolph & Robinson, 2015; Gottlieb, 2007; Spencer et al., 2009; Withagen & van der Kamp, 2010). For example, Karen Adolph, one of the leading contemporary infant motor development researchers, states, "This unified 'developmental systems' view of neurobehavioral development emphasizes the multiple resources underlying development and provides a framework for addressing more specific questions about the roots of behavioral change" (Adolph & Robinson, 2013, p. 427).

The study of virtually any aspect of lifelong human development is inquiry into *change*. For change to be labeled developmental, it must have a successive character. For example, changes seen at a later time are at least influenced in part by the changes that occurred earlier. In essence, the study of development implies systematic and successive changes over time.

Developmentalists study two kinds of change: quantitative and qualitative. **Quantitative change** is a change in number or amount, such as height, weight, or reaction time. **Qualitative change** refers to a change in structure or organization, as marked by the emergence of a new behavior—for example, change in the process characteristics of balance and walking.

Objective 1.2

Lifelong motor development is a vital part of the field of human development over the life span. In general terms, **motor development** is the study of change in motor behavior resulting from the interaction of biological processes and the environment.

Basic to a comprehensive understanding of this field of specialization is knowledge related to the characteristics and principles of *growth* (change in size), *development* (change in level of functioning), and *motor behavior* (performance). Closely tied to these terms is *maturation*, which refers to the timing and tempo of progress toward the mature biological state. Underscoring the significance of these terms is the notion that development is not explained by age alone. Although age gives a rough estimate of when a specific behavior appears, it tells little about why a particular behavior emerges at a specific time. Traditionally, this area of inquiry was studied by developmental psychologists primarily interested in the childhood stages of development. In more recent years, however, the scope of motor development has been extended in recognition that the developmental process is continuous and observable from conception to the final stage in human life. This **life-span perspective** is based on the theory that the developmental process extends beyond puberty and young adulthood. Significant physiological and motor behavior changes occur during older adulthood and are important to our understanding of the full scope of human development. Hughes and Noppe (1991) state, "To examine only isolated segments of the life span is equivalent to studying isolated scenes from a film or play" (p. 6).

think about it

Why is it important to have a general understanding of human development in order to gain insight into lifelong motor behavior?

Objective 1.3

Along with the promising trend to view motor development from a life-span perspective has emerged the practice of studying behavioral change using an integrated **multidisciplinary approach**; that is, it is generally accepted that behavior in any domain (cognitive, affective, and psychomotor) is the product of many influences. To have a fuller understanding of human development, one should consider the full range of possible influences. Perhaps the strongest support for this point of view has been seen among those interested in child development from a total development perspective; professionals from such fields as developmental psychology, neuroscience, exercise physiology, medicine, biomechanics, and sociology have provided data adding to our understanding of total human development and behavior.

focus on change

One of the primary goals of the developmentalist is to describe the causes of *change*.

Objective 1.4

Developmental specialists seek to accomplish five major goals: (a) to determine the common and characteristic changes in behavior, function, and appearance across the life span; (b) to establish when these changes occur; (c) to describe what causes these changes; (d) to determine whether change can be predicted; and (e) to find out whether these changes are individual or universal.

THE PRIMARY DETERMINANTS OF MOTOR BEHAVIOR

Objective 1.5

At this point in the discussion, a relevant question is "What determines motor development?" More specifically, what factors influence growth, development, and motor performance across the life span? Figure 1.1 illustrates the interrelated nature of human development as supported by the developmental systems view—that is, how one's biological characteristics (heredity, maturation, and self-organizing properties) interact with environmental contexts (ecological systems and affordances) to determine, in large part, motor development and behavior at any given point in time. Each of these terms is defined in the following pages.

GENERAL TERMINOLOGY

Objective 1.6

As with any specialized field of science or education, motor development has established its own terminology and adopted words from related disciplines. The study of motor development cuts across several disciplines and subareas within the study of movement behavior and therefore uses a considerable amount of the general terminology of these related fields. Familiarity with this terminology will be important in developing a clear understanding of the developmental perspective.

Heredity refers to a set of qualities fixed at birth that accounts for many individual traits and characteristics. The cells of normal humans possess 46 chromosomes arranged in 23 pairs. These chromosomes are made up of thousands of genes that influence such traits as eye and hair color, personality, intelligence, height, muscle fiber type, and general body build. Although these traits are strongly influenced by genetic structure, they may be modified by environmental factors.

Growth, often used interchangeably with development and maturation, refers to observable *changes in quantity*; in this context, growth represents an *increase in body size*. Although maturation may be a factor in the growth process, environmental factors may also contribute.

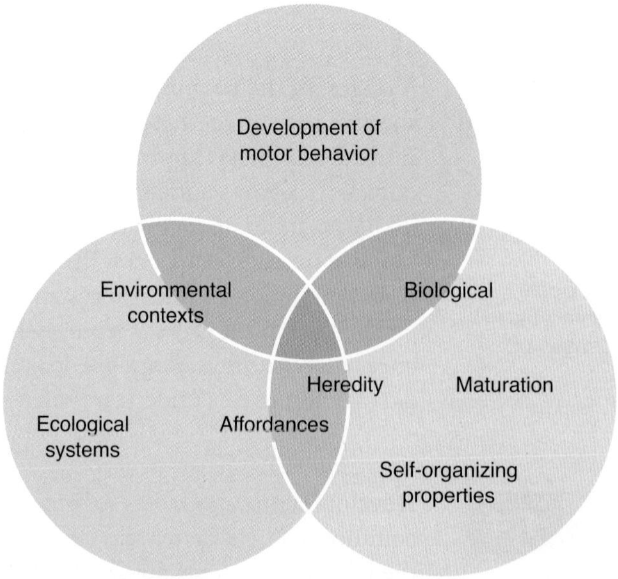

Figure 1.1 The determinants of motor behavior.

Development is a term that can be applied to several human behaviors. Basically, development refers to the process of *change in the individual's level of functioning*. Those changes may be either quantitative or qualitative in nature. Development is a product of growth as well as of heredity, maturation, and experience.

Maturation refers to when specific biological events occur. It is the underlying timetable of developmental events. From another perspective, it is progress toward the mature biological state. Examples are age at menarche (first menstrual flow in females) and the onset of the adolescent growth spurt. As mentioned earlier, maturation is tied to growth, development, and motor behavior, all of which are dynamic processes.

Motor behavior is the product of biological characteristics and environmental influence and refers to observable changes in the learning and performance of a particular movement or motor skill (e.g., balance, walking, and running).

In its purest sense, the term *motor* refers to the underlying biological and mechanical factors that influence movement (or observable action), although the terms *movement* and *motor* are frequently used interchangeably. As noted earlier, motor (or movement) performance is influenced by several integrated factors. Learning, integrated with growth and basic developmental factors, is a primary influence.

Learning is a relatively permanent change in performance resulting from practice or past experience. Although learning cannot be observed directly, it can be inferred from a person's motor performance. The term *motor learning* refers to a relatively permanent change in the performance of a motor skill, also resulting from practice or experience. Another term used frequently in the movement literature is *motor control*, referring to the area of study concerned primarily with the underlying processes involved in movement and how various movements are controlled. The focus of motor control study is on understanding specific neural, physical, and behavioral aspects of human movement.

Cephalocaudal and *proximodistal* are general terms used to describe the rather predictable sequences of growth and motor control. **Cephalocaudal development** is growth that proceeds longitudinally from the head to the feet. Complementing this physical growth is a gradual progression of increased muscular control, moving first from the muscles of the head and neck to the trunk and then to the legs and feet. **Proximodistal development** is growth that proceeds from the center of the body to its periphery—that is, growth and motor control occur in the trunk region and shoulders before the wrists, hands, and fingers. These developmental trends are typically observed in young children who exhibit greater coordination in the upper torso than in their legs and feet (cephalocaudal). Similarly, children will exhibit gross shoulder movements in their first attempts to draw long before their ability to make fine motor cursive forms is developed. As mentioned earlier, these terms reflect general observations; exceptions have been noted. For example, Galloway and Thelen (2004) reported that specific early motor behaviors need not develop in a strict cephalocaudal pattern; this is discussed in more detail in Chapter 8.

Environmental contexts are the circumstances, objects, or conditions by which one is surrounded. A key term related to this general description is *affordances*. **Affordances** are opportunities for action that objects, events, or places in the environment provide. Examples of affordances include toys, stairs in the home, and swimming pools. These affordances provide the stimulus for motor development.

WebLink
http://www.shapeamerica.org/

Developmentally appropriate refers to the instruction (program) and practice of activities appropriate for the level and needs of the individual. For example, the children of a specific kindergarten class very likely have different cognitive, emotional, and physical needs. Although an *age-appropriate* curriculum may fit most 5-year-olds, it does not have individual appropriateness. Refer to the Society of Health and Physical Educators (SHAPE America) WebLink for specific guideline documents.

Experience refers to conditions within the environment that may alter or modify various developmental characteristics through the learning process.

Learning is (as stated earlier) the relatively permanent change in performance that results from practice or past experience.

Readiness is the combination of maturation and experience that prepares an individual to acquire a skill or understanding.

Adaptation is the process of altering one's behaviors to interact effectively with the environment. The term is often used to describe the complex interplay between the individual and the environment.

The scope of motor development includes the study of biological change over the life span; therefore, the term *aging* has relevance to our understanding of the developmental process. **Aging** has been characterized as the deteriorated capacity to regulate the internal environment (e.g., cellular, molecular, and organismic structures), resulting in a reduced probability of survival. It may also be thought of as the process of growing old regardless of chronological age.

SIGNIFICANT OBSERVATIONS (ASSUMPTIONS) ABOUT DEVELOPMENT

Objective 1.7

Now that we have defined the field and talked briefly about primary goals, let's consider some basic assumptions. The following observations concerning human development have direct implications for the study of lifelong motor behavior and guide the general orientation of this text. In past years, and perhaps to some extent today, these points are considered somewhat controversial. However, although the degree of impact for each may be debatable, their presence in the developmental process is evident. Arguably, the most dramatic of observations is the interactive and dynamic roles that nature (biology) and nurture (environment) play in development. This assumption is described in the latter part of this section and represents the pervading theme in this text. Most of the following observations are discussed in greater detail in subsequent chapters.

1. *Human development is a continual and cumulative process from conception through older adulthood.* The only thing that is constant is change. Although development appears and may be described as stagelike at times, its bases are underlined by *continuity* of specific processes. Puberty, for example, although it appears to be an abrupt, discontinuous event, is actually a gradual process occurring over several years. Changes such as these are based on quantitative improvements. For example, as hormonal, neural, and muscle components gradually increase, various functional abilities may then appear such as menarche, walking, exhibiting strength, and coordination. With aging, the various systems steadily transform through periods of maturing and regression of function. Added to this is the daily effect of experience with our environment.

At times, theorists prefer to describe development as distinct stages in the life span. For example, Piaget and Erikson describe development in terms of **stages**, or periods, when common developmental milestones for each of us occur. This concept suggests qualitative differences in how individuals behave (e.g., think, move, and feel) at certain periods in their lives. Underlying this view, it appears that development undergoes rapid changes as one stage ends and a new one begins, which is then seemingly followed by a relatively stable period with minimal transition.

As readers of developmental literature, you will come across other terms in this and other texts that have meanings similar to the concept of stage, such as *sequence* and *phase*. However, in this context, a **phase** (or sequence) may also describe qualitative transitions over time that generally are not strictly affixed to specific age levels. The basic premise is that a specific behavior may be accomplished at varying age levels but generally in the developmental order identified. A phase underscores the relatively continual and overlapping characteristics of development. An example of this is illustrated in the following pages, which present the developmental continuum for motor behavior.

From a research (rather than descriptive) perspective, the problem appears to be one of identifying which developmental processes are controlled by continuous underlying constructs or mechanisms (continuity) and which processes are influenced only when experiential events or environmental forces interact with the individual.

2. *All domains of development are interrelated.* Although developmentalists often look separately at various domains of development (cognitive, perceptual, motor), each domain affects the others. For example, research supports the idea that all skills (including intellectual) are grounded in and supported by perceptual-motor activity.
3. *There is a wide range of individual differences in development.* Each child, from the start, is unique. **Individual differences** constitute the variation in human appearance and behavior. Children of the same age can be significantly different in, for example, height, strength, and motor skill. Heredity and the environment play major roles in our uniqueness.
4. *Environmental context plays a major role in development.* To understand motor behavior at any point in the life span, one must consider the impact of such things as the individual's history, culture, and opportunities for practice (affordances). Environmental context provides the nurturing effect that interacts with human biology (nature) to produce behavior (i.e., epigenesis).
5. *There are critical and sensitive periods in development.* A **critical period** refers to an optimal time for the emergence of certain developmental processes and behaviors. Recent research in early brain development complements this concept by suggesting that windows of opportunity exist in which neural networking (brain wiring) is optimal, based to some extent on environmental stimulation. These findings suggest that the general window of opportunity for critical wiring of movement is through the first 5 to 6 years of life, which has significant implications for early movement experiences and motor development programming. For example, suppose there is an optimal period between 4 and 8 months of age for the infant to acquire basic reach-grasp skills. If this assumption is correct, infants who do not have an opportunity to learn the skill during that critical period may never be as proficient as if they had acquired it during the optimal time period. Another example of a "window of opportunity" is the role of physical activity in bone development. Current research suggests that the most beneficial time for

exercise to pronounce its effect is in the early pubertal period (see Chapter 5). However, it also should be noted that humans have the astonishing ability to display considerable resilience to adverse conditions. For example, some children born into low socioeconomic conditions with lack of proper nutrition, education, and enrichment experiences achieve significant successes in their lives.

Although similar, a **sensitive period** reflects a time in the life span when individuals may be especially sensitive to specific influences. An example is possible exposure to teratogens—agents such as drugs, stress, and alcohol—that can cause fetal malformation. The embryonic and fetal periods have been reported as especially sensitive to teratogens.

6. *Development is aided by positive stimulation.* One of the cardinal principles of developmental psychology is that early experience has a profound effect on human development. An excellent example of this is in reference to research in early brain development. Scientists have found that to achieve the precision of adult neural circuit patterning, the brain must be stimulated. Deprived of a stimulating environment, a child's brain may suffer. Complementing these observations are comments that are rather common among leading researchers in the field, such as "experience is the chief architect of the brain" (Perry, 1997, p. 55). Fortunately for the field of motor development, research also shows that physical activity as a form of stimulation has significant developmental effects on the brain; this applies to older persons as well. This is just one example in the life span of how stimulation affects development. Other strong cases for support have been shown for the effects of exercise on muscle and bone development.
7. *There is much plasticity in human development.* Humans have a dramatic capacity for change, or **plasticity**, in response to positive or negative life experiences at virtually all periods in the life span. This is especially evident with biological characteristics such as neural and bone development. In essence, some structures have the amazing ability to reorganize themselves, thus being somewhat plastic (flexible). Refer to the examples regarding critical and sensitive periods in development that link plasticity to positive and negative experiences such as injury and deprivation. Plasticity is discussed in more depth in Chapter 2.

focus on change

Acquisition and *change* in voluntary movement skill is based on our body's unique self-organizing system.

8. *Motor skill development is a multifaceted, dynamic phenomenon.* A central theme in contemporary motor development research is the idea that development of movement abilities is not tied predominantly to a predetermined (genetic) process that emerges simply as one matures. Becoming motorically skillful is generally a process that reflects the interaction of certain biological traits, environmental influences, and task constraints. An assumption complementing this perspective is that individuals acquire certain skills and behaviors based on the unique dynamics of their *self-organizing properties* and *affordances* provided by the environment. Current views of motor development strongly emphasize the roles of exploration and selection in finding solutions to new task demands.
9. *With advanced aging, it is inevitable that most abilities will regress.* Certain aspects of advanced aging, such as the decline in vision and hearing, loss of muscular strength, and general psychomotor slowing, are undesirable and inevitable. One of the exciting possibilities of development, however, is that certain undesirable aspects may be reversed or modified to be less detrimental in their effects. Scientists are becoming increasingly confident that someday, even purely biological deterioration may be reversed by techniques developed through research and a better understanding of the mechanisms underlying the aging process. Aging takes its toll on almost every facet of physiological function, but the quality of life among individuals can be extremely variable.

As noted earlier, the guiding assumption and pervading theme of this text is that *biology and environmental context play vital interactive roles in development*. Human development stems from the dynamics of biological and environmental systems. This relationship provides the resources for individuals to achieve their potential because the interplay of these factors is unique to each person. In the past, focus appeared more on the issue of nature versus nurture and which has the most influence on development. A common example of this is whether children naturally crawl at 6 months and walk at 12 months because of what they have learned from the environment or because of some unfolding biological process. These are the types of questions on which theories are based. However, after considerable discussion and research, the only possible conclusions are that both nature and nurture contribute to all behavior traits and that the extent of their contribution cannot be specified for any trait. Therefore, it is understanding the interplay of the two factors that is more meaningful.

think about it

What is another example of motor behavior to which both nature and nurture contribute, and how does each effect contribute?

PERIODS OF LIFE-SPAN DEVELOPMENT

Objective 1.8

Closely associated with the life-span approach to studying the various aspects of motor development are designated **periods of life-span development** representing approximate chronological age behavior. The following stages compose the framework for addressing each aspect of motor development.

Prenatal (from Conception to Birth)

This is where the story of human development begins. The *prenatal period* is one of immense physical change that begins with genetic transmission and continues through a number of cellular and structural variations. Development of the embryo and fetus is genetically predetermined, but there are several environmental influences on prenatal development. Significant stages of growth and development within this period are the *embryonic period* (up to 8 weeks) and the *fetal period* (8 weeks to birth).

Infancy (from Birth to 2 Years)

The first month of *infancy* is known as the *neonate period*. This period of development has become a popular area for specialized study because of the possibilities for observing initial motor responses and infant survival characteristics. Infancy is a time of extensive dependency on adults. It also marks the beginning of many motor and psychological activities such as language, symbolic thought, and sensorimotor coordination.

Childhood (from 2 to 12 Years)

Due to the large number of developmental milestones reached during this period, *childhood* is divided into two stages:

1. *Early childhood (from 2 to 6 years)*. This period corresponds roughly to the time in which the child prepares for and enters school. It represents a significant stage in the development of fundamental motor skills, perceptual-movement awareness, and the ability to care for oneself.

2. *Later childhood (from 6 to 12 years).* Sometimes called the *elementary school years*, this is a period of fundamental motor skill refinement and the mastery of certain academic skills. Physical growth slows substantially, and thought processes are usually more concrete than in the adolescent period.

Adolescence (from 12 to 18 Years)

The term *adolescence* comes from the Latin verb *adolescere* which means "to grow into maturity." With this period begin the physical changes relating to one of the major landmarks in human development: puberty. Some of the dramatic changes associated with adolescence are accelerated growth in height and weight, the appearance of secondary sex characteristics, the ability to reproduce, and deepening of the voice. This is also a period in which the degree of logical and abstract thought increases as well as a concern about identity and independence.

Adulthood (18 Years and Older)

The period of *adulthood* has traditionally been subdivided into three stages:

1. Young adulthood (from 18 to 40 years)
2. Middle age (from 40 to 60 years)
3. Older adulthood (60 years and older)

With the increased interest in the physiological and motor behavior changes that take place with aging emerged a greater focus on the characteristics of adults who are from 30 to 70 years and older.

THE DEVELOPMENTAL CONTINUUM

Objective 1.9

Figure 1.2 illustrates the **developmental continuum** of life-span motor behavior by depicting the relationship of behavior to specific age-related stages and phases. The notion of a phase in this context is the relatively continual and overlapping characteristics of human development. Developmental stages are included to complement the overlapping relationship as related to motor behavior characteristics normally associated with chronological age categories. The general premise underlying this model reflects the primary assumption that development involves continuous and cumulative change from conception to older adulthood.

More detailed discussions related to characteristic behaviors associated with each of the phases follow in later chapters of this text. The following is a brief overview of the categories of motor behavior across the life span.

Reflexive/Spontaneous Movement Phase. The *reflexive/spontaneous movement phase* is the span of motor behavior that begins at about the third fetal month and continues after birth into the first year of life. Movements at this phase mirror the relative immaturity of the nervous system. As the system matures, reflexes (involuntary motor responses) and spontaneous movements (stereotypic rhythmic patterns of motion that appear in the absence of any known stimuli) are gradually phased out as voluntary control increases.

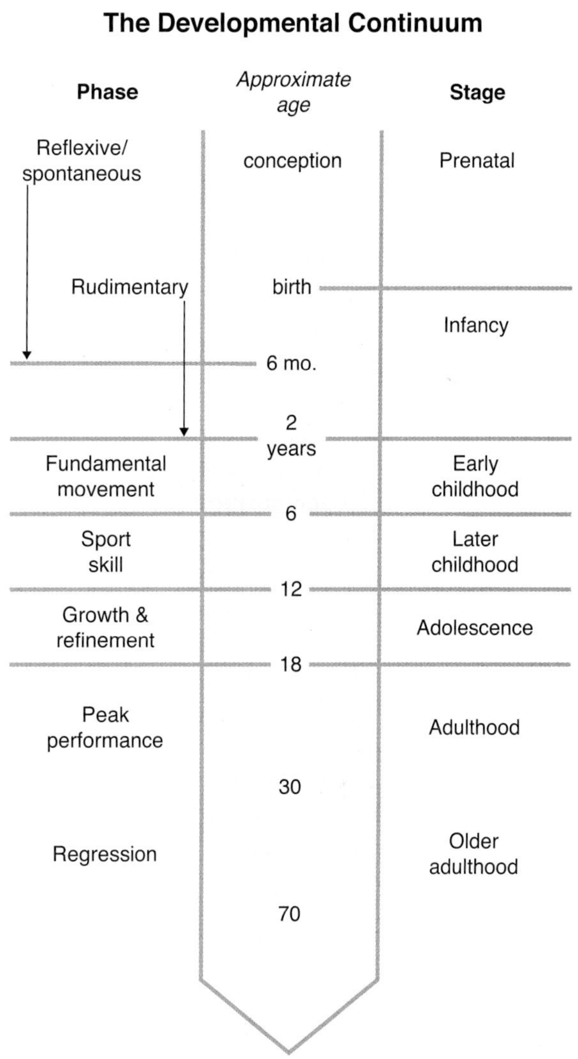

Figure 1.2 The continuum depicts the phases and stages of lifelong motor development.

Rudimentary Phase. The *rudimentary phase* corresponds with the stage of infancy (from birth to 2 years). Rudimentary behavior is voluntary movement in its first form. These movements are determined to a large extent by maturation and appear in a somewhat predictable sequence. Motor control generally develops in a cephalocaudal/proximodistal order and is characterized by such behaviors as crawling, creeping, walking, and voluntary grasping.

Fundamental Movement Phase. The *fundamental movement phase* is acknowledged as a major milestone of early childhood (from 2 to 6 years) and of life-span motor development. Considered an outgrowth of rudimentary behavior, this phase witnesses the appearance of a number of fundamental movement abilities: perceptual-motor awareness (e.g., body awareness and balance), locomotor skills (e.g., running and jumping), nonlocomotor skills (e.g., twisting/turning and stretching/bending), and manipulative skills (e.g., throwing and kicking). These abilities establish the foundation for efficient and more complex human movement in later phases of development. More than 30 characteristic movement skill abilities that emerge during the early childhood period have been identified.

Sport Skill Phase. The motor skills and movement awareness abilities the child acquires during the fundamental movement phase gradually become more refined and, in many instances, adapted to sport and recreational activities in the *sport skill phase*. The primary stimuli during this phase are the individual's increased interest in sport skill events and the ability to learn and practice these movements.

Growth and Refinement Phase. Growth may occur during all periods of development, but perhaps the most significant motor behavior change is seen at the time of puberty and the accompanying growth spurt that generally marks the first stage of adolescence. This is the *growth and refinement phase*. As the levels of hormones rise in the body, changes in muscle and skeletal growth provide a new dimension within which acquired motor skills can be asserted. During the later stages of adolescence, sex differences (mainly favoring males with regard to physical size) become more apparent due primarily to the increased amount of androgen hormones.

Peak Performance. Most sources have identified the time of *peak performance* (peak physiological function and maximal motor performance) to be between 25 and 30 years of age. As a general rule, females tend to mature at the lower end of the range (from 22 to 25 years) and males at the upper end of the range (from 28 to 30 years). This is especially evident in three of the most influential factors in motor performance: strength, cardiorespiratory function, and processing speed.

Regression. Although considerable variation among individuals is apparent after 30 years of age, most physiological and neurological factors decline at a rate of about 0.75% to 1% a year. During this phase, the phenomenon known as *psychomotor slowing* (primarily in speeded tasks) appears, and the earlier developmental process of differentiation begins to reverse, which results in similar performance characteristics among the very young and the older adult. The regression of motor behavior is generally characterized by decreases in cardiovascular capacity, muscle strength and endurance, neural function, flexibility, and increases in body fat. Although exercise training has not been shown to retard the aging process, it does allow the individual to perform at a higher level.

RESEARCH IN MOTOR DEVELOPMENT

Objective 1.10

The study of motor development has emerged as a full-fledged scientific endeavor only in recent years. Although researchers and the medical profession have been concerned with motor development as long ago as the days of Hippocrates, little scientifically designed inquiry was conducted until the 1930s. During that period, psychologists such as Bayley, Shirley, Gesell, Ames, and McGraw interested primarily in child development began to establish the database on which the life-span perspective was later formed. Motor development specialists then began to contribute to the literature, led by the pioneering efforts of such individuals as Wild, Espenschade, Eckert, Rarick, Glassow, Halverson, and Roberton.

Today, researchers across several disciplines are actively involved in the scientific study of growth and motor behavior across the developmental continuum. The science of motor development is supported by millions of dollars in research funds annually, and the results of that research are disseminated through numerous highly respected technical journals and instructional periodicals. Through the efforts of researchers in basic inquiry, educators and parents gain information with which to implement effective educational programs and understand the characteristics of human behavior. An excellent article by Jill Whitall (2009) discusses in some detail the evolution and status of motor development as a field of scientific inquiry (see "Suggested Readings" at the end of this chapter). Esther Thelen, who passed away in 2004, is regarded as the foremost researcher of contemporary motor development. Thelen's work had a major impact on how parents and practitioners view child development. Her work in dynamical systems continues to influence scholars in several disciplines. Several contributions of her work are referenced in this textbook.

WHY STUDY MOTOR DEVELOPMENT?

The importance of studying motor development is tied closely to our need to understand the diverse nature of life and self. From conception until death, physical growth and motor behavior are integral parts of human development.

To fully understand human behavior, we need to gather knowledge of all the determinants of existence. Some important reasons for studying motor development are summarized in the following statements:

1. To interact effectively with other individuals, we need to be aware of what they can and cannot do—motorically, cognitively, and socially.
2. If we understand what constitutes the normal range of motor development, we can better understand and guide individuals who may be developing abnormally.
3. We can use our understanding of motor development to improve health and optimize motor performance.
4. Our understanding of motor development contributes to a more comprehensive body of knowledge that, in turn, enables us to better understand ourselves.

METHODS OF STUDY

Part of the quest to understand motor behavior across the life span is the goal of explaining *change*. We change with age, but we do not change because we get older. Instead, we change because we are affected by the dynamics of the body and environmental influences that occur as we age. So, how can researchers identify the factors related to change? They do this through scientific methods of study.

As mentioned, the study of motor development has evolved into a legitimate and contributing field of research. It is important to have knowledge of the way researchers gather their data for drawing conclusions about the way motor development takes place. Although a discussion of the numerous experimental and statistical techniques is beyond the scope of this text, it helps to have a general understanding of those research designs and data collection methods used most frequently.

As shown in Figure 1.3, investigators use the scientific method to answer questions about human development. For example, the investigator first formulates a *hypothesis*, which is a hunch, guess, or prediction about some aspect of motor development. The hypothesis (or research question) is then tested by collecting evidence in the form of data and analyzing the information to determine whether

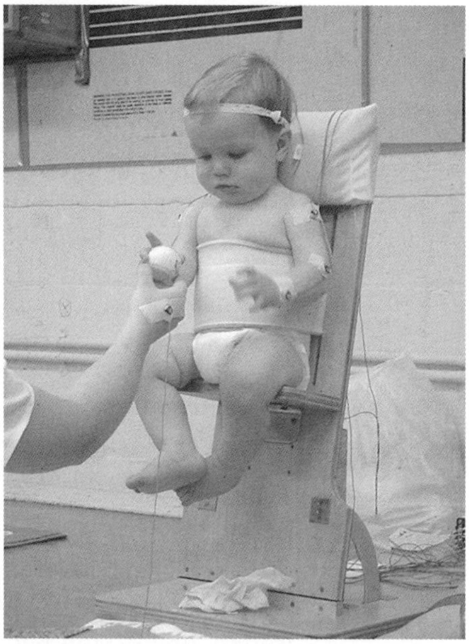

Figure 1.3 Using the scientific method, researchers record kinematics (angle and velocity of movements) during infant reaching.

it supports or rejects the original assumption. In most cases, the study is repeated with different subjects to further confirm the original findings.

In addition to the study of individuals of similar age (e.g., 5-year-olds), a special interest of developmentalists is investigations that focus on the relation of increasing age to some other variable. The primary types of research designs used to address this interest are cross-sectional, longitudinal, microgenetic, and sequential.

Cross-Sectional Design

The vast majority of research studies in motor development have a *cross-sectional design*. Investigators observe age differences by selecting individuals who represent different age groups and measuring their behaviors. In the cross-sectional study, subjects are chosen carefully so individuals in the different age samples are as nearly alike as possible in all ways other than age. The primary value of this design is that it permits a developmental change to be detected in a fairly short period of time. However, it has its limitations. Researchers cannot be certain that the behavioral differences are due to age because individuals and age groups (*cohorts*) grow up under different circumstances, such as those related to education, nutrition, and habits of physical activity. These circumstances are referred to as *cohort effects*.

Longitudinal Design

One of the most popular and perhaps the most reliable type of research designs is the *longitudinal design*. In this method, data are collected on the same individual over an extended period of time, usually across several years. One strength of this design is that development is observed directly and not implied, as with the cross-sectional and cross-cultural methods. It may be one of the best designs, but the

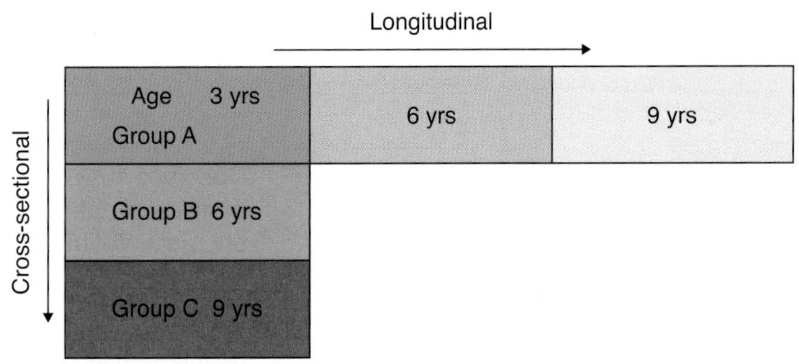

Figure 1.4 Cross-sectional and longitudinal designs.

method has weaknesses. Over a long period of time, subjects may move away, testing personnel may change, and the cost of the study in time and money may be a problem. Repeated testing of the same subjects may also be a problem. The individual's performance may improve with repeated test sessions because of increasing familiarity with the task (the "practice effect") rather than because of increased maturity. The shorter the span of time and the fewer the number of measurement sessions, the easier it is to conduct a longitudinal study. Figure 1.4 compares cross-sectional and longitudinal designs.

Microgenetic Design

A unique modification of the longitudinal approach is the *microgenetic design*. With this approach, change is tracked over a series of sessions from the time it begins until it stabilizes, as subjects master an expected or novel task. This method can be quite effective for observing behavior that emerges over a relatively short period of time, such as specific reflexes and initial infant reaching. It offers the potential for unique insight into the developmental process.

Sequential Design

The *sequential design* offers some improvement over the longitudinal and cross-sectional strategies. This method includes elements from each of these other two designs in that it allows the researcher to study several different-aged samples over a period of years. An advantage of the design is that subjects with different characteristics (e.g., age and background) can be compared at the same chronological age to identify existing behavioral differences. Another advantage is that a study of this type can be conducted in a relatively short span of time. Table 1.1 presents a summary of developmental research design characteristics.

Regardless of the design used, data must be collected. Systematic observation is perhaps the most popular method for collecting data, and it is the basic tool of any science. If researchers wish to focus on naturally occurring spontaneous behavior in a natural setting (e.g., at home, at play, and at school), the method is known as *naturalistic observation*. *Structured observation* requires the researcher to manipulate the environment in some way, as is the case when the study is conducted in a laboratory setting or in a familiar environment in which new elements are presented. Known as the *experimental method*, it is the most powerful design for explaining change by cause and effect.

TABLE 1.1 Strengths and Limitations of Developmental Research Designs

Design	Description	Strengths	Limitations
Cross-sectional	Observes subjects of different ages at one point in time	Detects change in a short period of time	Differences may be distorted because of cohort effect.
Longitudinal	Observes subjects repeatedly at different ages	Shows individual differences in development and relationships between early and later events and behaviors	Age-related changes may be distorted because of biased sampling, subject dropout, and cohort effects; it also can be lengthy and expensive.
Microgenetic	Tracks change from the time it begins until it stabilizes, as subjects master a novel or an everyday task	Offers unique insights into the processes of development	Requires frequent observation of subjects' behaviors; the time required for change is difficult to anticipate.
Sequential	Follows groups of subjects born in different years over time	Permits both longitudinal and cross-sectional comparisons; reveals existence of cohort effects	May have the same problems as longitudinal and cross-sectional designs

In other techniques, the individual is questioned directly. The *case history* provides an in-depth analysis of background information on the individual. The *interview* generally does not provide as much background information, but it is especially valuable if the goal is to obtain a lot of information in a short period of time. In the interview, researchers actively probe the individual's ideas, feelings, and motives; the data come in the form of words rather than observed actions, as is also true of the case history. The *survey* (questionnaire) is similar to the interview except the researcher seeks written responses to a series of questions.

think about it

In addressing the limitation of correlation research, how many different explanations are there for the observation that children who watch more television have more body fat?

Information gathered in this manner, or in combination with direct measurement of some type, is often analyzed using a *correlational method*. The goal is to describe the strength of the relationship between factors. For example, are children who watch more TV (parent survey) fatter (as measured by skinfold or body weight)? Obviously, a limitation of this method is that it does not determine cause-and-effect factors.

One of the most commonly used methods of collecting information about motor development is through the use of *standardized tests*. These tests are widely available and offer researchers a source of objective data. Chapter 13, which describes assessment, includes a detailed discussion of motor development tests and makes recommendations for their use.

To design an investigation that conforms to the scientific method, the researcher must make a series of choices. Experts agree there is no single appropriate investigative method. The choice should depend on the research question under investigation, the available resources, and the investigator's judgment.

MEASURING BRAIN STRUCTURE AND FUNCTION

Much of the progress made in contemporary brain behavior and development research can be attributed to the advances in brain imaging techniques (see "Developmental Cognitive Neuroscience" on page 27). Examples of these techniques can be found in several studies mentioned throughout the text. Brain imaging technology has enabled researchers to see inside the living brain and help them (a) understand the relationships between specific areas of the brain and what function they serve, (b) locate areas of the brain affected by neurological disorders, and (c) develop new strategies to treat brain disorders. The following is a brief description of selected techniques commonly used in growth and motor development research to measure brain *structure* (anatomical) and *function* (typically a derivation of blood—e.g., oxygen, glucose—and electrical activity).

> **focus on change**
>
> Advances in technology afford a more in-depth and precise interpretation of *change*.

Magnetic Resonance Imaging and Functional Magnetic Resonance Imaging

Magnetic resonance imaging (MRI) uses the detection of radio frequency signals produced by displaced radio waves in a magnetic field. It provides an anatomical view of the brain. It has several advantages over the other techniques described (e.g., it is safe and painless, and no special preparation is required); however, it is also expensive and cannot be used with claustrophobic patients (the participant lies in a body-length capsule).

For movement-oriented research, functional MRI (fMRI) is quite effective. This technique detects changes in blood flow to particular areas of the brain. It provides both an *anatomical* and a *functional* view of the brain. In the brain, blood perfusion is presumably related to neural activity, so fMRI can be used to find out what the brain is doing when subjects perform specific tasks or are exposed to specific stimuli.

> **WebLink**
>
> http://www.jove.com/; see *Measuring Brain Activity in Infants* and YouTube for demos.

Electroencephalography

Electroencephalography (EEG) measures changes in brain *function*. Electrodes are strategically placed on the scalp which record electrical activity, as shown in Figure 1.5. Often associated with use of EEG is event-related potentials (ERP). ERP is an average of EEG responses that represent the time related to the processing of stimuli (an event such as attention, memory, movement).

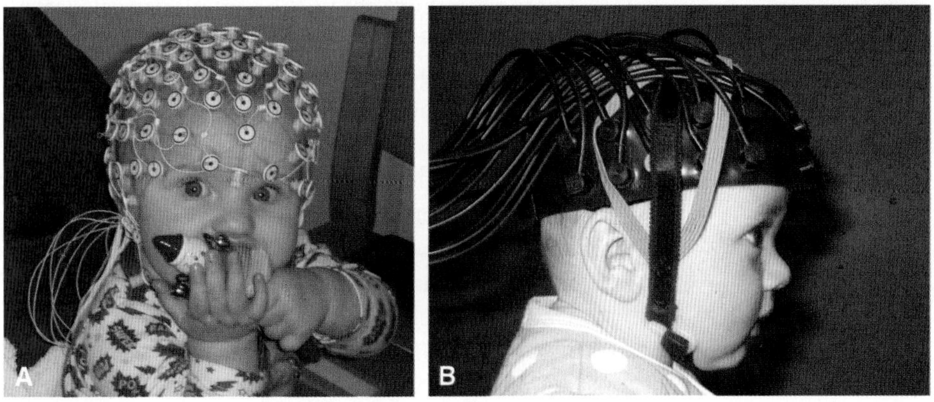

Figure 1.5 Brain imaging has opened up new frontiers in understanding the relationship between brain and motor function. EEG **(A)** and functional near-infrared imaging (fNIR) **(B)**, shown here.

SOURCE: **B**, Courtesy of Baby Research Center, Nijmegen, Netherlands.

Magnetoencephalography

Magnetoencephalography (MEG) measures the magnetic fields produced by electrical activity in the brain (*function*). It uses a series of superconducting coils, fixed within a helmet, to record the tiny magnetic fields generated by active cortex. It requires little setting up time relative to EEG; however, it is detrimentally affected by head movement—which can be particularly problematic when working with young children. However, this technique is projected to be widely used in the future.

Functional Near-Infrared Imaging

Because positron emission tomography (PET) and fMRI require the participant to lie motionless as possible for an extended time, they can be less effective with infants and young children. *Functional near-infrared imaging* (fNIR) is one of the more recent technological creations that works relatively well with those populations. It is a spectroscopic imaging method for measuring the level of neuronal activity (*function*) in the brain. The technique is based on neurovascular coupling; that is, the relationship between metabolic activity and oxygen level (oxygenated hemoglobin). This technique shows promise with studying the brain–behavior relationship.

Transcranial Magnetic Stimulation

Transcranial magnetic stimulation (TMS) uses brief high-intensity magnetic fields to stimulate corticospinal neurons. Weak electric currents are induced in the tissue by rapidly changing magnetic fields. This technique is used to assess the excitability (*function*) of the central nervous system (CNS). TMS has been used, for example, to measure function of the CNS beginning at infancy.

THEORETICAL VIEWS

Objective 1.11

In the field of developmental psychology, theories are used to describe various patterns of behavior and to explain why those behaviors occur. From this perspective, a *theory* may be defined as a set of concepts and propositions that allows the theorist to organize, describe, and explain some aspects of behavior. To gather a comprehensive and meaningful understanding of motor development, it is essential to know something about the way individuals learn and react to their environment. Theories that have earned respect for describing some aspect of behavior enrich our knowledge of the complexities of human development.

In the early years of developmental psychology, much of the information reported, especially on motor development, was of a descriptive nature. That is, researchers viewed and explained development through a systematic cataloging of growth norms and age-related behaviors. One of the primary views was that maturation (i.e., maturational theory) rather than learning (or the environment) was the main impetus for developmental change. In recent years, contemporary views of development have taken a much more comprehensive and explanatory perspective of developmental change. These theories consider the *environmental context* in which development occurs and try to explain the mechanisms and processes accounting for change (growth, development, and behavior), thus attempting to provide a more comprehensive explanation of the dynamic interaction between the organism and its environment.

As noted in the chapter introduction, as a general philosophical view of human and motor development, this text supports the *developmental systems perspective*. This approach underscores the dynamic interaction between the multilevel biological and environmental systems (Fig. 1.1, page 6); that is, the changing relationship between the developing person and his or her changing environmental contexts. The discussion that follows provides a brief description of the prominent approaches and theories that fit this perspective; they are grouped for convenience as *environmental context theory*, *biological systems theory*, and an *applied (combined) model*. This is not to say that select theories do not recognize the importance of other domains because most contemporary models do; it is their primary contribution to this discussion that justified the grouping. Each theory provides information that helps us understand the complex mechanisms, processes, and factors involved in life-span changes in motor development. These theories are described in greater detail in relevant sections of the text.

Before the discussion of the theories most directly relevant to the determinants of motor development and the developmental systems perspective, a brief mention of three other *contributing views* is warranted. Although these approaches may seem more indirect to our focus, each continues (as is the case here) to be used to explain specific aspects of the developmental process with relevance to motor development.

focus on change

Biological and environmental theory help us understand *change* from several perspectives.

In addition, no dialogue of life-span development would be complete without comment on theories of advanced aging. Although most treatises on this subject focus on the biological aspects of advanced aging, evidence also suggests that an individual's longevity and quality of life are influenced by environmental factors. Selected theories are described in Chapter 11 with the discussion of regression. Chapter 14 discusses some views on how an individual's perspective on aging and social experiences may influence the aging process. It is hoped that with this information, the reader develops a better understanding of the aging process as influenced by nature and nurture.

CONTRIBUTING VIEWS

Maturation View

Gesell's (1925) *maturation theory* played a significant role in the evolution of the study of child development during the 1930s and 1940s. Gesell was a pioneer of systematic observation; his timetables detailing when most children achieve certain developmental milestones are still widely used today. Basically, Gesell's theory contends that development is the result of inherited factors and requires little, if any, stimulation from the external environment. The maturational view of development emphasizes the emergence of patterns of development of organic systems, physical structures, and motor capabilities under the influence of genetic forces. Gesell believed that growth of the intellect and of the motor functions was tied closely to growth of the nervous system, a perspective that underlies our fundamental understanding of phylogenetic and ontogenetic motor behavior. Unless certain neurological and biological characteristics are sufficiently developed (matured), it may be futile to practice certain phylogenetic skills. On the other hand, learning and experience (practice) are necessary for the existence of ontogenetic behavior. For example, maturational theory is illustrated in those developmental charts that show how human locomotion develops in the infant from rolling to walking.

Although maturation plays an important role in early development, more contemporary views contend that the sequence of developmental milestones is not fixed and due as strongly to heredity.

Learning-Behavioral View

Bandura (1986, 2009) is one of the main architects of contemporary arguments associated with *observational learning* and social learning theory. Observational learning contends that virtually all of what individuals (children) learn comes from observing others. Bandura suggests that through observational learning (also called *modeling*), we cognitively represent the behavior of others and then are likely to adopt this behavior ourselves. For example, a boy may adopt the competitive manner of his father (as seen while golfing) and display such behavior when observed with the boy's peers. Positive behaviors may also be adopted, for example, after observing peers or family members participating in healthy physical activity.

think about it

Think of a few major role models in your life and describe how they have affected your development—in general and with regard to motor development.

The application of behavioral learning theory plus cognitive processes to the development of learning is known as *social learning theory*. This view emphasizes behavior, the environment, and cognition as key factors in development, with each factor influencing the other factors.

Both the behavioralist and social learning views may be criticized for lack of elaboration on the biological determinants of children's development, especially the fact that children mature at different rates. For an excellent contemporary review and analysis of this perspective, see Rosenthal and Zimmerman (2014).

Cognitive-Developmental View

Of the theories of cognitive development, Jean Piaget's efforts have perhaps had the single greatest effect on modern developmental psychology. Piaget (1963, 1985) believed that the individual discovers solutions to problems primarily through interaction with the environment. According to *Piaget's theory of cognitive development*, the child is not a passive recipient of events (as most behaviorists propose), but, rather, the child seeks out experiences. Piaget's studies focused on the structure of cognitive thought and its orderly sequence of development. Although Piaget did not deny the significance of maturation in the development of the intellect, he did not view all of development as the unfolding of biological processes, as maturational theory contends. Piaget instead viewed the developmental process as the interaction of biological maturation and environmental (the more contemporary term is *contextual*) experience.

One of Piaget's lasting contributions to developmental psychology was the notion of stages. Many of Piaget's writings make references to movement activities and the *importance of play*. Piaget believed that through play (both structured and free), the child has the opportunity to test novel physical, cognitive, and social behaviors that cannot otherwise be accommodated in the real world. Once the behaviors are tested through play, they become part of memory; hence, from a cognitive perspective, play is a medium for intellectual development. In general, several of Piaget's ideas are mentioned with credibility in contemporary dynamic systems theory literature. Perhaps most notable is the use of the classic Piagetian task, A-not-B error, which is described in Chapter 6. This task has been used to test the notion that movement is not separate from cognitive processes. This is an issue that has drawn considerable interest in recent years among developmentalists. Piaget's broad distinctions among four basic periods of development from infancy through adolescence also continue to be used.

ENVIRONMENTAL CONTEXT THEORY

A term closely linked to the developmental systems perspective and this determinant of motor development is *developmental contextualism*. Lerner (2002, 2012), one of the originators, describes this view as part of the more general developmental systems perspective. As bases for behavior and developmental change, both focus on the integrative dynamic relationship between the developing person and the changing context within which he or she lives. However, whereas the developmental systems model is more comprehensive, with equal attention paid to the contributions of biological and environmental systems, contextualism gives more attention to how context influences personal development.

Two prominent theories that provide considerable insight into this determinant of motor development are *Bronfenbrenner's bioecological systems theory* and *Gibson's ecological perspective*. The first provides an excellent framework for studying and understanding the various multilevel ecological systems. Gibson's model gives insight into an important question in motor development: How do individuals perceive and act on the environment in the form of *affordances*?

Bioecological Systems Theory

One of the most extensive models of the contextual approach is the **bioecological systems theory** proposed by Bronfenbrenner (1986, 2005). This perspective emphasizes the broad range of situations and contexts individuals may encounter. These characteristics continue to be affected and modified by the individual's contextual surroundings. Bronfenbrenner describes the settings or environments (contexts) in which individuals develop as five distinct systems: the microsystem, mesosystem, exosystem, macrosystem, and chronosystem (see Fig. 1.6).

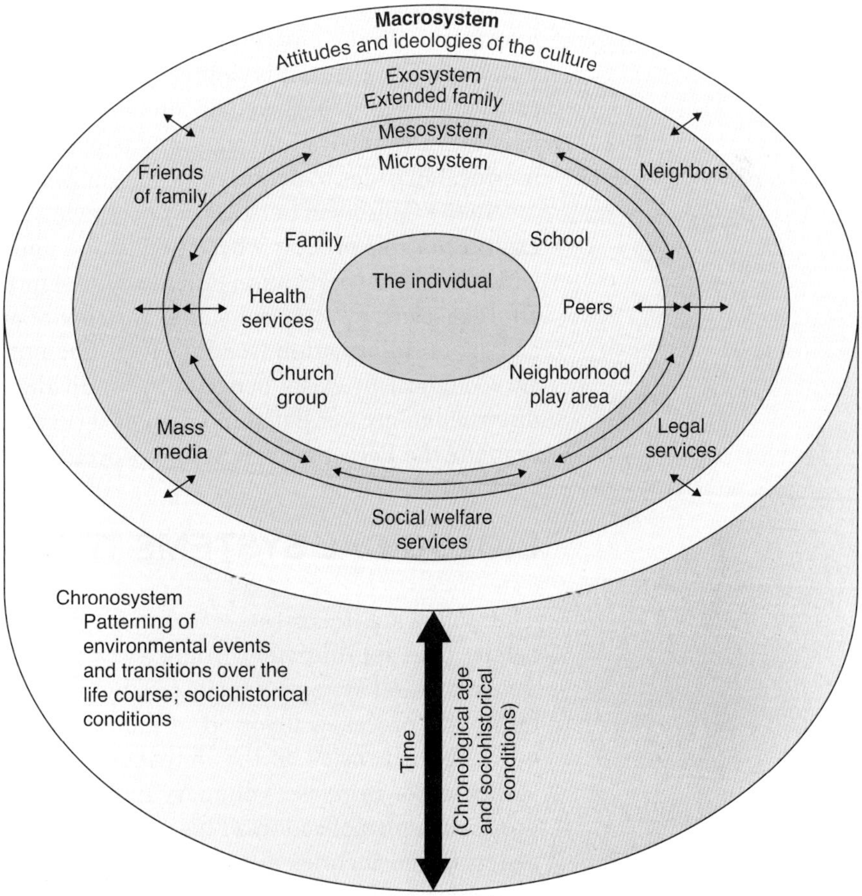

Figure 1.6 Bronfenbrenner's bioecological systems theory of development.

In brief, the *microsystem* is the setting in which the individual lives; the contexts include the person's family, peers, school, and neighborhood. The *mesosystem* is concerned with the interrelationships among the various settings within the microsystem; for example, the relationship of family to school experiences or of family to the community. When experiences in another social setting in which the individual does not have an active role influence what the individual experiences in an immediate context, the setting is the *exosystem*. An example of this is city government (parks), which is responsible for the quality of play and recreational opportunities. The *macrosystem* involves the culture in which the individual exists. In many instances, behavior patterns, beliefs, and other products of a particular group are passed from generation to generation. In many cultures, sport and dance are integral parts of the setting, thus providing the individual with the refinement of such behaviors. The final contextual influence is the *chronosystem*, which involves the patterning of environmental events and transitions over the life span, that is, the sociohistorical contexts. For example, females of today are much more likely to participate in athletic endeavors than they were 40 years ago.

think about it

How have your environmental surroundings influenced the physical (including motor skill proficiency) person you are today?

With the idea of providing a more applicable model with focus on the person (biological), Bronfenbrenner (1995) introduced the Process–Person–Context–Time (PPCT) model. In recent years, this model has garnered the attention of the research community. This model is described in Chapter 14.

Gibson's Ecological Perspective

As noted earlier, **Gibson's ecological perspective** provides insight into an important question in motor development: How do individuals perceive and act on information in the environment? Proposed by Eleanor Gibson (2001) and James Gibson (1979, 2014), this view contends that infants, for example, can directly perceive information in the environment and act with a reasonable response. This is in contrast to the traditional constructivist notion suggesting that past experience is critical in order to act on information in a meaningful manner.

In the Gibsonian perspective, perceiving is experiencing; the infant is an active explorer in this process where perception and motor action are coupled. That is, we cannot study perception independent of movement. The environment provides affordances (e.g., toys and stairs) that invite and challenge the child to perceive and act on information (see Fig. 1.7). The notion of affordances emphasizes that an ecological fit exists between the individual and the situation. This theory is discussed in greater detail in Chapter 6 (Perceptual Development) as we begin to examine the Perception → Action process.

BIOLOGICAL SYSTEMS THEORY

The following theories—*information processing* (programming) and the three perspectives appropriately grouped as *developmental biodynamics*—complement the developmental systems perspective by providing unique insight into the mechanisms and processes involved in the development and regression of coordinated movement. In brief, as the individual perceives information and desires to act with a motor response, voluntary movement requires the formulation of a motor program (a plan of action). This plan includes control of the perceptual and motor systems. The theories discussed here and in Chapter 7 address the control processes involved and their developmental unfolding.

Focus on Application

Using the Bioecological Model in Sport and Physical Activity

Aside from more recent work on affordances and motor behavior, comparatively little has addressed one of the primary determinants of lifelong motor development: environmental context. Researchers today are closing that gap by using Bronfenbrenner's bioecological systems model (Fig. 1.6), described in this chapter and in Chapter 14. Furthermore, in some very diverse and interesting ways, the model has been used to study the development of sports talent and expertise (e.g., Krebs, 2009; Wattie et al., 2015) and physical activity/health behaviors (e.g., Merritt & Snyder, 2015; Nichols et al., 2015). To illustrate its use, Salmon and Timperio (2007) conducted a review of the literature regarding the environmental effects on children's physical activity. Their findings were that several contextual factors have been reported. For example, safety concerns (e.g., road safety, crime and concerns about strangers), social interaction (e.g., child peers, neighborhood relationships, other children live in neighborhood close by), and urban design (e.g., connectivity of streets, access and availability of public open spaces and sports facilities). Furthermore, they recommended that "there is a need for conceptual models that take such complexities into account, and need for multilevel study designs that incorporate individual-level influences, proximal social influences and influences within the broader environment in order to better understand physical activity behavior" (p. 196).

Given that the obesity problem in the United States is arguably one of our greatest health concerns, how could you apply this model to understand and create change?

Sources:

Krebs, R. J. (2009). Bronfenbrenner's bioecological theory of human development and the process of development of sports talent. *International Journal of Sport Psychology*, *40*(1), 108–135.

Merritt, D. H., & Snyder, S. M. (2015). Correlates of optimal behavior among child welfare-involved children: Perceived school peer connectedness, activity participation, social skills, and peer affiliation. *American Journal of Orthopsychiatry*, *85*(5), 483–494.

Nichols, M., Newman, S., Nemeth, L. S., & Magwood, G. (2015). The influence of parental participation on obesity interventions in African American adolescent females: An integrative review. *Journal of Pediatric Nursing*, *30*(3), 485–493.

Salmon, J., & Timperio, A. (2007). Prevalence, trends and environmental influences on child and youth physical activity. Medicine and *Sport Science*, *50*, 183–199.

Wattie, N., Schorer, J., & Baker, J. (2015). The relative age effect in sport: A developmental systems model. *Sports Medicine*, *45*(1), 83–94.

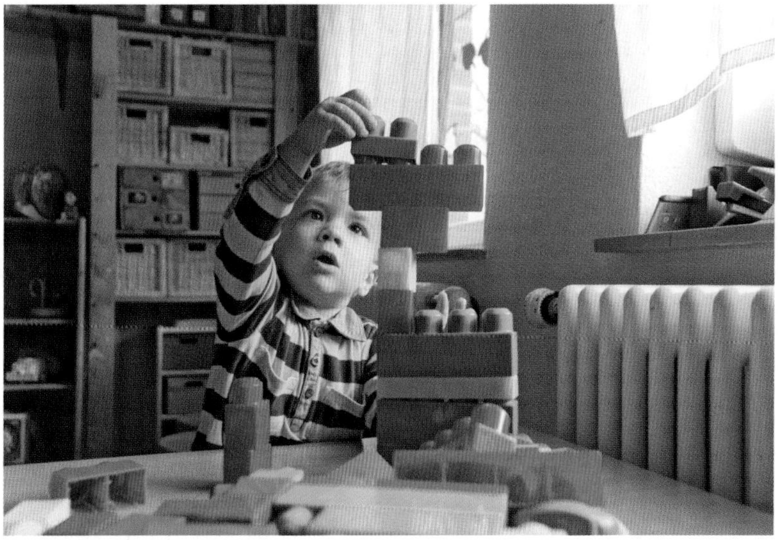

Figure 1.7 Affordances challenge the infant to act on the environment and develop skills.

Information-Processing View

Since its introduction in the 1970s, the **information-processing view** has been one of the dominant approaches in the field of cognitive psychology and motor behavior (Halford & Andrews, 2011; Siegler, 2006). The information-processing approach depicts the mind as a system through which information flows. Scientists who support this approach have drawn close analogies between the human mind and a computer. That is, the brain and CNS are the *hardware*, and the mental processes (such as attention, perception, memory, and problem solving) are the *software*. Like computers, human minds have a limited capacity for processing information. With development, changes in the capacities of cognitive structures, including critical strategies, occur. The primary challenge for researchers is to provide an understanding of how individuals' thinking change as they develop across the life span. Schmidt and Lee (2014) note that the information-processing perspective studies movement from the point of view of the human as a processor of information; it focuses on storage (memory), coding, retrieval, and programming, with the result of production of an outcome (movement). Unlike Piaget, many information-processing theorists insist that cognitive development is not stagelike; instead, mental programs develop gradually over time and involve quantitative rather than qualitative change.

Developmental Biodynamics

Developmental biodynamics is an umbrella term used here to describe theories and scientific approaches to explain the psychobiological characteristics of voluntary motor coordination and control. In essence, the primary attempt is to describe and explain the intimate connection between the brain and body. This approach represents a vast improvement from the more traditional maturational approach, which described change in a descriptive series of developmental milestones. Although this approach is just beginning to address the challenges associated with a developmental synthesis of the brain-body phenomenon, researchers have already made significant contributions toward a better understanding of the problem. A thorough scientific examination of the topic is beyond the scope of this section and text, but a brief description of the basic tenets of the approach should be useful in understanding the merits of an interdisciplinary view of the research problem. Chapter 7 addresses this approach in greater detail in reference to *coordinative structures*, *dynamic systems theory*, *and neuronal group selection theory*.

Bernstein (1967) introduced the term *biodynamics* in his writing on the genesis of motor coordination. The researcher's basic premise was that coordination and control emerged from continual and intimate interactions between the nervous system (brain) and the periphery (body). This idea prevails with contemporary views and research.

COORDINATIVE STRUCTURES

The central question Bernstein (1967) asked was "How can the brain control individually all the diverse elements (e.g., neurons, muscles, and joints) and multiple linkages associated with the production of movement?" To address the problem, Bernstein introduced the notion of *synergies*—classes of movement patterns involving collections (groups) of muscle or joint variables that act as basic units in the regulation and control of movement. Bernstein also proposed that there must be an inseparable relation between the brain and associated movement components (e.g., hands, arms, and legs), and they must act and develop collectively. This basic premise set the agenda for the efforts of different disciplines to address the interface between perception and action.

This basic theme—interaction between perception and action—and variations have been addressed using, for example, mathematical techniques of nonlinear dynamics, principles of biomechanics, neural modeling, and, as previously mentioned, considerations of the context in which the development and behavior occur. In addition to computer modeling and the use of robotics and animals, experimental observations have included humans (usually infants) performing a variety of upper-limb (reaching and grasping), locomotor (walking), and reflexive/spontaneous movements.

DYNAMIC SYSTEMS THEORY

Dynamic systems theory is an applied branch of developmental biodynamics that continues to stimulate considerable inquiry. Originating from Bernstein's problem with brain and body control, Kugler et al. (1980, 1982) introduced the dynamic systems approach, which focuses on the developmental perspective; that is, the emergence, or unfolding, of motor behavior. Most traditional views on how human movement evolves have been based on the descriptive-maturational perspective; that is, the orderly and sequential emergence of behaviors linked to development of the nervous system (e.g., spontaneous/reflexive behavior, crawling, and walking). Although this type of research has contributed to the understanding of when motor skills emerge and what they look like, one criticism has been that it falls short in explaining *how* motor behavior emerges (i.e., the processes of change). The dynamic systems perspective suggests that coordination and control emerge as a result of the dynamic properties of the muscle collectives (i.e., coordinative structures). This view of development emphasizes the importance of the *dynamic* and *self-organizing properties* of the motor system to the individual's developing motor competencies. Along with biological considerations, this perspective (as a feature of biodynamics) suggests that change is stimulated by characteristics of the environment and demands of the specific task (contexts). Since its inception, dynamic systems research has done much to provide a better understanding of how motor behavior emerges.

NEURONAL GROUP SELECTION THEORY

Whereas the coordinative structures and dynamic systems approaches focus primarily on motor control with muscle units as the key feature, *neuronal group selection theory* addresses organization of the CNS in motor behavior; that is, wiring of the system from brain structure to muscle (motor) unit.

DEVELOPMENTAL COGNITIVE NEUROSCIENCE

This scientific "field" has emerged in recent years as one of the more promising for the study of change in motor behavior. Furthermore, it shows promise in shedding light on classic developmental questions related to the mechanisms subserving developmental *change*. As you have gathered, developmental cognitive neuroscience (DCN) complements the various developmental biodynamic approaches. Researchers in this field aim to identify linkages and relations between the developing brain, behavior, and genes. This field in general addresses the question: What are the interrelations between developmental *changes* in the brain (e.g., morphology, connectivity) and developmental *changes* in perceptual and motor behavior? DCN offers a means to study both associations and dissociations using both behavioral and neuroscientific techniques.

Areas of focus are varied (e.g., memory, attention) but underscore the perceptual and cognitive mechanisms for action processing and execution. According to Adele Diamond (2016), a prominent researcher in this field, DCN is an interdisciplinary field devoted to understanding how children's minds *change* as they grow up, interrelations between that and how the brain is *changing*, and environmental and biological influences on that. DCN is an interdisciplinary scientific field situated at the boundaries of neuroscience, cognitive science, genetics, psychology, and movement sciences.

One of the primary reasons for the scientific acknowledgment of this field is technological advances (and use of) electrophysiology (e.g., EEG, MEG) and brain imaging (e.g., fMRI, PET) associated with, among several brain aspects, action processing. In addition to studying the developmental change of typically developing persons, with these innovations there is the increasing trend for studying atypical groups (autism, developmental coordination disorder, cerebral palsy). In 2007, a special issue of the journal *Developmental Review* was published in recognition of this field's emerging potential (see articles by Luciana, 2007, 2010; Pennington et al., 2007). Subsequent to that publication, other prominent scientific journals devoted space to acknowledge this promising field (e.g., *Developmental Psychobiology*; Astle & Scerif, 2008). For an updated review of this promising field see Johnson and de Haan (2015).

Constraints Model

The **constraints model** (Newell, 1986) is an excellent approach to observing, assessing, and studying motor behavior across the life span from an ecological perspective. This model has strong implications for both teachers and clinicians. While incorporating the developmental systems elements of the *individual* (biological factors) and the *environment*, emphasis is also given to a third factor, the *task*, as part of the environmental context. The underlying notion is that the qualitative and quantitative aspects of movement emerge from these factors. Newell described these elements as *constraints* that may influence developmental change; that is, they interact to constrain the control of motor tasks.

This general model has been adopted in a wide range of life-span research. To illustrate, for many older adults, there are "constraints" in their ability to move independently within the context of constantly changing task demands and environmental contexts. In essence, although these individuals can manage (walk) independently within their home environment, when presented with a different set of contextual factors, such as standing on a moving bus, walking up and down stairs, or moving across unfamiliar surfaces, their level of mobility may be significantly hindered. This same general scenario is applicable to the infant learning to walk. In these examples, postural stability and leg strength (individual constraints) and task constraints would apply. This model and its applications is described in greater detail in Chapter 7.

think about it

Why is there no single theory that can explain all aspects of human development? If you had to pick two to study motor behavior, which would they be?

Obviously, no single theory described in the chapter entirely explains the complexity of lifelong motor behavior. As mentioned earlier, each in its own particular way casts some light on explaining what influences change. With this in mind, you are encouraged to use an *eclectic theoretical perspective* when viewing behavior broadly, an orientation that does not follow any one theory but incorporates what seem to be the best or most useful elements from various approaches. This method, of course, depends on the perspective desired and goal of observation. Is the goal to explain multiple influences on behavior, or is it to delineate change due to a specific factor? With today's advanced scientific technology for observing motor behavior, new theories are emerging that, in most cases, require developmentalists to rethink their original perspective. Table 1.2 provides a summary of the organization and main features of the theories described.

TABLE 1.2 Summary of Theoretical Views of Motor Development

View	Main Features	
Contributing	Maturation view	Development is tied predominantly to biological maturation.
	Learning-behavioral view	Learning comes from observation of others and the environment.
	Cognitive-developmental view	Children are not passive learners; they seek experiences. In the process of developing the cognitive domain, play is important.
Environmental systems	Bronfenbrenner's bioecological systems theory	Individual development may be modified by five distinct ecological systems.
	Gibson's ecological perspective	Individuals can directly perceive information in the environment and act with a reasonable response. The environment provides affordances.
Biological systems	Information-processing view	Development is described in the context of a computer that has hardware and software, which operate in the form of input, central processing (planning), and output (motor response).
	Coordinative structures	The question of how the brain controls muscle and joint movements is addressed. Control is executed by collections (groups) of muscles and joint variables that act as basic units of movement (synergies).
	Dynamic systems theory	The emergence (unfolding) of movement patterns as a dynamic and self-organizing process is described.
	Neuronal group selection theory	Wiring and control of motor control from the brain to the muscle (motor) unit are explained.
Applied (environment/ biology)	Constraints model	This applied model describes three analytical features (constraints) to motor performance: the performer, the environment, and the task.

CAREERS IN MOTOR DEVELOPMENT

Objective 1.12

As a course of study and as a research field, motor development has experienced considerable growth in recent years. With this growth, a wide variety of professional career opportunities have emerged. In addition to the common higher education setting (teaching and research), excellent opportunities may be found, for example, in hospitals, business/industry, government agencies, professional education associations, private research facilities, and a variety of schools, where practitioners can address a wide range of ages. Figure 1.8 shows one example of these career opportunities.

It is becoming more common for developmentalists to work for business/industry as consultants and researchers on projects such as play environments for children, toy development, educational publications (publishing companies), and media programming (e.g., TV and the Internet). Developmentalists can also be found working for state education divisions and with federal agencies such as the National Science Foundation, National Institutes of Health, Centers for Disease Control and Prevention, and Department of Education. A considerable part of our federal government's current social policy related to education and research is devoted to early childhood and the older adult, suggesting that the future is bright for individuals who wish to focus on this field as a career. A program of study in motor development also provides an excellent background for those who wish to pursue professional schools, such as those for physical and occupational therapy and medicine.

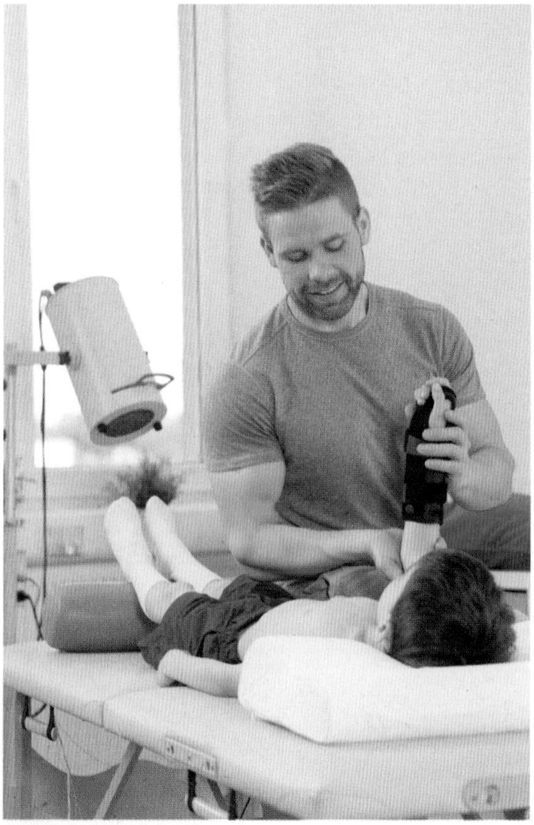

Figure 1.8 Physical therapy is just one of the exciting professions that use the study of motor development.

Summary

Motor development is a field of specialized study that examines change in motor behavior resulting from the interaction of biological processes and the environment. With the development of a lifelong perspective has emerged the multidisciplinary approach to studying associated behavioral change. The major objective of the developmentalist is to identify and explain the characteristics associated with change across the life span. To understand the factors that influence change, the developmental systems perspective is appropriate. This view recognizes the changing relationship (interaction) between the developing person and changing multilevel environmental context. In general, development is a dynamic and self-organizing process.

Several fundamental observations (assumptions) have relevance to motor development. In brief, development appears stagelike, but its bases are underlined by processes that are likely continual and cumulative; all domains are interrelated; a wide range of individual differences exist; environmental context plays a major role in development; there are critical and sensitive periods in development; development is aided by positive stimulation; there is much plasticity in development; motor skill development is a dynamic and self-organizing process; with advanced aging, regression of most skills is inevitable; and primary to this text is the observation that biological and environmental systems are interactive factors in development.

From a descriptive view, complementing the age-related periods of life span development are phases of motor behavior. This developmental continuum provides an outline for the study of lifelong growth, development, and motor performance.

Motor development is a scientific and applied discipline. Through motor development research, we learn to better understand the capabilities of individuals in order to guide their development and improve their health and performance. The scientific method of studying human development and performance may employ a variety of research designs. The most popular method for collecting information and the basic tool of any science is systematic observation. This can be conducted in either a natural or a structured setting.

Whereas earlier theoretical approaches to explaining development were more descriptive, more contemporary approaches attempt to explain the mechanisms and processes accounting for change. Included in the comprehensive study of lifelong development are considerations of the biological systems and environmental context in which development occurs.

For those who wish to pursue motor development as a career, there are promising opportunities as teachers, researchers, consultants, and medical professionals.

think about it

1. **Why is it important to have a general understanding of human development in order to gain insight into lifelong motor behavior?**
2. **What is another example of motor behavior to which both nature and nurture contribute, and how does each effect contribute?**
3. **In addressing the limitation of correlation research, how many different explanations are there for the observation that children who watch more television have more body fat?**

4. **Think of a few major role models in your life and describe how they have affected your development—in general and with regard to motor development.**
5. **How have your environmental surroundings influenced the physical (including motor skill proficiency) person you are today?**
6. **Why is there no single theory that can explain all aspects of human development? If you had to pick two to study motor behavior, which would they be?**

■ LEARNING ACTIVITIES

Objective: To learn more about your chosen future career. First, search on the Web for a national organization representing your chosen field. Write a brief summary of the subfields/specializations within. Then, select one or two, find out a bit more about the field(s) and write on why you made that selection.

Objective: To consider how life-span motor development information might be important in my career. Think of your career goals, explore what is available on the Web about that career, and then list five ways that this course may have application. You may want to look ahead at the chapter content.

WebLinks

MAJOR ORGANIZATIONS AND CAREER INFORMATION

American Academy of Pediatrics
https://www.aap.org/en-us/Pages/Default.aspx

Society of Health and Physical Educators
http://www.shapeamerica.org/

American College of Sports Medicine
http://www.acsm.org/

Centers for Disease Control and Prevention
http://www.cdc.gov/

National Association for the Education of Young Children
http://www.naeyc.org/

National Institute on Aging
https://www.nia.nih.gov/

National Institute of Child Health and Human Development
https://www.nichd.nih.gov/Pages/index.aspx

American Physical Therapy Association
http://www.apta.org/

American Occupational Therapy Association
http://www.aota.org/

Society for Neuroscience
https://www.sfn.org/

part two

Biological Growth and Development

part two provides information related to the structural and functional changes of human development and motor behavior. Keep in mind that these topics are strongly interrelated. Chapters 2 and 3 focus on the hereditary, neurological, and physical aspects of human development typically manifested as structural growth. Chapter 4 builds on that information in discussing change related to functional processes. Finally, Chapter 5 describes the variety of other factors that may influence growth and development such as prenatal care, nutrition, environmental agents, hormones, and physical activity.

Chapter 2

Heredity and Neurological Changes

OBJECTIVES

Upon completion of this chapter, you should be able to

2.1 Define the term *heredity* and describe its primary characteristics.

2.2 Identify the three primary functions of the nervous system.

2.3 Outline the basic structure of the central and peripheral nervous systems and briefly describe their functions.

2.4 Explain the basic structure and function of a neuron and identify the various types of neurons.

2.5 Describe a *motor unit*.

2.6 Describe how nerve impulses are conducted.

2.7 Outline and describe the sequence of early developmental changes in the central nervous system.

2.8 Identify the primary developmental changes that occur in the brain.

2.9 Explain brain lateralization in terms of both brain structure and its effect on motor behavior.

2.10 Outline and briefly describe the primary neurological changes that occur with advanced aging.

KEY TERMS

heredity
genotype
phenotype
central nervous system (CNS)
peripheral nervous system (PNS)
motor unit
nerve conduction velocity
integration
differentiation
synaptogenesis
pruning
myelination
critical periods
brain plasticity
brain (hemispheric) lateralization

HEREDITY

Objective 2.1

focus on change

Heredity is viewed as the foundation of *change*, one that interacts with the environment to form development and behavior.

Heredity is the total set of characteristics biologically transmitted from parent to offspring. From the moment of conception, two primary factors interact to determine the developmental characteristics of the individual: genetic makeup and the environment. Thus, from the start, heredity and the environment are interrelated. The environment, even during prenatal development, modifies and interacts with heredity to shape the individual and to control the extent to which maximal potential will be realized. The *nature–nurture* relationship suggests the significant influence of these two factors. Today, behavioral scientists know that nature (heredity) and nurture (the environment) both contribute continually and inseparably to an individual's development. There is no organism in which one part is influenced only by genes and another segment only by the environment. The capacity of a living thing to respond to experiences in the environment is as genetically determined as the maturation of its neurological system. However, a gene is only a probability for a given trait, not a guarantee.

A *gene* is the basic unit of heredity found within a chromosome. Each human cell contains 46 chromosomes (in 23 pairs) in its nucleus. Each *chromosome* consists of hundreds of genes strung together in a chainlike formation. Genes are located on molecules of DNA, which are packed tightly into the cell nucleus. During normal cell division, or *mitosis*, the DNA molecule unzips, breaking its rungs and forming two separate strands. Each strand becomes part of a new DNA molecule. In this fashion, all 46 chromosomes of the single cell reproduce themselves.

The DNA molecule contains the genetic code that determines what hereditary information is to be transmitted from one generation to the next. The genetic code provides the directions for creating a new individual with his or her own unique combination of characteristics, such as intelligence, height, blood type, and eye color. To get from blueprint to creation, information in the DNA molecules is transcribed into molecules of RNA. These molecules take the code from the DNA into the cytoplasm of the cell, which contains the raw material for making proteins. It is out of the proteins, made according to instructions from the RNA, that the functioning parts and capabilities of each human being are developed.

Not long ago, researchers believed the human body consisted of about 100,000 genes. However, due to the incredible work of the Human Genome

WebLink
https://www.genome.gov/

Project, the estimate is now 20,000 to 25,000 genes (Human Genome Project). The project undertook one of the great feats of exploration in history—the complete mapping of all the genes of human beings, known as the *human genome*. This project has greatly advanced our ability to identify which genes control specific traits or behaviors.

The **genotype** is all of an individual's genetic inheritance. The actual expression of the genotype as the person's visible characteristics and behavior is referred to as the **phenotype**. The phenotype depends not only on the individual's genetic makeup but also on all the environmental elements that affect the person from the moment of conception. The observable characteristics of a phenotype include physical traits such as height, eye color, and skin pigmentation, and psychological characteristics such as intelligence, creativity, and personality. Heredity also influences aging, puberty, time of tooth eruption, muscle fiber type ratio, body fat, and the development of skeletal age. Although body weight and aging are primarily the product of heredity, both can be significantly affected by environmental factors such as diet and exercise.

think about it

List some of your phenotype characteristics and from which parent you inherited them. Can you think of ways the environment affects phenotype over time?

Much of our information about the genetic component of behavior has come about through the comparison of identical and nonidentical twins. Because identical twins have the same genetic material, variability in their behavior is due, in theory, primarily to environmental factors such as learning. Although the answers are far from complete, data such as these suggest that selected motor performance activities are significantly influenced by genetic factors.

Table 2.1 shows the estimated genetic contribution of selected biological components. Subsequent chapters give additional attention to specific genetic contributions relevant to the topic being discussed.

TABLE 2.1 Estimated Genetic Contribution

Component	Genetic Contribution (Approximate) (%)
Anaerobic performance	50
Body fat	25–40
Body weight	40
Bone mass	80
Maximum heart rate	50
Muscle fibers: types I and II	45
Physical working capacity	70
Physique	40
Regional fat distribution	50
Stature	60
VO_2max (aerobic performance)	50

SOURCE: Modified from Malina, R., Bouchard, C., & Bar-Or, O. (2004). Genetic regulation of growth, maturation, and performance. In *Growth, maturation, and physical activity* (2nd ed.). Champaign, IL: Human Kinetics; McArdle, W. D., Katch, F. I., & Katch, V. L. (2015). *Exercise physiology* (8th ed.). Philadelphia, PA: Wolters Kluwer Health; and Burnham, J. M., & Leonard, M. B. (2008). Bone mineral acquisition in utero and during infancy and childhood. In R. Marcus, D. Feldman, D. A. Nelson, & C. J. Rosen (Eds.), *Osteoporosis* (3rd ed., pp. 705–742). San Diego, CA: Academic Press.

NEUROLOGICAL CHANGES

Objective 2.2

Of all the systems of the human body, the nervous system is one of the most important. Everything that takes place consciously or unconsciously, voluntarily or as a reflex, has its primary initiation within the nervous system. Growth, development, and motor behavior all depend on the efficient functioning of this system. The effectiveness of a motor response is significantly influenced by the quality and capability of the nervous system and the brain. The nervous system has three primary functions: (a) a sensory function; (b) an integrative function, which includes the memory and thought processes; and (c) a motor function.

Basic Structure and Function

Objective 2.3

A basic review of the anatomy of the nervous system is important to the further discussion of the neurological changes that occur across the life span. The nervous system has two major parts: the **central nervous system (CNS)**, which consists of the spinal cord and brain, and the **peripheral nervous system (PNS)**, which is made up of all the nerve fibers that enter or leave the brain stem and spinal cord to supply the sensory receptors, muscles, and glands. Essentially, the PNS represents the lines of communication, whereas the CNS is the center of coordination and the mechanism that determines the most appropriate response to incoming impulses.

CENTRAL NERVOUS SYSTEM

focus on change

Neurological *changes* underscore (drive) motor performance *changes* across the life span.

The structures of the CNS basically function to transmit information about the environment and the body to the brain, where it is recorded, stored in memory, and compared with other information (Fig. 2.1). The CNS also carries information from the brain to muscles and glands, thus producing motor responses and the body's adaptations to environmental demands. The following discussion provides a brief description of selected parts of the CNS deemed most relevant to the study of motor development.

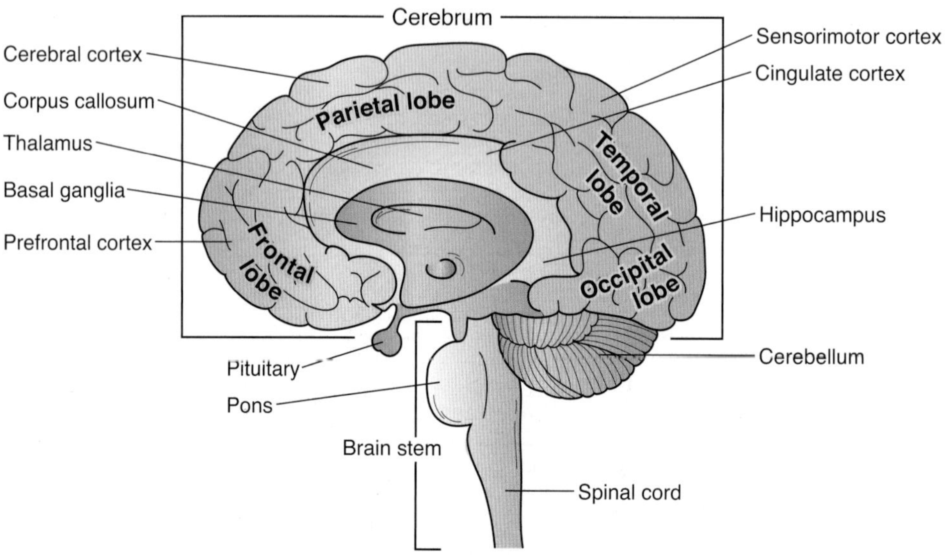

Figure 2.1 Parts of the brain (side view).

Spinal Cord. The spinal cord has an essential role in the input and response phases of information processing and motor behavior. Its primary function is to act as a transmission pathway; it carries to the brain all sensory information from the body and all motor commands sent down from the brain to muscles (and glands). The spinal cord also has an important function in reflex behavior.

The Brain. The brain is the principal integrative area of the nervous system. It is the location where memories are stored, thoughts are developed, emotions are generated, and complex control of motor behaviors is performed.

The *brain stem* is that part of the brain primarily responsible for several involuntary (reflexes), metabolic functions, and the regulation of posture. The brain stem also sets the rhythm of breathing and controls the rate and force of breathing movements and heartbeat. Several important fiber tracts pass both upward and downward through the brain stem, transmitting sensory signals from the spinal cord mainly to the thalamus and transmitting motor signals from the cerebral cortex back to the spinal cord. The major structures of the brain stem are the pons, midbrain, medulla, diencephalon, and reticular formation. The *medulla* contains a number of sensory tracts for carrying information to the brain and motor tracts for carrying information to the muscles and glands. The medulla serves primarily to regulate vital internal processes such as respiration, blood pressure, and heart rate. The ventral and dorsal parts of the *pons* contain several nerve tracts that allow for coordination and involuntary influences on automatic movement and posture. The *midbrain* is involved with reflex movements caused by visual and auditory stimulation. The *diencephalon* consists of two areas: the thalamus and hypothalamus. The *thalamus* is an important integration center through which most sensory information passes. The *hypothalamus* is the structure where neural and hormonal functions work to create a constant internal environment (body temperature). The *reticular formation* plays an important role in attention and activation of the individual for cognitive and motor activity.

The *cerebral cortex* is the outermost layer of the cerebrum and is composed of an estimated 75% of the total neurons in the CNS. It is the functional head of the nervous system in its responsibility for higher order critical thinking and information processing. Basically, the cortex mediates (a) the reception and interpretation of sensory information, (b) the organization of complex motor behaviors, and (c) the storage and use of learned experiences. The motor areas of the cortex (*motor cortex*) play an integral role in planning and executing coordinated movements. The motor cortex occupies the posterior half of the frontal lobe and consists of the primary motor area, premotor area, and supplementary motor area. In general, this structure controls the specific fine motor muscles (e.g., muscles of the hand, fingers, feet, and toes). The *primary motor area* is responsible for the actual execution of movements. In addition, this structure has a critical role in the control of speed and force of actions. The *premotor area* is linked to working memory, making it possible to plan and guide movements. The premotor area also plays an important role in advance planning and coordination of complex movement sequences. The *supplementary motor area* is involved in the preparation for movement, especially when the actions to be executed are internally generated as opposed to being elicited by sensory events. For example, the supplementary motor area is engaged when imagining (using motor imagery) before executing.

The *basal ganglia* area of the brain is made up of a group of nuclei located in the inner layers of the cerebrum. The basal ganglia integrate the sensory motor centers and are involved with unconscious behavior such as the maintenance of muscle tone required in upright posture. It also plays an important role in planning and coordinating movements. A major function of the basal ganglia is to control very fundamental gross body movements, whereas the cerebral cortex plays prominently in the performance of more precise movements of the arms, hands, fingers, and feet.

The *cerebellum* is an important part of the motor control system. Although it is located far away from both the motor cortex and the basal ganglia, it interconnects with both of these areas through special nerve pathways. It also interconnects with motor areas in both the reticular formation and spinal cord. Its primary function is to determine the coordinated sequence of muscle contractions during complex movements. Its functions are also associated with vestibular awareness (balance), postural adjustments, and reflex activity.

It should be stressed that the emerging motor behavior resulting from the processes described earlier is the outcome of an interaction among the many subsystems within the CNS. This interaction is further shaped by the goals of the task and environmental constraints.

PERIPHERAL NERVOUS SYSTEM

The PNS is a branching network of nerves. It is so extensive that hardly a single cubic millimeter of tissue anywhere in the body is without nerve fibers. The PNS is divided into two systems: the somatic and the autonomic. The *somatic system* controls all the skeletal muscles (contracted through voluntary initiation); the *autonomic system* is primarily responsible for regulating the automatic functioning of the smooth muscles of internal organs such as the heart, liver, lungs, and endocrine glands. The activities of the autonomic system are seldom subject to voluntary control.

PNS nerve fibers are of two functional types: *afferent fibers* for transmitting sensory information into the spinal cord and brain and *efferent fibers* for transmitting motor impulses back from the CNS to the peripheral areas, especially to the skeletal muscles. The peripheral nerves that arise directly from the brain itself and supply mainly the head region are called *cranial nerves*. The remainders of the peripheral nerves are spinal nerves.

Objective 2.4

Neuron. A *neuron* (nerve cell) is the basic structural unit of the nervous system. There are billions of neurons in the nervous system; the average neuron is a complex structure that has thousands of physical connections with other cells. Nerve impulses travel along neurons to relay information from one cell to another (and through the nervous system). The junction between two cells across which the information must pass is called a *synapse*. The three basic parts of the neuron are the cell body (soma), dendrites, and axon (Fig. 2.2).

The *cell body* (soma) is the metabolic center of the cell. It contains the nucleus, which is responsible for regulating the various processes of the cell. Neuron cell bodies are located mostly within the CNS. Within the CNS, clusters of cell bodies are called *nuclei*. A *dendrite* is a nerve fiber that extends from the cell body. Each neuron can have from one to thousands of dendrites. Dendrites are the receiving part of the neuron, serving the important function of collecting information and orienting it toward the cell body. Although many dendrites branch from the cell body of a neuron, there is only one axon. The *axon* is the nerve cell structure that carries information away from the cell

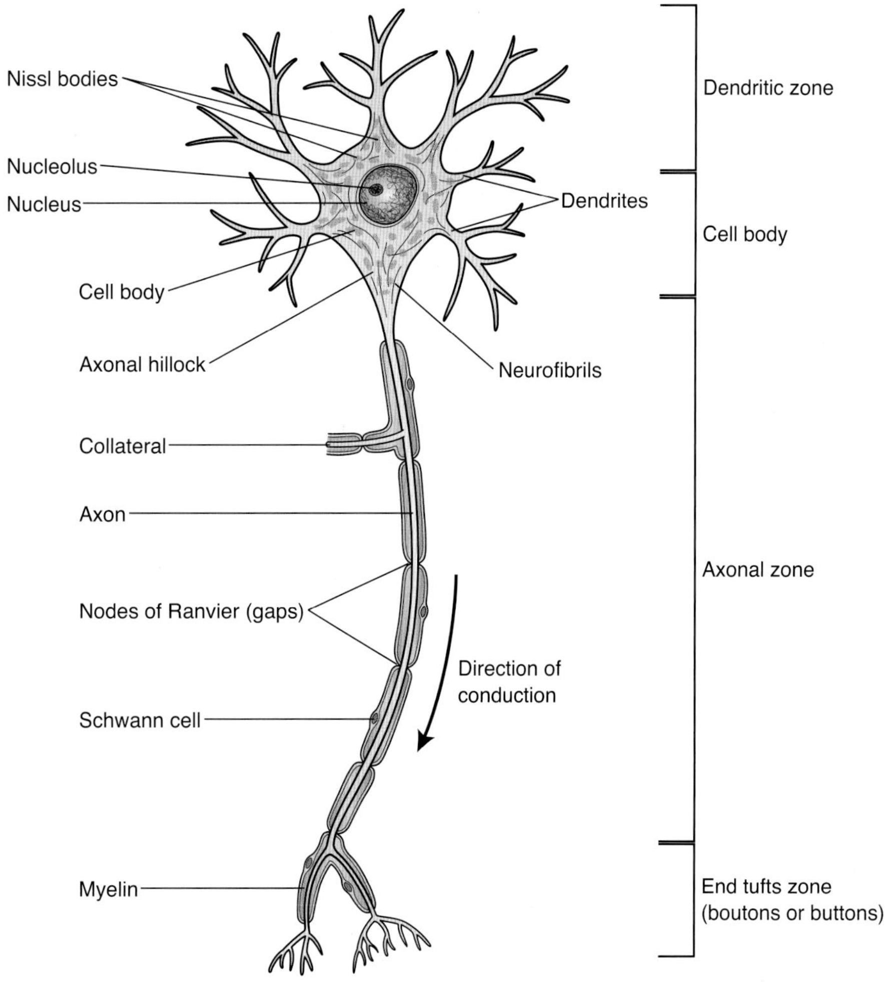

Figure 2.2 The basic parts of a neuron.

body to other cells. As previously noted, nerve impulses travel along neurons to transmit information. An impulse is an electrochemical process that travels in a chainlike sequence from the dendrite or cell body of one neuron to its axon, to the dendrite or cell body of another neuron, and so on, through the length of the nerve tract. The functional connection between the axon and another neuron is the *synapse*.

Neurons are generally classified according to their function. *Afferent neurons*, also referred to as sensory neurons, carry nerve impulses from the sensory receptors into the spinal cord or brain of the CNS. *Efferent neurons* transmit impulses from the CNS to the muscles and glands. Efferent neurons passing impulses to muscles are commonly called *motoneurons*. More than 95% of all neurons are classified as *interneurons*. This type of neuron originates and terminates solely within the CNS.

Along with the neuron, the other basic types of nervous system tissues are supporting and insulating cells. These cells have the important function of holding neurons in place and preventing signals from spreading between the neurons. In the CNS, these cells are collectively called *neuroglia* and referred to specifically as *glial cells*. In the PNS, they are referred to as *Schwann cells*. Schwann cells wrap myelin sheaths around the large nerve fibers, thus insulating the pathway for an electrochemical nerve impulse.

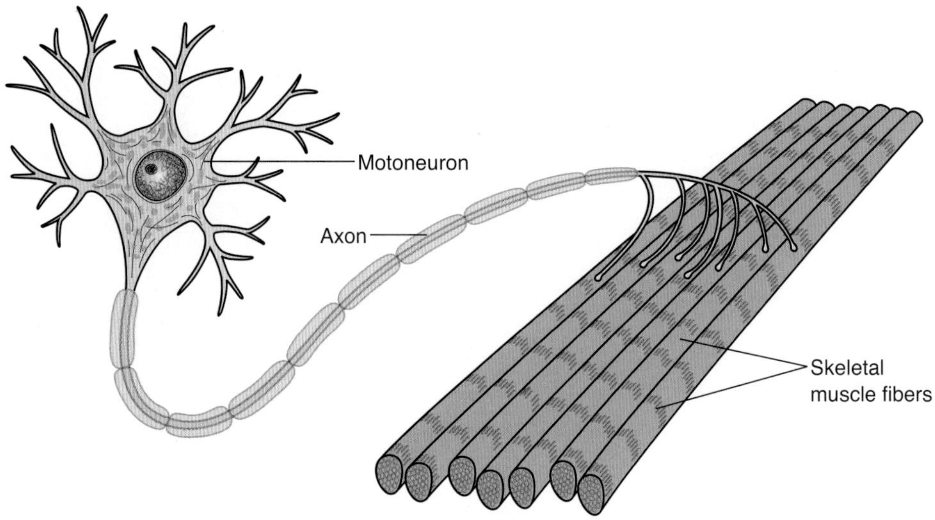

Figure 2.3 A motor unit.

Objective 2.5

The Neuromuscular (Motor) Unit. Each motoneuron axon branches into several synaptic terminals, and each of these terminals provides the nerve supply to a muscle fiber. A neuron and all the muscle fibers innervated by it are referred to as a **motor unit** because all the muscle fibers contract as a unit when stimulated by the motoneuron (Fig. 2.3). Each of the muscle fibers making up the small delicate muscles of the eye may be supplied by a motoneuron, but larger postural muscles may only have one motoneuron to supply as many as 150 muscle fibers.

Pathways. The nerve tracts of the spinal cord together with the spinal nerves provide a two-way line of communication between the brain and parts of the body outside of the nervous system. The tracts that conduct sensory impulses "to the brain" are called *ascending tracts*. Tracts that conduct motor pulses "from the brain" to motor neurons that control muscles are the *descending tracts*. Both tracts are composed of axons. Typically, all the axons within a given tract originate from neurons located in the same part of the nervous system and end together in some other part. For example, a spinothalamic (ascending) tract begins in the spinal cord and carries sensory impulses associated with pain and pressure (touch) to the thalamus of the brain. Another neuron then relays the information to the cortex. The corticospinal (descending) tract originates in the cortex and carries motor impulses downward via the spinal cord and spinal nerves. These impulses control skeletal muscle movements. Ascending tracts are also referred to as afferent or sensory pathways, whereas descending tracts are associated with efferent or motor pathways.

Objective 2.6

Impulse Conduction. Neurons send information through their axons in the form of brief impulses, or waves, of electricity in the form of single electrical clicks called *action potentials*. **Nerve conduction velocity** is the speed at which information travels; this rate is greatly affected by the presence or absence of a material called *myelin* around the axon. Myelin is a fatty material that forms a sheath around many axons both within and outside of the CNS. The myelin sheath is formed from a type of insulating cell called a *Schwann cell*. These cells wrap around the axon and form a jelly-roll-type structure that serves as an effective insulator of electrical currents. The myelin sheath is interrupted every millimeter or so by gaps called *nodes of Ranvier* (see Fig. 2.2 on page 41). The neuron membrane is active only at the nodes, so the impulse is conducted when the action potential jumps from one of these nodes to another. This type of impulse conduction is known as *saltatory conduction* and is significantly faster than conduction in non-myelinated axons.

Saltatory conduction also requires less metabolic energy, enabling myelinated axons to fire nerve impulses at higher frequencies for longer periods of time. Research has also indicated that there is higher conduction velocity, lower threshold, shorter latency, and higher amplitude coincident with the time of appearance and the degree of myelination. Another factor in conduction velocity is the size of the axon. Basically, the larger the cross-sectional diameter, the faster the speed of conduction. Apparently, axon conduction velocity is related to the urgency of the information it is called upon to transmit. Axons that have greater speed potential are concerned with the control of movement, especially in the mediation of rapid reflexes; axons that transmit visceral information are small, generally unmyelinated, and slow.

Early Developmental Changes

Objective 2.7

A mature brain contains more than 100 billion neurons intricately connected with one another in ways that make possible the amazing functions that underlie our behavior. Perhaps most remarkable is the precision of neural circuitry (wiring) that develops between connections that occur; each neuron links up with thousands of others to form trillions of connections. The total length of wiring between neurons is estimated at 62,000 miles (Coveney & Highfield, 1995). It was once believed that the wiring diagram for each person was predetermined by one's genetic blueprints. However, the contemporary perspective is that although the main circuits may be prewired for responses such as breathing, control of heartbeat, and reflexes, stimulation from the environment can shape the trillions of finer connections that complete the architecture of the brain. This critical effect, which has profound implications for our nature–nurture theme and motor development in general, is discussed in the latter part of this section.

Normal CNS development appears to follow a dynamic sequence of integrated biological events; these include the processes of *cell proliferation*, *migration*, *integration and differentiation*, *myelination*, and *cell death*. Basically, the developmental process begins with immature neurons (cell proliferation). These cells become specified regarding their function and location within the system. When their location has been determined, the different cell types migrate to various sites and integrate with other cells. At the site of integration, neurons begin to elaborate axons and dendrites in preparation for establishing the functional connection (synapse) between cells (differentiation). In their final stage of morphological development, most nervous system pathways become coated with myelin to allow them to transmit impulses more effectively. Many neurons are eliminated during early development of the nervous system (cell death), which is believed to be a normal part of the development process.

WebLink

http://developingchild.harvard.edu/—see *Experiences Build Brain Architecture* and YouTube

It should be reemphasized that although the developmental sequence is rather exact, it is also a complex and intricate process. The sequence described only represents highlights in the process. The following discussion elaborates in greater detail significant events that occur within the sequence of early neurological development.

CELL PROLIFERATION AND CHANGES

Neurons first appear in the brain during the second prenatal month, and virtually all of the *cell proliferation* process (growth in number) is completed by birth. At this time, a baby's brain contains about 100 billion neurons and a trillion glial cells, which form a honeycomb that protects and nourishes the neurons. Not only do neurons multiply very rapidly during early development but they also grow in size. The period of dramatic increase in neuron size seems to occur from the sixth prenatal month through the first year of life.

Beginning around the third trimester of gestation and continuing into at least the fourth year is a period of rapid brain growth and development called the *brain growth spurt*. The general period also includes development in terms of cell proliferation, myelination, dendritic and synaptic growth, and refinement of certain enzyme systems. A considerable body of evidence suggests that the brain has a critical period for laying down its foundation (wiring of circuits) for optimal development. After this critical period, there are limits to the brain's ability to reorganize (plasticity). It is also important to note that the timing of the growth spurt cannot be altered; the time line for development is predetermined genetically. However, as will be discussed later, the extent of development is *activity-dependent*; that is, it is significantly affected by experience and stimulation. This fact points to the importance of prenatal care and a stimulating postnatal environment, especially during the early years (Fig. 2.4).

The genetic structure of the cell nucleus plays a primary role in controlling cell proliferation and differentiation. About half of the body's total genes are involved in forming and maintaining the CNS. Although their role during growth is vital to the wiring of basic functional circuits, there are simply not enough of them to specify the trillions of finer connections made after birth.

Along with the process of cell proliferation, several developmental changes occur in the axon and dendrite structures. Once the neurons have *migrated* to their

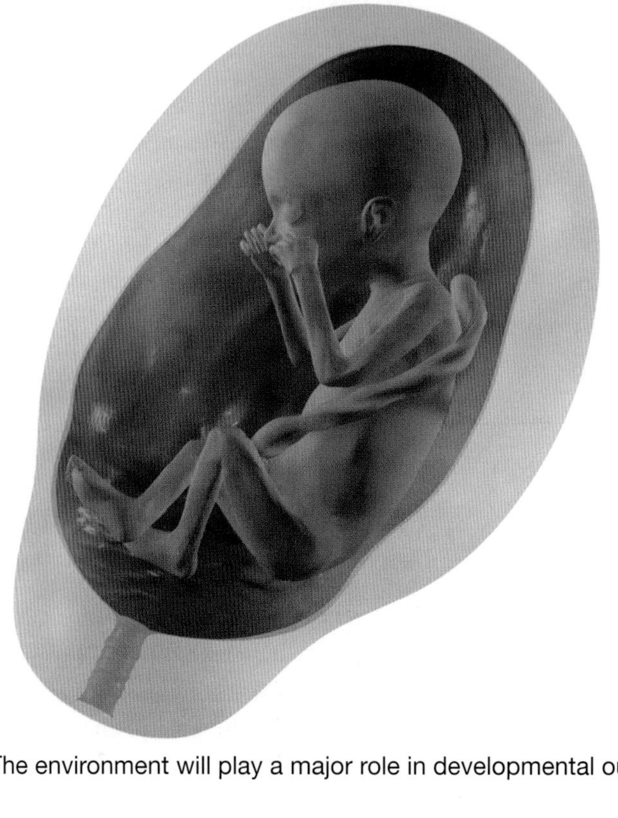

Figure 2.4 The environment will play a major role in developmental outcome.

final location in the CNS, they begin to elaborate their axon and dendritic structures in readiness to accept impulses through synaptic interconnections. Again, neurons may be categorized as sensory (afferent, sending signals to the CNS), motor (efferent, sending signals from the CNS to the muscles), or central (originating and terminating in the brain or spinal cord; also known as *interneurons*). This specification is likely biochemically set. The axons of sensory neurons must often travel relatively long distances to reach their synaptic conjunction.

Terminal targets of motor neurons do not appear to be as specific as those for sensory neurons, but complex specificity is still evident in the growth process. The growth of the axon of a motor neuron is guided somewhat by the chronological order in which it matures and differentiates as well as by its biochemical properties. When a motor neuron innervates a muscle, the axon makes contact and induces biochemical specificity into the muscle, thus allowing the two structures to match up biochemically. Once specificity of the neuromuscular junction is established, sensory and central neurons form their synaptic connections.

One of the major events in cortical neuronal differentiation is the elaboration of dendritic structures. Dendrites are important because they are the main receptors for the neuron. At the synaptic junctions, the dendrites of each neuron can receive signals from literally thousands of other neurons. It has been estimated that dendrites of cortical neurons provide more than 95% of the targets for transmitting information through the system. Not until approximately the eighth fetal month do the first signs of thick dendrites that have conspicuous spines start to appear on cells in the visual cortex. Although the motor cortex is noted as more advanced in dendritic development than the visual cortex at that time, the appearance of dendritic spine development is not as evident. At around 30 weeks of gestation, the dendritic spines show obvious immaturity; they are few in number and irregular in shape. But by 8 months (postnatal), the number of well-formed, lollipop-shaped, stubby spines has multiplied. Dendrite growth is a major reason that brain weight increases significantly from birth to age 2 years. Figure 2.5 represents the various stages of dendritic development in large pyramidal neurons (Lund, 1978).

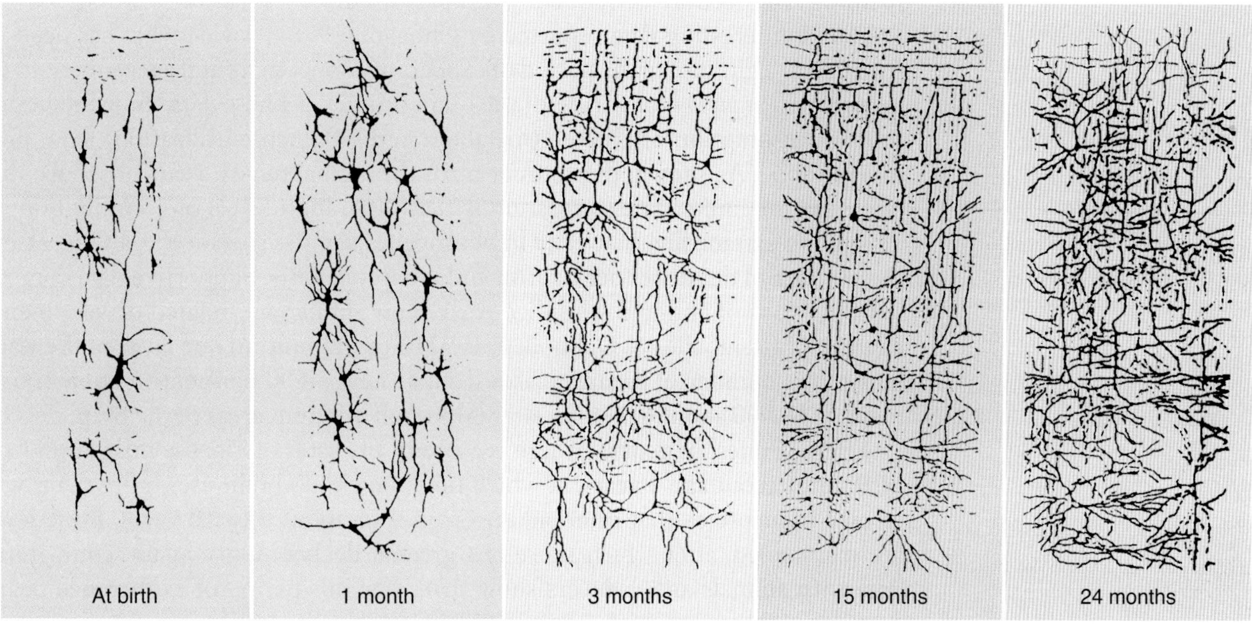

Figure 2.5 Representation of dendritic development.

INTEGRATION AND DIFFERENTIATION

As cells begin to multiply, migrate to their final location, and elaborate, they also undergo the concurrent processes of **integration** and differentiation (i.e., wiring of the brain). Integration refers to the intricate interweaving of neural mechanisms toward their target destination. **Differentiation**, on the other hand, is the process by means of which structure, function, or forms of behavior become more specialized. This term also refers to the progression of motor control from gross, poorly controlled movements to precise, complex motor behavior. Differentiation cannot occur until **synaptogenesis** has taken place (i.e., the synapses between neurons have formed).

Estimates for the average number of neuronal connections range from 1,500 to 15,000, depending on the type and function of the neuron, producing trillions of connections. The formation of synapses occurs at different times and in different parts of the brain, with the sequence tied with the emergence of various functions and skills. Neuronal connections begin to form during embryonic development, when each differentiating neuron sends out an axon (the transmission lines of the nervous system) tipped at its leading point by a growth cone. The cone migrates through the dense environment to its synaptic targets. Current theory suggests that the growth cone navigates itself (at times, relatively long distances) to the target using guidance mechanisms (cues) involving various chemical attractor and repulsion processes. By the time of birth, the infant's brain has already formed trillions of neuronal connections (synapses). Areas already wired prior to birth include functions for breathing, circulation, heartbeat, reflexes, and basic (spontaneous) movement. In the first months of postnatal life, the number of connections will increase 20-fold. Synaptogenesis begins in the motor cortex at about 2 months of age—a time when basic reflexes (e.g., startle and rooting) begin to phase away and purposeful movement emerges (e.g., reaching). Tied closely to this event is synaptic formation in the visual cortex at about 3 months, allowing the infant's eyes to focus on an object. Shortly after, the brain, in a phase of biological exuberance, begins to produce trillions more connections than it can possibly use. Around the age of 10 years, the brain selectively eliminates (also referred to as **pruning**) connections infrequently or never used.

Some interesting data reported by Chugani (1998) provide what has been referred to as a glimpse of the period of exuberant connectivity and a testament to the general *critical period* for wiring of the brain (Fig. 2.6). These data show the human brain's consumption of glucose (metabolic rate of glucose utilization) from birth to adulthood. As shown, the rates at birth through about 10 years are more than twice that of adults. The suggestion is that these high levels of consumption are devoted to extraordinary activity in neurogenesis, more specifically, an increase in the number of dendrites per neuron and synaptogenesis. Supportive data comparing the brains of children who died early show similar age-related developmental change (Huttenlocher & Dabholkar, 1997). For example, in one layer of the visual cortex, the number of synapses rises from around 2,500 per neuron at birth to as many as 18,000 about 6 months later. Although different areas of the brain develop at different rates, in general, there is a rise in the rates of glucose utilization from birth until about age 4 years, at which time the child's brain uses more than twice as much glucose as that of an adult. From 4 to about 9 to 10 years, these levels are maintained, after which there is a gradual decline. Once again, comparative data with animals and cadavers show that after this period of exuberance begins a pruning phase, in which surviving neurons show a decline in synaptic density. Hypothetically, neurons stimulated adequately during the critical period show less

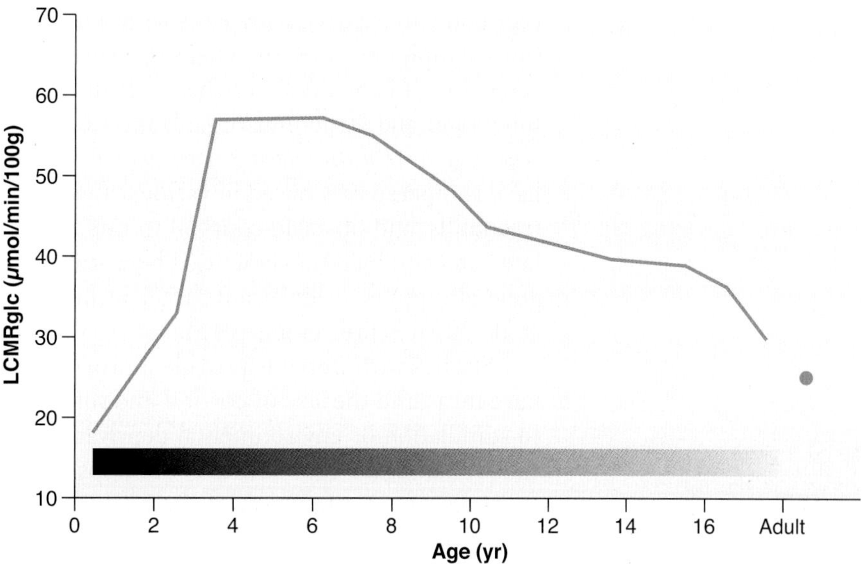

Figure 2.6 Average glucose utilization levels in four areas of the cortex.

SOURCE: Adapted from Chugani, H. T. (1998). A critical period of brain development: Studies of cerebral glucose utilization with PET. *Preventive Medicine*, *27*, 184–188.

elimination and support the idea of activity-dependent stabilization. Correlations between regional glucose consumption and behavior provide much of the basis for what has become known as the optimal windows of opportunity for wiring and efficient learning.

The Effects of Early Experience. As alluded to in Chapter 1 and in this section, scientists now believe that to achieve the precision of the mature brain, neural function and stimulation during infancy and early childhood are necessary. That is, optimal development is *activity-dependent*. Dr. Bruce Perry, a noted researcher in this field, provides a classic statement still supported today, "Experience is the chief architect of the brain" (*Time*, February 3, 1997).

The general notion is that although genetics plays a major role in determining the main neural circuits of the brain, positive stimulation significantly influences the trillions of finer connections made after birth. Experience appears to exert its effects by strengthening synapses; that is, stimulation from the environment produces a signal that forms various connections. Connections that are not made, or are weak, are pruned away. If the neurons are used, they become integrated into the circuitry of the brain. Thus, due to differences in experience, not even identical twins are wired the same.

How do scientists know this? They invasively examine (invade the tissue of) the brains of animals after experimental manipulation and noninvasively study infant brain structure and activity using sophisticated neuroimaging techniques. Most research on this topic has been conducted with regard to development of the visual system in mammalian species (cat, rat, and ferret). Although the measurement techniques are more sophisticated, several modern studies have followed the general experimental manipulation popularized by Hubel and Wiesel in the 1970s; that is, either one or both eyes of the animal are deprived of stimulation prenatally or postnatally for a period as long as several weeks. Scientists then make comparisons of anatomical and physiological changes to those of control animals, or they compare visual cortex areas within the animal. Common observations include (for example) number of synapses, neuron and axon size, and biochemical characteristics. The general conclusion from these experiments suggests that optimal functional and structural organization of the brain (wiring of the visual system) *requires a level of stimulating experience*. In addition, several interesting experiments have compared rats raised in various environmentally enriched settings (e.g., toys, treadmills, and obstacle courses) to rats kept in deprived environments (e.g., isolated and confined movement). These studies also confirm that stimulation (of this general type) is a significant factor in brain development (see review by Berardi et al., 2015; Scholz et al., 2015).

Studies with humans provide a provocative parallel. For example, researchers have measured the size of cortical and subcortical areas of a child's brain, as related to stimulation or environmental deprivation. These studies, in general, found that the human brain grows in size, develops complexity, makes synaptic connections, and modifies as a function of the quality and quantity of sensory experience. For example, brain imaging studies of children who grew up in a deprived environment (orphanage) show depressed brain activity (Reeb et al., 2009). It is speculated that during infancy and early childhood, exercise and play provide vital sensory and physiological stimulation resulting in increased nerve connections.

Without question, this line of research has added a great deal to our understanding of brain development, and the future looks quite promising. However, at this point, it is still quite unclear as to the specific types of experience and how much is optimal to stimulate the formation of particular neural connections. For an excellent review of research on the effects of early experience on development, refer to Fox and Rutter (2010).

DOES THE BRAIN DEVELOP NEW NEURONS AFTER BIRTH (IN ADULTHOOD)?

Recall from our discussion of neuron proliferation that virtually all neurons are present at the time of birth. A long-standing belief was that neurons were produced only during the embryonic and fetal periods and for only a short time after birth, if then. However, due in large part to new techniques for observing brain processes, that belief has changed dramatically. Researchers now know the brain does indeed generate new neurons on a rather regular basis throughout much of the life span. The number of neurons is relatively small, and the location appears to be limited to the hippocampus, which is involved in memory and learning processes. Most interesting, however, is compelling evidence that environmental manipulations affect adult neurogenesis and improve learning (Merritt & Rhodes, 2015; Shors, 2014). This has been shown in animal studies as evidenced by exercising mice (running on a treadmill) that produce 2.5 times the growth of new neurons compared to animals housed in more sedentary conditions. This line of research supports the theory discussed earlier that environmental manipulations may affect neurogenesis in a positive manner.

think about it

Can parents do anything to optimize brain development in babies? If yes, what?

MYELINATION

The developmental process of **myelination** has been one of the most extensively examined indicators of neurological growth. Much of the early growth in brain size and weight can be attributed to myelination. Evidence has already been presented to show that neurons have slower transmission rates before myelination, are more prone to fatigue, and are more limited in their rate of repetitive firing.

Focus on Application
Running Enhances Neurogenesis

As noted in this section, research has shown that exposure to an enriched environment (with movement) increases neurogenesis in the dentate gyrus of adult mice. Environmental enrichment, however, typically consists of many components, such as expanded learning opportunities, increased social interaction, more physical activity, and larger housing. In what is considered pioneering efforts in this area, van Praag and associates (1999) wanted more specific movement-oriented information so they assigned adult mice to various conditions: water-maze learning (learner), swim (swimmer), voluntary wheel running (runner), enriched (enriched), and standard housing (control) groups. Neither maze training nor swimming had any effect on positive cell number. However, *running doubled the number of surviving newborn cells,* in amounts similar to enrichment conditions. Thus, the results demonstrate that voluntary exercise (running) increases cell proliferation, survival, and neuronal differentiation in the hippocampus of adult mice. Although the results in this case are specific to mice, newer studies suggest that exercise in humans may also produce positive results.

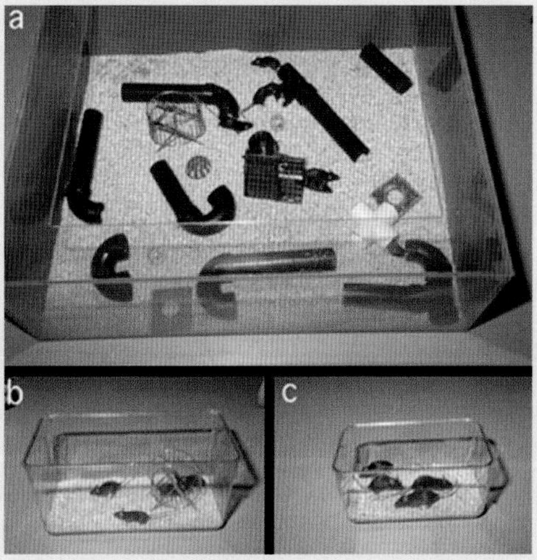

Example of environments: **A.** Enriched. **B.** Setup for voluntary exercise (running). **C.** Standard cage

Sources:
van Praag, H. (2009). Exercise and the brain: something to chew on. *Trends in Neurosciences*, *32*(5), 283–290.
van Praag, H., Kempermann, G., & Gage, F. H. (1999). Running increases cell proliferation and neurogenesis in the adult mouse dentate gyrus. *Nature Neuroscience*, *2*(3), 266–270.

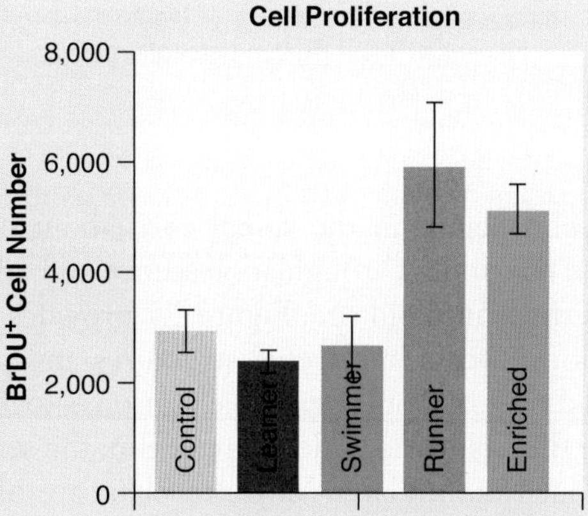

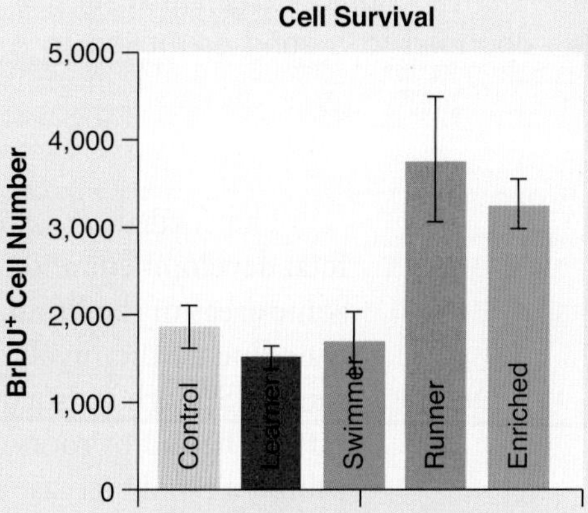

A. Total number of cells 1 day after. **B.** Total number after 4 weeks (survived).

The relative rates of myelination in different areas of the brain give a rough estimate of when these areas reach adult levels of functioning. The degree of myelination is also closely related to maturation (and readiness) in acquisition of motor skills during early childhood. The ages at which myelination begins and ends seem to vary from one brain structure to another, as does the time required for the myelination process itself.

Focus on Application

Movement Influences the Wiring of Rhythm in Infants

Phillips-Silver and Trainor (2005) found that having 7-month-old babies move with their mother to various beats influenced rhythm perception. It was suggested that movement played an important role in helping wire babies' brains to hear rhythm. The researchers tested the infants by having them listen to music made by a snare drum and sticks that had an ambiguous rhythm—no accented beats. Half of the mothers bounced their infants on every second beat, in a marchlike rhythm, and the other half bounced their infants on every third beat, in a waltzlike rhythm. Then the researchers played the music again, this time with the beats accented in either the march or waltz pattern. The infants preferred to listen to the pattern that matched how they had been bounced. The researchers concluded that the perception and development of musical rhythm comprise a multisensory experience that likely reflects a strong interaction between auditory and vestibular (movement) information in the human nervous system.

Underscoring the importance of movement in developing rhythm, the researchers contend that how we move may influence what we hear. Early development of the vestibular system and infant delight at vestibular stimulation when bounced to a song or rocked to a lullaby suggest a strong vestibular-auditory interaction critical for the development of human musical behavior. It has long been known that infants are attracted to music and responsive to its emotional content. This work provides evidence that the experience of body movement plays an important role in musical rhythm perception.

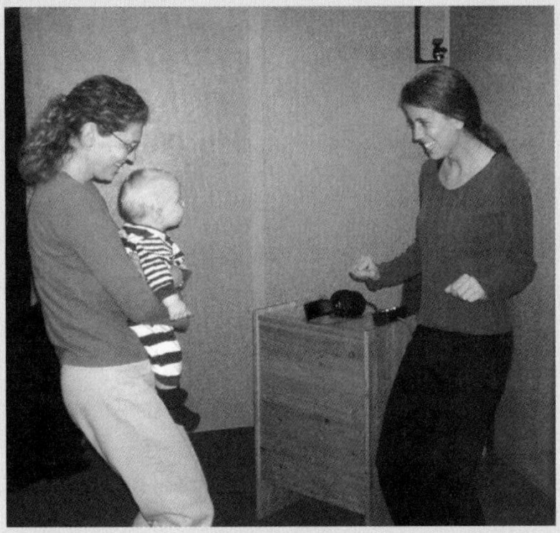

Source:
Phillips-Silver, J., & Trainor, L. J. (2005). Feeling the beat: Movement influences infant rhythm perception. *Science*, *308*, 1430.

The formation of myelin begins in the spinal cord about halfway through fetal development and then continues through adolescence and adulthood and, in some areas of the brain, perhaps into old age. Figure 2.7 provides an approximate time line of the myelination process in selected structures and pathways within the CNS. Both sensory and motor roots begin myelination 4 to 5 months before birth. The motor roots are the first parts to develop myelin; the sensory structures exhibit a rapid increase about 1 month later. Motor mechanisms of the spinal cord appear fully myelinated and functional by the end of the first month after birth. Once again, the sensory mechanisms lag behind somewhat and do not show significant myelin growth in the cord until approximately 6 months after birth.

The primary sensory tracts to the cortex appear to mature at slightly different times during the life span. The myelination of the visual pathways (optic mechanisms) begins around the time of birth. However, once the developmental process of the visual pathways begins, it proceeds very rapidly and is completed sometime during the first 5 months of postnatal life. The higher somesthetic pathways related to touch show myelin growth around the eighth prenatal month, and by birth, these pathways are myelinated through to the cortex. Evidence of this level of development is exhibited by newborns who are normally quite sensitive

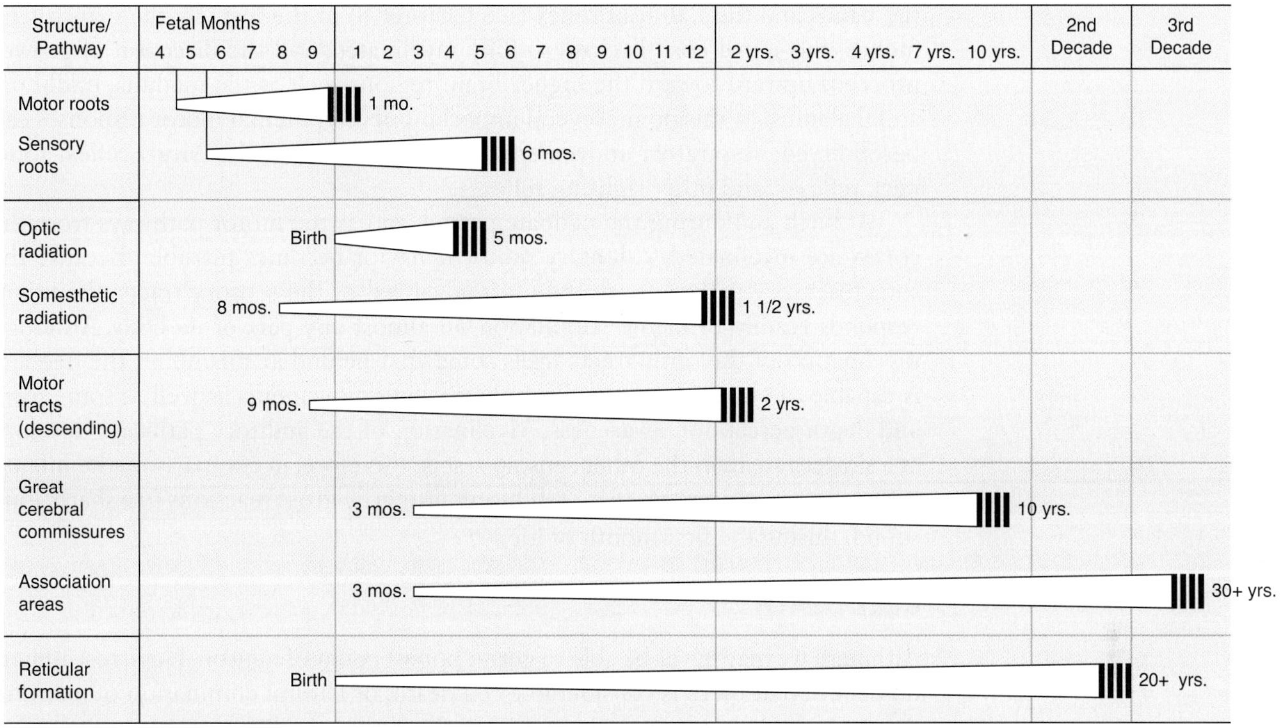

* Width and length of bars indicate increasing density of myelination; blacked-in areas at end of bars indicate approximate age range of completion of myelination process.

Figure 2.7 An estimated time line of the myelination process.

to touch stimuli. Significant growth continues in the somesthetic pathways until approximately 2 years of age.

The descending motor tracts, the major efferent pathway from the motor cortex, begin myelination a month before birth. Although the pathway does not achieve full maturity for about 2 years, it is probably functional by 4 to 5 months, when intentional (voluntary) motor behavior can be observed in the infant. The part of the brain that integrates information (cerebral commissures) exhibits a rapid increase in myelin about the third month after birth, and this process continues until approximately age 10 years. The reticular formation associated with the attention processes begins a period of rapid myelination at birth and continues to mature in an individual until sometime after the second decade. This observation has led to the belief that a person's capability to selectively attend to a task is still being modified until early adulthood. Last to undergo myelination are the areas of the brain associated with memory. These structures, called *association areas*, begin to show significant myelin growth that starts around the third month after birth and continues into and beyond the third decade of life.

The development of myelin and the characteristics of early motor behavior present an interesting developmental parallel. Prior to the initiation of voluntary motor control, movement is primarily exhibited in the form of neurogenic and reflex behaviors. After the appearance of myelin in the spinal cord at about the third or fourth fetal month, movement can be elicited through the motor neuron's connection with the muscle. This type of behavior, which is affected by neural structures, is called *neurogenic behavior*. When myelination is more complete in the spinal cord, *reflex arcs* appear, meaning that the fetus can receive sensory input and reflexively translate the information into a behavior or motor response. Touch stimulation can elicit such movement behaviors as the primitive grasp reflex of the hands and the Babinski reflex (see Chapter 8) of the feet. By the eighth fetal month, the spinal cord is close to fully myelinated, and the direction of growth proceeds upward toward the higher brain regions such as the medulla, midbrain, and thalamus. At this point, several important developmental motor responses can be observed: respiratory movements, primitive sucking, the Moro reflex, tonic neck reflexes, and other righting reflexes.

At birth and during the neonate period, and as the motor pathways from the cortex are myelinated, voluntary motor behavior becomes possible. Because the somatosensory pathways are the most advanced of the sensory tracts, the infant responds readily to tactile stimulation on almost any part of its body. Although myelination of the optic tracts trails somewhat behind at this point, the neonate is capable of visual fixation and simple tracking movements as well as some form and depth perception awareness. Myelination of the auditory pathways develops at a slower rate than the other sensory tracts; therefore, in comparison, the infant's responses are less mature (e.g., exhibiting primarily gross reactions to a sharp, loud sound) during the first month of life.

CELL DEATH

Although we may never be able to get an honest count of neuronal loss, researchers do believe that there is considerable cell death, or natural elimination of neurons, during early development and as we age. During early development, some structures may lose 40% to 75% of neurons initially generated. Cell death of neurons in this instance is believed to be a normal part of the developmental process of establishing synaptic connections (i.e., differentiation), first in a phase of synapse overproduction, followed by selective elimination (i.e., pruning) or preservation to yield a more specific neural connection. It has been hypothesized that proliferating cells compete with each other for a limited number of synaptic sites or for some function that is vital to their existence. Table 2.2 provides a summary of the sequence of early neurological development.

TABLE 2.2 Summary of Developmental Events Associated with the General Sequence of Early Brain Neurogenesis

1. With proliferation, the brain produces many more neurons than it needs and then eliminates the excess neurons.
2. These neurons migrate to their final location.
3. Once cells have reached their target destination (integration), they spin out axons that connect to other neurons via dendrites (synaptogenesis). Spontaneous bursts of electrical activity strengthen some of these connections, whereas others die.
4. During this process, myelination (insulation of the neural pathway) and differentiation (greater specialization of function) occur.
5. After birth, the brain experiences a second growth spurt (in neuronal size) reflected by an explosion in the number of dendrites; that is, new connection sites. Additional sensory stimulation fine-tunes the brain's circuitry by making and strengthening new connections.
6. Connections not made or stimulated adequately are pruned away.
7. Cell death is a natural, lifelong process.

CRITICAL PERIODS (WINDOWS OF OPPORTUNITY)

think about it

From this discussion, describe the role of biology/environment in early brain development. If you were designing a motor development program for 3- and 4-year-olds, what would it look like based on this information?

One of the strongest implications of the research described is the observation that during the developmental period of exuberant connectivity, there is a relatively high degree of *brain plasticity*. That is, there are **critical periods** in neuronal development in which experience may be most effective in forging connections (wiring the brain). From another perspective, these critical periods have more recently been referred to as *windows of opportunity*, the theory that nature opens certain windows for the experience effect starting before birth and then "narrows" each opportunity, one by one. In theory, a series of windows exists for developing motor control, vision, language, feelings, and so on. With increasing age, the brain's plasticity declines. The child who misses an opportunity may not develop the brain's circuitry to its full potential for a specific function. However, keep in mind that genetics and individual differences also play a significant role.

Most relevant to our discussion is the general window of opportunity estimated for motor development. For basic gross motor skills, it appears to be from the prenatal period to around the age of 5 years. Keep in mind once again that this is a period in which experience is vital to forging the foundation of brain circuits dedicated to motor control. Other factors such as myelination are also important. The main circuits for reflex (involuntary) behavior are wired prenatally. The window for the primary circuits that control posture and general movement, housed in the cerebellum, is open for about the first 2 years. It is during this time that children begin to gain considerable experience in the world as they move about in the environment. Once again, this suggests that physical activity may be a strong determinant in early development of the brain, not just motor control. In regard to finer muscle control and timing (which follow gross-motor development), it seems reasonable that the general window would be open from shortly after birth to about age 9 years. Evidence from brain activity research (mentioned earlier) suggests that the general closure of the window of opportunity is around the age of 10 years, especially for second-language development. This is the period when the balance between synaptic connectivity and pruning abruptly shifts.

Changes in Major Brain Structures

***Objective* 2.8**

Throughout brain growth from early periods, the appearance of function approximates maturation in structure. Keep in mind that structure is influenced by experience, therefore making age predictions gross estimates. However, general trends have been documented. The adult brain weighs about 3.5 pounds, and although it makes up only about 2.5% of the total body weight, it requires 15% of the body's blood supply and about 25% of all the oxygen consumed. From 2 to 8 weeks following conception, the nervous system begins to develop as a long, hollow tube on the back of the embryo. As the system develops, brain size increases into a mass of neurons, losing its primitive tubular appearance. At birth, the infant's brain weighs about one-fourth of its adult weight. After birth, nerve cell size increases, other supporting cells called *neuroglia* are formed, and the myelin develops, causing the brain to double in volume. By age 3 years, the brain has reached nearly 90% of its adult size, and by age 6 years, it has basically achieved its full size. In contrast, total body weight at birth is just 5% of young adult size, and by age 10 years, body weight is only 50% of the weight that will eventually be attained.

think about it

What scientific measurement techniques provide us with information about development of the brain? Furthermore, what can they tell us?

The part of the brain most fully developed at birth is the midbrain. As previously mentioned, the midbrain is the part of the CNS that controls much of the early reflex behavior. After the midbrain (in developmental progression) comes the cerebrum and, considerably later, the cerebellum.

Growth and differentiation of the cortical regions of the brain are landmark features in the functional maturity of the CNS. As previously noted, the cortex is composed of an estimated 75% of the total neurons found in the brain; this is an estimated 75 billion, interconnected by thousands of miles of axons and dendrites. Yet in actual size, the cortex accounts for only a very small portion, forming the outermost layer of the cerebrum—about ¼ inch in thickness. Although thickness of the cortex normally reaches adult levels by approximately 2½ years of age, functional maturity of the cortical areas in general is usually not achieved until later early childhood.

As a general observation, two clear gradients of development occur during early brain development. First is the order in which *general structural areas develop*, and second is the order in which *specific functional localizations advance* within the areas. The rate of development among the cerebral lobes is quite varied. Each lobe has its own rate of development, each area in each lobe has its own developmental rate, and each layer of those areas has different rates of development. In order of increasing maturity, the occipital lobe (visual functions) matures first, the parietal lobe (somatosensory functions) matures next, and the temporal (auditory and memory functions) and frontal (memory and motor functions) lobes are the slowest to reach full maturity. The most advanced part of the cortex is the primary motor area, which is involved in the execution and control of movement. Next is the primary sensory area, then the primary visual area in the occipital lobe, and then the primary auditory area in the temporal lobe. The association areas lag behind the corresponding primary areas.

Following the basic principle of cephalocaudal development within the motor area, control of the legs generally evolves later than the capabilities for upper body movements. The same is generally true in the sensory area. By about 2 years, the motor and sensory areas are similar in maturity and the association areas add considerably to function. The cerebellum, the area of the brain primarily responsible for controlling coordinated motor responses, lags behind the midbrain, areas of the spinal cord, and the cerebral cortex in development. Closely linked to its functional maturity is myelination of the tracts between it and the cortex, which reaches potential about age 4 years.

Brain Plasticity. Amazingly, the brain has the ability to learn new motor skills, language, and musical creation—all of which is associated with **brain plasticity**. Plasticity, also referred to as *neuroplasticity*, is the lifelong ability of the brain to reorganize neural pathways based on new experiences. As we learn, we acquire new information and skills through experience or instruction. In order to learn or memorize a fact or skill, there must be persistent functional changes in the brain that represent the new knowledge. To illustrate, when we learn a new dance form or new language, the neural circuitry in the brain reorganizes in response to experience or sensory stimulation. Significant plasticity may occur in three conditions: (a) during normal brain development when the immature brain first begins to process sensory information through adulthood, (b) in events of learning, and (c) in case of brain injury to compensate for lost functions or maximize remaining functions. And, as our general development theme complies, in addition to biology, the environment plays a key role in influencing plasticity. An illustration was given in the earlier "Focus on Application" involving how movement influences the wiring of rhythm in infants. Work, using functional magnetic resonance

think about it

We talked about critical periods for "basic" motor skill connectivity, what about connectivity for general dance? Select a dance and consider what is activated.

WebLink

See Discovery Channel—"Brain Plasticity" on YouTube.

focus on change

The brain has the ability to *change* (plasticity) throughout the life span.

imaging revealed that musical training with young children resulted in brain structure plasticity that was correlated with improvements in musically relevant motor skills (Hyde et al., 2009). Similar training effects have been reported in dancers (see review by Karpati et al., 2015). In regard to plasticity after brain trauma, one of the most amazing cases is that of a young girl who had her left brain "removed" (the procedure is called a *hemispherectomy*) due to constant epileptic seizures. Although the left brain is organized to control the right half of the body, amazingly, the young girl's brain reorganized itself to allow the girl to walk again within a relatively short period of time.

One of the more common demonstrations of plasticity is after a stroke. As in the case of the young girl, healthy brain cells reorganize to take over the functions of damaged brain cells. This means that certain lost functions, such as speech and language, may reemerge as the result of intensive rehabilitation.

Brain Lateralization and the Corpus Callosum

Objective 2.9

Although the two hemispheres of the brain appear symmetrical, in functional terms, they are quite different. Each hemisphere has its own specialized functions (i.e., functional asymmetries), a characteristic known as **brain (hemispheric) lateralization.** In most humans, the left hemisphere is associated with the governance of language, logic, and sequential processing, whereas the right hemisphere is specialized for nonverbal, visuospatial functions (e.g., music awareness, map reading, and figure drawing). Of more direct relevance to motor behavior is that the cortex of the right hemisphere controls muscular activity in and receives sensory input from the left half of the body (Fig. 2.8), whereas the left hemisphere has a complementary role in conscious movement on the right side of the body.

Dividing and connecting the two hemispheres of the brain is a tough band of myelinated tissue called the *corpus callosum*. One of its primary functions is to provide the link for shared information between the two hemispheres, in essence allowing the right hand to know what the left hand is doing. Thus, the corpus callosum is important for the functional integration of the two cerebral hemispheres

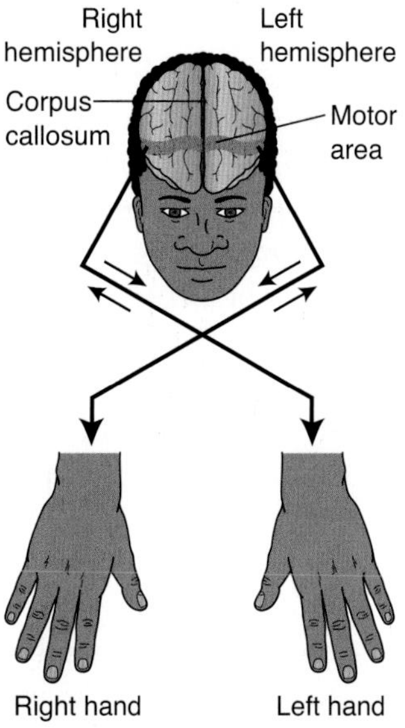

Figure 2.8 The concept of lateral dominance of limb control.

and possibly for the manifestation of functional asymmetries. The callosum undergoes marked growth in overall size and myelination during postnatal development, and by 5 years, its development is fairly advanced. However, behavioral studies of the development of interhemispheric communication (also known as "cross-talk") linked to corpus callosum function suggest that development continues over the first 10 years of life. Further discussion of this topic is provided in Chapters 8 and 9 in relation to theoretical and applied considerations of functional (motor) asymmetries (i.e., the development of handedness, footedness, and eye preference).

Neurological Changes with Advanced Aging

Objective 2.10

focus on change

Change in brain structures during older adulthood has significant implications for daily living skills and, in some case, independence.

There are considerable individual differences in aging of the brain. In addition, the many components of the brain itself vary in degree of age-related change. The loss of neurons in various regions is accepted as a significant part of the aging process. It is estimated that this loss is about 5% to 30% by old age. The brain loses about 7% of its weight from the time when we are younger adults. This amount could be substantially more if some form of organic brain disease or other secondary aging element (e.g., drugs, diet, alcohol, or health of the cardiovascular system) is present. It is generally believed that the brain has such remarkable recovery capabilities (plasticity) that, although significant neuron loss may occur, the brain may only lose a small portion of its ability to function. In fact, to compensate for losses, older brains literally rewire themselves for a given task.

In addition to a significant loss of neurons, other important changes appear to be occurring within the neurons themselves. One of the most critical of these changes involves the gradual shrinking and withering away of the dendrites (density) and axons (i.e., interconnectivity among neurons), whereas other mutations may include the cell body. Process deficits normally associated with advanced aging include a decrease in neuron connectivity, delay in new axon growth and myelination, decrease in neuron excitability, and estimated twofold increase in synaptic delay. Several of the characteristics listed have been associated with the older adult phenomenon known as *psychomotor slowing* (to be discussed in greater detail in Chapters 7 and 11).

In general, aging may be constituted by a proliferation of abnormal material and functions referred to as vacuoles, plaques, and tangles. *Vacuoles* are thick granules surrounded by fluid. Although they are most common in diseased brains, vacuoles show up in three-fourths of the brains checked from people older than 80 years of age. *Senile plaques*, collections of debris consisting of cells, silicone, and macrophagic elements, are frequently found in the frontal and occipital lobes of the brain. *Neurofibrillary tangles*, tangled clumps of double-helical strands of protein, appear in older brains, but no one clearly understands their effect. Tangles tend to be particularly prominent in the cerebral cortex as a whole and in the thalamus, basal ganglia, and spinal cord. Studies have also noted that as neurons and dendrites deteriorate, neuroglia (the connective tissue that fills the spaces between neurons) increase in number. Bodies of astrocytes, star-shaped neuroglia, get larger in the aging brain and may prevent neurotransmitters from building up between nerve cells.

One of the most dramatic decreases in basic neurological function related to motor behavior is the deterioration of vestibular awareness (balance). Neurons in one layer of the cerebellum die off fairly rapidly after the age of 60 years. With this decrease is an estimated 40% loss of vestibular hair and nerve cells by 70 years. As previously noted, the cerebellum functions to coordinate voluntary motor behavior and vestibular awareness. Balance as measured by speed-of-return-to-equilibrium

TABLE 2.3 Selected Basic Neurological Changes with Advanced Aging

Neurological Structure	Function
Brain weight	Decreases
Number of neurons	Decreases
Dendritic density	Decreases
Nerve conduction velocity	Decreases
Connectivity	Decreases

think about it

Name some reasons why large individual differences exist in brain function of the elderly.

and body sway deteriorates significantly during old age (Shumway-Cook & Woollacott, 2012). The topic of balance in older persons is discussed in Chapter 11.

Another basic neural process crucial to motor behavior is nerve conduction velocity. This function also declines with increasing age. The loss appears more prominent in the distal segments of the body and in the lumbosacral regions. The results of such a loss have been evidenced by several studies showing how reaction and movement time slow with increased age. In general, the decline of both functions tends to occur most rapidly in the lower parts of the body and in areas of most frequent use, such as the fingers. The general rate of decline appears to be affected by the complexity of the task.

Table 2.3 presents a summary list of selected neurological functions that normally show signs of deterioration with advanced aging.

Summary

The blueprint for our heredity is contained in the genes found within the 23 pairs of chromosomes of a human cell nucleus. Heredity influences numerous developmental factors such as aging, puberty, general body type, height, muscle fiber type, and skeletal age. These factors can also be affected by the environment as evidenced by the documented effects of diet and exercise on body weight and aging.

The nervous system serves three primary functions: (a) sensory, (b) integrative, and (c) motor. The basic function of the CNS is to transmit information about the environment and the body to the brain, and to carry information from the brain to muscles and glands, thus producing motor responses and bodily adaptations to environmental demands. The PNS is a branching network of nerves, including the somatic system that controls all the skeletal muscles.

The basic parts of a neuron are the cell body, dendrites, and axon. Dendrites are the receiving part of the neuron, whereas the function of the axon is to carry information away from the cell body to other cells. The functional connection between the axon and another neuron is called a synapse. The ascending and descending motor pathway systems provide the channels through which nerve impulses travel. How fast the information travels depends to some degree on the presence of myelin, which forms an insulating sheath around many axons.

Development of the CNS can be described in a sequence of six integrated biological events: cell proliferation, migration, integration, differentiation,

myelination, and cell death. The process of proliferation is virtually completed by birth. As proliferation occurs, cells migrate to their final location and elaborate, which is evidenced by the developmental changes that take place in the axon and dendrite structures. Neurons are also involved in an intricate interweaving process to target cells (integration) and, in turn, become more specialized (differentiation). A significant influence in the wiring process is stimulation provided by the environment. During this general process, the development of myelin (myelination) also transpires. A normal part of the developmental process is cell death.

The brain undergoes several rapid structural and developmental (level of functioning) changes during the first few years. During the course of development, each hemisphere establishes its own specialized functions; this is referred to as lateralization. Related to this concept is the notion that hand and foot motor control on one side of the body is controlled by areas of the brain in the opposite-side hemisphere.

Several neurological changes occur during the latter stages of aging. Along with the loss of neurons and brain weight, important functional changes are also evident. Among the most affected are vestibular awareness (balance) and nerve conduction velocity (a slowing of movement).

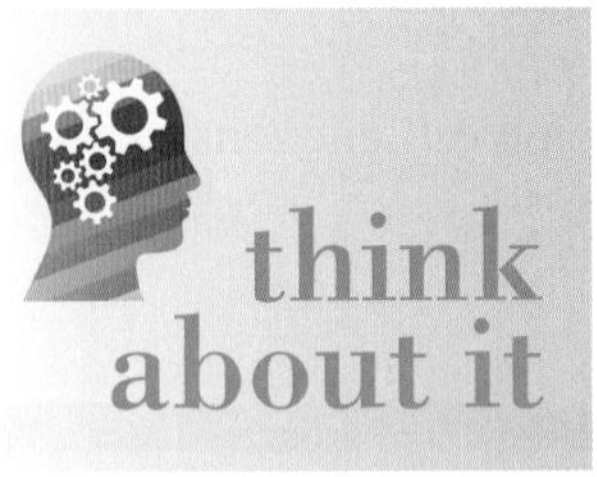

1. **List some of your phenotype characteristics and from which parent you inherited them. Can you think of ways the environment affects phenotype over time?**
2. **Can parents do anything to optimize brain development in babies? If yes, what?**
3. **From this discussion, describe the role of biology/environment in early brain development. If you were designing a motor development program for 3- and 4-year-olds, what would it look like based on this information?**
4. **What scientific measurement techniques provide us with information about development of the brain? Furthermore, what can they tell us?**
5. **We talked about critical periods for "basic" motor skill connectivity, what about connectivity for general dance? Select a dance and consider what is activated.**
6. **Name some reasons why large individual differences exist in brain function of the elderly?**

■ LEARNING ACTIVITIES

Objective: To design appropriate programs to optimize brain development. Considering the information and *Think About It* questions pertaining to early brain development and "windows of opportunity," and what you can find on the Web, formally design a program for:

1. Parents to optimize brain development in babies (up to 2 years)
2. 3- and 4-year-olds

Objective: To consider the functional implications due to an aging brain for elderly persons. For example, what are some of the possible declines in daily living (functional) skills? Report on at least two research papers supporting your points.

Suggested Readings

Sanes, D., Reh, T., & Harris, W. (2011). *Development of the nervous system* (3rd ed.). New York, NY: Academic Press.

Schaie, K. W., & Willis, S. (Eds.) (2015). *Handbook of the psychology of aging* (8th ed.). New York, NY: Academic Press.

Chapter 3

Physical Growth Changes

OBJECTIVES

Upon completion of this chapter, you should be able to

3.1	Provide a brief summary of the major changes in physical growth that take place over the course of the life span.
3.2	Define the terms *physical anthropology*, *anthropometry*, and *growth curve*.
3.3	Outline and briefly describe the significant growth and development events that occur during the prenatal period.
3.4	Discuss the major characteristics and changes associated with the pubescent (adolescent) growth spurt.
3.5	List and briefly describe the major changes in body proportions and physique that take place during normal growth and development.
3.6	Discuss how height and skeletal growth measurements typically change during development.
3.7	Identify the major changes in body mass that accompany lifelong development and the methods used to assess those changes.
3.8	List and briefly describe the various ways of estimating physical maturity.
3.9	Discuss maturity variations among developing individuals.
3.10	Explain secular trend.
3.11	Discuss the implications for motor performance of change in physical growth characteristics.

KEY TERMS

anthropometry	ossification
growth curve	body mass
pubescent growth spurt	chronological age
menarche	biological age
growth hormone (GH)	secular trend
somatotype	

In the previous chapter, you learned about the growth and development characteristics of the basic neurological structures. This chapter focuses on changes in physical growth over the life span. Specific discussions cover a general overview of physical growth, prenatal development, the adolescent growth spurt, body proportions and physique, height and skeletal growth, and body mass. Methods of estimating maturity level and maturity variations are also examined.

AN OVERVIEW OF PHYSICAL GROWTH AND DEVELOPMENT

Objective 3.1

The new perspective on lifelong human development stresses the fact that the developmental process evolves along a continuum from conception to physical death. This perspective is supported through the observation of physical growth changes. Although the first two decades of life are a period of significant growth increases, marked changes also occur during later stages of the aging process.

focus on change

Heredity (Chapter 2) affects *change* in physical growth. However, the environment plays a vital role.

In regard to the determinants of body size in general, there is little doubt that a number of factors act independently or in concert to modify individual outcome. As discussed in Chapter 2 (see Table 2.1 on page 37), the genetic contribution to physical growth characteristics can be considerable. However, the overall contribution varies with environmental circumstances, such as diet and physical activity. For example, children who have similar genotypes and who would likely reach similar adult height under ideal conditions may turn out quite differently due to environmental influences.

Growth begins in a general cephalocaudal and proximodistal pattern. With the cephalocaudal pattern, growth (especially during the prenatal stage) first occurs in the head and gradually proceeds downward to the neck, shoulders, and trunk. At the same time, proximodistal growth proceeds from the center of the body and moves toward the extremities (e.g., the hands and fingers). Individuals grow at a faster rate during gestation and the first year after birth than they will at any other time in their lives. During the early childhood years, physical growth progresses at a relatively uniform and steady rate. In middle and late childhood, growth is a relatively slow, consistent process that may be characterized as the calm before the dramatic biological change that occurs during early adolescence and the onset of puberty. The pubescent growth spurt represents a landmark in physical growth with regard to sex differences and motor performance. Later in early adulthood, physical development usually begins to slow down. And as people age, they generally get shorter, lose muscle mass, experience a change in body proportions, and get heavier. Interestingly, in old age, individuals tend to become lighter than they were during middle adulthood due in large part to losses in bone and muscle mass.

Objective 3.2

WebLink
http://www.cdc.gov/

The field of *physical anthropology* provides information and scientific procedures related to the study of biological growth and development. Physical anthropology is basically concerned with the meaningful understanding of the nature, distribution, and significance of biological variation in humans. The branch of science concerned with biological growth and body measurement is referred to as **anthropometry**, which is one of the basic tools used in growth studies. This chapter includes a description of anthropometric measurement techniques. For detailed descriptions, refer to the Centers for Disease Control and Prevention (CDC) WebLink; also refer to Howley and Thompson (2012). For the latest growth charts for head circumference (birth to 36 months), height, weight, and body mass index (BMI) (2 to 20 years), refer to the student resource for your text *thePoint*.

Anthropometric data used to assess growth take the form of mean value comparisons, percentile rankings, and growth curves. Perhaps a less known but frequently used procedure in growth studies is to plot the pattern of physical change in individuals or groups on a **growth curve**. One type of curve is called a *distance curve*, which is used to plot growth from one year to the next. The distance curves for males and females exhibit a gradual height increase before a leveling off occurs, as shown in Figure 3.1. It depicts typical individual height curves based on data from many individuals. If the values of only one individual were plotted, the graph would be unlikely to show such a smooth curve.

Another anthropometric technique is to measure the rate of growth using what is known as a *velocity curve*. This type of measurement better reflects the

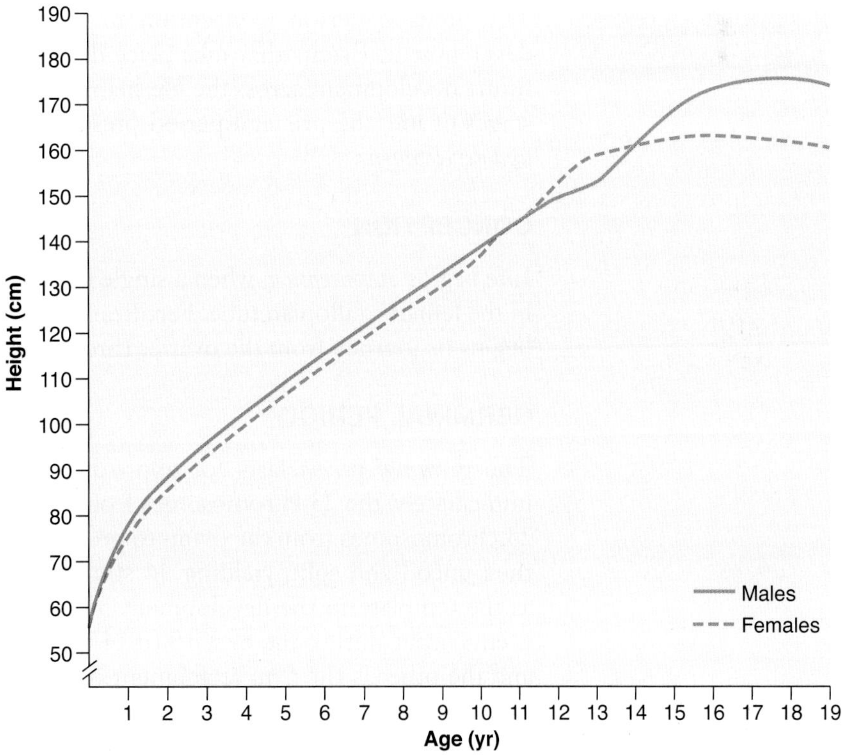

Figure 3.1 Typical distance curves for change in height.

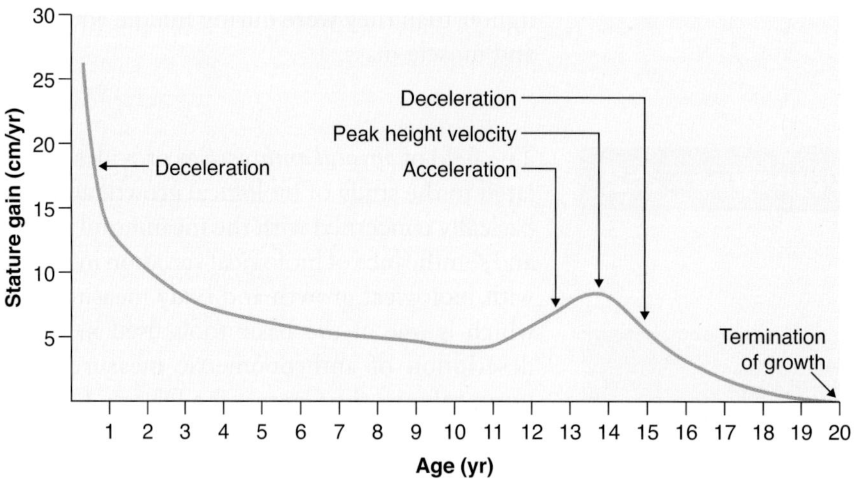

Figure 3.2 An example of a velocity curve for height, indicating the different phases of growth.

individual's growth state at any particular moment than it does the distance or change in growth achieved in preceding years. The velocity of growth refers to increments in growth value from year to year and is represented by points of deceleration or acceleration. Figure 3.2 illustrates a hypothetical velocity curve that has different phases of growth rate for height.

This next section highlights the two most prominent periods in physical growth: prenatal development and the adolescent growth spurt.

Prenatal Development

Objective 3.3

The prenatal period (conception to birth) plays a significant role in human development. Events that take place during this period forge the foundation for future development across the life span. In comparison to the other developmental stages of life, the prenatal period presents the *greatest variation in human growth and development.*

CONCEPTION

Life begins at *conception*, when a single male sperm cell unites with the ovum (egg) in the female's fallopian tube. Fertilization occurs within several days after the egg begins its journey from the ovaries through the fallopian tubes to the uterus.

GERMINAL PERIOD

The *germinal period* lasts for approximately 14 days after conception. Almost immediately, the 23 chromosomes from the sperm cell nucleus combine with the 23 chromosomes from the ovum to produce 46 chromosomes. The chromosomes then uncoil and split, yielding 46 strands of deoxyribonucleic acid, which serve as the template in the development of the individual. Two major developmental events occur during the next 10 to 14 days. One is continued cell differentiation, and the other is the firm attachment of the ovum to the wall of the uterus. During this time, the divided cells gradually form a spherical mass, which separates into inner and outer segments. The outer segment eventually forms part of the mother–fetus barrier, and the inner segment becomes the fetus.

EMBRYONIC PERIOD

By 2 weeks after conception, the embryonic disk has folded and formed the distinct layers of cells called an *embryo*. The *embryonic period* lasts from about 2 to 8 weeks after conception. During this period, human form begins to take shape. Although the embryo after 8 weeks is only about 1 inch (2.5 cm) long and weighs only half an ounce (14 g), the basic parts of the body—the head, trunk, arms, and legs—can be identified. Some of the finer features such as the eyes, ears, fingers, and toes are also discernible. The central nervous system (CNS) is relatively developed, and the internal organs (e.g., the heart, lungs, reproductive organs, liver, and kidneys) are beginning to function to some degree. All of these developments take place according to a master blueprint that dictates that development starts at the head, then moves to the trunk, and then to the lower extremities, in cephalocaudal order. This developmental blueprint also calls for development to proceed proximodistally from the midline of the body (centering around the spine and heart) outward to the extremities (the shoulders, arms, and hands).

FETAL PERIOD

The *fetal period* of development begins about the eighth week, when the embryo becomes a recognizable human being, and lasts until the time of birth.

By the third month, the fetus is about 3 inches (7.5 cm) long and weighs approximately 1 ounce (28 g). The sex organs are developed to the point where sex can be determined, and a number of physical and anatomical features are better defined. The forehead is more prominent, and the eyelids, nose, and chin are clearly distinguishable. Although the process may have begun during the embryonic period, it can now be seen that flexible cartilage is replaced by bone in a process called **ossification**. The fetal period also marks the time at which the first muscle movements in the mouth and jaw probably occur. By the ninth week, the muscles of the arms and legs are capable of responding to tactile stimulation.

> **think about it**
>
> In the study of motor development, why is this period so relevant?

The fourth month (16 weeks) of fetal development is a period of significant growth. The fetus will increase in length to about 6 inches (15 cm) and in weight to approximately 4 ounces (110 g). Although a considerable amount of growth has already occurred in the upper body, there is now a growth spurt of the lower parts of the body in the cephalocaudal direction. The toes and fingers have separated, and fingerprint and footprint patterns begin to emerge.

By the end of the fifth month (20 weeks), the fetus is approximately 12 inches (30 cm) in length and weighs about 1 pound (450 g). Features of the skin have become more differentiated, and distinctive fingernails and toenails are present.

During the sixth month (24 weeks), the eyes and eyelids are completely formed, the eyelids open for the first time, and a fine layer of hair has begun to form on the head. At this point, the fetus weighs approximately 2 pounds (900 g) and is about 14 inches (36 cm) long.

The seventh month (28 weeks) is sometimes called *the age of viability*—meaning that the fetus has matured enough to have a good chance of surviving outside of the womb if birth comes prematurely. Although not a certainty for all, due to medical advances in neonatal care, many babies survive born at 25 weeks with body weights of less than 3 pounds. The internal organs are functioning, and the brain now can regulate breathing, body temperature, and swallowing. The fetus is about 16 inches (40 cm) long and weighs close to 3 pounds (1,350 g).

The eighth and ninth months are a period of rapid weight gain. The fetus gains about half a pound per week for a total of 5 pounds (2,250 g) for the 2-month period, on the average. Just a few weeks prior to birth (and at delivery), the average fetus is 20 inches (50 cm) long and weighs about 7 pounds (3.2 g). During these months, fatty layers are developing that will help to nourish the fetus after birth.

Table 3.1 summarizes the major physical growth changes that occur during the prenatal period.

TABLE 3.1 Major Physical Growth Changes from Conception to Birth

	Age	Height	Weight	
Period	**(wk)**	**(cm)**	**(g)**	**Notable Characteristics**
Germinal	(0–2)			Cell differentiation begins.
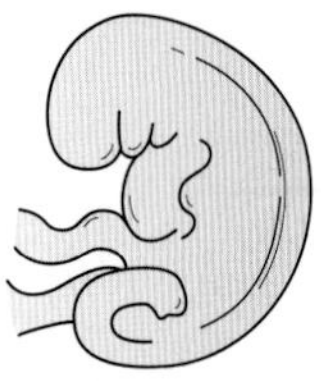				Inner and outer mass formed.
Embryonic	(2–8)	2.5	14	CNS relatively developed.
				Human form takes shape (ears, eyes, arms, legs).
				Internal organs begin to develop (heart, lungs, reproductive, liver, kidneys).
Fetal	12	7.5	28	*Movement*
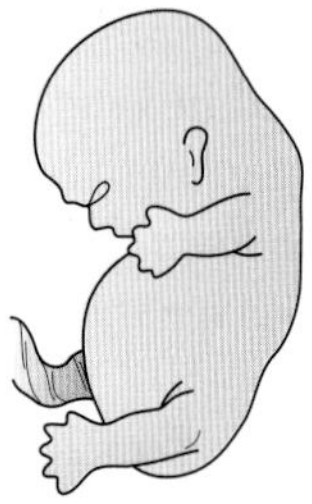				Sex can be distinguished.
				Bone replacing cartilage
				Head growth, facial features
	16	15.0	110	Growth spurt in lower part of body
				Fingerprints and footprints emerge.
	20	30.0	450	Skin structures form.
				Fingernails and toenails present.
	24	36.0	900	Eyes, eyelids formed.
				Head hair forming
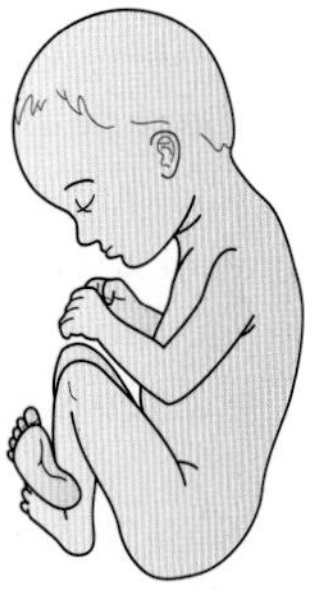	28	37.5–40.0	1,110–1,350	Internal organs functioning
				Age of viability
	32–36	40.0–50.0	1,800–3,600	Rapid weight gain
				Layer of fat forming beneath skin
				Bones of head are soft.

The Pubescent (Adolescent) Growth Spurt

***Objective* 3.4**

Next to the period of prenatal growth, the **pubescent growth spurt**, which occurs during early adolescence, has been described as the life span's *most dramatic period of biological change*. This period also has landmark significance for the evolution of motor performance and sex (biological) differences. These are discussed in detail in subsequent chapters.

At the beginning of adolescence, a number of rapid changes occur in physical maturation and growth. This period of biological development is known as *puberty*, hence, the term *pubescent growth spurt*. These changes are controlled primarily by genetic factors and hormones. About two-thirds of the variation in age of puberty is genetic. Along with rapid changes in body size and proportions, sexual maturation is one of the most prominent aspects of the pubertal process. In this context, puberty is referred to as the *stage of maturation* in which the individual becomes physiologically capable of sexual reproduction.

The pubescent growth spurt generally begins at about 10 to 13 years of age in females and 12 to 15 years of age in males, and it lasts for 2 to 3 years. Females also go through the pubertal period in a somewhat shorter time than males and, thus, are typically about 2 years ahead of males in maturity (see Fig. 3.18 on page 80 with regard to height). Add to this the wide range of ages at which individuals enter puberty, and the general picture of the possible variation in individual differences becomes quite evident (Fig. 3.3).

In females, the growth spurt usually designates the beginning of sexual maturity, when breasts and pubic hair also first appear. This period of development is highlighted by a universal maturity landmark known as **menarche**, or the time of the female's first menstrual flow. The average age at menarche is about 12½ years; for many girls, the event may occur as early as the age of 10 years or as late as 15½ years. A major influence on the onset of puberty in females is body fat. Obese girls tend to reach menarche earlier than small girls (Currie et al., 2012; Oh et al., 2012). The issue of being too small to achieve menarche is discussed in greater detail in Chapter 5.

focus on change

Puberty is a period of dramatic biological *change*.

Maturity indicators for males include the appearance of pubic and facial hair, a change in voice, and an increase in the size of the reproductive organs.

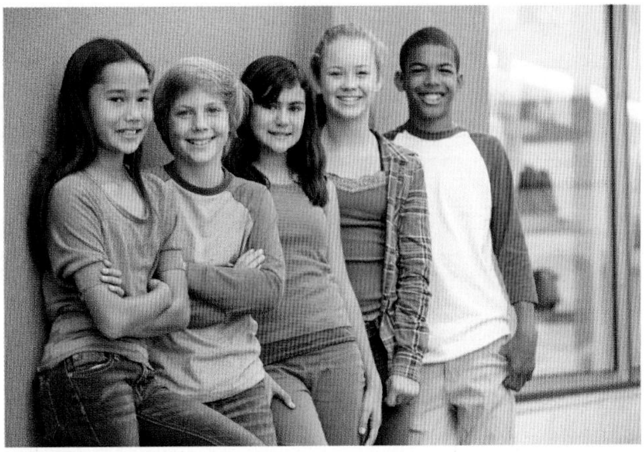

Figure 3.3 Although the boys and girls in this photo are the same age, the girls are similar in height.

HORMONAL INFLUENCE

Hormonal change is another prominent feature of the adolescent growth spurt. Primary agents of this change are the hypothalamus (a part of the brain) and the pituitary (master) gland, which regulates the endocrine system. The other primary glands include the gonads (sex glands), thyroid gland, and adrenal glands (which play a supportive role). Figure 3.4 illustrates the general location of these structures. In addition to regulating the endocrine system, the pituitary produces **growth hormone (GH)**, one of the primary agents that stimulates the adolescent growth spurt.

How does this complex system work (Fig. 3.5)? Basically, puberty begins as increased levels of hormones (via the endocrine system) enter the bloodstream in response to signals from the hypothalamus. These signals instruct the pituitary to release GH and stimulate production of thyroxine (from the thyroid) and sex hormones (from the gonads). Together, GH and thyroxine contribute strongly to the tremendous gain in body size and the completion of skeletal maturation during puberty. In addition to stimulating growth in most tissues, GH also is one of the major regulators of metabolism.

Perhaps as significant is the interaction between GH and androgens produced by the gonads. Throughout childhood, the male and female bodies

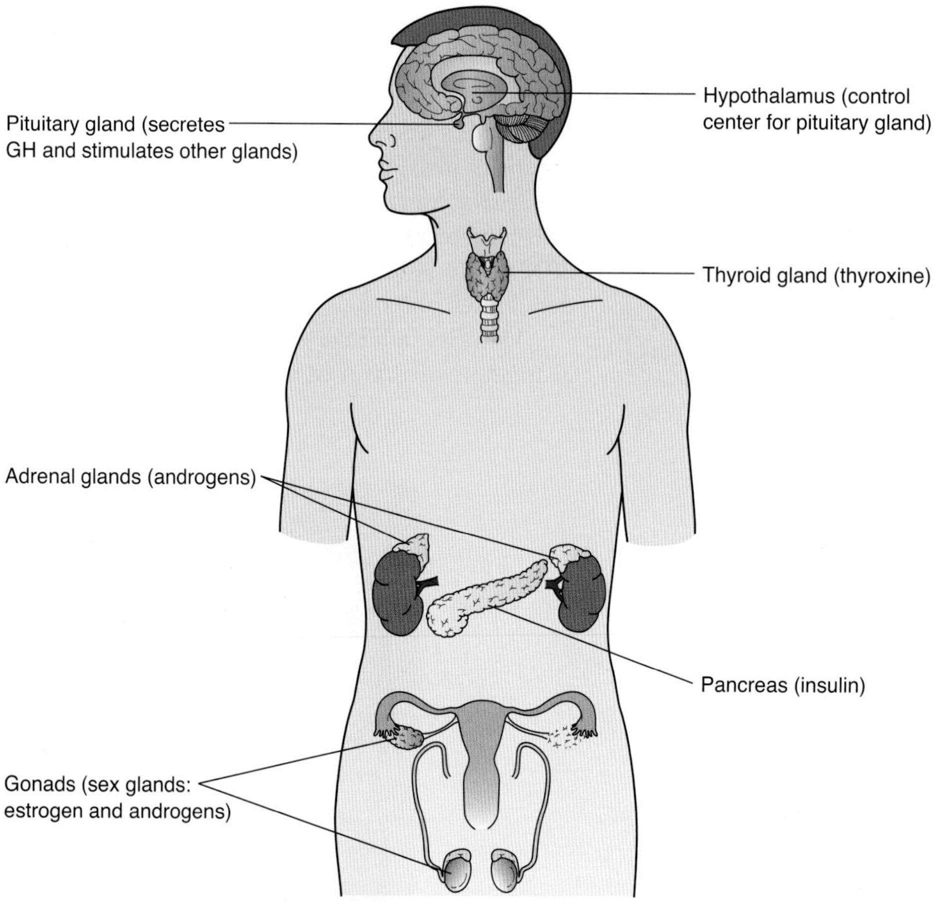

Figure 3.4 General location of major hormonal structures.

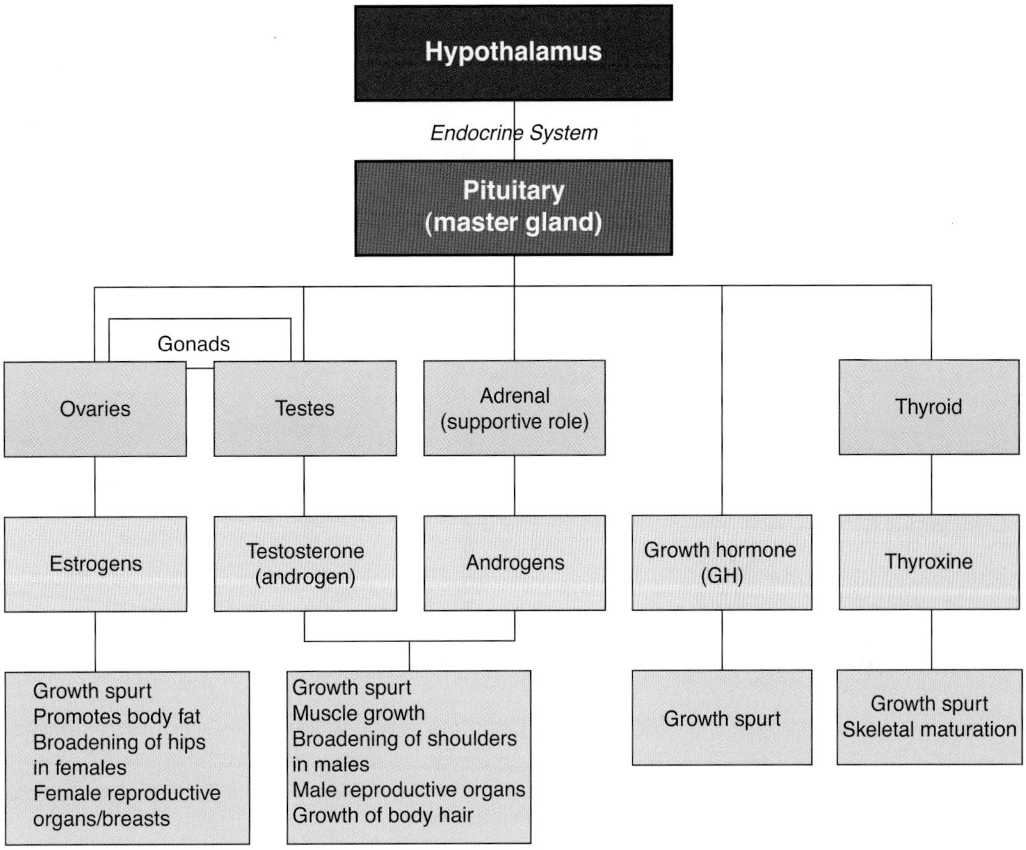

Figure 3.5 Hormonal influence on the body at puberty.

produce approximate levels of estrogens and androgens. After a signal from the hypothalamus, the pituitary sends a signal via *gonadotropins* to stimulate the production of estrogen in the ovaries (female) and androgens (mostly testosterone) in the testes (male). When secretions of these hormones reach critical levels, the pituitary produces more GH; the result is the growth spurt in both sexes.

Androgens play a significant role in hastening the fusion of epiphyseal growth plates in the bones and stimulating the protein synthesis required for the development of muscle tissue. A summary of research studies indicates that testosterone levels increase 10-fold in boys but only twofold in girls during puberty; in contrast, estrogen levels increased 10-fold in girls but only twofold in boys. Note that both hormones are present in both sexes, but that testosterone dominates in the male. Thus, it appears that adolescent boys experience larger growth spurts than girls primarily because of significantly greater testosterone levels. Estrogen, although important to the growth spurt and bone development in females, promotes the accumulation of body fat. Although females may continue to develop muscle tissue (due to the presence of GH and androgens), the effects of estrogen may account for the greater amount of fatty tissue in comparison to males. In addition, estrogens cause a quicker closure of the epiphyseal (bone) plate than testosterone; as a result, females usually do not reach the same height. With regard to androgens produced by the adrenal glands, recent thoughts are that the androgens play a secondary (supportive) role to

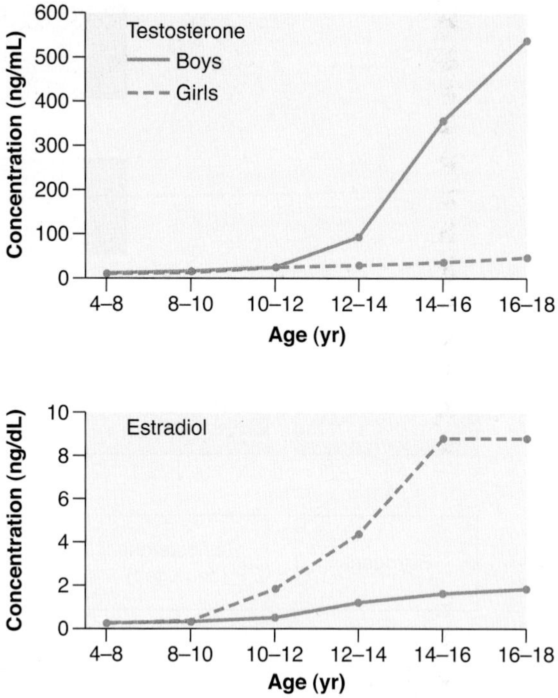

Figure 3.6 Changes in age in serum levels of testosterone and estradiol (estrogen) in children.

SOURCE: Adapted from Malina, R. M., & Bouchard, C. (1991). *Growth, maturation, and physical activity*. Champaign, IL: Human Kinetics.

think about it

Consider some ways the phenomenon of puberty can influence participation in sports. Include possible, if any, differences between males and females.

other hormones in promoting the development of muscle and bone. Figure 3.6 shows changes in testosterone and estrogen levels with age. The consensus of the medical community is that hormone interactions are more influential than the effect of any single hormone.

Table 3.2 provides a list of selected anatomical gender differences that emerge during the adolescent growth spurt due to genetic and hormonal influence. This information is useful in coming chapters that describe motor performance changes as age increases.

TABLE 3.2 Selected Anatomical Gender Differences

Height and weight: males: taller and heavier
Shoulder width: males: wider, more rotation torque
Forearm length: males: longer, more lever torque
Hip shape: insertion of femur more oblique in females
Elbow and knee joints: males: parallel; females: shaped
Leg length: relatively longer in males
Chest girth: greater thoracic cavity in males
Center of gravity: males: higher; females: lower
Fat-free weight: males: more muscle, bigger bones

Focus on Application

Growth Hormone Therapy for Children

For children determined to be too small (short in stature) for their age, GH therapy has been recently approved by the U.S. Food and Drug Administration for children 4 years of age and older to promote growth. Studies are now reporting very encouraging effects on adult height gains, especially in children who started GH therapy early, at least 2 years prior to the onset of puberty. Long-term GH treatment normalizes adult height above −2 SDs in 85% of children, and 98% of children achieve adult height within their target height range. The benefits are in terms of not only height but also body composition.

Who qualifies for this type of therapy? Typically, the marker is a child of short stature: 2 to 2.5 SDs below the mean for his or her age. One of the target populations includes children who are born small for gestational age (SGA) and who frequently fail to catch up. SGA is one of the most common causes of childhood short stature, accounting for 20% of all cases. If an SGA child has not shown catch-up growth by 3 years, they are unlikely to do so and adult height will be short.

As with any relatively new drug associated with growth, the risk of side effects needs to be monitored, and potential long-term complications examined. Furthermore, there are ethical questions because the majority of short children are otherwise healthy. For example, some people use GH therapy to increase height for athletic enhancement, rather than medical concerns. Incidentally, synthetic GH is very expensive, usually costing $20,000 to $40,000 a year, depending on the dosage.

Sources:

Ong, K., Beardsall, K., & de Zegher, F. (2005). Growth hormone therapy in short children born small for gestational age. *Early Human Development*, *81*(12), 973–980.

Ross, J., Czernichow, P., Biller, B. M., Colao, A., Reiter, E., & Kiess, W. (2010). Growth hormone: Health considerations beyond height gain. *Pediatrics*, *125*(4), e906–e918.

CHANGES IN BODY PROPORTIONS AND PHYSIQUE

Objective 3.5

Although the development of the human body follows a relatively consistent cephalocaudal/proximodistal pattern of development, specific body parts show varying rates of growth. During the course of development from birth to adulthood, the head size will double, trunk length will triple, the length of the upper limbs will quadruple, and the length of the lower limbs will quintuple. Along with these differential growth rates, observable changes in body proportions and general body build (physique) can be noted.

Body Proportions

BODY PROPORTION CHANGES RELATIVE TO THE HEAD

Figure 3.7 shows general postnatal body proportion changes with age. Most notable are the proportional changes of head size in relation to total body length. The head of the newborn accounts for approximately one-fourth of its total height, and its legs make up only about three-eighths of its stature. In comparison, the adult head accounts for about one-eighth of total height and leg length accounts for approximately half of stature. The principle of cephalocaudal development is clearly evident here. Also interesting to consider is that in the newborn, head width is very close to that of the shoulders and hips, whereas head width of adults is only about one-third of shoulder width. After birth, shoulder width is generally greater than

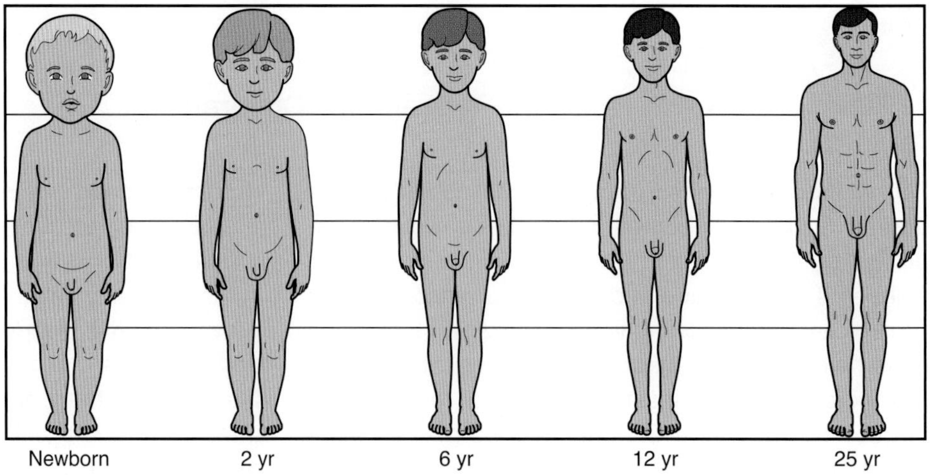

Figure 3.7 Postnatal body proportion changes.

hip width. During postnatal development, the legs grow at a faster rate than other body parts in moving toward the adult model of body proportions.

Head circumference is a common anthropometric measurement and is used to estimate the rate of brain growth among infants and young children. The head circumference measurement is taken at the level of the plane passing just above the bony ridge over the eyes and the most posterior protrusion on the back of the head (Fig. 3.8). Normal head circumference values fall within a relatively narrow range for any given age group, with the variance remaining almost constant for the entire growing period. Although there are slight sex differences, with males having a greater circumference, the difference generally does not exceed 1 centimeter at any age. Table 3.3 provides information on average head circumferences for individuals from birth to 20 years of age.

During the early months of postnatal life, growth in head circumference is very rapid and then begins to decelerate. During the first 4 months, there is an increase of about 5 centimeters which doubles by the end of the first year. From that point until age 18 years, head circumference only increases another 10 centimeters. Head circumference norms, apart from being used as an estimate of brain growth, are also used to identify significant abnormal trends such as hydrocephalus. As noted earlier, refer to *thePoint* for the latest growth charts. Charts such as these are frequently used in clinical settings to examine changes in the rate of growth over a specific period of time.

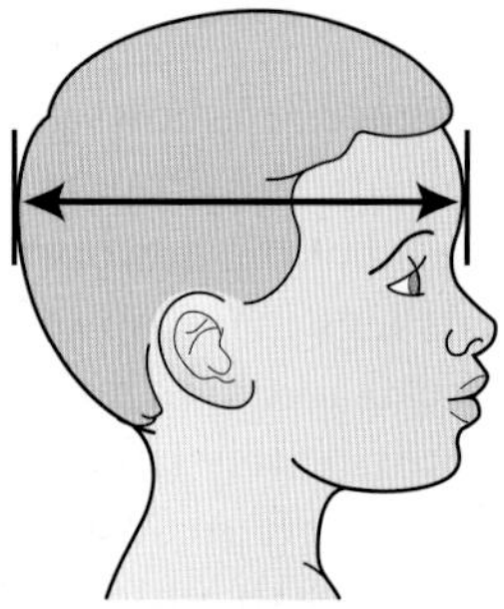

Figure 3.8 Measuring head circumference.

TABLE 3.3 Average Head Circumference

	Mean			Mean	
Age	**Inches**	**Centimeters**	**Age**	**Inches**	**Centimeters**
Birth	13.8	35.0	5 y	20.0	50.8
1 mo	14.9	37.6	6 y	20.2	51.2
2 mo	15.5	39.7	7 y	20.5	51.6
3 mo	15.9	40.4	8 y	20.6	52.0
6 mo	17.0	43.4	10 y	20.9	53.0
9 mo	17.8	45.0	12 y	21.0	53.2
12 mo	18.3	46.5	14 y	21.5	54.0
18 mo	19.0	48.4	16 y	21.9	55.0
2 y	19.2	49.0	18 y	22.1	55.4
3 y	19.6	50.0	20 y	22.2	55.6
4 y	19.8	50.5			

SOURCE: Data from Lowrey, G. H. (1986). *Growth and development of children* (8th ed.). Chicago, IL: Year Book Medical; and Centers for Disease Control and Prevention. (2000). *Physical activity and good nutrition: Essential elements to prevent chronic diseases and obesity*. Atlanta, GA: Author.

Head size in the very young may have biomechanical implications for motor skill performance. It would seem quite possible that even if the newborn were neurologically ready to attempt walking, a top-heavy body would present problems in maintaining balance. Another commonly seen example is that of a 4- to 5-year-old attempting to perform a backward roll. Due to the larger proportional head size of younger compared to older children, the task of completing a smooth roll over the back of the head often presents difficulty. Few, if any, research findings have shed real light on performance differences attributable to proportional diversity among children.

CHANGES IN RATIO OF SITTING HEIGHT TO STATURE

The ratio of sitting height to stature measures the contribution of the legs and trunk to total height. Sitting height is measured as the height from the seat of the chair in which a person is sitting (with spine erect) to the vertex or top of the head (Fig. 3.9). Measures of the change in head and trunk height can then be compared with measures of total stature, which includes leg length.

Sitting height is typically 60% to 70% of total body length in the early years and decreases to about 50% when mature height is reached. The most noticeable changes occur in the legs and trunk; the head actually contributes very little to height change after birth. Figure 3.10 depicts the ratio of sitting height to stature for individuals up to 18 years. The rapid growth of the legs is evidenced by the decrease in the ratios over time. The ratio is highest in infancy and declines throughout childhood into adolescence. Females reach the lowest ratio point around 12 to 13 years, whereas males hit theirs about 2 years later (from age 13 to 15 years). Until approximately 12 years of age, 55% to 60% of overall height gains for both sexes are attributed to leg growth, because males and females experience almost identical increases in sitting height (trunk length). Prior to adolescence, males

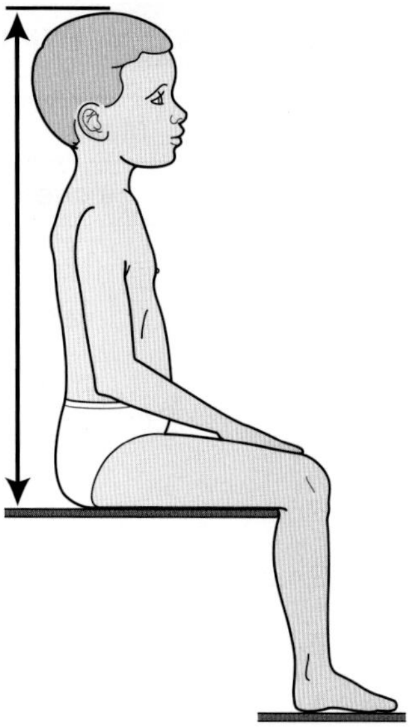

Figure 3.9 Measuring sitting height.

and females are proportionately similar in terms of relative leg and trunk length. However, after that point in time, females exhibit, for an equal stature, relatively shorter legs than males.

think about it

What is the relationship between specific body proportions and motor performance after pubertal change?

CHANGES IN SHOULDER AND HIP WIDTH

The shoulder/hip ratio serves as a basic descriptor of proportional growth in the human body. It also provides information with biomechanical implications for motor performance. The shoulder/hip ratio is determined from two measurements: (a) biacromial breadth (or shoulder width)—the distance between the right and left acromial processes (Fig. 3.11) and (b) bicristal breadth (or hip width)—the distance between the right and left iliocristales.

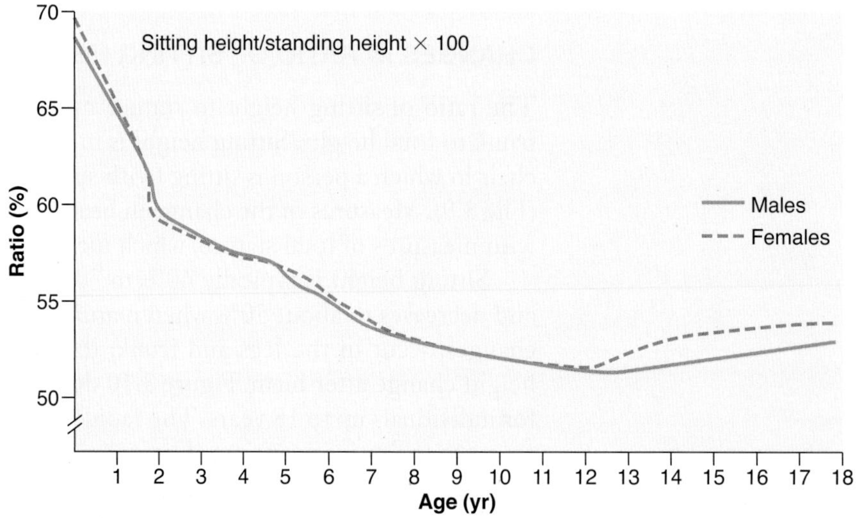

Figure 3.10 Ratios of sitting height to stature.

SOURCE: Data from Hansman (1970), as reported by Malina, R. M. (1984). Human growth, maturation, and regular physical activity. In R. A. Boileau (Ed.), *Advances in pediatric sport sciences: Biological issues* (Vol. 1). Champaign, IL: Human Kinetics.

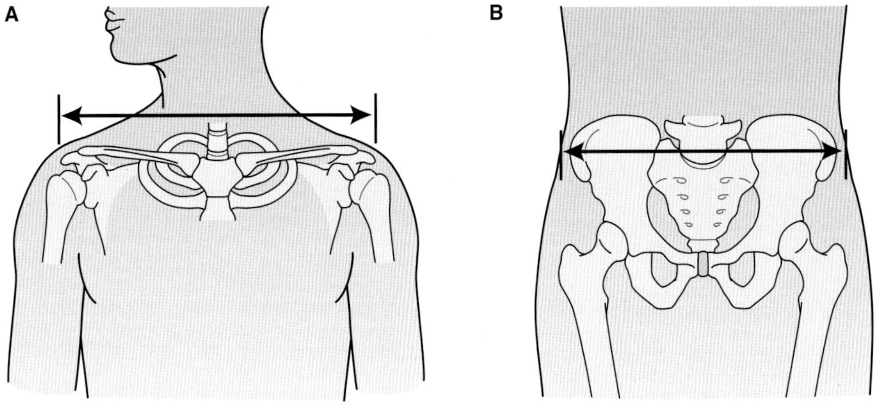

Figure 3.11 **A.** Measuring biacromial (shoulder) width. **B.** Measuring bicristal breadth (hip width).

Although hip and shoulder width appear almost equal in the newborn (see Fig. 3.7 on page 72), shoulder width is typically greater than hip width for all individuals. Figure 3.12 illustrates shoulder (biacromial) and hip (bicristal) width values for males and females from 6 to 17 years of age. Although there are differences between the sexes prior to adolescence, the variances are generally minimal. Beginning with the pubescent growth spurt, the obvious broadening of the shoulders relative to the hips is characteristic in males, whereas females experience greater hip breadth gains relative to the shoulders and waist. The biacromial/bicristal ratio remains relatively constant in males from ages 6 to 11 years and then exhibits a marked increase that continues up to around 6 years. This increase is due primarily to the fact that shoulder breadth is increasing at a more rapid rate than hip breadth is. After peaking at approximately 12 years of age, the ratio for females steadily declines as a result of increased hip growth relative to shoulder breadth (Fig. 3.13).

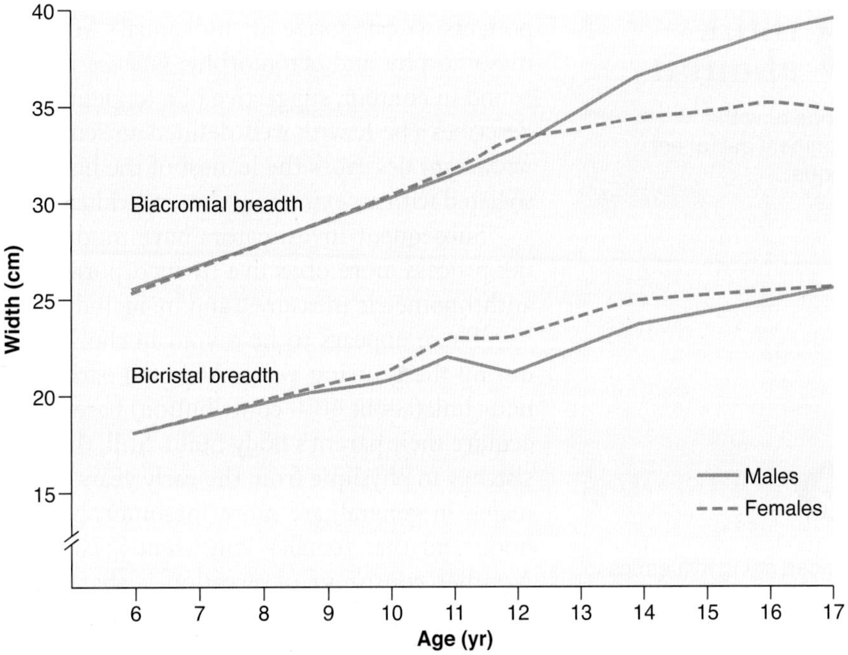

Figure 3.12 Shoulder and hip width values.

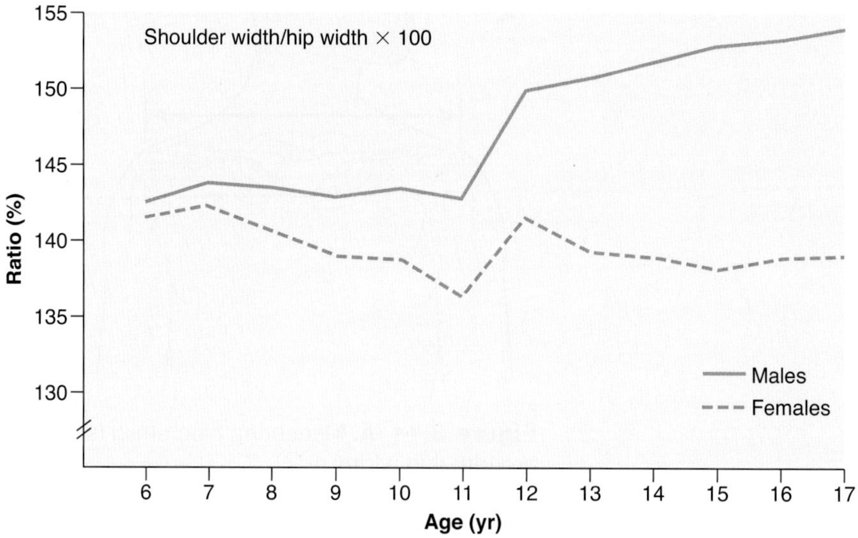

Figure 3.13 Shoulder and hip width ratios.

PHYSIQUE

Also referred to as *body build*, physique is a composite of body proportion relationships and body composition characteristics. An informal assessment of body build is made when an individual is identified using terms such as stocky, lean, muscular, or soft-bodied. Various ratios of body mass (weight) to height have been used to provide a simple and convenient estimate of physique; however, several limitations have been noted. Because body proportions change with growth and lifestyle (diet and exercise), it is very difficult to develop a scheme of body typing for use over the life span.

The Sheldon method (Sheldon et al., 1954) uses three general body build components to categorize an individual's **somatotype**, or body build: endomorphy, mesomorphy, and ectomorphy. *Endomorphy* describes a body type that is soft and round in contour, suggestive of a tendency toward fatness and obesity; *mesomorphy* describes a body with well-defined muscularity and balanced body proportions; and *ectomorphy* describes the leanest of the body types, with characteristics typically associated with an extremely thin individual.

think about it

Describe how the environment can affect physique.

Subsequent investigators have modified Sheldon's method to make the rating process more objective by incorporating data on body composition, by using anthropometric measures, and by including children and females (Carter, 2002).

There appears to be a void in the literature related to changes in physique during the growing years. As noted earlier, some evidence suggests a strong genetic link (about 40% contribution) based on the high percentage of children who acquire their parent's body build. Still, there is no strong evidence indicating consistency in physique from the early years to maturity. There have been reports that males, in general, are more mesomorphic from preschool through young adulthood and that females consistently exhibit more endomorphic characteristics. A rather consistent observation is that considerable variation exists within sex, racial, and geographic groups in children and adults. For an excellent discussion on this topic, refer to Malina et al. (2004).

focus on change

Advanced aging influences *change* in growth and motor behavior.

Changes with Advanced Aging

As individuals reach middle age, mesomorphic characteristics tend to diminish due to loss of muscle mass; consequently, more endomorphic and ectomorphic traits are exhibited. As a result of bone tissue loss along with a decrease in total height, changes in body proportions also tend to occur with aging.

STRUCTURAL DEVELOPMENT

Height

Objective 3.6

The measurement of body length is one of the simplest and most common measures of structural growth. Height is determined by measuring the individual while either lying down or in a standing position. Until the infant can stand erect without assistance, total body length is measured in the supine position from the vertex (top of head) to the heel, referred to as *recumbent length*. A special slide ruler (Fig. 3.14) or anthropometer is used to measure the distance to the nearest ⅛ inch (0.1 cm). The preferred measurement of body length is standing height (stature), which is the distance between the vertex and the floor. To gain greatest accuracy, measurements are taken without shoes, using a sliding headboard (Fig. 3.15).

We learned earlier that the embryo at about 8 weeks begins to take human form and has a body length of approximately 1 inch (2.5 cm). During the remainder of prenatal development, a phenomenal rate of growth produces an average length at birth of 20 inches (50 cm). The growth rates that occur during the 9 months preceding birth and the first year of life are the fastest the body will experience. A typical child will increase its birth length by 50% at 1 year. After age 2 years, the growth rate slows somewhat to average about 2 inches per year until the onset of the pubescent growth spurt. It is not uncommon for children to experience a midgrowth spurt in height around the age of 7 years, although this change is usually less dramatic than the adolescent spurt. Growth accelerates before and during puberty, with peak rates of between 3 and 4 inches per year. Until puberty, males on the average are slightly taller than females; however, there is a large overlap, with some females taller than males. Females generally enter the height growth spurt 2 years earlier than males do and typically complete the process in a shorter period of time (Fig. 3.16); however, the age of onset and completion can vary considerably.

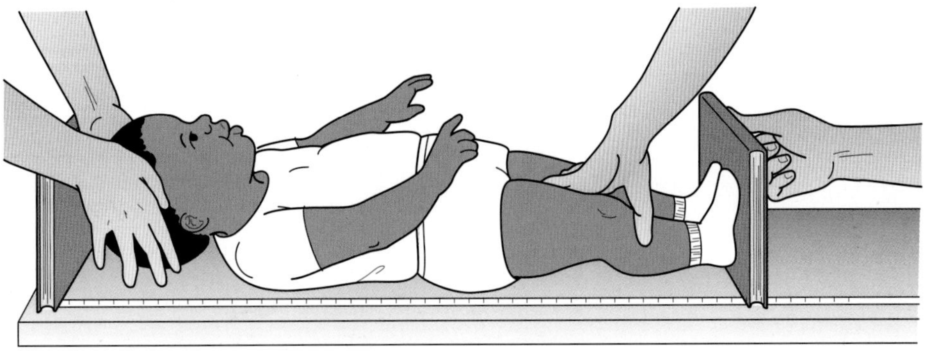

Figure 3.14 Measuring recumbent length in infants.

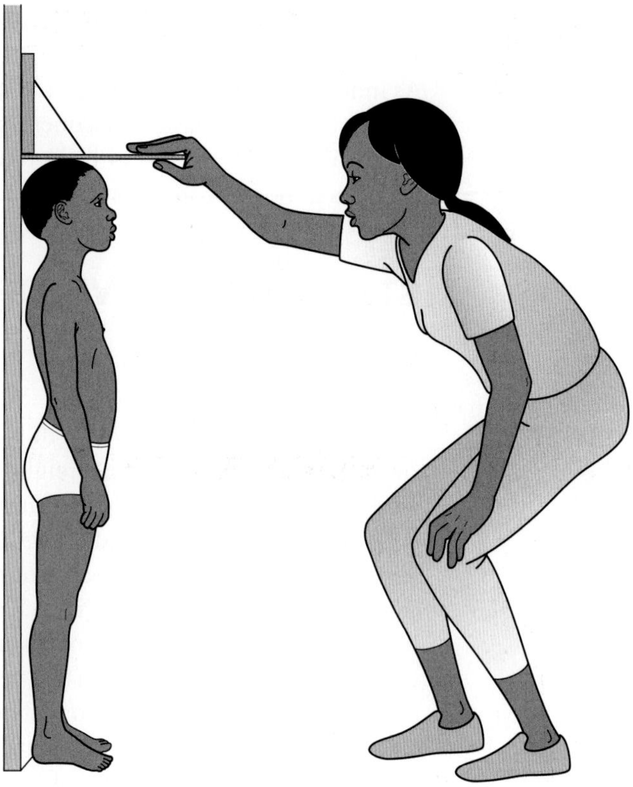

Figure 3.15 Measuring standing height (stature).

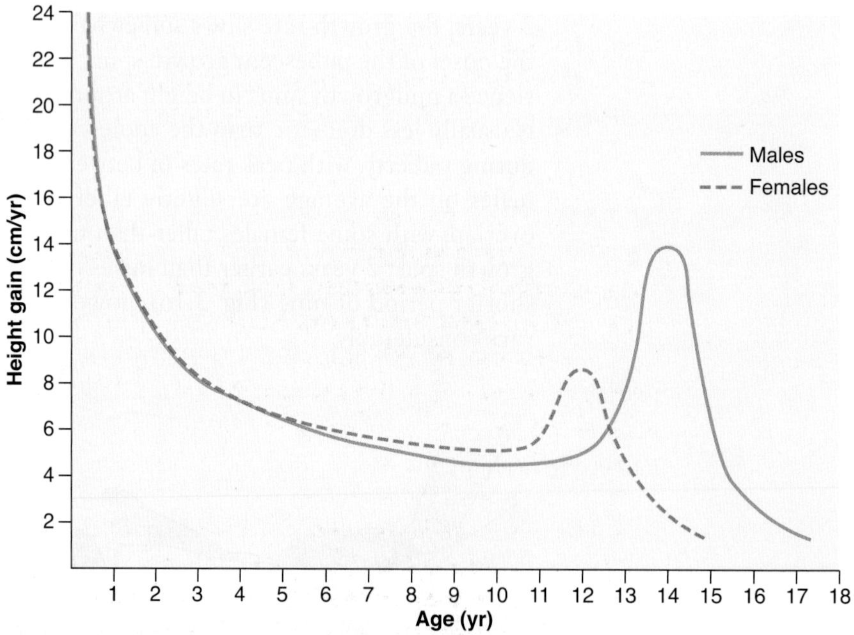

Figure 3.16 Typical velocity curves for males and females, illustrating height gain per year.

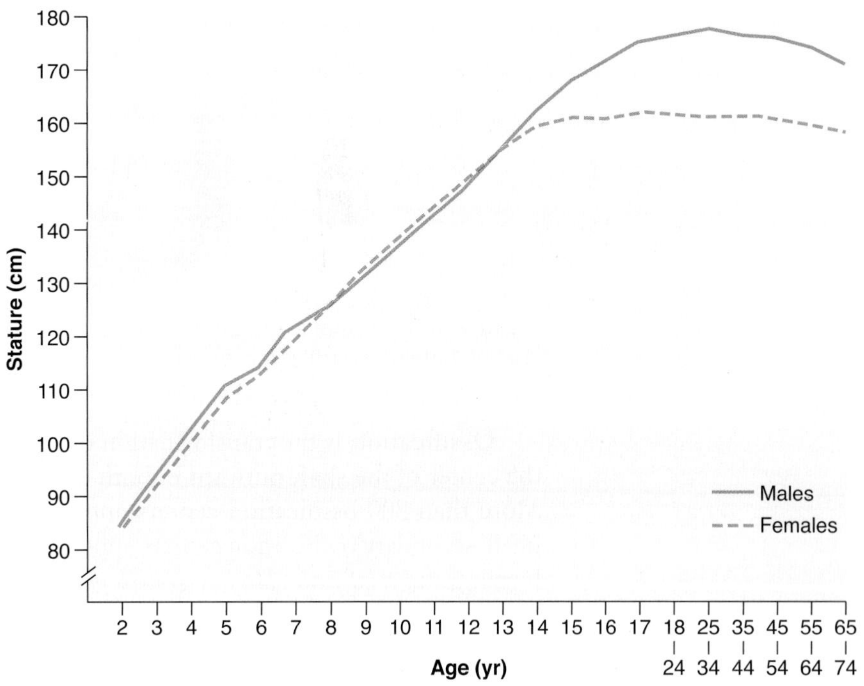

Figure 3.17 Distance curves for stature.

Females, on the average, complete their peak growth period by 16½ years of age, whereas males continue to gain in stature for another 2 years or so. Males are typically 4 to 6 inches taller than females when they reach mature height. According to Tanner (1990), maximum growth of the long bones may not be reached until about age 25 years and of the vertebral column until approximately 30 years, at which time an individual may add ⅛ to ¼ inch to his or her height. As illustrated in Figure 3.17, height remains relatively stable until sometime after the third decade of life, when total height begins to regress. Refer to *thePoint* for growth charts for ages 2 to 20 years.

Skeletal Growth

Bone mass, a composite measure of bone size and density, is a determinant of bone strength and depends on the mass acquired during skeletal growth and development. Heritability estimates for bone mass range up to 80%. However, individual variance depends on (for example) gender, nutrition, physical activity, and obesity. The process of bone growth and development that will lead to skeletal maturation begins with the formation of mesoderm cells in the embryo about 16 days after fertilization. Approximately 5 to 6 weeks after conception, the first ossification centers appear in the jawbones and collar bones. This is also the approximate time that the long bones of the upper arm and leg appear in a cartilage form. Soon after the cartilage takes the shape of a long bone at about 2 months (fetal age), a ring of true bone begins to form. At the same time, primary ossification centers begin to appear in the midportion (*diaphysis*) of the long bones. In most bones, the primary ossification center appears by the third month of fetal life. The developmental status of a human fetus skeleton at 18 weeks is shown in Figure 3.18 on page 80.

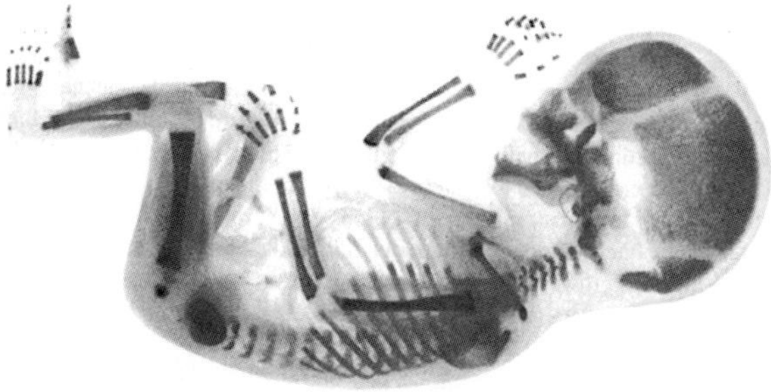

Figure 3.18 A fetal skeleton at 18 weeks; dark areas denote ossified portions and spaces between cartilage models.

Ossification is the transformation of cartilage to true bone. It proceeds from the center of the shaft outward in both directions until the entire shaft is ossified. More than 800 ossification centers appear in the body after birth. Shortly after birth, secondary ossification centers appear at the end of the shaft (epiphyseal area), forming the *epiphyseal plate*, or *growth plate*. Basically, cartilage cells are nourished by the blood in a reservoir next to the epiphysis. They begin to increase in size in the proliferating zone before moving on to the hypertrophic zone where the cells arrange themselves in vertical columns. At that point, the cartilage cells erode, and true bone begins to grow as collagen is secreted by *osteoblasts* (the bone cells engaged in producing true bone). *Osteocytes*, the principal cells of mature bone, become trapped in the tissue matrix and collect calcium and phosphorus. Essentially, bone is a matrix composed primarily of collagen fibers and noncollagenous proteins. When full maturity is completed, the epiphysis fuses to the *metaphysis* (the area between diaphysis and epiphysis), and the growth plate is erased (Fig. 3.19).

The mechanism controlling bone girth (appositional growth) is not as complex as the cartilage replacement processes responsible for growth in length. New rings of bone are added in circular layers on top of the layers formed earlier. The bone has a compensating mechanism that controls thickness. As new rings are added, old layers are removed from the inner circumference of the bone sleeve, permitting the shell to become thicker. This process continues until each of the long bones reaches full maturity in late childhood to early adulthood.

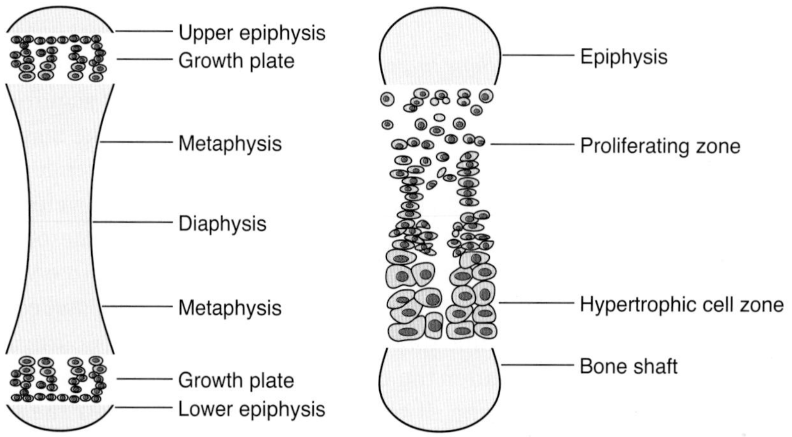

Figure 3.19 Long bone with upper and lower epiphyses **(left)**. General process of bone formation **(right)**.

SOURCE: Modified from Tanner, J. M. (1990). *Fetus into man: Physical growth from conception to maturity*. Cambridge, MA: Harvard University Press.

Another important mechanism of long bone growth is modeling resorption. At birth, the bone shaft tends to flare out at its ends, hence creating a thinner middle. As the bone grows in length, the end becomes wider and the shaft heavier. The mechanism for maintaining the linear form of the bone is called *modeling resorption*. As the ends become increasingly thick, the excess bone tissue is removed by a process of resorption or breakdown, thus permitting the bone to maintain its linear shape while it is growing longer.

During the growth of short bones of the wrist and fingers, the core of the bone in the center of the cartilage steadily enlarges. At the same time, the original cartilage itself is growing appositionally, as more cartilage is deposited on its surface. Growth of new bone tissue proceeds faster than growth of cartilage; thus, more and more bone is added to the developing structure. This continues until the bone matures fully.

Epiphyseal plate closure, indicative of long bone maturity, generally starts somewhere between 13½ and 18 years of age, beginning at the distal humerus. Most of the long bones reach maturity from about 16 to 18 years of age in females and 18 to 21 years in males. Cranial development follows a different postnatal growth curve. The majority of growth is completed by 3 years, with 50% attained by the ninth month. There are areas of the braincase, however, that do not reach maturity until well into adulthood.

Females, from birth, typically have a more developed skeleton than males. Females are approximately 20% more advanced in skeletal maturity than boys, which in practical terms is a difference of about 2 months at age 1 year and 2 years at age 10 years. There are also indications that there is less variability in rate of ossification for females. Greater size in the male after puberty is due to the longer growing period (approximately 2 years) and the increased production of adrenal androgens and testosterone. As will be noted later in the discussion of maturity estimates, skeletal age may precede or lag behind chronological age by as much as a year.

Changes with Advanced Aging

Normal aging causes the bones to lose mass and the total height to decrease. Women begin to lose bone mineral at about age 30 years and men at approximately 50 years of age. Stature decreases with age because of an increase in postural kyphosis (rounding of the back), compression of intravertebral disks, and deterioration of vertebrae. Estimates of height decreases from 40 to 80 years of age are 1 to 3 inches. Figure 3.20 illustrates height changes from 20 to 80 years of age (Sorkin et al., 1999).

The loss of bone mass presents a more complex problem, especially in women. Bone loss in women begins slowly during the third decade (0.75% to 1% per year) and can increase to a higher rate (2% to 3% per year) shortly before and after menopause. The total bone mineral mass loss by age 70 years is approximately 25% to 30%. Bone loss estimates for men at age 70 years are about half of what women experience (12% to 15% by age 70 years). The amount of bone loss is specific to the individual and varies considerably in different types of bone. Age- and sex-related changes in the width of cortical bone are illustrated in Figure 3.21. Figure 3.22 depicts loss of spine and femur bone density in females with advanced aging.

Osteoporosis has become a familiar term to the general public; it refers to the loss of total bone mass to such an extent that the skeleton is unable to maintain its mechanical integrity. The development of this condition is a complex process

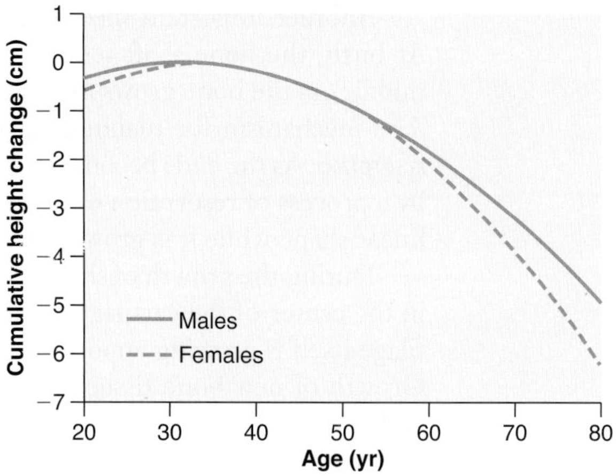

Figure 3.20 Cumulative height change in men and women from young to older adulthood.

SOURCE: Adapted from Sorkin, J. D., Miller, D. C., & Andres, R. (1999). Longitudinal change in the heights of men and women: Consequential effects on body mass index. *Epidemiologic Reviews*, *21*, 247–260.

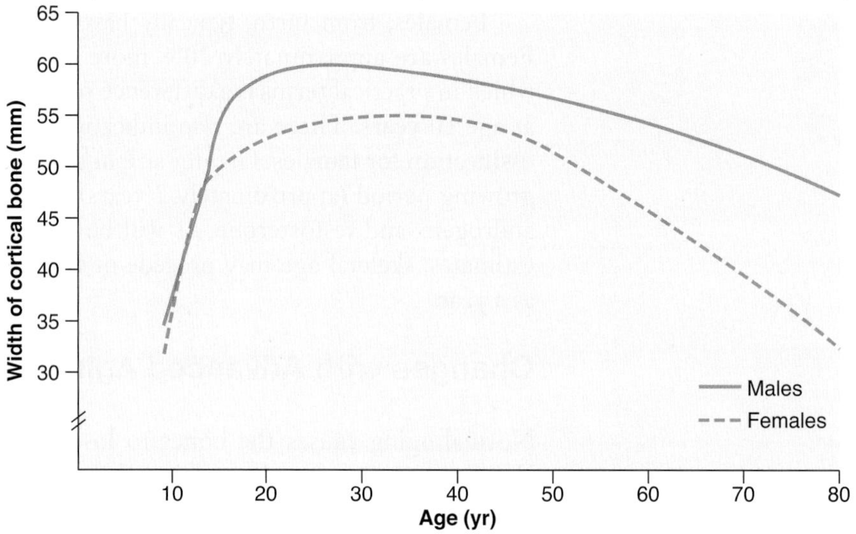

Figure 3.21 Age changes in width of cortical bone (second metacarpal).

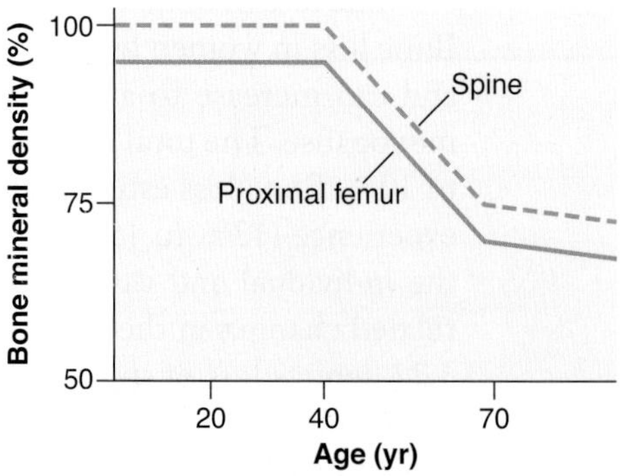

Figure 3.22 Loss of bone density in females.

influenced by a variety of nutritional (related primarily to calcium), physical, hormonal (primarily estrogen), and genetic factors. In the scientific community, there is some debate concerning the dividing line between normal aging of bones and the more pronounced brittleness of bones generally associated with osteoporosis. As a result of osteoporosis, bones tend to break more easily, which increases the risk of fracture. Almost one-half of all women older than the age of 60 years are affected by osteoporosis.

BODY MASS

Objective 3.7

Body weight and *body composition* are terms frequently used to describe an individual's **body mass**. Body weight is a general descriptor of total body mass that is a composite of all tissue components. Body composition, in contrast, is a description of the various independent tissue components—namely, lean body mass (fat-free weight) and body fat. Thus, body weight equals lean body mass plus fat. The following discussion of body composition focuses on skeletal muscle tissue (lean body mass) and body fat. It should be noted, however, that lean body mass (for body weight measures) encompasses all of the body's nonfat tissues including skeleton, muscle, water, connective tissue, organ tissues, and teeth. The growth and development of cardiac (heart) muscle tissue is discussed in Chapter 4.

Body Weight

The assessment of body weight is the most common anthropometric measure used to estimate body mass. Instrumentation is relatively simple in that the individual stands on clinical scales (preferably beam type) without shoes and dressed in as little clothing as possible (preferably briefs or bathing suit). Infant scales and bed scales are typically used for the disabled, elderly, or other individuals not capable of standing without aid. Weight is measured to the nearest 10th of a kilogram (or quarter of a pound).

The embryo at 8 weeks weighs about half an ounce (14 g); by the end of the fifth month, the fetus weighs about 1 pound (450 g). The last 2 months of prenatal life is a period of rapid weight gain. The fetus gains about half a pound (225 g) a week for a total of 5 pounds (2,250 g) on the average. Just a few weeks before birth (and at delivery), the average fetus weighs about 7 pounds (3.2 g). Females, on the average, are about half a pound smaller than males at birth.

Total body mass generally decreases during the first few days after birth due to transition factors such as maternal milk supply and level of physiological stress. However, birth weight is usually regained within 2 weeks. Body weight typically doubles after 3 to 4 months and triples at 1 year. Although environmental factors play a determining role, many children will reach one-half of their mature body mass by age 10 years. Figure 3.23 illustrates a distance curve for body weight among individuals 2 to 74 years of age.

The pubescent growth spurt for body weight is similar to the height curve except that it generally continues for a longer time. Female growth patterns reveal a particularly rapid weight gain between the ages of 12 and 13 years. As in the growth pattern for height, males begin the growth spurt later than females do and add more body size. Males increase their body mass by about

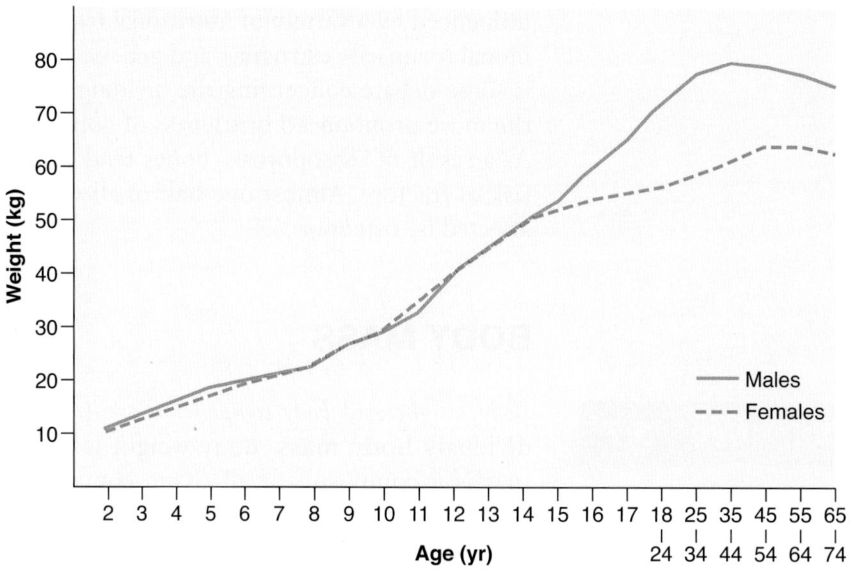

Figure 3.23 Distance curves for body weight.

45 pounds (20 kg) and females by approximately 35 pounds (16 kg) by early adulthood. Mature body weight is about 20 times that of birth weight. Total body mass begins to decline with aging as a reflection of bone and muscle tissue losses. Refer to *thePoint* to compare individual growth values using percentile charts (from ages 2 to 20 years).

Body Composition

Body weight is a general measure of body mass and therefore does not break down the contribution of different tissues making up this collective measurement. A measure of body composition, however, independently assesses two types of tissue: muscle tissue (lean body mass) and body fat. A variety of measurement techniques are available to estimate total body fatness, lean body mass, or both. All of the measurements are only estimates because they are indirectly determined. The only direct way of taking the measurements is by making a biochemical analysis of cadavers.

Some of the more common measurement techniques include underwater (hydrostatic) weighing, anthropometric dimensions (skinfolds), bioelectrical impedance, dual-energy X-ray absorptiometry (DXA) scan (X-ray), and BMI. Here, are descriptions of the two most commonly used techniques: BMI and DXA scan, the latest technology. For detailed discussions of these and other methods, refer to Howley and Thompson (2012).

BMI is a calculation of body fat based on height and body weight:

$$\text{BMI} = \text{body weight (kg)} / \text{height (m)}^2$$

This method, which is the worldwide standard, is a reliable and practical tool. The predictive accuracy of this equation as an estimate of body fat has not been extensively studied. The existing data indicate that it warrants only a fair rating and is less accurate than the triceps skinfold method. The basic limitation of BMI is that it ignores the possibility that muscle tissue rather than fat may contribute to excessive body weight relative to height. Refer to *thePoint* for BMI percentile values from 2 to 20 years.

Even with its limitations, the user-friendly BMI has received considerable worldwide attention in recent years due in large part to increasing obesity rates. This topic is discussed in greater detail in Chapter 5. As a reference to the BMI graphs, overweight is defined as a BMI of 25 to 29.9, obese as a BMI of 30 to 39.9, and a BMI above 40 is extremely obese.

DXA scan. DXA scan is an enhanced form of X-ray technology that is used to measure bone mineral density, as well as body fat and muscle proportions (percentages) (Fig. 3.24). It is considered the gold standard for body fat and bone density assessment. It involves noninvasive imaging that is appropriate for children and adults. In addition to measuring changes in growth over time, DXA has significantly applications with, for example, bone decrement and other tissue loss during adulthood. Compared to estimates using BMI, DXA is obviously more expensive and not as practical for large-scale studies. However, DXA provides significantly more detail and accuracy.

On the average, males at all ages have greater body densities and greater lean body mass than females (Malina et al., 2004). Although the differences are closer during the childhood years, females have greater amounts of body fat across the life span. This difference is magnified as adolescence approaches and continues on through development. Figure 3.25 on page 86 shows selected body composition values for ages 7 to 70 years. During the pubescent growth spurt, males experience a rapid increase in lean body mass and a decrease in percentage of fat. Females also experience an increase in lean mass, although less than males do, and an increase in body fat. Figure 3.26 depicts estimated changes in fat-free mass, fat mass, and relative percentage of fat during the first 20 years.

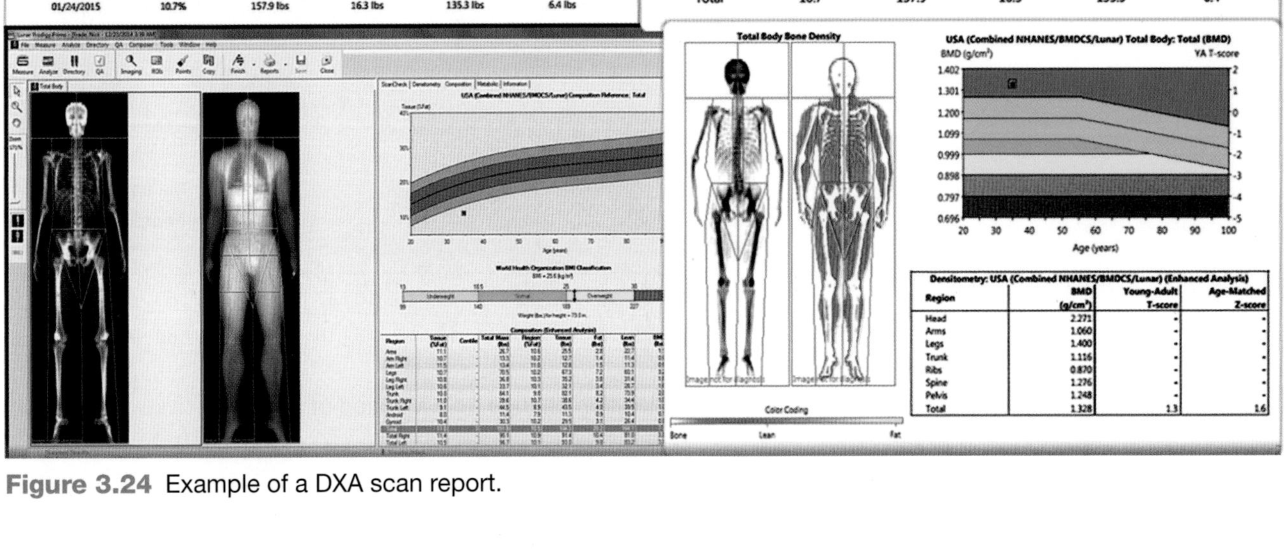

Figure 3.24 Example of a DXA scan report.

Focus on Application

Anorexia Nervosa: What Constitutes Too Small?

With the national epidemic and focus on obesity, physicians, educators, and parents are concerned with overweight and how to assess it. However, there is another problem showing an increasing trend—being too small (underweight). Chapter 5 talks about underweight and nutrition and its effects on development, but as a growth question, what is too small?

First of all, from a growth perspective, too small is a BMI of less than 18.5 or less than fifth percentile on growth charts. Commonly associated with this condition is anorexia nervosa, an eating disorder characterized by refusal to maintain a minimally acceptable body weight and a fear of weight gain. The exact cause of anorexia is not known, but social attitudes toward body appearance are believed to play a major role. Some experts also suggest that conflicts within a family may contribute to the problem. For example, a child may want to draw attention away from marital problems to bring the family back together. The condition usually occurs in adolescence or young adulthood. Some estimates say only about 1% of American girls and women have anorexia. Other studies suggest that up to 10% of adolescent girls have this condition.

Unfortunately, bone loss is a well-established consequence of anorexia. Key studies have found significant decreases in bone density in anorexic adolescents. For example, *anorexic teens have been shown to have a spinal density 25% below that of healthy teens*. Up to two-thirds of teens who have the disorder have bone density values more than 2 SDs below the norm. As noted in this chapter and Chapter 11 (aging), bone density is important to overall motor behavior.

Sources:

National Institutes of Health. (2016). *NIH Osteoporosis and Related Bone Diseases—National Resource Center*. Retrieved from http://www.niams.nih.gov/Health_Info/Bone/

Mayo Clinic. (2016). *Anorexia nervosa*. Retrieved from http://www.mayoclinic.org/diseases-conditions/anorexia/home/ovc-20179508

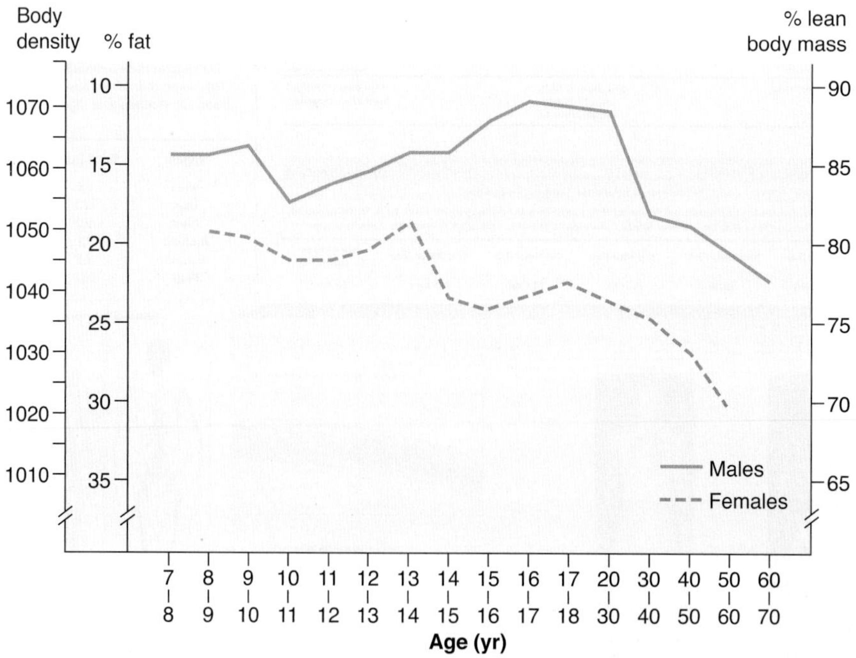

Figure 3.25 Body composition change as a function of age.

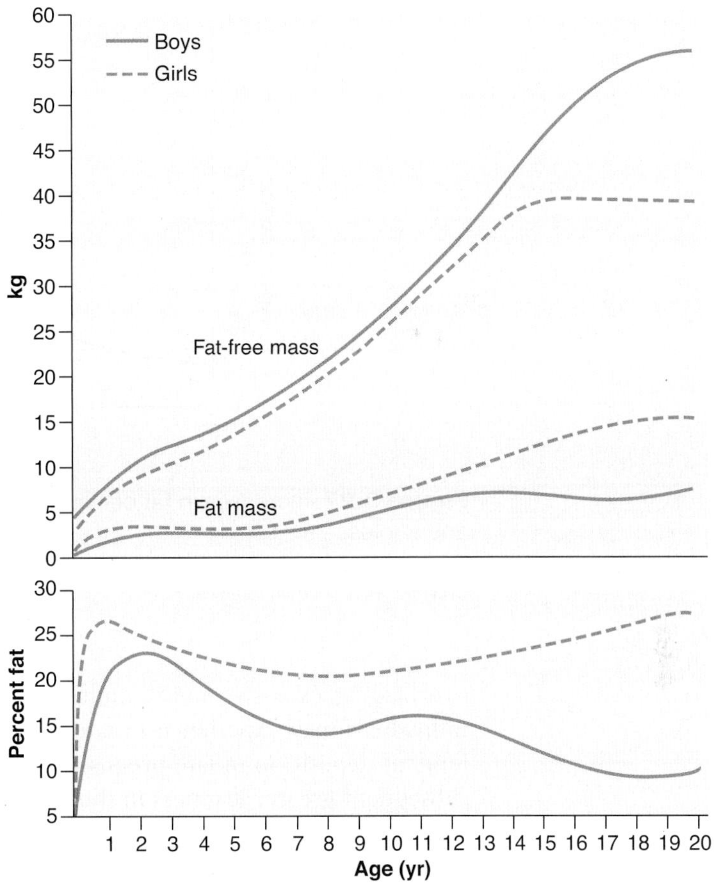

Figure 3.26 Body composition across age for boys and girls.

BODY FAT GROWTH

Body fat layers appear in the fetus between the seventh and eighth prenatal months. Between birth and 6 to 9 months, body fat mass will increase 10% to 20% before tapering off to a plateau that may last from 5 to 7 years. On the average, percentage of body fat increases from about 16% at birth to between 24% and 30% at 1 year. Some individuals will experience an increase during the midgrowth spurt of 5½ to 7 years, which generally ceases after that period in males but continues in females through the adolescent years. As noted earlier, females have more body fat (absolute and relative) than males at all ages, with differences more apparent during and after puberty.

Fat and muscle cells grow both in number (hyperplasia) and in size (hypertrophy). The adult of average body size has between 25 and 50 billion fat cells. Obese individuals may have 75 billion or more (McArdle et al., 2015). The size of fat cells in children up to 1 year is about one-fourth that of adult fat cells. Fat cell size triples during the first 6 years and then remains relatively stable until the onset of puberty.

By the end of the first year of life, the number of fat cells is about 3 times what it was at birth. It is believed that most of the fat cell production takes place during the last trimester before birth. After the first year, the number of cells increases gradually until the onset of the pubescent growth spurt, at which time the number increases significantly (Fig. 3.27). Although the evidence is not decisive, there is speculation that overfeeding and a high-fat diet during the early stages of life promotes overmultiplication of fat cells. Relationships have been drawn between

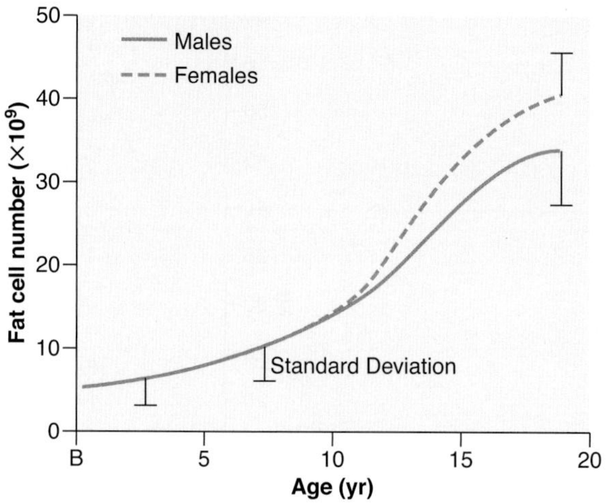

Figure 3.27 Increases in fat cell number in males and females during childhood and adolescence.

SOURCE: Adapted from Malina, R. M., & Bouchard, C. (1991). *Growth, maturation, and physical activity*. Champaign, IL: Human Kinetics.

overfeeding, excessive fat cell multiplication, and the weight control problems that individuals may experience in later life. There are also indications that reduced fetal fat deposition in late pregnancy (i.e., less intake by the mother) may lead to subsequent greater leanness in the infant (Dietz, 1997).

Although there is some disagreement, it is generally believed that by adulthood (or perhaps before), the number of cells becomes fixed and increases in size only, except in cases of extreme obesity. When individuals gain fat tissue as a result of overeating, their fat cells enlarge but no new cells are created. Complementing this line of information, Dietz (1997) describes three critical periods for the development of obesity: the prenatal period, between 4 and 6 years of age, and adolescence (especially in females). As noted in Chapter 2, about 25% of the variation among people in percentage of body fat is genetically determined; thus, there is considerable environmental effect.

SKELETAL MUSCLE TISSUE GROWTH

Muscle fibers develop in the premuscular mesodermic tissue. After the 16th week of fetal development, the first muscle fibers can be identified. Growth of voluntary muscle during the prenatal period is both hyperplastic and hypertrophic. The hyperplastic phase continues until shortly after birth, after which cell growth is predominantly achieved by increasing cell size hypertrophy. The increase in mass of a skeletal muscle of up to 50 times during postnatal development is due almost exclusively to a massive increase in the size of individual fibers. Protein, the essential element in muscle composition, increases gradually during the fetal period and, by birth, reaches a level very near that found in adults. Approximately 15% of total body mass of the fetus halfway through its development consists of skeletal muscle tissue. This percentage increases progressively to about 25% of birth weight for both sexes. Approximately 40% to 50% of body mass in the adult male are skeletal muscle. Females generally do not show a significant increase in lean body mass during puberty; and at maturity, they have only about 60% of the muscle mass and force characteristics of males.

The differentiation of fiber types and sizes is frequently used to describe muscle growth and development. Basically, in the adult, *type I fibers* (described as slow twitch) are relatively fatigue-resistant and are associated with the performance of aerobic endurance activities (e.g., long-distance running and cycling). *Type II fibers*, in contrast, are fast twitch and have the capacity to contract 5 to 10 times faster and more forcefully, but they also fatigue rapidly. Fast-twitch fibers are associated with the performance of short-duration (anaerobic) activities (e.g., sprinting, jumping, and weight lifting). At birth and through childhood, type I fibers constitute approximately 50% of all muscle fibers. During this same period, only about 25% of type II fibers are found. The amount of undifferentiated (transitional) fibers at the same time is also about 25%. By adulthood, there are very few, if any, undifferentiated fibers and the average distribution is about 50–50 for slow and fast fibers.

think about it

What type of training (specifically) do you think might change transitional fibers?

Studies that have investigated muscle fiber changes during adolescence have noted the possible significant effects of pubertal hormones on growth and differentiation. Researchers have found a relatively high percentage (7% to 13%) of transitional fibers in adolescents. In *transitional fibers*, the functional features of the enzyme system may develop as either aerobic (type I) or anaerobic (type II), depending on the physical training to which the fibers are treated. These fibers supposedly develop after infancy due to the influence of pubertal hormones. Such factors may have implications for motor programming and training with adolescents.

With regard to muscle fiber size, the typical adult has a fiber diameter of 50 to 60 micrometers. At birth, the size is approximately 12 to 15 micrometers, and by the end of the first year, the fiber size will be about 30% of adult size; at 5 years, it will reach approximately 50%. It should be noted, however, that size (and type) of muscle fiber can vary considerably in individuals of the same age. There does not appear to be any major differences between upper and lower extremities or proximal and distal muscles, or any significant variance between the sexes. Although several hypotheses have been proposed concerning how muscle growth and differentiation take place in both the prenatal and neonatal period, the strongest is that the pattern is inherited and genetically coded (45% contribution) in the nucleus of the muscle cell.

Changes with Advanced Aging

think about it

Using a velocity curve format, illustrate the major physical growth (weight and body weight) milestones across the life span. Then, briefly summarize each event.

Significant changes in body fat and lean muscle mass take place with aging. Although height decreases with age, weight increases steadily beginning in the third decade and continues until 55 to 60 years of age when it declines. An increase in body weight is usually accompanied by gains in body fat and a decrease in lean body mass. After age 60 years or so, total body weight decreases despite the increase in body fat due in part to *loss of muscle and bone mass*. By the end of adolescence, the average male is 23% fat and by 60 years increases to about 31%. Females change from about 32% body fat at 17 years to approximately 42% at 60 years. These values can vary to quite an extent depending on lifestyle and tend to be less in individuals who are physically active. According to the CDC (2016), these figures reflect the continued trend of overweightness in the United States.

As individuals age, the distribution of body fat also tends to change. With advanced aging, there is an increased general tendency for a large proportion of the total body fat to be located internally rather than subcutaneously. As females age, they tend to accumulate fat in the hip, thigh, and breast region, whereas in males, the abdomen is the specified site. As noted earlier, these patterns of distribution are inherited at a contribution of about 50%.

Lean body (fat-free) mass tends to decrease with age. This overall effect is due primarily to the loss of bone mass (15% to 30%) and the reduction of muscle mass.

TABLE 3.4 Summary of Physical Growth Changes with Advanced Aging

Physical Growth Characteristic	
Stature	Decreases
Bone mass	Decreases
Body weight	Increases/decreases (after 60 y)
Percentage of body fat	Increases
Lean body (muscle) mass	Decreases
Muscle fibers	Greater loss of type II (fast-twitch)
Distribution of fat	More internal

Most individuals experience a marked deterioration in muscle mass with aging. For people older than 60 years of age, the loss of muscle mass can be as high as 30% to 50% of that in young adults. This age-related reduction of muscle mass is caused mainly by a loss of muscle fibers, especially type II (fast-twitch) fibers. Overall lean body mass loss approximates losses in muscle and bone. Table 3.4 summarizes physical growth changes with advancing age.

MATURITY ESTIMATES

Objective 3.8

Because maturation is a qualitative process, it can be a challenge to determine in quantitative terms how far an individual has progressed along his or her road to full maturity. Level of maturity is generally estimated from chronological age and biological (developmental) age characteristics.

Chronological age refers to the age of an individual in relationship to standard calendar days. Estimating level of maturity using this method alone is of limited value because of the wide variance in growth and development possible at any single age. An accurate calculation of chronological age does provide the basic factor with which measures of growth and development are compared when estimating level of maturity. The measurement of **biological age** generally provides a better method for estimating maturity by providing information that may be compared with the individual's age. Characteristics commonly used in a measurement of biological age include estimates of morphological age, dental age, sexual age, and skeletal age.

think about it

What are the implications of advanced age-related declines in motor behavior for daily living activities?

Morphological Age

The term *morphology* refers to the form or structure of an individual. Morphological age is usually estimated from height. A measure of height is easy to attain, and there are several height percentile charts that indicate where an individual ranks for a given age and sex. A frequently used general assessment of a person's maturity might indicate that he or she is above or below average for age and sex. A measure of height alone, however, is not a good estimate of maturity because individuals differ in mature height. To be assessed as above average in height at a specific time in a child's life may signify either a rapid pace of growth or an average rate of growth for a child who will be above average in height as an adult.

focus on change

Heredity and the environment *change* maturity characteristics over time (secular trend).

Dental Age

The age at which teeth erupt may also provide information on approximate level of maturity. Eruption of both deciduous (temporary) and permanent teeth in most individuals occurs fairly predictably. The deciduous dentition erupts from 6 months to 2 years; permanent teeth generally appear from about 6 to 13 years of age. One limitation of using dental age to gain a complete perspective of full maturity is the lack of available information on dentition growth between the ages of 2 and 6 years and after age 13 years. Recent research has focused on dental calcification seen in X-rays as a promising indicator of dental age.

Sexual Age

This biological estimate of sexual age refers to the assessed maturity of primary and secondary sexual qualities. Subjective maturity rating scales are often used to evaluate the status of sexual development in the reproduction organs, pubic hair, and breast development and menarche in females. Of the sexual characteristics of females, the age of menarche (first menstrual flow) is the most common standard of maturity.

In most cases, menarche occurs relatively late in the adolescent growth period, after growth in height has peaked. Approximately 96% of females experience menarche between the ages of 11 and 15 years. It can also be estimated from this data that most females will have their first menstrual flow between 12 and 13 years of age. Although menarche indicates maturity in uterine development, it does not always denote full maturity of the female reproductive system. Initially, menstrual cycles may be very irregular, and it may be several years after periods begin that a female becomes fertile. Figures 3.28 and 3.29 illustrate the normal range of the development of selected sexual characteristics in males and females.

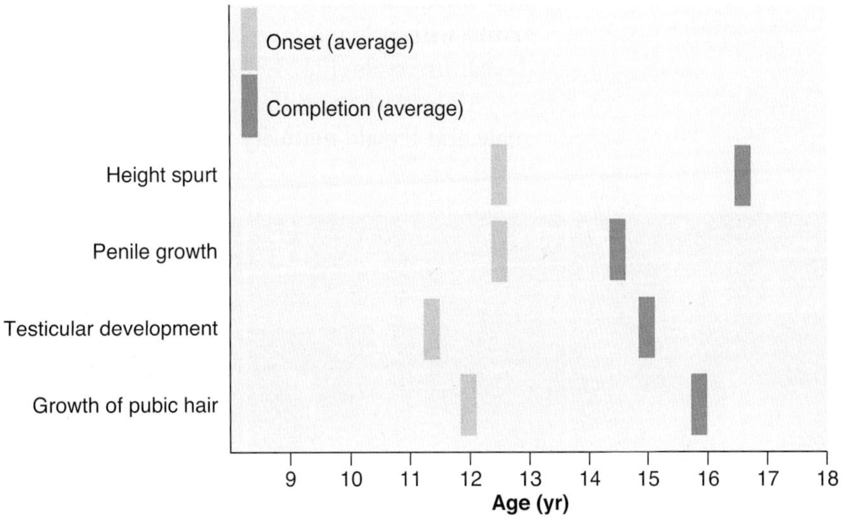

Figure 3.28 Average age and range of sexual development in males.

SOURCE: Tanner, J. M. (1990). *Fetus into man: Physical growth from conception to maturity*. Cambridge, MA: Harvard University Press.

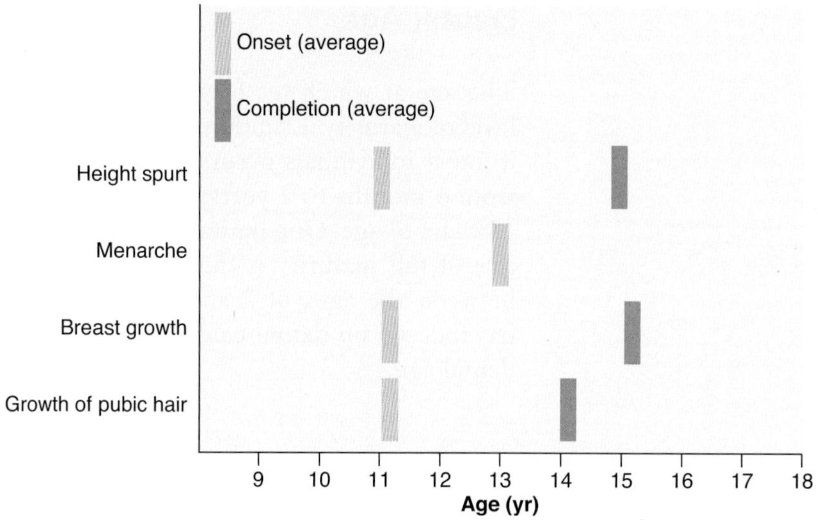

Figure 3.29 Average age and range of sexual development in females.

SOURCE: Tanner, J. M. (1990). *Fetus into man: Physical growth from conception to maturity*. Cambridge, MA: Harvard University Press.

Skeletal Age

The best method of maturity estimate is derived from evaluating the successive stages of skeletal growth as seen in X-rays. Also referred to as *bone age*, skeletal age provides a good estimate of maturity because its development spans virtually the entire period of active growth and maturation. All normally developing people, regardless of whether they are early, average, or late maturing, will eventually reach a stage of complete skeletal maturity. Skeletal maturity is usually measured by X-raying the bones of the left wrist and hand complex, which consists of some 29 separate ossification centers. The hand and wrist, however, only provide useful information for individuals who are about 18 months of age and older. Other parts, such as the leg, knee, and foot, have also been recommended for measuring the skeletal age of younger and older populations. The progressive enlargement and change in shape of ossification centers can be detected on an X-ray and compared with other X-rays standardized to represent skeletal ages at 6-month and 1-year intervals (Fig. 3.30).

Along with the differences in skeletal growth, these X-rays can differentiate the male and female maturity rates. Females, in general, are more biologically mature

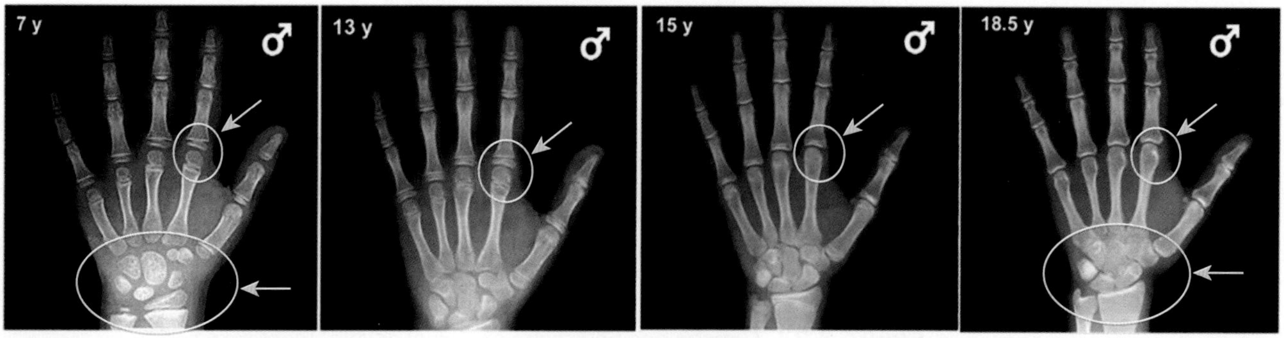

Figure 3.30 Bone development shown for males 7 to 18 years of age.

SOURCE: Courtesy of University of California, Los Angeles Radnet.

than males. Areas that appear as spaces between the wrist and fingers (black or grayish in appearance) are cartilaginous bone not yet calcified. As the bone matures, or ossifies, it becomes more dense and, thus, is more visible in the X-ray. Females are approximately 20% more advanced in skeletal maturity than males are. In practical terms, the difference is about 2 months at age 1 year and 2 years at age 10 years. Popular atlases of skeletal maturity include those developed by Tanner and associates (2001) and the latest, Gilsanz and Ratib (2012).

MATURITY VARIATIONS

Objective 3.9

Although diet and other health factors may influence the rate of maturity, the biological clock within the individual sets the pace of maturation. Individuals are generally grouped into categories of early, average, and late maturers, according to where they fit on various maturational scales. We are often concerned with the development of individuals who appear to be late maturers or early maturers. As noted earlier, it can be difficult to quantify a rather qualitative aspect of growth and development. However, the extremes can be established with more accuracy than levels in the midrange of maturity.

Early maturers are those in whom the maturity characteristics are in advance of their chronological age, whereas late-maturing individuals are behind in relation to the standard. For example, an individual who has a chronological age of 10 years and a skeletal age of 13 years is categorized as ahead (early maturing) of the normal maturation pace. A female who experiences menarche at 10 years (when the average is 12½ years) is also an early maturer. In contrast, a female who does not experience menarche until her 15th birthday is considered late maturing, as is the female who is 8 years old and has a skeletal age of 6 years.

> **think about it**
>
> What might be some advantages of being a late-maturing person?

What is early or late? A relatively common view suggests that when comparing chronological age with skeletal age, a 20% difference from mean skeletal age should be considered early or late, respectively. For example, if a 10-year-old is average maturing, he or she has a skeletal age of 10 years; a skeletal age of 8 years is considered late maturing, and a skeletal age of 12 years is early maturing. These, however, are arbitrary cutoffs, and clinical practice often uses up to 1 to 3 years on either side of chronological age. Another method is to state that (using one example) the child is 22 years behind or 12 years ahead. Early maturers, on the average, take 4 to 5 fewer years to achieve full skeletal maturity and tend to complete the pubertal growth period faster than late maturers do.

Although differences in maturity levels are apparent prior to the pubescent growth spurt, they appear to be most pronounced during adolescence. Early maturers are generally taller and heavier for their age than late-maturing peers are. Late maturers, however, catch up to early maturers in stature during late adolescence or early adulthood. Various maturational rates also may affect body build. Early-maturing males are generally more mesomorphic, and early-maturing females are more endomorphic. Later-maturing males and females tend to have less weight for stature, whereas early maturers of both sexes generally have more body fat during adolescence.

In terms of interaction with peers, early maturation appears to be advantageous. Early maturers are more likely to be elected to class offices, rated as popular, and excel in athletics. The superior size and advanced physiological characteristics (e.g., strength and speed) associated with early maturing are in accord with male sex-role expectations. For an excellent discussion of maturity-associated variation, refer to Malina et al. (2004).

Focus on Application
Girls' Early Puberty

As noted in the text, average menarche is about 12½ years. So, what about those who begin "early." Before menarcheal stage, girls begin the onset of breast development; so an indicator of early maturation. Recent figures indicate that about 16% of girls enter puberty by the age of 7 years and about 30% by the age of 8 years. Recent research indicates that one of the influencing factors is obesity—heavier girls tend to enter puberty earlier. Girls are 10 times as likely to have precocious puberty as boys. Other factors also play a role, such as genetics, atypical hormonal development, and medical problems. With that said, researchers have noted the following associations.

Stress. Even when it's happening to average 12-year-olds, puberty can be a stressful time. For example, they might feel awkward about their appearance (breast development). Early-maturing girls may also feel unsettled with early menstruation.

Physically less active. One study found that early-maturing girls at age 11 years had subsequent lower physical activity levels at age 13 years; that is, compared to late-maturing girls. In addition, earlier puberty was associated with lower psychological well-being. Such psychological and emotional stress has been linked to participating in risky behaviors like alcohol use and smoking.

Increased animal protein intake. Higher total protein and meat intake in young children is associated with earlier menarche, compared to diets that are higher in vegetable protein intake. It has been suggested that high-protein intake elevates hormones (namely, IGF-1) that promote growth. As noted in the press, there is also speculated that the consumption of select meats and dairy products may contain chemicals that stimulate early growth.

With each of the factors noted, there are suggests for parent education and school programs designed to address self-esteem/consciousness and the promotion of physical activity. Obviously, there is considerable variation in how individual girls react to early puberty, but awareness of the potential problem is important.

Sources:

Benaroch, R. (2015). *Early puberty: Causes and consequences*. Retrieved from http://www.webmd.com/children/guide/causes-symptoms

Fuhrman, J. (2011, May 6). Girls' early puberty: What causes it, and how to avoid it. *The Huffington Post*. Retrieved from http://www.huffingtonpost.com/joel-fuhrman-md/girls-early-puberty_b_857167.html

Objective 3.10

think about it

Considering the secular trend, speculate on the difference between the 15-year-old of today and the 15-year-old of the year 2050. What type of research design would you use to study this?

These maturational differences are *individual differences*. As a group, today's population is taller and heavier and matures earlier than the population of generations past. These observations are referred to as **secular trend**. Today, the average female reaches adult height 2 years earlier than females at the turn of the century. Figure 3.31 illustrates the secular trend for menarche. Note that menarche occurred around age 17 years for Norwegian girls in 1840, compared with just older than 13 years of age in 1969; the average for American girls today is 12½ years. The mean age of menarche has been declining an average of about 4 months per decade. Thus, due primarily to improved health conditions and nutrition, females are maturing earlier (sexually).

Most males today reach adult stature by age 18 or 19 years, whereas about 75 years ago, most males did not reach maximal height until age 25 or 26 years. Since 1900, children from average households have increased in height between the ages of 5 and 7 years by approximately 1 to 2 centimeters each decade. Secular differences in stature appear to be most evident during the adolescent growth period due to the faster rate of maturation in more recent generations. The difference between a 15-year-old male of 1880 and 1960 was approximately 5½ inches (14 cm). The difference in maximal adult height during that same period was of a lesser magnitude—about 3 inches (8 cm) (Eveleth & Tanner, 1990).

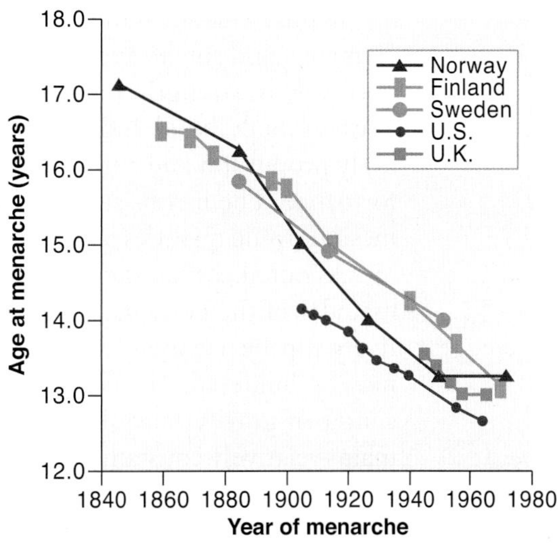

Figure 3.31 Secular trend for menarche.

It has been suggested that secular trend in size and maturation in individuals from developed countries has leveled off in recent years. Speculation is that the factors associated with secular trend, in general, such as improvement in nutrition, reduction in the incidence of disease, better health practices, and greater genetic hybridization, have been maximized. A negative secular trend noted in recent years is that children carry more body fat than their counterparts of the 1960s (CDC, 2015). In addition, there is evidence that after the age of 11 years, society in general is less physically active. These topics are discussed in greater detail in Chapter 5.

IMPLICATIONS FOR MOTOR PERFORMANCE

Objective 3.11

All of the physical growth characteristics described in this chapter are related in some manner to motor performance. Although research has produced few conclusive findings, especially with young populations, some generalizations can be offered.

A common finding of investigations has been that infants who are longer for their weight tend to walk at an earlier age in comparison to shorter and fatter babies. However, follow-up studies have revealed that delayed groups usually catch up quickly and that initial walking patterns of the early group are quite immature. Similar inconclusive findings concerning young populations have also been reported concerning the relationships between body size, body mass, body fat, selected anthropometric measures, and strength-related tasks.

With school-age and older populations, research has demonstrated rather clearly an inverse relationship between excess body fat (using BMI, for example) and performance on tasks that require the body to be propelled (e.g., running, and jumping), particularly in endurance activities (e.g., D'Hondt et al., 2014). For example, Okely et al. (2004) found that boys and girls (age 9 to 16 years) who were not overweight were 2 to 3 times more likely to possess advanced locomotor skills than those who were overweight. In tasks requiring that an object be propelled or force be applied, increasing body size (fat-free mass) usually has a positive effect on performance. It should be noted, however, that the overall contribution of age, stature, and body mass to variation in motor performance is generally low to moderate at best.

Similar relationship levels have also been found in regard to strength performance and somatotype. In general, mesomorphy and endomorphy are related positively to strength, whereas ectomorphic characteristics are not. Relationships between body build and motor performance (especially with activities involving body propulsion and agility) are generally low between endomorph and task performance. The inconsistency here is that correlations between individuals having mesomorphic qualities and motor performance are generally positive but low.

As noted earlier, the proportion of the infant's head in relationship to the remainder of the body may influence motor performance. Because infants are relatively top-heavy, their ability to balance and perform such tasks as body rolling may be hindered. As body proportions change during childhood, an individual's center of gravity may also vary considerably. Although the center of gravity remains relatively constant in proportion to total height with age, the center of gravity is higher in children because they carry a greater proportion of weight in the upper body. In general, females have a lower center of gravity than males, which contributes to the better performance of females in tasks requiring balance.

The structural and anatomical changes that occur during adolescence also may contribute to motor performance differences between the sexes. As a result of the pubescent growth spurt, males generally become taller and heavier, develop wider shoulders and longer legs and forearms, and gain in lean body weight. Females during this period will develop a lower center of gravity.

The implications of these characteristics for performing motor tasks are not decisive but warrant consideration from a biomechanical perspective. The female's lower center of gravity and shorter legs contribute to better balance. Shorter leg length and wider hips, however, are disadvantageous in running (especially sprinting) and jumping events, when compared to the performance of males whose legs are proportionately longer and whose hips are narrower. The male's longer arms and wider shoulders also may provide a mechanical advantage for motor tasks involving throwing and striking, for example. As emphasized earlier, one should keep in mind the fact that there is considerable variation across and within sexes.

Summary

Characteristic of the changes in lifelong physical growth are the cephalocaudal and proximodistal patterns of development. The study of these changes can be measured using a variety of instruments and techniques.

Individuals grow faster during gestation and the first year after birth than at any other time in the life span. After conception, three major periods of physical growth are associated with the rapid changes that occur before birth: the germinal period, the embryonic period, and the fetal period.

Next to the rapid changes in growth that appear during the prenatal stage, the growth spurt that takes place with puberty represents the life span's most dramatic period of biological alteration. In males, puberty is characterized by significant sexual, anatomical, and physiological changes. For females, the changes are less dramatic, but a major milestone reached during this period is menarche—the first menstrual flow and the universal indicator of sexual maturity. One of the primary mechanisms at work in the changes associated with puberty is the endocrine system and the increased levels of hormones it releases.

Specific body parts undergo dramatic changes during the course of physical growth and development. Along with a doubling of head size, there are also comparable changes in limb length (especially the legs), trunk length, and shoulder and hip width. Prior to puberty, males and females appear to have similar body builds; however, noticeable differences occur thereafter.

A typical child will increase birth length by 50% at 1 year of age and reach approximately one-half of mature height at 2 years of age. Most females complete their peak growth period by age 16½ years, whereas males continue to gain in stature for at least another 2 years.

The elaborate process of bone ossification begins shortly after conception and continues until maturity, when epiphyseal plates and fusion areas are closed. Although growth of the long bones is generally complete by the early 20s, portions of the braincase do not reach maturity (or become fused) until well into adulthood.

With advancing years, significant losses may occur in stature, bone mass (especially among females), and lean body mass (muscle).

Estimating the level of physical maturity is best accomplished using measures of biological age rather than chronological age. Of these methods, skeletal age, which is derived from comparisons of radiographs, is perhaps the most accurate estimate of physical maturity.

Individuals are often categorized as early, average, or late maturers, according to where they fit on various maturational scales. In general, early maturers are taller and heavier for their age than their late-maturing peers. However, late maturers often catch up to others during late adolescence or early adulthood.

Observations of the secular trend indicate that today's population is maturing earlier and is taller than past generations. The explanation for this trend is complex but includes the factors of improved nutrition, reduced incidence of disease, and better health practices. Negative trends are increased body fat and reduced levels of physical activity.

Although few conclusive findings have been reported, several generalizations can be made about the implications of change in body size for motor performance. For example, it appears that excess body fat hinders the development of several fundamental locomotor skills.

think about it

1. **In the study of motor development, why is this period so relevant?**
2. **Consider some ways the phenomenon of puberty can influence participation in sports. Include possible, if any, differences between males and females.**
3. **What is the relationship between specific body proportions and motor performance after pubertal change?**
4. **Describe how the environment can affect physique.**
5. **What type of training (specifically) do you think might change transitional fibers?**
6. **Using a velocity curve format, illustrate the major physical growth (weight and body weight) milestones across the life span. Then, briefly summarize each event.**

7. **What are the implications of advanced age-related declines in motor behavior for daily living activities?**
8. **What might be some advantages of being a late-maturing person?**
9. **Considering the secular trend, speculate on the difference between the 15-year-old of today and the 15-year-old of the year 2050. What type of research design would you use to study this?**

LEARNING ACTIVITIES

Objective: To develop skills in measuring and interpreting anthropometric data. Select a male and female adolescent (ages 12 to 17 years) who are similar in age. Using the measurement descriptions provided in this chapter, collect anthropometric information on the physical characteristics in the following list. After data collection is complete, use the interpretative tables and figures provided in the chapter and on *thePoint* to assess each person. Provide a report of their characteristics using percentile rank.

Anthropometric characteristics

Height
Body weight
BMI
Sitting height
Shoulder width
Hip width
Somatotype (use Sheldon's method or estimate subjectively)

Objective: To create a hypothetical growth (velocity) curves with the aim of visualizing change over time

a. Using the stature-for-age charts shown on *thePoint* (distance curves) for males and females, illustrate on one graph velocity curves for both genders across ages 2 to 20 years; use the 50th percentile and show growth patients at 2, 5, 10, 15, and 20 years.

b. Do the same for BMI.

Suggested Reading

Spirduso, W. W., Francis, K. L., & MacRae, P. G. (2005). *Physical dimensions of aging* (2nd ed.). Champaign, IL: Human Kinetics.

Chapter 4

Physiological Changes

OBJECTIVES

Upon completion of this chapter, you should be able to

4.1 Outline and briefly describe the basic structure and functions of the cardiorespiratory system.

4.2 Identify significant growth and development changes that occur during the part of the life span prior to puberty.

4.3 Distinguish between the terms *aerobic power* and *anaerobic power* and describe the lifelong developmental changes that take place in these characteristics.

4.4 List the major changes that occur over time in heart rate, cardiac output and stroke volume, and vital capacity and pulmonary ventilation.

4.5 Identify significant differences between children and adults in *thermoregulation*.

4.6 Describe the ways in which the body's blood characteristics change as individual's age.

4.7 Define *basal metabolic rate* and briefly note how it changes over the life span.

4.8 Distinguish between the various types of muscular strength and describe how their characteristics may vary through the lifelong developmental process.

4.9 Discuss what determines flexibility and its developmental characteristics.

4.10 Describe the effects of advanced aging on each of the basic physiological functions in both general and specific terms.

KEY TERMS

maximal oxygen uptake (VO_2max)	thermoregulation
aerobic power	basal metabolic rate (BMR)
anaerobic power	muscular strength
cardiac output	muscular endurance
vital capacity	flexibility

focus on change

Physiological *change* underscores lifelong motor performance, physical fitness, and quality daily living.

think about it

How can health-related components of fitness be considered constraints to motor performance?

Important to any comprehensive discussion of lifelong motor development is an understanding of the basic physiological changes associated with exercise and motor skill performance. In the context of this aspect of developmental exercise physiology and motor development, this chapter focuses on the cardiovascular and respiratory systems, basal metabolic rate, muscular strength, and flexibility. Along with the functions of the central nervous system, these components provide the basis for motor skill performance and lifelong physical fitness. In recent years, the term *health-related fitness* has been used to describe those aspects of physical fitness related to functional health and preventive medicine (aerobic fitness, muscular strength and endurance, flexibility, and optimal body composition) rather than motor performance (speed, power, agility, and coordination).

This chapter discusses the particular effects of physical activity and exercise on the basic physiological components of change outlined in the following pages. For a more detailed discussion of lifelong physiological change as a result of various intensities of exercise, refer to Kenney et al. (2015); McArdle et al. (2015); Rowland (2005); and Taylor and Johnson (2008).

CARDIORESPIRATORY DEVELOPMENT

The term *cardiorespiratory* in this discussion refers to selected aspects and functions of the cardiovascular and respiratory (pulmonary) systems. Early system growth and development, as well as the developmental aspects of selected functions and capabilities of these systems, will be covered.

Basic Structure and Function

Objective 4.1

The *cardiorespiratory system* consists of the heart; its cardiovascular network of arteries, capillaries, and veins; and the respiratory (pulmonary) system. The heart is a four-chambered muscular organ that weighs less than 1 pound yet has the power to beat approximately 40 million times per year. The heart may be viewed as two separate pumping units. The chambers that compose the right side of the heart receive blood returning from all parts of the body and then pump blood to the lungs. The left side of the heart receives oxygenated blood from the lungs and pumps it into the aorta for distribution throughout the body by way of the circulatory system.

The heart is composed of three layers: the pericardium, the outer layer composed of fibrous and adipose tissues; the myocardium, the middle layer composed of cardiac muscle tissue; and the endocardium, or inner layer. Cardiac muscle tissue differs from skeletal muscle tissue in that cardiac muscle is involuntary. The individual fibers of cardiac tissue are multinucleated cells that are interconnected

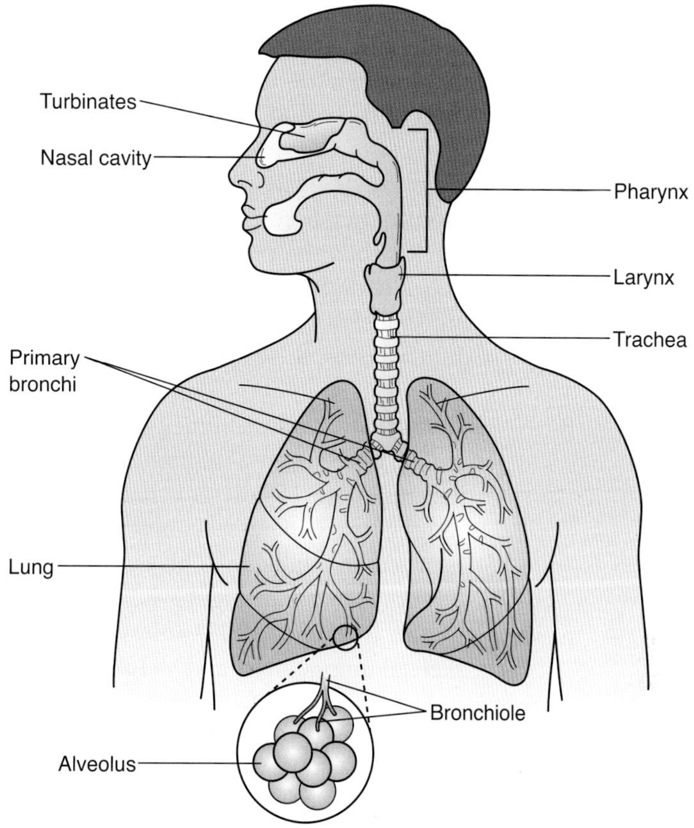

Figure 4.1 Basic structure of the respiratory system.

in a close network. Consequently, when an individual cell is stimulated, the action potential, or impulse, speeds through the entire heart and causes it to function as a unit.

The process by which air is brought into and exchanged with the air in the lungs is referred to as *pulmonary (respiratory) ventilation*. Air enters through the nose and mouth and flows into the ventilation system, where it is adjusted to accommodate body temperature. The air is then filtered and humidified as it passes through the trachea. The inspired air then passes into two bronchi, the large tubes serving as primary conduits in each of the lungs. The bronchi further subdivide into numerous bronchioles that conduct the air to be mixed with existing air in the alveoli, or terminal branches of the respiratory tract (Fig. 4.1).

Early Growth and Development

HEART GROWTH

Objective 4.2

The heart begins its development as a single tube. Its first pulsations may occur as early as the third week after conception, although there is no blood for the heart to circulate because the fetus is getting oxygen through the umbilical cord. By 12 weeks, the circulatory system is operating. By sometime between the fourth and fifth fetal months, the heartbeat is regular and strong enough to be heard using a stethoscope. Heart weight doubles during the first year and has increased 6 times by age 9 years. From 9 to 16 years of age, the heart undergoes a second phase of rapid growth that parallels the general growth rate during that period.

All of the functional mechanisms found in the adult electrocardiogram are also evident in the fetus after about 5 weeks.

In the fetus, the vessels that develop from the main trunk of the heart grow in direct proportion to the parts of the body supplied. This indicates that a relationship exists between caliber of growth and the volumes or weights of the regions supplied. At birth, the right ventricular muscle outweighs the left, but by the fifth month, they become equal in weight. By 7 years of age, the left wall is 2 to 3 times thicker than the right, as it is in the adult.

The thickness of the walls of the major veins doubles between the time of birth and puberty, and cavity size increases approximately 2.5 times by early maturity. In newborns, the total blood volume of the heart, one indicator of size, is approximately 200 milliliters. By the end of the first year, this value doubles, and at the time of maturity, blood volume is 5,500 milliliters for males and 4,200 milliliters for females. There is little difference between the sexes until puberty; after that, the male heart is about 15% larger than the female heart is, even with adjustment for body weight. As a general rule, heart size is related to body size, so children have smaller hearts than adults do. This accounts for much of the endurance performance differences observed. Figure 4.2 illustrates change in heart mass from 5 to 17 years of age. Rowland (2005) notes that the changes are remarkably similar to those of skeletal muscle mass and VO_2max.

Respiratory Component Growth

By the sixth fetal week, the trachea, bronchi, and lung buds are evident, and migration toward the thoracic region begins. By the third fetal month, the journey is almost complete, and thereafter, the lungs gradually begin to descend into their destined location. At birth, the larynx is approximately one-third of its adult size, but it is about the same size in relation to the rest of the body as it is in the adult. At the time of delivery, the trachea is roughly one-third (about 4 cm) of its adult length; by puberty, both its anteroposterior and lateral diameters will increase nearly 300%.

Anatomical growth of the lungs follows individual patterns for each of the major ventilatory components. Development of the lungs begins as a lung bud protrusion that appears between the third and fourth fetal week. Growth proceeds when this protrusion branches, and by about the 16th fetal week, the bronchial

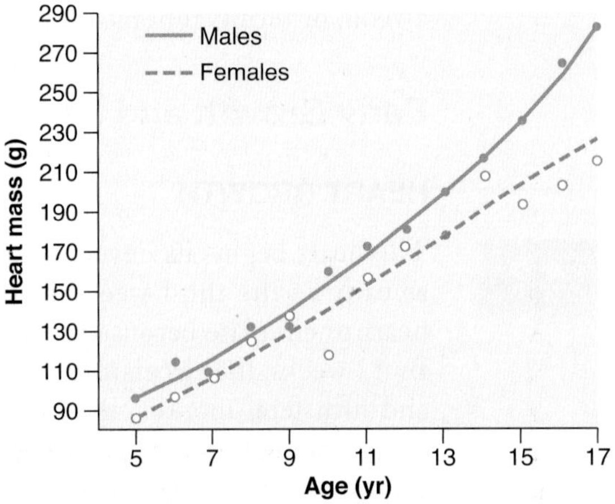

Figure 4.2 Change in heart mass during childhood and adolescence.

focus on change

Change in physiological performance is closely tied to biological maturity and experience (stimulation).

think about it

What does it mean by *independent existence*? And, more important, what are the medical implications?

tree is completely formed. Shortly thereafter, the airways canalize, and a little later, alveoli develop from the distal branches of the airway. Bronchial cartilage begins to form at 10 weeks; by 25 weeks, its distribution resembles the adult model. By 15 weeks, bronchi sensory and motor nerves can be detected along the pathways to the most distal passages. Capillaries appear about the 20th week and multiply rapidly near the developing airways when the alveoli begin to grow. Development of the alveolar-capillary interface for the exchange of oxygen and carbon dioxide is essential for *independent existence* after birth; this process is seldom complete before the sixth fetal month.

The weight and capacity of the lungs double in the first 6 months, triple by age 1 year, and increase approximately 20-fold by maturity. There also will be an increase of 2 to 3 times in the diameter of the airway. The diameter of the bronchi doubles by age 6 years and that of the bronchioles and trachea by approximately age 15 years. About 20 million primitive alveoli are present at the time of birth. During the first 3 years after birth, the increase in lung size primarily is due to increases in the number of alveoli. By age 8 years, there are about 300 million alveoli—about the same number found in the adult. After age 8 years, the alveoli begin to increase in size until the chest wall ceases growing.

Aerobic Power

Objective 4.3

Sometimes referred to as maximal oxygen consumption and maximal aerobic power, **maximal oxygen uptake (VO_2max)** is the maximum amount of oxygen an individual can use per unit of time. This amount usually is expressed in liters or milliliters of oxygen per minute. Maximal oxygen uptake is considered the best measure of cardiorespiratory fitness, as indicated by graded maximal working capacity tests using either a cycle ergometer or a treadmill.

The association between VO_2max and aerobic power lies with the energy sources of the body. For the body to do mechanical work, it depends on the splitting of adenosine triphosphate (ATP) to release energy for muscle contraction. This can be supplied from (a) limited stores of phosphagens; (b) glycolysis, which produces lactic acid; or (c) the conversion of substrates to carbon dioxide and water in a phase of carbohydrate breakdown called the *Kreb's cycle*, which is coupled with the electron transport system. The first two sources are considered anaerobic processes because additional oxygen is not required. Muscle contractions that result from anaerobic sources generally cannot be sustained longer than 40 or 50 seconds. Motor performance activities considered more anaerobic are sprints, jumping, weight lifting, and other movements where the required power intensity is high and the duration relatively short. In contrast, the third conversion method requires oxygen, meaning that it uses **aerobic power**. Muscle contractions that use oxygen as an energy source can last several minutes and, in trained individuals, several hours. Activities primarily, although not exclusively, associated with aerobic power include long-distance running, cycling, cross-country skiing, and swimming. These activities also involve anaerobic processes to a degree.

Figure 4.3 illustrates the relationship between maximal oxygen uptake and age. As a general trend, maximal oxygen uptake increases with growth through childhood; both sexes have similar values until approximately 12 years of age. Maximal oxygen uptake in males continues to increase until about age 18 years, whereas females show little improvement beyond age 14 years. The increase in VO_2max for males in puberty appears to correspond with the peak increase in height and with

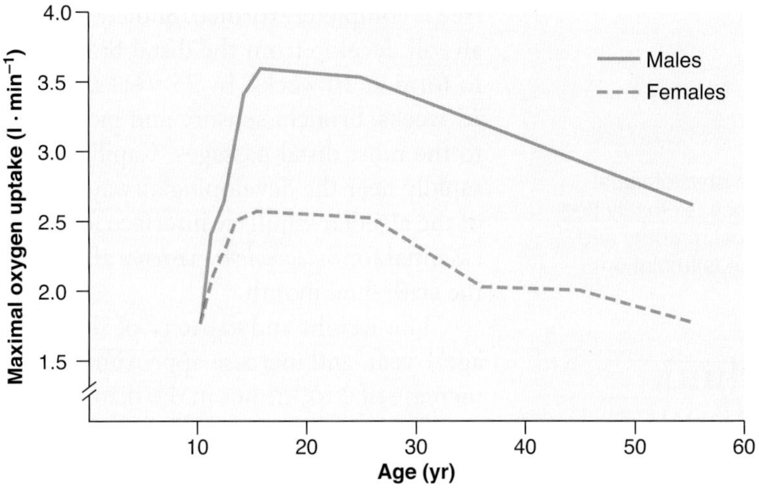

Figure 4.3 Maximal oxygen uptake as a function of age.

the time when androgen secretion increases dramatically. After about age 25 years, capacity declines steadily. Both children and adults have shown improvements in aerobic capacity through training; average increases range from 5% to 20%.

Maximal oxygen uptake is strongly related to lean body mass, which accounts to a great extent for the difference between the sexes after puberty. As noted earlier, lean body mass formation that follows puberty tends to level off in females as additional mass, primarily in the form of body fat, is added. Males, in contrast, continue to gain lean body mass. Approximately 70% of the individual differences in VO_2max can be explained simply by differences in body mass (McArdle et al., 2015). Values for young adult females are typically 15% to 30% lower than those for males. Among trained athletes, the difference ranges from 12% to 20%. Although aerobic capacity has been shown to increase with growth through childhood, when expressed relative to body mass, aerobic capacity remains the same or decreases with age.

WebLink
http://www.pbrc.edu/heritage/

Along with training and physical characteristics, maximal oxygen uptake also is influenced by heredity. Based on the findings that genetic factors appear to influence the growth of body size and mass as well as muscle fiber type, the heritability estimate for maximal oxygen uptake (which itself accounts for about 50%) is believed to be more than 90%. Supporting the relatively strong genetic contribution are results from the HERITAGE Family Study (e.g., Green et al., 2004; also see WebLink noted). This unique study was designed to evaluate the role of genetic and nongenetic factors linked to responses to aerobic exercise training. One interesting finding regarding VO_2max is that part of the gene component for this trait expresses itself only in response to an active lifestyle. Results from the HERITAGE Family Study have important implications for understanding human variation in a variety of physiological variables and risk factors for common chronic diseases.

Body weight is the major physical determinant in maximal oxygen uptake capacity; however, several other factors are also related. These factors include cardiac output, vital capacity, heart rate, stroke volume, and the oxygen-carrying properties of the blood, including blood volume and hemoglobin. Differences between the sexes are primarily related to differences in the values associated with these factors and differences in heart size. Table 4.1 indicates adult gender differences in maximal oxygen uptake.

TABLE 4.1 Gender Differences in Maximal Oxygen Consumption (50th Percentile)

Age (y)	Males	Females
20–29	40.0	31.1
30–39	37.5	30.3
40–49	36.0	28.0
50–59	33.6	25.7
>60	30.0	22.9

SOURCE: From Pollock, M. L., Wilmore, J. H., & Fox, S. M. (1978). *Health and fitness through physical activity*. New York, NY: Wiley. Copyright © 1978 John Wiley & Sons, Inc., New York.

Anaerobic Power

In contrast to the characteristics of aerobic power, **anaerobic power** is the maximum rate at which metabolic processes can occur without additional oxygen. Sustained aerobic activity depends on a continuous transport of oxygen to the working tissues, as measured by VO_2max. However, when exercise continues longer than a few seconds, more energy for ATP resynthesis must be generated through the anaerobic reactions of *glycolysis*. More intense, all-out activity requires levels of energy that far exceed what the respiratory processes alone can generate. Consequently, the anaerobic reactions of glycolysis predominate, and large amounts of lactic acid accumulate within active muscle and in the bloodstream. The level of lactic acid in the blood is the most common indicator of anaerobic activity. As the intensity of exercise increases and VO_2max is reached, the amount of lactic acid in the blood increases quickly. Under these conditions, work can be maintained only for a few minutes. Anaerobic power generally is measured in tests requiring that a supramaximal exercise be performed for a minute or less. Popular tests include sprinting up a flight of stairs (Margaria-Kalamen power test), arm or leg cranking on a cycle ergometer (Wingate anaerobic test), jumping-power tests, and short sprints.

think about it

What factors contribute to making a great sprinter and long-distance runner (biology/environment)?

Anaerobic power increases with age up to early adulthood no matter whether the values are expressed absolutely or relative to body weight (Rowland, 2005). In anaerobic tests that last 1 minute or less, children exhibit significantly lower scores than adolescents and adults do. Although maximal aerobic power generally does not change and may even decrease relative to body weight, anaerobic power increases progressively with growth. Figure 4.4 compares anaerobic power for age 7 years, age 12 years, and adults. Note the age difference over the first 2 minutes.

The differences in anaerobic power cannot be accounted for by muscle tissue mass. The markedly lower capacity of young children reflects, to a great extent, a qualitative deficiency in the muscle. The major age-related difference appears to be in glycolytic capacity—the resting concentration of glycogen and the rate at which lactate is produced with its utilization. Although exercise lactate levels rise progressively during childhood, they are lower than in older populations. The level of acidosis at which the muscle still can contract also is used as an indicator of anaerobic capacity. Following a pattern similar to glycolytic capacity, children do not reach the levels of acidosis of which adolescents and young adults are capable. Regardless of measured values, maximal acidosis also increases with age.

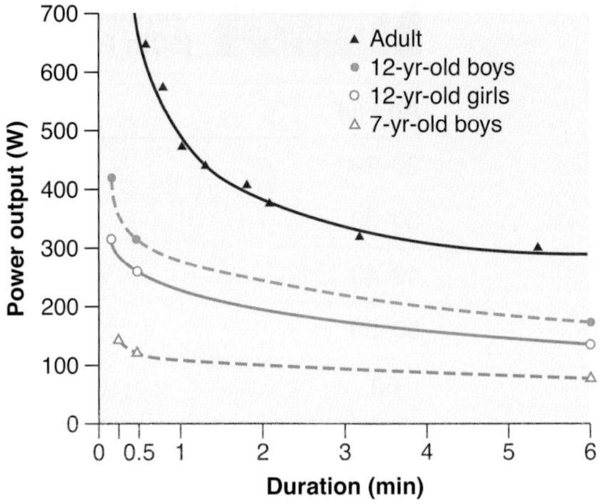

Figure 4.4 Anaerobic power values for children and adults while cycling.

As an overall concluding statement, this information suggests that as children grow older, they experience a progressive increase in the ability to overcome fatigue during physical work.

Females, in general, do not have the anaerobic power of males, especially after puberty. However, gender-related differences cannot be explained merely by differences in body size. Although unclear at this time, the explanation likely is based in part on qualitative factors such as hormonal variation, muscle characteristics, or the nature of motor unit activation. As noted previously, individual differences can be explained in large part by genetic influence (about a 50% contribution).

Heart Rate

Objective 4.4

Due to the relative ease of monitoring, *heart rate* has been one of the most commonly used measures of cardiovascular response to exercise and of energy expenditure. Because heart rate is the major determinant in cardiac output (the amount of blood pumped per unit of time), it is also an important factor in maximal oxygen consumption. Heart rate measures can be taken at rest, at a given rate of exercise (submaximal), and at maximal level of exercise (for maximal heart rate). A rough estimate of maximal heart rate can be obtained by subtracting a person's age from 220. A more direct and accurate measure is obtained by measuring the highest heart rate during a treadmill test that pushes the individual to maximal oxygen uptake.

Resting heart rate levels decrease with age; females average 5 bpm higher than males (Table 4.2). A similar pattern exists for heart rate at a submaximal exercise level—namely, that submaximal heart rate also declines with age and that females exhibit higher rates. Under these exercise conditions, it is not unusual for a preadolescent child to have a heart rate 30 to 40 bpm higher than a young adult performing the same task. The difference is due in part to the greater relative exercise intensity performed by the younger individual and the physiological compensation for a lower stroke volume.

The reported reasons for the higher rates for females are not conclusive. A possible reason, at least among adults, is the lower blood hemoglobin levels of women. However, the hemoglobin levels of preadolescents are similar, and females still exhibit greater heart rates. Another explanation has been related to stroke

TABLE 4.2 **Average Heart Rate at Rest**

Age	Average Heart Rate[a]
Birth	140
1 mo	130
1–6 mo	130
6–12 mo	115
1–2 y	110
2–4 y	105
6–10 y	95
10–14 y	85
14–18 y	82
20–29 y	66
30–39 y	65
>40 y	64

[a]Female values are an average 5 bpm higher than male values are.
SOURCE: Data recalculated from Lowrey, G. H. (1986). *Growth and development of children* (8th ed.). Chicago, IL: Year Book Medical; and Pollock, M. L., Wilmore, J. H., & Fox, S. M. (1978). *Health and fitness through physical activity*. New York, NY: Wiley.

volume differences between the sexes. Increased heart rate may compensate for the lower stroke volume and cardiac output of females.

Londeree and Moeschberger (1982) conducted a comprehensive review of existing information on maximal exercise heart rate among sampled individuals from 5 to 81 years of age. The review showed that maximal exercise heart rate declines with age and that as age increases the decline accelerates slightly. It was also reported that no significant differences between the sexes and categories of race for maximal exercise heart rate are apparent. Although this general trend is evident in updated reports, there are indications that rates are more stable throughout the childhood and early teen years and decrease across the life span.

Cardiac Output and Stroke Volume

Cardiac output is the major indicator of the functional capacity of the circulatory system. Output refers to the rate blood is pumped by the heart (heart rate) and the quantity of blood ejected with each stroke (stroke volume). As previously noted, cardiac output is the primary determinant of maximal oxygen uptake.

In general, as heart volume increases with growth and age, maximal cardiac output gradually increases, much like the pattern of development in maximal oxygen uptake (see Fig. 4.3 on page 104). Children have a significantly lower stroke volume than adults at all exercise levels and thus a lower cardiac output. This is compensated for by higher heart rates. Males have a higher stroke volume than females at all levels of exercise (although the difference is not dramatic) partly due to the biological advantage of a larger heart that has greater volume and pump capabilities, especially after puberty.

Vital Capacity and Pulmonary Ventilation

Vital capacity refers to the total volume of air that can be expired voluntarily following maximal inspiration. Vital capacity consists of the tidal volume, the air moved during inspiration or expiration, plus the available reserve volumes. The movement of air in and out of the pulmonary system is called *ventilation (breathing)*.

The growth pattern of vital capacity indicates that as males and females age and grow larger in body size, their vital capacity increases (Fig. 4.5). Vital capacity is strongly linked to body size. Males and females experience similar increases until the onset of puberty, when the larger body size of the male allows for greater absolute values. At 20 years of age, males have approximately 20% greater vital capacity than females. Because females enter puberty earlier than males (from 10 to 12 years of age), body sizes are relatively equal at that time and their vital capacities are much closer to equal.

As with vital capacity, the absolute volume for pulmonary ventilation increases with age and body size until young adulthood. An average 6-year-old may have a maximal ventilation of 30 to 40 liters per minute, whereas a young adult can reach 100 liters per minute easily. However, children's maximal ventilation values are not significantly different from adolescent and adult values when expressed relative to body weight. Once again, due to body size differences, maximal ventilation is normally higher in males. Interestingly, however, due to the smaller lung capacity in children, their respiratory rates are markedly higher than that of adults when performing a submaximal exercise task. Ventilation at any given oxygen uptake is higher in children, and the ventilatory breaking point, which signifies the onset of blood lactate, appears earlier than in adolescents and adults. During a submaximal test, a child of 6 years can have a ventilation value 50% higher than that of an individual of 17 years. In fact, children breathe more rapidly than adults, with a decline in maximal rate observed during childhood. Although not conclusive, research related to ventilatory equivalent, a numerical expression of ventilatory efficiency, suggests that it decreases with age. This indicates that children are less efficient at ventilating.

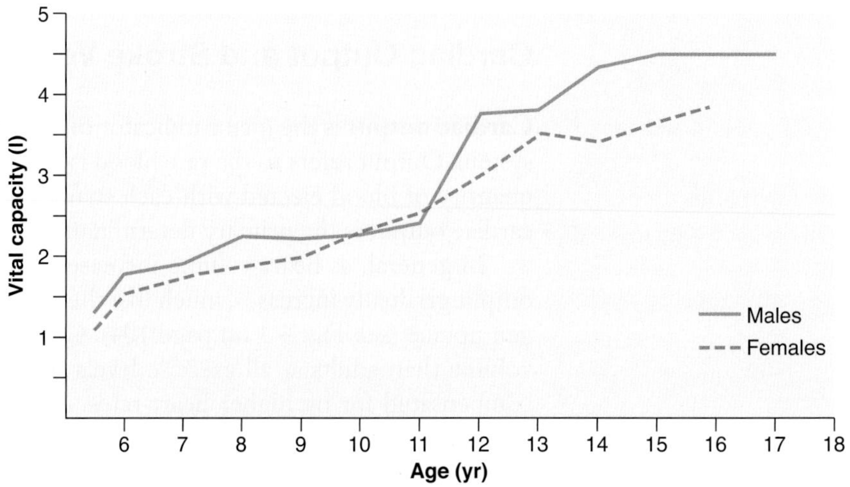

Figure 4.5 Vital capacity in relation to age.

Thermoregulation

Objective 4.5

Thermoregulation refers to the body's ability to regulate heat, in the context of this discussion, during exercise. As heat levels rise during physical activity, heat must be dissipated. Otherwise, there is a rise in the body's core temperature, which is a condition that may result in decreased performance and risk of internal injury. Heat is dissipated (a) by increasing blood flow to the skin for convective heat loss and (b) by increasing sweat rate for evaporative cooling, which is more effective. Both processes are expected to elevate stress levels on the cardiovascular system. From a developmental perspective, two characteristics differentiate children from adults: (a) Children typically tolerate exercise in the heat less efficiently than adults, and (b) children create more heat relative to their body mass during exercise than older persons.

In regard to the primary mechanism at work—sweat glands—the number appears to be fixed early in infancy. Thus, the density of sweat glands actually decreases on the skin surface with growth. Therefore, explanations of sweat rate efficiency refer to an expression of increased output per gland. Output is controlled in the brain (peptic area) in response to increased body heat. Adult men have a 40% greater output rate than prepubertal males. Females tend to sweat less than males during childhood, with the difference increasing substantially at puberty. For example, the sweat rate of an adult male may be three times greater than that of a mature female. Related to this outcome is the observation that children generate more heat per body mass than adults when performing the same workload. Given that sweat rate is significantly lower in children, this causes younger persons to rely more on the less effective process of convective heat loss (blood flow to the skin).

Although sweating is an efficient way to cool the body, too much sweating leads to another potential problem—dehydration. A review of studies comparing children and adults suggests that the magnitude of danger is similar in both groups; that is, in regard to water losses during exercise. See American College of Sports Medicine and American Academy of Pediatrics for heat stress guidelines for exercising children and young athletes.

WebLink
http://www.acsm.org/; https://www.aap.org/en-us/Pages/Default.aspx

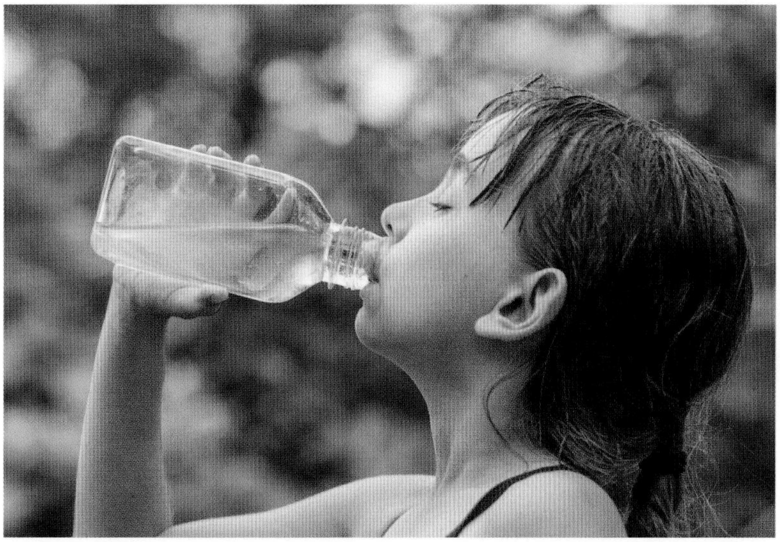

Figure 4.6 Proper hydration is important to thermoregulation.

BLOOD CHARACTERISTICS

Blood Volume

Objective 4.6

The increase in total blood volume maintains a relatively constant relationship to growth in body weight. The average newborn infant has a blood volume of 85 milliliters per kilogram relative to body weight. This increases to about 105 milliliters shortly after birth and then decreases during the first few months. Thereafter, the average blood volume is 75 to 77 milliliters per kilogram, which is maintained through adolescence and adulthood. Males' larger body mass, especially after puberty, results in a greater total and relative blood volume than that of females. The relative difference is approximately 10 milliliters per kilogram.

Red Blood Cell Content

The red blood cell is one of the most specialized cells in the body. Red blood cells contain the compound hemoglobin, which accounts for more than 95% of the total protein and for about 90% of the dry weight of the cell. The function of hemoglobin is to combine reversibly with oxygen, which allows red blood cells to collect oxygen from the lungs and deliver it to the tissues.

By the second week of gestation, the developing embryo begins to produce red blood cells. The production of these structures outside of the skeletal system peaks at about the fifth fetal month. Thereafter, production takes place in the bone marrow. Red blood cell count at birth is about 4.7 million. The life span of a red cell lasts about 90 days, compared to 120 days in adults. After this period, cell production increases gradually throughout childhood and adolescence.

The number of red blood cells and, consequently, the amount of hemoglobin are closely related to growth in body mass and blood volume (Fig. 4.7). Values in

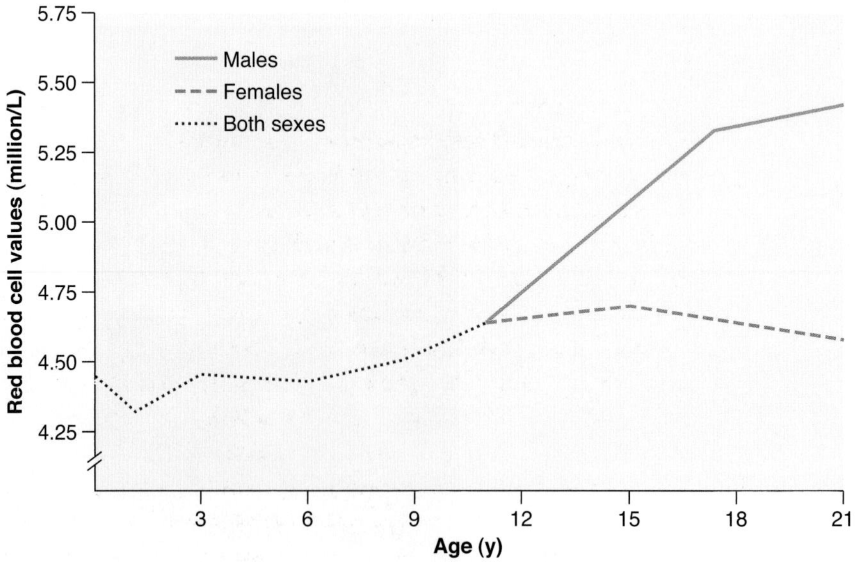

Figure 4.7 Mean red blood cell values in relation to age.

males and females first begin to diverge during adolescence. In the female, the gradual increase starts in preadolescence, continues into early puberty, and then levels off. In contrast, increases in the male appear to be related to sexual and physical maturity. The higher values of androgens in males after puberty have been associated with higher concentrations of hemoglobin. During adolescence in males, blood levels vary with sexual maturity. Higher hemoglobin levels in males help to explain higher anaerobic capacity.

Basal Metabolic Rate

Objective 4.7

think about it

What circumstances and processes count for significant metabolic activity over the first 2 years? (You may want to refer back to Chapter 2.)

Basal metabolic rate (BMR) refers to the amount of heat produced by the body during resting conditions. This physiological process reflects the minimum level of energy required to sustain the body's vital functions in the waking state. BMR usually is determined indirectly by measuring submaximal oxygen consumption and is recorded in terms of the heat produced per square meter of body surface. Individuals are measured after they have fasted for at least 12 hours to avoid the increase in metabolism due to the energy required to digest food. The BMR frequently is used to establish an energy baseline for constructing programs of weight control.

Basically, BMR declines continuously after infancy to old age (Fig. 4.8). The BMR per kilogram of weight in an infant is more than twice that of an adult. Males have slightly higher values than females do at all ages; the values for adult females are 5% to 10% lower than those for adult males. This difference is largely because females generally have more fat tissue, and fat is metabolically less active than lean body tissue. This difference between sexes is nearly eliminated when BMR is expressed relative to fat-free or lean body mass. The hormonal effects of increased androgens in males also have been mentioned as a possible contributing factor in sex differences. Overall, the decline can be explained by a decrease in the relative size of the major organs contributing to resting energy metabolic expenditure (Rowland, 2005).

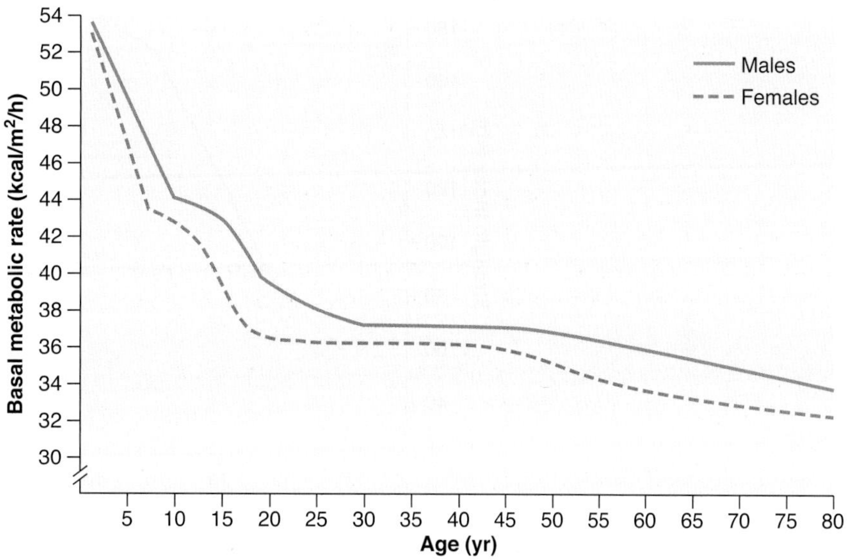

Figure 4.8 Basal metabolic rate as a function of age and sex.

Muscular Strength

Objective 4.8

Previous discussions regarding muscles have focused on their neurological structure and tissue development. This section provides information concerning the force characteristics of a muscle and their relationship to motor performance. **Muscular strength** refers to the maximum force or tension generated by a muscle or muscle groups. Tension of the muscle in partial or complete contraction without any appreciable change in length is identified as *isometric* contraction. This type of muscular force is referred to as *static strength* and is generally measured using a dynamometer and tensiometer. If the muscle varies its length when activated to produce force, the contraction is *isotonic*. Isotonic force is also known as *dynamic strength*. It is usually determined by a one-repetition maximum, which refers to the maximum amount of weight lifted one time. Some exercise physiologists also refer to isokinetic contraction. This is a muscular contraction in which the muscle shortens at a constant velocity. For training purposes, isokinetic machines can be set to move at various specified velocity rates and resistance levels.

Most past descriptive studies of children have documented the development of static strength using either a hand-grip dynamometer or, for other parts of the body, a cable tensiometer. With more recent advances in scientific instrumentation and the emergence of microprocessor technology, it is now possible to update this body of information (especially with younger populations) by quantifying more accurately the muscular forces generated during a variety of movements.

Figures 4.9 and 4.10 show means of strength characteristics (absolute and relative to body weight) for individuals from 10 to 59 years of age. Basically, muscular strength increases with age in both sexes and reaches a peak between 25 and 29 years of age. There is, however, considerable variability within and between the sexes. The development of strength is basically symmetrical on both sides of the body, although the dominant side is slightly stronger. The legs contribute approximately 60% to total body strength.

Reports of the development of strength during childhood show that both sexes demonstrate strength increase with age, with the values for boys slightly

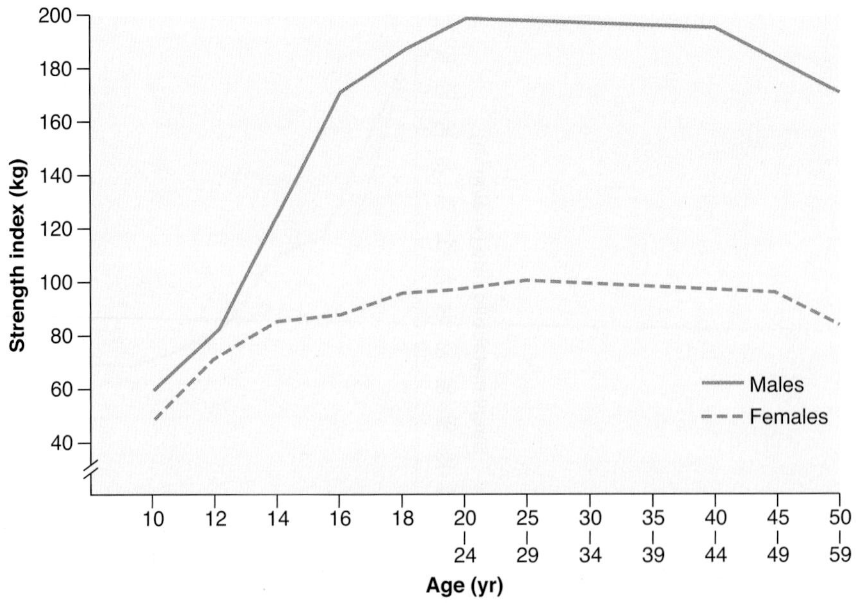

Figure 4.9 Strength index (mean) of grip of right and left arm.

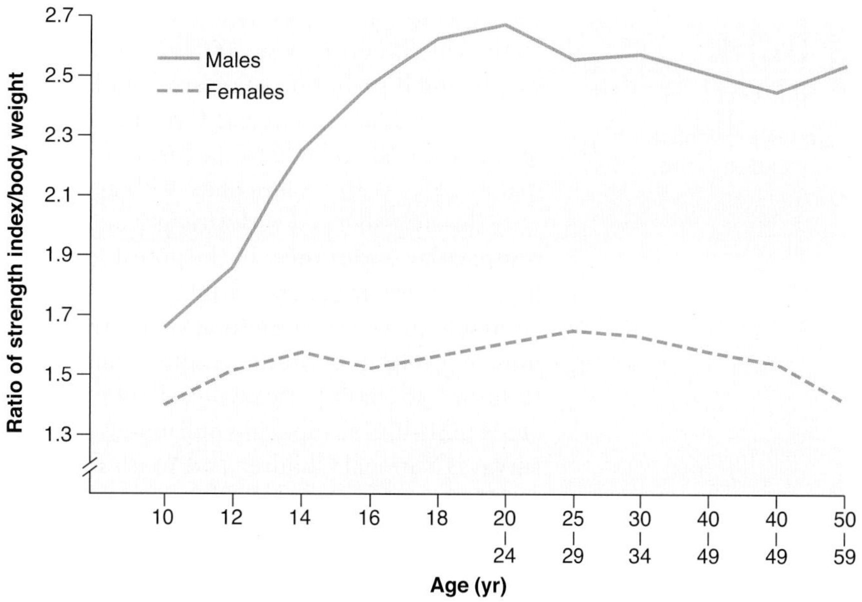

Figure 4.10 Ratio of strength index to body weight.

WebLink

http://www.cdc.gov/; refer to NYFS (2012).

think about it

Recently, there has been controversy regarding weight training by prepubescent children. What do you suppose is the issue? Furthermore, what would be safe for increasing strength?

greater (Rowland, 2005). More recent findings from the 2012 National Youth Fitness Survey (NYFS) (see CDC website) for grip strength, core strength, and maximal knee extension, indicate no significant differences between boys and girls aged 6 to 11 years. As expected, older boys (12 to 15 years) surpassed younger boys and girls of all ages. Some of that difference is attributed to the onset of puberty. The significant physiological and structural changes associated with the adolescent growth spurt are reflected in both capacity and differences between the sexes. However, as noted throughout this text, motor performance is strongly influenced by sociocultural and other environmental factors (e.g., physical activity level, health, and support).

When evaluating the differences between the sexes, three approaches may be taken: (a) relative to muscle cross-sectional area, (b) on an absolute basis as total force, and (c) relative to body weight or lean body mass. Regardless of sex, human skeletal muscle, based on cross-sectional analysis, generates approximately 3 to 4 kilograms of force per square centimeter (McArdle et al., 2015). Here, the difference is related to the size of the muscle cross-section; for the same-size muscle section, there is little difference.

When strength is compared on an absolute basis, males usually are considerably stronger than females (Fig. 4.8 on page 111). Males are typically 30% to 50% stronger than females are in most muscle groups. The difference is generally less when comparing the strength of the trunk and legs, as opposed to the shoulders and arms. As noted earlier, much of this difference, especially after puberty, is related to higher androgen levels and larger lean body mass in males. Researchers also have noted that the greater levels of androgens are an advantage in muscle hypertrophy, an increase in muscle size in response to training. Adult males have about 10 times the amount of androgens as prepubescent children and women do.

When strength values are expressed relative to body weight, males are generally still stronger (Fig. 4.9). This difference is due in part to the fact that the measurement of body weight reflects total body fat and lean body mass. Because females have more body fat and less lean body mass than males do, their strength per unit of body weight is lower. When strength is calculated relative to lean body weight,

think about it

What are the implications of weak muscles in the elderly?

the large absolute differences are reduced considerably. This information has led to the conclusion that sex differences are a function of differences in lean body weight and distribution of muscle and fat in the body segments.

The decline in muscular force production after it peaks (from 25 to 29 years of age) is closely related to the loss of muscle mass. A decrease in mass of approximately 25% to 30% takes place with aging.

Closely associated with strength and the ability of the muscle to produce force is **muscular endurance**. In the purest form, muscular strength refers to maximum force or tension generated by a muscle or muscle group in a single maximum contraction. Muscular endurance, on the other hand, is the ability of a muscle or muscle group to perform repeated contractions. That is, endurance is the ability to sustain strength performance. Commonly used tests of muscular endurance include push-ups, sit-ups, and pull-ups. According to two nationwide physical fitness surveys (National Children and Youth Fitness Study I [NCYFSI], 1985; NCYFSII, 1987), children gain steadily in sit-up and pull-up performance from 6 to 9 years of age; males generally continue to increase through adolescence, and females show indications of leveling off around the time of puberty. Figure 4.11 illustrates this pattern with bent-knee sit-ups. Part of that finding was supported in the newer 2012 NYFS noted earlier. That is, girls displayed no significant improvement in modified pull-ups from ages 6 to 11 years to early adolescence (12 to 15 years).

Other gross motor activities such as running, swimming, bicycling, and gymnastics require varying levels of muscular endurance. The primary component in the initiation of any muscular endurance task, however, is muscular strength.

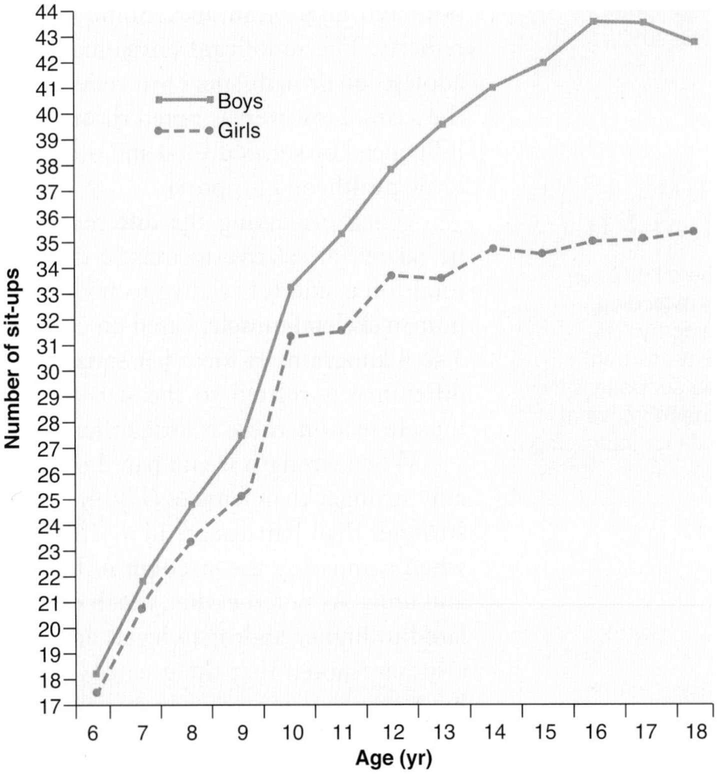

Figure 4.11 Average scores on bent-knee sit-ups (60 seconds) for ages 6 to 18 years.

SOURCE: As reported by Ross, J. G., & Gilbert, G. G. (1985). The National Children and Youth Fitness Study: A summary of findings. *Journal of Physical Education, Recreation, & Dance*, *56*(1), 45–50; and Ross, J. G., & Pate, R. R. (1987). The National Children and Youth Fitness Study II: A summary of findings. *Journal of Physical Education, Recreation, & Dance*, *5*(9), 51–56.

FLEXIBILITY

Objective 4.9

Flexibility is the degree of ability to move body parts through a range of motion without undue strain. This is an essential component of health-related fitness for optimal performance of motor skills and for preventing muscle injury. Research on the basic tenets of flexibility has produced the following conclusions: (a) Flexibility is specific to each joint, (b) flexibility is not related to the length of limbs, (c) strength development need not hinder range of motion, (d) activity levels are a better indicator of flexibility than age is, and (e) females tend to be more flexible than males.

Most flexibility tests are classified as relative or absolute measures. Relative tests measure flexibility relative to the length or width of a specific body part; thus, the movement and influencing body parts are measured. Tests that measure only the movement are referred to as *absolute*. The most commonly used instruments for testing flexibility are various types of flexometers and goniometers (linear or rotary measuring devices) and the sit-and-reach box. In recent years, the sit-and-reach test, which is an absolute measure of hamstring, lower back, and hip flexibility, has been used extensively in field studies.

In a comprehensive review of the literature, Clarke (1975) concluded that general range of motion increases steadily through childhood, with males starting to decline around age 10 years and females beginning to decrease at about age 12 years. This conclusion is not decisive, however, because several other reports have indicated both earlier or later initial declines. This is not surprising considering that flexibility is joint-specific, rather than a general attribute, and these studies have not measured the flexibility of the same body parts. It also has been speculated that activity levels are a better indicator of flexibility than age.

think about it

Take a position that males are as flexible as females. What proof can you provide?

When considering the best single test, the sit-and-reach task, it appears that flexibility begins to decline in the late teens with the trend continuing through adulthood. A rather consistent finding complementing this trend is that, in general, females are more flexible than males from age 5 years to adulthood. Explanations for the difference only have been speculative but include relative differences in physical activity patterns, limb length, body size, and specific body composition and hormone levels. Another suggestion is that as body surface area increases, flexibility decreases; thus, during adolescence, males would be at a disadvantage. This seems plausible, providing that the males do not participate in exercises that stimulate range of motion.

Before we begin the discussion of changes with advanced aging, which are given more attention in Chapter 11, Table 4.3 summarizes the key differences

TABLE 4.3 **Summary of Key Physiological Differences Between Children and Adults**

- Heart size is related directly to body size, so children have smaller hearts and thus lower stroke volume and cardiac output.
- Absolute aerobic capacity is lower in children; however, when expressed to reflect body size, there is little or no difference.
- Anaerobic capacity is lower in children due in large part to a lower glycolytic capacity.
- Children are more susceptible to heat stress.
- Prepubescent children can increase muscle strength with resistance training, primarily through neural recruitment. However, significant increases are difficult due to relatively low androgen levels (see Chapter 5).

Focus on Application
Is Marathon Running Okay for Children?

It is generally well accepted that running is good for the cardiorespiratory system, and it promotes fitness in children and adults. But how young and how much running is okay? Children as young as 5 years of age have run a full 26.2-mile competitive marathon. However, with the training required, which is usually time-consuming and intense, there are issues for children worthy of consideration. For example, the American Academy of Pediatrics (AAP) suggests that sporting activities should be geared to meet the developmental level of children and adolescents in regard to their physical abilities, cognitive capacities, initiative, and interest. Furthermore, the AAP warns against intense training and sports specialization in young athletes. As such, many would question the suitability of marathon training for the child. Psychological concerns include emotional burnout and feelings of failure and frustration when the demands, both physical and cognitive, exceed their internal resources. In regard to physical issues, researchers point out possible dangers related to heat stress and overuse injuries affecting the feet, legs, and hips.

In 1996, the AAP recognized that children younger than 18 years require shorter distances of triathlon competition and specific guidelines to protect them from harm in competitions and activity initially designed for adults. Should the recommendation apply to the 26.2-mile marathon? Obviously, placing an age limit and distance limit are difficult. They depend on the physical and mental maturity of the individual. However, given the concerns raised, most experts would agree that the marathon is not developmentally appropriate for the prepubescent and early adolescent child.

Sources:

American Academy of Pediatrics. (2000). Intensive training and sports specialization in young athletes. *Pediatrics*, *106*, 154–157.
American Academy of Pediatrics. (1996). Triathlon participation by children and adolescents. *Pediatrics*, *98*, 511–512.
Washington, R. L., Bernhardt, D. T., Gomez, J., Johnson, M. D., Martin, T. J., Rowland, T W., . . . Li, S. (2001). Organized sports for children and preadolescents. *Pediatrics*, *107*, 1459–1462.

between children and adults, as derived from Kenney et al. (2015), McArdle et al. (2015), and Rowland (2005).

CHANGES WITH ADVANCED AGING

Objective 4.10

focus on change

Change with advanced aging is highly influenced by activity level and lifelong health practices.

Physiological maturity and motor performance peak between the approximate ages of 25 and 30 years. In the age span of 30 to 70 years, most physiological functions decline at the rate of 0.75% to 1.0% per year. After age 70 years, the decline can be much steeper. The rate of decline in some functions depends to some degree on lifelong health practices, including physical activity. The difference between physiological age and chronological age may be considerable. Figure 4.12 shows hypothetical curves of physiological function of an active and sedentary person across the life span. This figure is discussed in detail in the broader context of performance peak and regression in Chapter 11. Excellent reviews of change with advanced aging are found in McArdle et al. (2015) and Taylor and Johnson (2008).

Change in Cardiorespiratory Function

Maximal oxygen uptake follows a clear trend of decline with a drop of approximately 30% between 30 and 70 years of age (see Fig. 4.3 on page 104). Sedentary persons have nearly a twofold faster rate of decline in VO_2max as they age. The closely

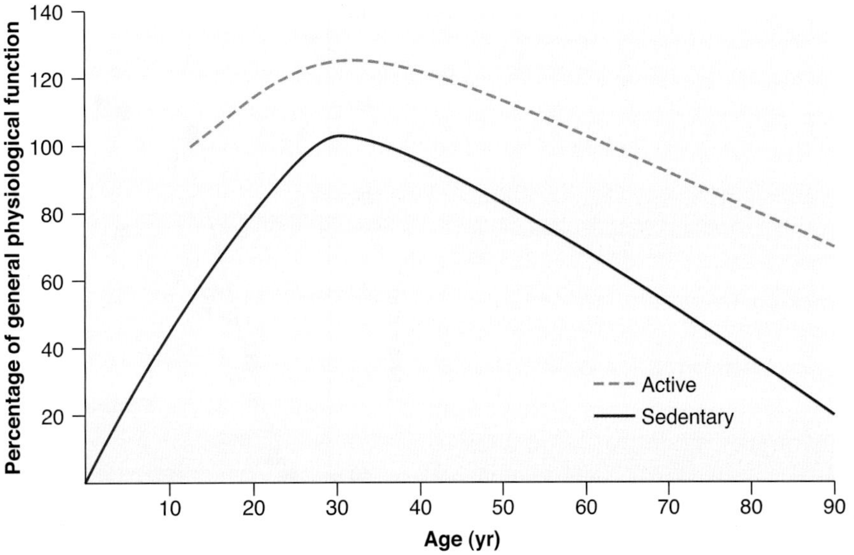

Figure 4.12 A hypothetical curve representing physiological function of an active and sedentary person over the life span.

related function of cardiac output, which consists of stroke volume and maximal heart rate, also declines about 30% over this time span. It should be noted that resting cardiac output (stroke volume and resting heart rate) is not affected markedly by age. Parallel to the loss in aerobic capacity is a slightly greater decline in anaerobic power—about 40% by age 70 years. With this is a slower clearing of blood lactate in older adults, which may partially explain age-related decrements in endurance. Although there is little change in diastolic blood pressure, systolic values may increase significantly. Aging also produces an increased resistance to blood flow due, in part, to a stiffening of the blood vessels and/or fatty deposits on the vessel walls.

Respiratory function, in general, also declines with age. The main outcome of the aging process in terms of lung function is the reduction of the amount of oxygen delivered from the outside air to the arterial blood. Along with changes in the cardiovascular and muscular systems, the effects of aging in the respiratory structures compound the limitations on the ability to perform physical work. Vital capacity may diminish up to 40%, whereas residual lung volume (the amount not expired) increases 20% to 50%. The aging process also has been associated with a decrease in the surface area available for the exchange of gas between the alveoli and capillaries, due primarily to loss of functioning alveoli and the associated capillary network. Perhaps the most significant functional change with aging is a decline in the static-elastic-recoil force of the lung and the decreased resistance of the chest wall to deformation. Under normal conditions of respiratory function, the lung recoils inward and the chest wall expands outward, in balance, at the end of expiration. As the lung expands inspiration, the elastic-recoil force (pressure) increases, thereby assisting in expiration. The loss of recoil force means that less pressure by the chest wall is needed to produce a change in lung volume. In practical terms, this change means that an older individual performs about 20% more work to overcome the elastic resistance compared to a young adult. Loss of pulmonary elasticity also is related to impaired ventilation due to the premature closing of the airways. Figure 4.13 shows pulmonary ventilation values at maximal exercise (keep in mind that ventilation refers to the volume of air breathed per minute). Note the decrease with advanced aging and the slower recovery in older untrained persons.

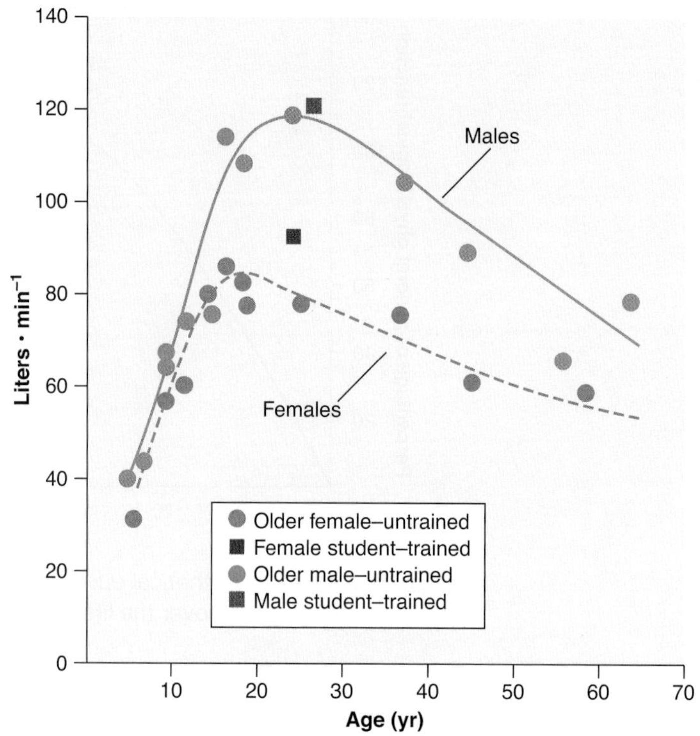

Figure 4.13 Pulmonary ventilation values at maximal exercise.

Change in Basal Metabolic Rate

Closely associated with the decline in work capacity and muscle mass is the decreased ability of the individual to function within the environment. This decline affects BMR with a decline of about 10% to 15% during adulthood (see Fig. 4.7 on page 110).

Change in Muscular Strength

With aging comes a deterioration in muscle mass of approximately 25% to 30%. Accompanying this loss are decreases in the size and number of fibers and the functioning of individual motor units. As this takes place, less contractile force is available when a motor unit is recruited for muscle contraction, and the action potential of the muscle is decreased. In addition, the number of type II muscle fibers, which are associated with strength and power, is reduced. These fast-twitch fibers are thought to atrophy because the motoneurons that activate the muscles themselves atrophy, and the muscle fibers die because of the loss of innervation. After the period of peak strength between the ages of 25 and 29 years, it is not surprising to see muscular force decrease by about 25% to 30% with aging, thus matching the loss in muscle mass. Figure 4.14 depicts longitudinal data for strength and power for men ages 20 to 80 years. Power in this case represents the speed at which force is exerted during cycling. These data show that over time, power declines to a greater extent than strength does (Metter et al., 1997).

Change in Flexibility

Flexibility generally declines across adulthood, but after about age 50 years, the trend appears more significant. In specific areas, such as the lower back (extension),

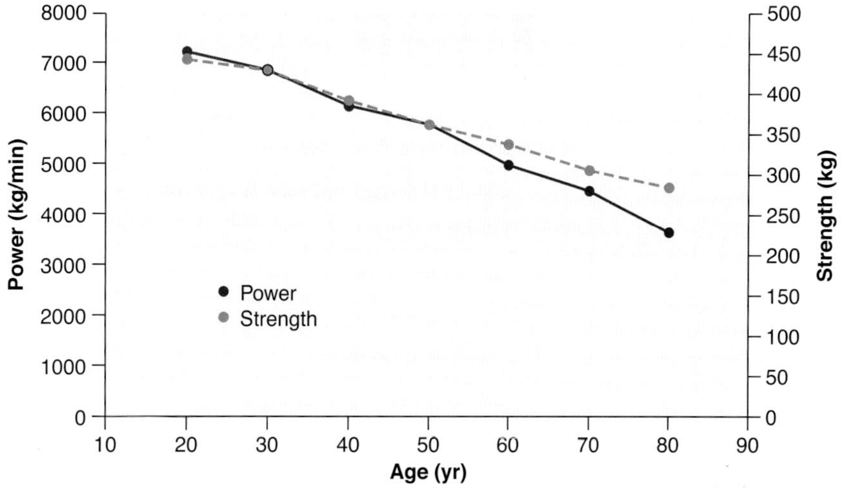

Figure 4.14 Longitudinal data for strength and power for males.

SOURCE: Adapted from Metter, E. J., Conwit, R., Tobin, J., & Fozard, J. L. (1997). Age-associated loss of power and strength in the upper extremities in women and men. *The Journals of Gerontology Series A: Biological Sciences and Medical Sciences, 52*(5), B267–B276.

significant loss can occur much earlier; Einkauf and associates (1987) found sharp declines between 30 and 49 years (Fig. 4.15). Closely linked to decreased flexibility and range of motion with aging are changes in the joints and muscles and the presence of degenerative joint diseases. The smooth functioning of the body's joints is made possible by the strength and elasticity of the tendons and ligaments and the condition of the synovial fluid. As individuals age, their joints become less stable and their mobility diminishes as collagen fibers and synovial membranes degrade and the viscosity of synovial fluid decreases. As a result, the joints become stiff, which possibly decreases their range of motion. However, there is no conclusive evidence that biological aging inherently causes decreases in flexibility. A considerable amount of research also links loss of flexibility with degenerative joint diseases such as osteoarthritis and osteoarthrosis. Osteoarthritis affects more than 80% of individuals older than 65 years of age, and more females than males have the disease.

think about it

Considering all of the changes (regression) that occur with advanced aging, what daily living activities are more likely to be profoundly affected?

Table 4.4 summarizes changes that occur with advanced aging. This includes topics covered in the last three chapters; topics for this chapter are bolded.

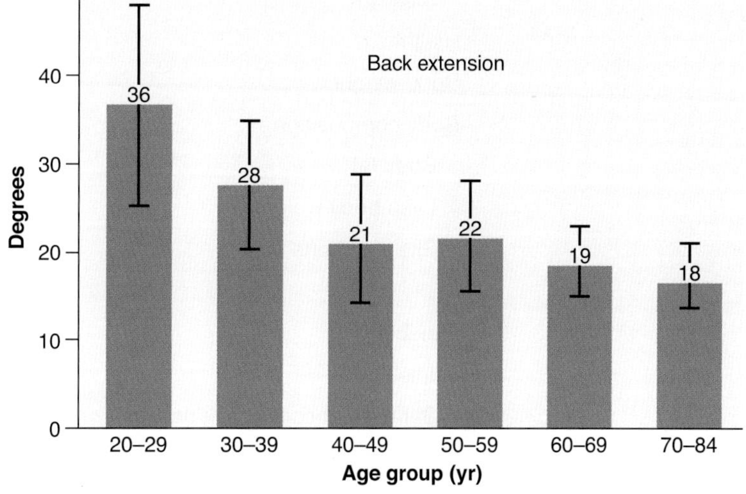

Figure 4.15 Decline in lower back flexibility (extension).

TABLE 4.4 Summary of Changes with Advanced Aging after Peak Maturity (30 Years of Age)[a]

	Decrease (↓) Increase (↑)	
Cardiorespiratory system		
Maximal oxygen uptake (VO_2max)	↓	30%
Cardiac output	↓	
Stroke volume	↓	
Heart rate (max)	↓	
Anaerobic power	↓	40%
Blood pressure (systolic)	↑	
Elasticity of blood vessels	↓	
Blood flow (resistance)	↑	
Respiratory		
General pulmonary function	↓	
Vital capacity	↓	40%
Lung residual volume	↑	20%–50%
Functioning alveoli	↓	
Ventilation	↓	
Basal metabolic rate	↓	10%–15%
Nervous system		
Brain cells	↓	
Synaptic delay	↑	
Motor unit size	↓	
Nerve conduction velocity	↓	10%–15%
Reaction time	↑	Slows
Muscle		
Mass	↓	25%–30%
Fiber number/size	↓	
Biochemical capacity	↓	
Strength	↓	25%–30%
Height	↓	
Body weight	↑	↓ after age 60 y
Body composition		
Body fat	↑	
Lean body weight	↓	
Skeletal (bone loss)	↓	female 30%
		male 10%–15%
Flexibility	↓	
Joints		
Stiffness of connective tissue	↑	
Accumulated mechanical stress	↑	

[a]Overall decline of functional capacity is 0.75%–1.0% per year.

Summary

Growth and development of the cardiorespiratory system begin with a single, noncirculating heart tube and the appearance of respiratory buds during the early stages of fetal development. From these beginnings, the system experiences tremendous growth and development prior to birth that continue across the life span.

Maximal aerobic power increases through childhood. Much of the difference between individuals can be explained by variations in body mass. Peak capacity occurs around age 25 years and declines steadily thereafter. Anaerobic power also rises steadily to early adulthood.

Resting and submaximal heart rate levels normally decrease with age; females have slightly higher levels than males have. Maximal heart rate also decreases with advancing age.

Cardiac output is the major indicator of the functional capacity of the system and a primary determinant in maximal oxygen uptake (aerobic power). In general, as heart volume increases with age, maximal cardiac output also increases. The trend is similar to that associated with maximal oxygen uptake; it increases until early adulthood and declines shortly thereafter. Vital capacity tends to increase as body size increases. As with a number of other physiological functions, the measured values of both sexes are similar until after puberty, after which the larger body size of males produces the greater absolute values found.

The production of red blood cells begins by the second week of gestation and increases, with only a slight interruption, throughout adolescence. As body weight increases, comparable increases in total blood volume take place. With this increase come higher numbers of red blood cells and higher levels of hemoglobin, which collect oxygen from the lungs and transport it to the tissues.

BMR declines continuously from birth to old age; males have slightly higher values at all ages. The gender difference is due primarily to greater levels of fat tissue in females, which is metabolically less active than lean body tissue is.

Muscular strength normally increases with age and peaks between 25 and 29 years of age. Due largely to higher levels of androgen and larger lean body mass after puberty, males are typically 30% to 50% stronger than females are in most muscle groups. Decline in strength after the peak years is closely related to the loss of muscle mass.

The literature on flexibility is perhaps the most inconclusive of all the developmental characteristics discussed. In general, range of motion increases steadily through childhood. Then, during early adolescence, it begins the continued life-span trend of decline.

After peak physiological maturity between the approximate ages of 25 and 30 years, functions begin to show a decline at the rate of 0.75% to 1.0% per year between the ages of 30 and 70 years. Although there are wide differences among individuals due to factors such as physical activity, the effects of age are evident. By age 70 years, substantial losses are observable in cardiorespiratory function, basal metabolic rate, muscle mass and muscular strength, and joint mobility (flexibility).

think about it

1. **How can health-related components of fitness be constraints to motor performance?**
2. **What does it mean by *independent existence*? And, more important, what are the medical implications?**
3. **What factors contribute to making a great sprinter and long-distance runner (biology/environment)?**
4. **What circumstances and processes count for significant metabolic activity over the first 2 years? (You may want to refer back to Chapter 2.)**
5. **Recently, there has been controversy regarding weight training by prepubescent children. What do you suppose is the issue? Furthermore, what would be safe for increasing strength?**
6. **What are the implications of weak muscles in the elderly?**
7. **Take a position that males are as flexible as females. What proof can you provide?**
8. **Considering all of the changes (regression) that occur with advanced aging, what daily living activities are more likely to be profoundly affected?**

LEARNING ACTIVITIES

Objective: To create a statement from the perspective of your chosen career (e.g., physical education teacher, physical/occupational therapist, trainer). Using the information presented in this chapter, prepare a two-page statement that could be submitted to a congressional committee in support of promoting physically active lifestyles.

Objective: To discover that health-related fitness components are constraints. Expand the *Think About It* question regarding "How can health-related components of fitness be constraints to motor performance?" Select two fitness-oriented activities and using the constraints model (Chapters 1 and 7), address individual constraints as it applies to your selected activities.

Chapter 5

Factors Affecting Growth and Development

OBJECTIVES

Upon completion of this chapter, you should be able to

5.1 List and briefly describe maternal factors that can affect prenatal development.

5.2 Identify the principles of teratogenic effects and describe associated environmental agents.

5.3 Discuss the role of nutrition on postnatal development.

5.4 Identify the possible effects of physical activity on growth, development, and motor performance after birth.

5.5 List and briefly describe the possible effects of hormones on growth and development over the life span.

KEY TERMS

teratogen
sensitive periods
fetal alcohol syndrome
low birth weight (LBW)
preterm
catch-up growth
stunted growth
obesity
female athlete triad
neural (motor) recruitment
growth hormone (GH)
thyroxine

A variety of factors and conditions may affect the normal course of human growth and development, including motor behavior. Common to the research and discussion in this field of study are the risk factors that are either suspected or have been proven to negatively affect prenatal development. This information is vital to a comprehensive understanding of the genetic and environmental influences on early development and has profound implications for physical growth and motor behavior. Other factors come into play to affect the growth and development processes after the birth process; the most important of these factors are nutrition, exercise and physical activity, and hormones.

PRENATAL DEVELOPMENT

Objective 5.1

Several factors and conditions can affect the normal development of an unborn infant. Some of these are classified as *internal (maternal) factors* because they are linked with genetic influences or the maternal conditions of the prenatal environment.

Although the fetus is well protected by the placenta, it is not impervious to the outside environment. Through this membrane, the fetus is affected by *external (environmental) factors*—by what the expectant mother eats, breathes, drinks, or smokes. Certain substances are known to penetrate the placenta and cause negative reactions in the form of physical deformities and behavioral dysfunctions. An environmental agent that can cause a birth defect or kill the fetus is called a **teratogen**. Fortunately, about 97% of all babies are born without serious defects or deficiencies; human beings have a strong tendency to develop normally under all but the most damaging conditions.

focus on change

A variety of prenatal and postnatal factors and experiences can affect *change*.

PRINCIPLES OF TERATOGENIC EFFECTS

Objective 5.2

Although the effects on the developing organism vary with the specific teratogen, several general principles appear to apply to most of them.

1. Teratogens affect prenatal development by interfering with basic biochemical processes.
2. The susceptibility of a developing organism to a teratogenic agent varies with the organism's developmental stage at the time of exposure. In general, once the different body systems have begun to form, each is most vulnerable at the time of its initial growth spurt; this is associated with a sensitive period in development.
3. Each teratogenic agent acts in a specific way on specific developing tissue, therefore causing a particular pattern of abnormal development.
4. Not all organisms are affected in the same way by exposure to a given amount of a specific teratogen. Reaction depends to some degree on the organism's and the mother's genotype and on the mother's physiological state (e.g., age, nutrition, and hormonal balance).
5. In general, the greater the concentration or longer the exposure to the teratogen, the greater the risk of abnormal development.
6. Levels of teratogens that can produce defects in the developing organism may affect the mother only mildly or not at all. For example, some diseases and drugs that have minimal effect on the mother can lead to serious abnormalities in the developing organism.
7. Some teratogens may cause temporary delays in development with no long-term negative consequences, whereas others will cause problems late (sleeper effects) in development.

As you will recall from Chapter 1, a basic assumption of this text is that there are **sensitive periods** in human development when an organism is most sensitive to certain environmental influences, such as teratogenic agents. Most experts agree that, in general, the entire prenatal period could be considered a sensitive period. However, it seems that during the embryonic period (weeks 2 to 8), when most organs and body parts are rapidly forming, the individual is most vulnerable to damage. Once an organ or body part is formed, it becomes less susceptible to harm. However, some organ systems such as the eyes and central nervous system (CNS) can be damaged throughout pregnancy.

The following material discusses selected maternal influences and environmental (teratogenic) agents. Each of the influences discussed, to some extent, have been linked to motor development.

Internal (Maternal) Factors

MATERNAL AGE

Compared to 20 years ago, women today start having children later in life, often because they spend their early adult years in education and establishing careers. The age of the expectant mother appears to have some bearing on the ease of the birth process and the general well-being of the child. Females older than 35 years and younger than 16 years of age have a higher risk of infant defect, prematurity, and low birth weight, all of which can influence postnatal physical growth and motor development. Risks to older women include difficulties in conceiving and delivering, an increased probability of having a child with Down syndrome, and low birth weight. In girls, the reproductive system may not be mature and general prenatal care may be poor. The ages between 22 and 29 years are physiologically the best time to have a baby. However, we still have much to learn about this issue; proper exercise and nutrition may help prolong the efficiency of the reproductive system.

think about it

What does research tell us about exercising while pregnant? Are there any possible effects on the fetus?

NUTRITION

The development of the fetus can be affected by the quality of the expectant mother's diet both before and during pregnancy. Because the mother is the sole source of nutrients for the fetus, an adequate diet is vital. Several studies indicate a relationship between maternal diet deficiencies and low birth weight, prematurity, brain development, skeletal growth retardation, below-normal motor and neurological development, and poor mental functioning. The first trimester is an especially vulnerable time. However, the last 3 months also may be critical because this is a time of rapid brain growth. In addition to a well-balanced diet, recommended additives commonly include iron, calcium, and folic acid.

GENETIC ABNORMALITIES

Each year in the United States, approximately 125,000 infants (approximately 3% to 5% of births) are born with a genetic abnormality. Of the many types of abnormalities, Down syndrome (DS) is one of the most common.

DS, one of the most common genetic abnormalities, is caused by the presence of an extra chromosome in the 21st pair of chromosomes; thus, the zygote has 47 chromosomes instead of the normal 46 chromosomes. Individuals who have this condition generally have retarded mental and motor development, heart defects, short hands and feet, and distinctively abnormal facial features. This condition is not inherited. The risk that a woman will bear a child with DS increases markedly with the expectant mother's age, especially after the age of 35 years. DS appears approximately once in every 400 live births at age 35 years and 1 in 100 at age 40 years. This topic is discussed in more detail in Chapter 12 (Atypical Motor Behavior).

MATERNAL STRESS

Today, we know that an expectant mother's stress can be transmitted to the fetus. Due to psychological experiences, such as intense fear, natural disaster, and prolonged anxiety and depression, physiological changes can occur that may affect the developing fetus. For example, stress can produce hormonal changes, such as higher levels of adrenaline that restrict blood flow to the uterine area and possibly deprive the fetus of the normal flow of oxygen. Supporting a possible negative outcome of this event, several studies indicate that stress during pregnancy was a determinant of delay in motor development (Cao et al., 2014; King et al., 2012). However, it should be noted that moderate stress during gestation might not be bad. For example, DiPietro et al. (2006), in a follow-up study of one hundred 2-year-olds whose mothers reported some stress midway through pregnancy, found that the children scored higher on selected measures of motor development. Apparently, moderate stress stimulates blood flow, which in turn may stimulate neural development of the fetus.

think about it

Consider how maternal factors affect postnatal motor development.

External (Environmental) Factors

As noted earlier, although the fetus appears safe in its protective membrane, it is not impervious to the external environment. Although the placenta does a good job of filtering many contaminants, the fetus still can be affected by disease-producing bacteria and by what the expectant mother eats, breathes, drinks, smokes, or injects (teratogenic agents).

INFECTION AND DISEASE

Fortunately, several potentially dangerous infections have been minimized through preventive drugs (e.g., rubella [German measles]). However, other viral influences and diseases still can be a danger to the developing fetus, including cytomegalovirus disease, diabetes, and toxoplasmosis.

No infections are more common, and few are more hazardous than sexually transmitted diseases. *Syphilis* is a potentially dangerous disease that if undetected in an expectant mother can attack the nervous system of the fetus and thus produce complications. The disease has been linked to miscarriages, stillbirth, deafness, blindness, and congenital mental dysfunctions. The signs of damage from syphilis may not appear until the child is several years old. Another sexually transmitted disease that can harm the fetus in a manner similar to syphilis is *genital herpes*.

A condition receiving attention today is *HIV* and its potential outcome is *AIDS*. More and more children are born infected as a result of the mother's condition. In addition to causing death in some cases during the first few years of life, in others, there may be significant motor delays (Chase et al., 2000). Blanchette and colleagues (2001) reported significant motor delays and computed tomography scan abnormalities, particularly for motor control structures.

DRUGS AND CHEMICAL SUBSTANCES

This section addresses the potential effects of tobacco, alcohol, and drugs on the developing fetus. Included in the drug category are over-the-counter remedies, prescribed medicines, and illegal substances.

Smoking. Prenatal smoking is one of the most preventable causes of low birth weight and fetal growth retardation. The nicotine from tobacco has the same effects on the fetus as it does on the mother. But because the same amount of the drug is available to a much smaller body area, the effects of the drug on the fetus are much greater. The carbon monoxide produced while smoking is known to interfere with the oxygen-carrying capabilities of the hemoglobin and, therefore, to increase the risk of hypoxia, or oxygen deprivation. Cigarette smoking also has been associated with malformation of the heart, lungs, and other organs; low birth weight; and deficits in long-term physical growth (Fenercioglu et al., 2009; Wang & Pinkerton, 2008). Although not associated with the prenatal period, persistent smoking is also linked to reduced growth (weight) and body mass index (BMI) in adolescent females (Stice & Martinez, 2005).

Alcohol. Alcohol can have serious direct effects on fetal and neonatal development because the substance can cross the placenta. Because the fetus's liver is immature, the alcohol remains in its system for a long time. The fetus can be very sensitive to alcohol, and even in small amounts, alcohol has been shown to cause abnormalities in development. During the last trimester of pregnancy when brain development is rapid, alcohol may be extremely harmful.

Fetal alcohol syndrome (FAS) is a condition suffered by some infants exposed to alcohol during the prenatal period. The syndrome was first identified among infants born to pregnant women who drank heavily. Infants with this condition do not go through the normal catch-up period of growth after birth, and they exhibit signs of mental retardation and immature motor development. Other commonly found characteristics are low birth weight; facial, limb, and organ defects; and repetitive body motions associated with autistic behavior.

Unfortunately, the long-term outlook for children with FAS is not positive. Research indicates that these children will likely experience reductions in physical growth that persist through young adulthood (Carter et al., 2013). In addition, there are consistent findings that prenatal exposure has a negative effect on later motor skills, especially those involving fine motor tasks (see review by Doney et al., 2014). Barr and Streissguth (2001), using a longitudinal design, found that 4-year-olds whose mothers had consumed moderate levels of alcohol during their pregnancies showed deficiencies in fine motor control and balance. The researchers also reported that alcohol scores from the period prior to pregnancy recognition were the highest predictors of poor motor performance. Doctors at one time thought pregnant women could drink moderately without harming the fetus. However, more recent evidence has brought this assumption under serious question with reports suggesting that there may be no safe level of intake during pregnancy.

Drugs. Many drugs can cross the placenta barrier to have a direct effect on the developing fetus. Substances included in the category of drugs are prescribed medicines such as antibiotics; over-the-counter substances such as aspirin and cold remedies; and drugs such as heroin, cocaine, amphetamines, and marijuana. Drugs strike the fetus with such force for two primary reasons. First, a small amount of a drug for an adult may be a dangerously large amount for the tiny fetus. Second, the liver enzymes necessary for breaking down drugs do not develop until after birth. Therefore, just as with alcohol, drugs remain in the body of the fetus.

With the continued illegal drug use in our society, pregnant women addicted to heroin or cocaine are giving birth to infants with symptoms of addiction. *Cocaine* use constricts the blood vessels, reduces the flow of oxygen to the fetus, and increases fetal blood pressure. The number of these cases is growing at an alarming rate in the United States. And at present, we are experiencing an increase in *marijuana* use, which for the developing fetus, may also have detrimental effects similar to smoking. However, it should be noted that other factors such as low birth weight and poor rearing environment may contribute to these negative outcomes. The full impact of the influence of drugs of any type on fetal development is still being investigated. The general consensus in the medical profession is that expectant mothers should be very cautious about taking any medication (including aspirin) that is not prescribed.

As noted earlier, by no means is this discussion exhaustive. Numerous additional environmental agents may have teratogenic effects. Other considerations include specific prescription and nonprescription drugs and chemicals commonly found in paints, dyes, solvents, oven cleaners, pesticides, food additives, and cosmetic products. Table 5.1 presents a summary of effects of selected widely used drugs (based on a review by Ross et al., 2015).

think about it

Advances in science are telling us more and more about what affects prenatal development. Are you suspicious of any other (than the already described) agents that might affect prenatal development? Explain.

TABLE 5.1 Effects of Selected Widely Used Drugs

Cannabis (Marijuana)	Marijuana is the most commonly abused form of "illicit" drug in the United States. Fetuses may exhibit stunted growth, shorter gestation lengths, decreased birth weights, and deficits in other growth measures. Altered responses to visual stimuli and increased startles and tremors have been noted in newborns exposed to marijuana.
Methamphetamine	The most common effects in newborns: growth restriction, decreased weight, length, and head circumference. Effect in later life is weak fine motor function.
Amphetamine	Also known as *speed*. With use, there are higher odds of preterm birth and LBW.
Cocaine	Affects fetal physical growth and results in an increase of premature birth and generalized postnatal growth retardation, including decreased birth weight, shorter body length, and smaller head circumference
Opioids	The probability of premature labor, rupture of membranes, intrauterine growth retardation, and intrauterine death increases greatly with illicit opiate use during pregnancy.
Methylenedioxymethamphetamine (Ecstasy)	Premature births, a significantly increased risk of congenital defects, cardiovascular anomalies, and musculoskeletal anomalies. Use predicts poorer infant mental and motor development.

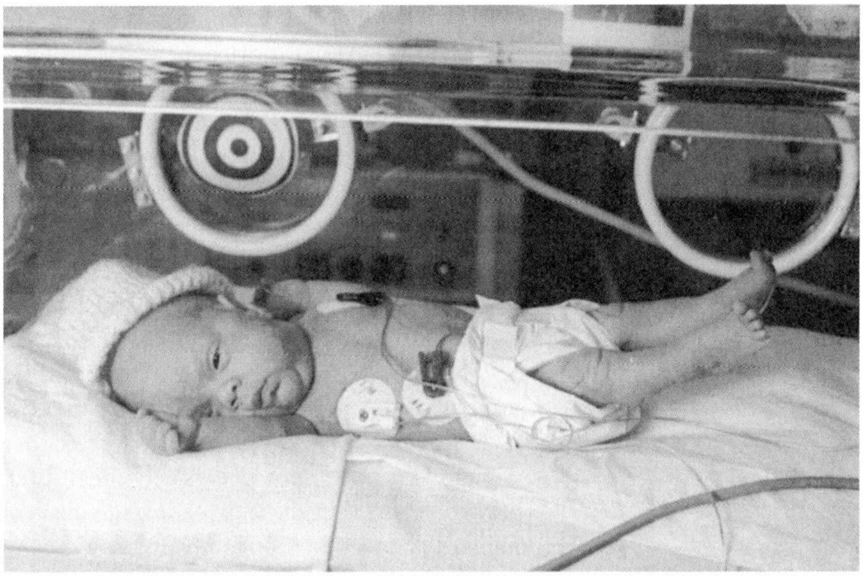

Figure 5.1 LBW and preterm birth may seriously affect later physical growth and motor development.

LOW BIRTH WEIGHT

A rather common symptom found among the prenatal influences described is **low birth weight (LBW)**, shown in Figure 5.1. LBW infants are born after a regular gestational period of 38 to 42 weeks, but they weigh less than 5.5 pounds (2,500 g). This condition is the chief contributor to infant illness and mortality and has implications for motor development. Closely associated with LBW are deficits in physical growth and motor behavior due in large part to impaired neurological and skeletal development. Babies born prematurely (**preterm**)—prior to 38 weeks after conception—often are of LBW and are high-risk as well. Influences mentioned that typically result in LBW and physical growth and motor deficits include mother's diet (nutrition), smoking, alcohol, and cocaine use. For example, pregnant smokers deliver infants who, on average, are 200 grams lighter than those of nonsmokers. Smoking is associated with a twofold increase in risk of LBW making it the single greatest contributor at approximately 25%. As a general observation, more LBW infants are born to a parent(s) of low socioeconomic status. This suggests that parent education—especially for the mothers—and prenatal care are important factors in preventing LBW.

WebLink
http://www.marchofdimes.org/

The spectrum of impairments associated with LBW/preterm includes a broad range of neuropsychological and cognitive outcomes, including motor behavior (e.g., Datar & Jacknowitz, 2009; de Jong et al., 2015). These infants are at risk for motor dysfunction and delay. For example, Wocadlo and Rieger (2008) reported that at age 8 years, one-third of their preterm sample (100/300) were identified as having developmental coordination disorder (see Chapter 12 for a description of this condition). One of the most frequently cited deficits is poor fine and visual motor integration (e.g., review by Gabbard et al., 2001). In addition to the direct perceptual-motor development concern, the literature provides a reasonable case that such deficits place this population at increased risk for poor academic performance and difficulties with specific daily living (self-help) activities.

Typically, infants and children born with very LBW (1,500 g) and extreme LBW (1,000 g) exhibit more deficits than the LBW group. For example, Husby and colleagues (2013) reported that motor skills at age 23 years differed between those born within normal levels and those born preterm/very LBW. Similar findings were reported by Poole et al. (2016) after tracking individuals from childhood to age 36 years. That is, those born extreme LBW had more difficulties than controls.

CATCH-UP GROWTH

As noted earlier, due to such factors as LBW and poor prenatal and postnatal care, some infants and young children experience lower than expected physical growth rates. However, some of those children will also experience catch-up growth. **Catch-up growth** is characterized by (for example) height and weight velocity above the limits of what would be expected for typically developing children for their age. This does not necessarily mean that those children would catch-up to what would have been their expected full growth, although some may. It is not possible to know whether catch-up growth is complete for an individual child, but if final height is within the target range, it can be considered that catch-up growth has probably been complete. With older children, catch-up growth is difficult to distinguish from the pubertal growth spurt. Interventions such as growth hormone therapy are sometimes used to help the child catch up. Studies indicate that growth hormone therapy can have a significant effect on growth of children of LBW. See "Focus on Application: Growth Hormone Therapy for Children" on Chapter 3.

NUTRITION AND PHYSICAL ACTIVITY DURING POSTNATAL DEVELOPMENT

Objective 5.3

The intake of essential nutrients and physical activity play influential and complementary roles in postnatal growth and health-related physical fitness across the life span. Children whose diets are unbalanced or are lacking in proper nourishment generally show below-average physical growth by age 3 years. Although diets lacking in protein and calories are by far the most common cause of growth failure during infancy and childhood, this problem is relatively rare in the United States and among other economically developed countries. We all know by now that the American diet consists of too much fat, refined sugar, and salt as evidenced by the high incidence of childhood obesity and by the link that has been established between diet and cardiovascular disease in adults. According to the latest statistics from the Centers for Disease Control and Prevention (CDC) (2016), overweight and obesity continues to be an important and disappointing health issue. About 69% of adults and one-third of children are overweight or obese. It has been estimated that physical inactivity and poor diet cause at least 300,000 deaths a year; only tobacco use causes more preventable deaths. Weight-related diseases (often associated with physical inactivity) cost the U.S. economy more than $150 billion every year. A sedentary lifestyle almost doubles one's risk for coronary heart disease, a condition that can begin to develop in childhood. Overall, the percentage of obesity in children has tripled in the last 30 years. A significant portion of overweight children grow up to be overweight adults.

WebLink

http://www.cdc.gov/; see Physical Activity/Obesity/National Youth Fitness Survey (2012).

think about it

What do you think is the greatest problem with children's health: lack of exercise or poor diet?

Type 2 diabetes, strongly linked to obesity in adults, was virtually unheard of in children during the 1990s. At that time, it accounted for less than 3% of all cases of new-onset diabetes in children and adolescents. The latest figures indicate that about 40% are obese and 80% are overweight (National Diabetes Education Program [National Institute of Diabetes and Digestive and Kidney Diseases, 2016]).

Focus on Application

Exercise Helps Teens Overcome "Obesity Gene"

Several people simply acknowledge that my whole family is overweight so I must possess the obese gene which makes it hopeless for me. The fact is, it might make it harder for you; however, research indicates as we have learned in this course that the environment plays a predominant role. Research indicates that physical activity, an hour a day, can negate the gene's effect. The study examined 752 male and female teenagers—some had no obese genes, others had one copy, and others two copies. Copies of the mutation were linked with higher BMI, higher percentage of body fat, and a larger waist. The take-home message (application) is "Be active. Try to do at least 60 minutes of moderate and vigorous physical activity every day—like playing sports."

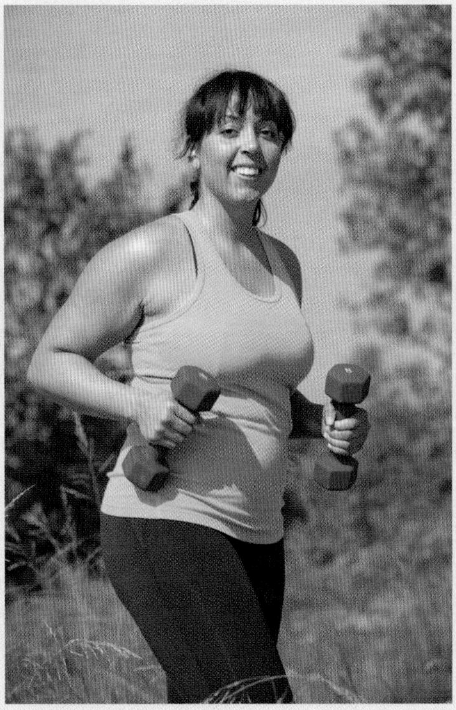

Source:

Ruiz, J. R., Labayen, I., Ortega, F. B., Legry, V., Moreno, L. A., Dallongeville, J., . . . Meirhaeghe, A. (2010). Attenuation of the effect of the *FTO* rs9939609 polymorphism on total and central body fat by physical activity in adolescents: The HELENA study. *Archives of Pediatrics & Adolescent Medicine*, *164*(4), 328–333.

A low physical activity level is characteristic of overweight/obese children and adults. Both groups watch too much electronic devices and are not physically active. Participation in all types of physical activity declines dramatically after age 11 years. Evidence of this is the observation that *only about 25% of youth (12 to 15 years) engage in the recommended number of minutes per day of moderate-vigorous physical activity, and 50% of adults are not physically active enough to reap any significant health benefits.* According to findings of the National Youth Fitness Study (National Center for Health Statistics, 2012), cardiorespiratory *fitness level decreased as body weight increased.* More on this topic is discussed in Chapter 10.

Nutrition and Development

Diet is perhaps the most potent environmental influence on growth and development. Regardless of age, individuals must have proper food for growth and for maintenance and repair of body tissues. Exciting research conducted over the last 15 years has revealed that the nutritional practices of infants and children also may have a marked influence on their health as adults. Because no standard for optimal growth has ever been defined and because individuals have varying nutritional needs based on differences in energy expenditure and bodily functions, it is difficult to determine what would compose the ideal diet for optimal growth. The following discussion focuses on information and research highlights regarding undernutrition, overnutrition, and breastfeeding.

UNDERNUTRITION

Undernutrition is the single most important cause of growth retardation worldwide. This is typically due to an inadequate intake of energy because of a lack of sufficient calories or quality protein; this is referred to as *malnutrition*. Although this condition is less common in the United States, forms of malnutrition exist due to deficiencies of vitamins, minerals, essential fatty acids and amino acids, and trace elements. A basic symptom of malnutrition is **stunted growth**. This condition results in below-average height, weight, bone mass, and brain development.

An inadequate intake of nutrients during prenatal development (especially during the last trimester) and in the early stages of life after birth can significantly affect brain weight, brain size, number of cells formed, and amount of myelin developed in the brain, which possibly results in impaired mental and motor behavior. Adequate nutritional intake is critical to sexual maturation and the development of bone and muscle tissue during the pubertal growth spurt. Potential consequences of an inadequate diet are smaller body mass and delayed menarche. To illustrate, in a longitudinal study of a large-scale, government-sponsored nutrition program in rural communities of Mexico, infants on the nutrition program showed better growth rates than a control group (Rivera et al., 2004). Data compiled by Malina et al. (2004) illustrate the growth difference. Figure 5.2 shows mean heights and weights of well-nourished and undernourished Mexican schoolchildren ages 5 to 17 years. Briefly, undernourished children are, on average, smaller, and their adolescent growth spurt is delayed by more than 1 year, compared to their well-nourished counterparts.

What is considered underweight? One marker is a BMI of 18.5 or 5th percentile on growth charts (refer to Chapter 3 for the discussion of BMI). Although obesity appears to be the focus of public health today, the problem of underweight is significant. According to the CDC figures for 2011 to 2012, an estimated 3.5% of children and adolescents were underweight. One concern in the sports community and society in general is the prevalence of eating disorders in females. Obviously, this problem extends to nonathletes (male and female) and older persons.

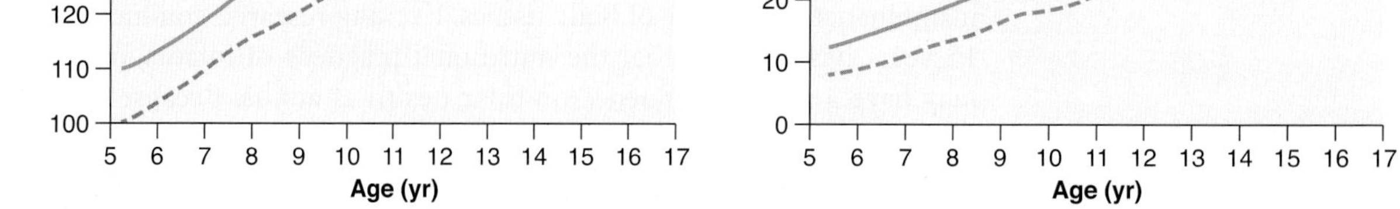

Figure 5.2 Mean heights and weights of well-nourished and undernourished Mexican schoolchildren.

SOURCE: Adapted from Malina, R. M., Bouchard, C., & Bar-Or, O. (2004). *Growth, maturation, and physical activity* (2nd ed.). Champaign, IL: Human Kinetics.

OVERNUTRITION

Overnutrition is consuming too much or the wrong kinds of food. Common outcomes are conditions of overweight and obesity—conditions aggravated by too little physical activity. A common standard for being overweight is a BMI of 25.0 to 29.9. **Obesity**, a condition of great concern in regard to public health, is defined as a BMI of 30. Another method, commonly practiced with children, is to use above the 95th percentile of U.S. growth charts.

Although heredity does play a role (25% to 40%), the environment has a significant influence on outcome, as reflected in eating and activity habits. Obese children and adolescents are more likely to become obese adults. This result may be a combination of heredity and lifestyle of the parents. Several studies show that the U.S. population of all ages eats too much fat, sugar, and low-nutrient food. Add to this the low physical activity levels of a large portion of the adolescent and adult populations (as noted in the previous section), and the outcome should not be too surprising. Part of the low physical activity levels is the increasing amount of time children and adolescents spend on the computer, mobile electronic devices, and watching TV. Studies report increases in body fat with increased electronic watching. Research also indicates that more viewing is related to smaller gains in bone mass (e.g., see review by Katzmarzyk et al., 2015; Okely & Janssen, 2015).

BREASTFEEDING

WebLink
http://www.cdc.gov/; see Breastfeeding.

For over a century, physicians have been preaching the medical benefits of breastfeeding. Today, the federal government (U.S. Department of Health and Human Services) and major health organizations (American Academy of Pediatrics [AAP] 2016, CDC, World Health Organization) support that claim with evidence-based initiatives. Breast milk contains valuable antibodies from the mother that may help the baby resist infections. According to CDC (2016), the beneficial effects of breastfeeding children include several medical conditions; for example, lower risk for ear and respiratory infections, gastroenteritis, type 2 diabetes, and sudden infant death syndrome. There are also several medical benefits to the mother.

The benefits of breastfeeding are also extended to physical growth and motor development. According to the same CDC (2016) report, there is a significantly reduced risk for overweight among children who were breastfed. Furthermore, studies indicate that children exclusively breastfed are less likely to have delays in motor development. Studies indicate better performance years later, compared to nonbreastfed controls, in motor planning, visual-motor performance, fine and gross motor development (see also Jwa et al., 2014).

So, what is the mechanism driving these positive effects? Although there is much to learn, breast milk is rich in docosahexaenoic acid, which is selectively concentrated in neuronal membranes and is thought to be necessary for optimal neurodevelopment. According to other latest figures (AAP, 2016), about 50% breastfeed up to 6 months, then the value drops to 27% at 12 months, which the AAP recommends.

Physical Activity

Objective 5.4

Physical activities are, in essence, the manifestation of the body's motor capabilities. The effects of physical activity on human development and behavior may be described from several perspectives. Two that are of direct bearing on the study of lifelong motor development are (a) the effects of physical activity and exercise on

focus on change

Physical activity can have a significant influence on *change* across the life span.

the structural aspects of physical growth and maturation and (b) the influence of physical activity on the physiological function of the human body.

Researchers and medical professionals generally agree that a minimum of physical activity is necessary for optimal biological growth and development. However, very little scientific information has been published on the subject, especially with respect to the long-term influence of habitual physical activity on human development. Much of the available information found in numerous dated physical education sources has been speculative. The difficulty in identifying the specific benefits of physical activity to growth and development from a scientific perspective lies primarily in the definition of terms. What is meant by the term *optimal growth*? And what level of activity is most beneficial to optimal growth?

Level of physical activity may be used to describe individuals as active or inactive, to identify those children who engage in play as normal, or to classify individuals who participate in regular physical training programs ranging in intensity from moderate to strenuous. Difficulty also lies in attempting to isolate physical activity in the growth process. An inherent weakness of almost any study of a topic that spans the growing years is how to explain the complex interaction of both genetic and environmental variables. In recent years, a considerable amount of information has been gathered on the specific effects of various types and intensity levels of physical activity on health-related fitness characteristics across virtually all ages. However, much work remains to be done to develop a clear understanding of how much physical activity is required to stimulate normal or optimal growth and development of other biological components.

Selected literature reviews and reports on the subject agree, in general, that a minimum of physical activity is apparently essential for specific aspects of normal growth and development to take place. One relatively clear example is that of bone mass (see the subsequent section, "Skeletal Growth and Development"). The phenomenon of accelerated maturation and the increased body size associated with secular trend over the last 100 years or so have given little mention to the possible contributions of exercise or physical activity. Instead, explanations speak more to better nutrition, improved health care and health status, and contributing genetic factors. It is probably best to view secular trend as an interactive result of several genetic and environmental factors, including the possible influence of physical activity.

The following discussion concerning the effects of physical activity on biological growth and development was derived from comprehensive reviews reported by Broekhoff (1986); Malina et al. (2004); Zauner et al. (1989) and more recent studies. In the context of this discussion, the term *physical activity* refers to practices that are *habitual* or additional to normal movement or irregular patterns of play and recreation. Included in this definition are regular physical training programs such as physical education in schools, swimming, running, youth sports, calisthenics or aerobics, and weight training. Although the topic of this section focuses on habitual physical activity, obviously extreme (intense) training could result in different outcomes; this is discussed further toward the end of this section and in Chapter 10.

STATURE

The vast majority of evidence based on studies using equivalent control groups of preadolescent and adolescent children indicates that regular physical activity has no apparent effect on stature. Although some earlier studies suggested that stature increases with physical activity, reviewers of that research have pointed out that the differences were usually quite small and the experimental procedures questionable. In some studies reporting increased growth in stature due to athletic training, the apparent increase was probably not as much the product of intensity of training as it was early maturity. One study of female swimmers found they were taller than the average in the years prior to the research; apparently, they had entered puberty earlier than the reference group with which they were compared. The same problem may have been prevalent among studies comparing young athletes with normal reference data. Note that the evidence does not indicate that training actually *promotes* significant growth in stature. It is clear, however, that the training has no *negative* effect on this aspect of physical growth.

BODY MASS

Although body composition changes considerably during normal growth, particularly during adolescence, it can be further modified by habitual physical activity. Regular physical activity is, in fact, an important factor in the regulation and maintenance of desirable body weight. Optimal change, however, occurs when diet also is controlled. Even during the growing years in which an increase in body weight is characteristic, and across the life span as well, individuals who engage in regular training programs tend to have more lean body mass and less body fat than their nontraining peers. Ample evidence exists to verify that carefully designed physical activity programs can be effective in reducing the percentage of body fat in children and adults. The magnitude of change, however, may vary considerably depending on the intensity and duration of the program. Changes in body composition are highly dependent on continued activity.

In one of the few longitudinal studies conducted with young children from 4 to 11 years of age, Moore et al. (2003) found that children in the top one-third of activity level had consistently smaller gains in BMI and sum of skinfold tests throughout childhood. Their conclusion underscores the notion that higher levels of physical activity during childhood lead to less body fat by the time of early adolescence. Evidence also suggests that individuals who maintain a program of habitual physical activity, especially endurance training, throughout adulthood have less tendency for increasing body fat with advancing age. The available information on individuals who began training in older adulthood provides mixed results. In some cases, minimal changes occurred in body fat, body weight, or lean body mass, whereas other studies reported significant losses of body fat. Further research is needed to arrive at more definitive conclusions.

Related to the fat cell theory mentioned in Chapter 3, the results of a series of experimental studies using rats indicates that there is a critical time in early infancy in which fat cell proliferation may be enhanced by overfeeding and a high-fat diet. This results in an abnormal number of cells that remain with the body for life. Evidence suggests that increased physical activity and control of diet initiated in the early stages of development can effectively limit fat cell proliferation and reduce body fatness in later life. These results, although not decisive, have some very practical implications for infant care and weight control.

BODY PROPORTION AND PHYSIQUE

In general, little evidence suggests that physical activity at any level of intensity affects body proportions or overall body shape. Interestingly, although there have been significant increases in the secular trend of height and other dimensions over the last 100 years or so, changes have been approximately proportional. Thus, if any alternation in body proportionality occurs, it is minimal. Studies that have focused on this aspect of physical activity and growth also indicate minimal influence due to training.

In one of the more comprehensive longitudinal studies of physical activity and growth, Parizkova and Carter (1976) found that boys who engaged in various levels of physical activity, from intense to untrained, over a 7-year span from 11 to 18 years of age, showed no significant difference in the distribution of somatotype ratings among the activity groups. It also was noted that individual ratings changed considerably over the period and occurred in a random manner among the groups, which suggests that such changes cannot be attributed to physical activity. All participants changed somatotype rating at least once, and the majority changed in component dominance.

The short-term benefits of training for muscular development through weight training to increase the mesomorphic component of the somatotype have been verified with numerous studies of teenagers and adults.

SKELETAL GROWTH AND DEVELOPMENT

Evidence currently suggests that regular physical activity has no apparent effect on skeletal maturity with regard to stature; however, it does enhance bone mass (skeletal mineralization and density). Numerous studies have suggested that greater skeletal mineralization and bone density and wider, more robust bones are associated with habitual physical activity. In fact, a growing number of studies support the notion that physical activity plays an important role in bone development. Furthermore, evidence has been presented suggesting that the most beneficial time (*critical period*) for physical activity to exhibit its effect on bone development is in early puberty and adolescence (Tolonen et al., 2015; Wang et al., 2005). It should be noted that studies of this nature typically compare active versus less active participants rather than athletes who have a training history.

Although several of the studies have been conducted with animals, observations on adult humans have indicated similar results. In general, the effects of prolonged activity provide localized results that are activity-related. For example, studies involving athletes have indicated that the more actively preferred limb of, for example, a tennis player, pitcher, or soccer player will exhibit greater mineralization and density than the nonpreferred limb. Studies that have observed bone density changes in runners relative to nonrunners also suggest greater values as a result of training. Similar findings have been reported on premenarcheal gymnasts and dancers compared to control groups (Bennell et al., 2000; Nickols-Richardson et al., 2000). The researchers suggested the results were due to the high-impact loading nature of the activities. As noted earlier, it has been suggested that these effects are related to regular physical training over several years' time.

think about it

What activities (not specific exercises) would you recommend for stimulating bone health, and why?

In regard to a training effect, theoretically, the pressure effects of physical activity can either stimulate growth or, in excessive amounts, retard linear growth. The difficulty lies in identifying and defining what is perceived as required, optimal, and excessive pressure. A theoretical notion known as *Wolff's law* may have implications for bone growth in general. The law simply states that bone structures will adapt to suit the stresses and strains placed on them. Obviously, more research and information are needed relative to the effects of varying levels of physical activity on growth plate genesis.

One of the more practical questions these data cannot answer clearly is whether active children have any skeletal advantages over relatively inactive children in later years. At this time, it appears that a lot more is known about the effect of physical inactivity on bone structure changes than about the effects of varying levels of physical activity.

In regard to adults (male and female), studies indicated that increased physical activity of a moderate level is associated with short- and long-term reduction in bone loss (Nilsson et al., 2012; Svejme et al., 2014).

SEXUAL MATURATION

As noted in Chapter 3, individuals today mature earlier than people did 100 years ago. The secular trend for onset of menarche has decreased approximately 4 months per decade since 1850. There is no evidence that this trend is linked to changes in physical activity patterns, or has there been any documentation in recent years that supports the theory that habitual physical activity has a positive influence on sexual maturation of the reproductive system. There have been indications that high-intensity physical training and athletic competition may be factors in delayed menarche, however. A consistent body of evidence indicates that selected athletes (e.g., gymnasts, long-distance runners, ballet dancers, and figure skaters), on the average, experience menarche later than the general population (Carlson, 2015; Czajkowska et al., 2015). Observations also indicate that the number of years of training as well as the level of competition, prior to maturation, are linked to delayed menarche. It should be noted that most of the data on this subject are limited, associative, and speculative and do not control for other factors that may have influenced the onset of menarche. It is generally agreed that it is difficult, at best, to design a study in which individuals are randomly assigned to athletic activities and then to isolate the training factor as the primary cause for delayed menarche. However, it is reasonable to suggest that overtraining, which varies in individuals, may play an important role in altering the reproductive system (Fig. 5.3).

Of the proposed theories related to the possible influence of intense physical training on the timing of menarche, one in particular is called the *critical-weight theory* (Frisch, 1991) and has received considerable attention. The researcher proposed

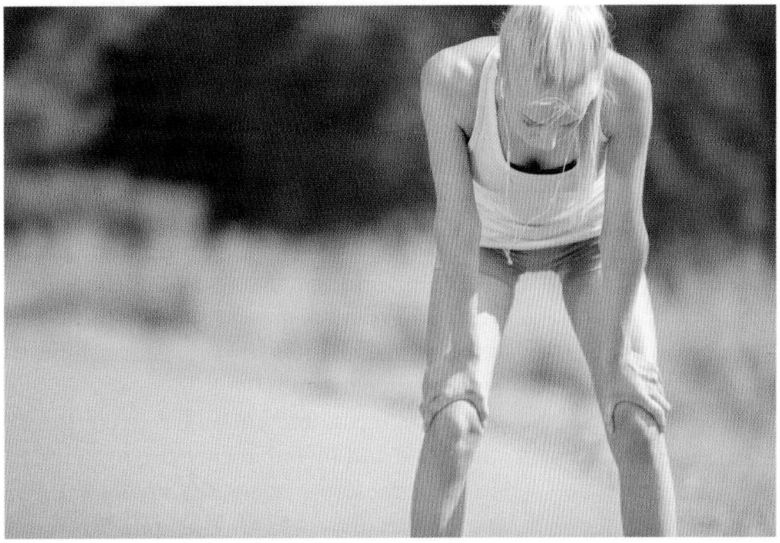

Figure 5.3 Overtraining, low body weight, and stress can interfere with the sexual maturation of some female athletes.

that a critical percentage of body fat (approximately 17%) must be reached before menarche can occur. It is also suggested that a body fat level of 22% is optimal for maintaining regular menstrual cycles. Thus, the association between female athletes who stay lean (i.e., less than 17% body fat) throughout their training and the incidence of amenorrhea (absence of menstruation) and delayed appearance of menarche provides the evidence to support this theory. The critical-weight theory has not found universal support, and the mechanisms by which intense strenuous physical training may affect the timing of menarche have not yet been clearly discerned.

There are indications that a relationship exists between the number of years of training prior to menarche and the time at which it appears. However, complementing the general idea of "critical weight" is a study reporting that most girls must weigh at least 100 pounds before experiencing their first period (Berkey et al., 2000). Studies show that delayed menarche occurs more frequently in gymnasts, figure skaters, and dancers than among other athletes. An inferred relationship can be drawn because females in these sports usually begin training early in life. Mean ages for menarche of slightly older than 15 years were found for those females who had extensive training before menarche; the average for the general population is around 12½ years.

Closely associated with the discussion of the physical growth issues in female athletes is a condition known as the **female athletic triad**. In recent years, numerous studies have addressed this condition with interest in gaining a better understanding of the potential "negative" effects of high-level athletic participation for females (Goolsby, 2014; Matzkin et al., 2015). Obviously, there is a widespread support and evidence for the positive effects of physical activity and sports participation. The female athlete triad refers to the relationship between three components: energy availability, menstrual function, and bone health. In certain sports, some named earlier (e.g., gymnastics, dance, running), one or more of the components are present. Concerns are, for example, low energy availability associated with eating disorders/lack of proper diet, menstrual dysfunction (delayed or irregularity), low and decreased bone mineral density. One or more of these conditions have been reported to persist in adulthood. Matzkin et al. (2015) estimate that as many as 50% to 60% of female athletes in certain sports will have at least one of the three components. As with most behaviors that we have discussed, causes can be multidimensional and interrelated. For example, diet, physical activity, genetics, and hormone levels can effect bone development across the life span. Most of the focus in recent years has been on prevention and understanding the long-term consequences of the female athlete triad.

MUSCULAR DEVELOPMENT AND STRENGTH

The evidence is overwhelming that specific strength training increases muscular force capabilities in adults and postpubertal children. Regular physical activity also results in some degree of skeletal muscle hypertrophy; the degree of hypertrophy varies with the intensity of training. The characteristics that generally accompany muscle hypertrophy are increases in enzymatic activity, myofibrils, contractile substances, and muscular strength. Muscles are strengthened by increasing their size and by enhancing the recruitment and firing rates of their motor units. Both of these processes are involved in the body's response to resistive physical activity, or exercise.

It appears that older males, prepubescent children, and females increase muscular strength primarily by **neural (motor) recruitment** (with some hypertrophy), whereas young males rely more on increases in muscle size. Neural recruitment refers to the recruitment of additional motor units to generate forces. An ongoing debate in exercise physiology is whether resistance training induces the muscle to both increase the number of muscle cells (hyperplasia) and increase the cells in size (hypertrophy). For a long time, the consensus was that muscles increased in size only after the hyperplasia period that ends shortly after birth. However, some recent, although controversial, evidence suggests that as a result of resistance training, muscle fibers may split as a means of increasing cell numbers. Even with this new hypothesis, it is generally agreed that the primary response to overload stress is muscle hypertrophy. Because the effects of intense (resistance) physical training on muscular development and increases in strength in postpubertal teenagers and young adults are well known, the remainder of this discussion focuses on the young and old.

We learned in Chapter 3 that adult men have approximately 10 times the androgens of children and adult women and that the bulk of this amount is produced during the adolescent growth spurt. At this time, the greatest changes in male strength seem to appear, and evidence strongly suggests that improvements in muscle force are related to greater testosterone levels. Often asked is whether prepubescent children can make significant gains in strength with training. Several studies confirm that prepubescent children are capable of making significant gains in strength, although they possess relatively low hormone levels.

Evidently, circulating androgens may not be the only primary influencing mechanism for strength development in this case. It is well documented that women, who also have low androgen levels, can make significant gains in strength without appreciable muscle hypertrophy. It appears that increases in strength in prepubescent children are probably the result of neural adaptions; that is, number of motor units recruited and their level of synchronization. It is also suggested that the risk of short-term musculoskeletal damage is minimal if training is supervised; the use of hydraulic machines reduces the risk even more. However, more research is needed with regard to the effects of resistance training on articular cartilage.

With regard to the effects of regular participation in sports, children and adolescents involved in youth sports on a regular basis typically are stronger than those individuals who do not participate. Although this result may be an indication of the strength-promoting benefit of sports, it also could be due to a weak comparison between groups because young athletes often mature early and thus are bigger for their age. It is reasonable to assume that any benefits to strength development depend primarily on the specific physical activities associated with a particular sport.

With regard to older individuals, it appears they are not able to improve their strength capacity to the same extent as young people are able to do; however, significant improvement from regular vigorous training can be expected regardless of age. Older persons who stay physically active generally are stronger than sedentary individuals. The reasons for the decrease in trainability with age are not well understood, but it has been speculated that they are due, in part, to the general decline in neuromuscular functions. As with prepubescent children, studies of older individuals indicate their strength increases not primarily by muscle hypertrophy but by increased neural stimulation, or motor unit recruitment. As discussed in Chapter 4, a general decrease of strength with age is expected because individuals generally experience a loss of muscle mass followed by a loss of motor unit fibers. A review of several studies suggests that significant gains in muscular strength can be achieved with vigorous training, at least into the ninth decade of life (McArdle et al., 2015).

Focus on Application
Strength Training for Children and Adolescents

Contrary to the traditional belief that strength training is dangerous for children, new views are that it can be a safe and effective activity, provided that the program is properly designed and competently supervised. However, strength training should not be confused with competitive weight training and powerlifting. Strength training should be one part of a well-rounded fitness program that also includes endurance, flexibility, and agility exercises. The following recommendations were written by a committee of experts convened by the American Academy of Pediatrics in 2008 (McCambridge & Stricker, 2008).

A medical evaluation should be given before commencing a formal strength-training program. Risks involved with the use of anabolic steroids and other body-building supplements are appropriate topics for discussion with any adolescent interested in getting bigger and stronger.

Young people who want to improve sports performance will generally benefit more from practicing and perfecting skills of the sport than from resistance training. If long-term health benefits are the goal, strength training should be combined with an aerobic training program.

Preadolescents and adolescents should avoid competitive weight training, powerlifting, body building, and maximal lifts until they have reached physical and skeletal maturity. Aerobic conditioning should be coupled with resistance training if general health benefits are the goal. Strength-training programs should include a warm-up and cool-down component.

Specific strength-training exercises should be learned initially with no load (resistance). Once the exercise skill has been mastered, incremental loads can be added. Progressive resistance exercise requires successful completion of 8 to 15 repetitions in good form before increasing weight or resistance. Exercises should include all muscle groups and be performed through the full range of motion at each joint. To achieve gains in strength, workouts need to be at least 20 to 30 minutes long, take place a minimum of two to three times per week, and continue to add weight or repetitions as strength improves. There is no additional benefit to strength training more than four times per week.

Any sign of injury or illness from strength training should be evaluated before continuing the exercise in question.

Source:
McCambridge, T. M., & Stricker, P. R. (2008). Strength training by children and adolescents. *Pediatrics*, *121*(4), 835–840.

CARDIORESPIRATORY DEVELOPMENT

think about it

This discussion noted the effects of normal habitual physical activity on development. What is your reaction to Olympic-style programs (e.g., 3 to 5 hours daily of swimming and gymnastics) for children?

There is little question today that regular vigorous physical activity produces physiological improvements regardless of age. However, just as in the case of muscular development, the magnitude of the potential improvement depends on several factors, including initial fitness level, type of training, and age. With regard to age, the situation is again similar to that describing the effects of training (physical activity) on strength development. Older teenagers and adults who engage in vigorous aerobic activity for 20 minutes or longer at least three times per week are likely to experience physiological changes that include an increase in heart volume and cardiac output, a lower resting heart rate, and a faster return to resting heart rate.

In Chapter 4, it was noted that the aging process can decrease general cardiovascular function by approximately 1% per year between the ages of 30 and 70 years. Along with the general decline in cardiorespiratory function as an individual ages, there also appears to be decreased trainability; that is, older individuals are not able to improve to the same extent as young people do.

Longitudinal studies of active men aged 25 to 70 years, indicate that physical training may delay the decline in maximal oxygen uptake (Jackson et al., 1995;

Kasch et al., 1990). Instead of the typical decline of 1% per year over the 20-year span, aerobically active men declined an average of only 12% over that time. As noted earlier, sedentary individuals typically have nearly a twofold faster rate of decline in VO_2max as they age, compared to aerobically active persons.

SKILL-RELATED FITNESS

The contention that regular instruction and practice of motor skills result in improved balance, coordination, speed, power, agility, and other skill-related fitness components is well documented. Such findings explain why regular participation in physical education programs is emphasized.

In addition to the issue of the extent to which habitual physical activity enhances growth and development is the concern over how competitive sports adversely affect prepubertal growth. Obviously, too much (intense) training in any sport could produce adverse effects. Psychological and physical stress and fatigue are not uncommon among young competitive athletes. And, as pointed out in the discussion of delayed menarche (sexual maturation), considerable individual differences exist within and between sports. With this in mind, Damsgaard and colleagues (2000) studied groups of competitive athletes from ages 9 to 13 years who represented swimming, tennis, team handball, and gymnastics. In addition to considering hours of training, the researchers considered genetic factors, birth weight, and early growth patterns. These factors were compared with the athletes' height, weight, pubertal development, and BMI. The overall conclusion was that prepubertal growth is not adversely affected by sport at a competitive level. However, it should be noted that most of the athletes studied trained less than 18 hours per week. Among top-level young performers in such sports as gymnastics and swimming, more than 20 to 30 hours per week, year-round, of training is not unusual. Some might consider this intense training. Daly et al. (2002) reviewed several studies of young high-level athletes and concluded that adolescents may be at risk of restricted growth and delayed maturation when intense training is combined with insufficient energy intake. One of the most evident findings, as noted in the sexual maturation section, was delayed menarche. The authors also reported that catch-up growth commonly occurs when training is reduced or ceased, suggesting that final adult outcome is unlikely to be compromised. However, the researchers were also quick to point out that, depending on the intensity, duration, and individual, adverse effects could be prolonged. As noted in the introduction, the inherent problem with studying this issue is the difficulty in discerning normal growth patterns from level of exercise or other factors that might influence growth (nutrition, genetics, and individual constitution [e.g., training tolerance]).

What are the recommended levels of physical activity? The CDC provides up-to-date recommendations for four groups: children 6 to 17 years, adults 18 to 64 years, older adults 65 years and older, and pregnant or postpartum women. In summary, children and adolescents need at least 60 minutes daily of aerobic, muscle strengthening, and bone strengthening activities. For adults, there are options with one being 2 hours and 30 minutes (150 minutes) of moderate-intensity aerobic activity per week and muscle-strengthening activities on 2 or more days per week. Recommendations are similar for older adults. The recommendation for healthy pregnant or postpartum women is at least 2 hours and 30 minutes (150 minutes) per week of moderate-intensity aerobic activity, such as brisk walking, during and after their pregnancy. For more specifics, see WebLink.

WebLink

http://www.cdc.gov/; see Physical Activity Recommendations.

GLANDS AND HORMONAL ACTIVITY

Objective 5.5

Hormonal activity has been discussed in terms of its relevance to the adolescent growth spurt. Although it is beyond the scope of this text to detail the endocrine system, a brief review of hormonal activity as it relates to more general growth and development across the life span is appropriate.

Remember from Chapter 3 (in reference to the adolescent growth spurt) that the endocrine system consists of several different glands that secrete hormones directly into the bloodstream. The endocrine glands regulate such vital functions as skeletal and muscle growth, sexual reproduction, metabolism, and the aging of cellular tissues. As with most physiological mechanisms in the human body, aging also affects the endocrine system. Characteristic of these changes are a decrease in the secretion of hormones, diminishing responsiveness of specific cells to hormones, a change in the chemical transmitters that carry hormonal messages into cells, and a change in the levels of enzymes that respond to hormones. Hormones, in general, are highly interactive and affected by numerous factors, many of which have not been identified; consequently, the study of the effects of hormonal activity on growth and development is a complex undertaking. For in-depth discussions of the endocrinology of growth, refer to Malina et al. (2004) and Wilson (2009). For a review of the general location of major hormonal structures, see Figure 3.4 on page 68.

Pituitary Gland

The pituitary gland is the master gland of the endocrine system. It produces one of the most important hormones involved in the process of human growth—the **growth hormone (GH)**. GH is necessary for normal growth from birth to older adulthood. The only major portion of the body not affected by this hormone, in terms of growth stimulation, is the CNS. The fetus has the capacity to synthesize GH by the end of the first trimester. Blood serum levels of the hormone in the neonate are significantly elevated above levels found during childhood. The importance of GH to the adolescent growth spurt is well documented; its relevance to fetal and infant growth is relatively unknown, although it has been determined that normal fetal development does occur in the absence of GH. Interestingly, the maximum production and secretion of GH occur in association with periods of deep sleep.

As noted in Chapter 3, GH promotes the incorporation of amino acids into tissue protein and stimulates the development of muscle and bone rather than fat tissue. GH also is known to stimulate DNA synthesis and cell multiplication. Its influence on increasing the number of cells in the body lasts from late infancy until adulthood, and its metabolic functions continue until death. The thyroid hormones and androgens interact with GH to perform functions vital to cell multiplication. As noted in Chapter 3, in recent years, the development and use of synthetic GH (GH therapy) has been quite effective in boosting the growth rate of children deficient in the hormone (see review by Ross et al., 2010).

Although the size and weight of the pituitary gland do not change with age, its blood supply gradually decreases after puberty. After about age 30 years, secretion of GH tends to decline, which in older adults is responsible in part for the decrease in lean body mass and bone density and thinning of the skin.

Focus on Application
Hormone Therapy for Being Too Tall?

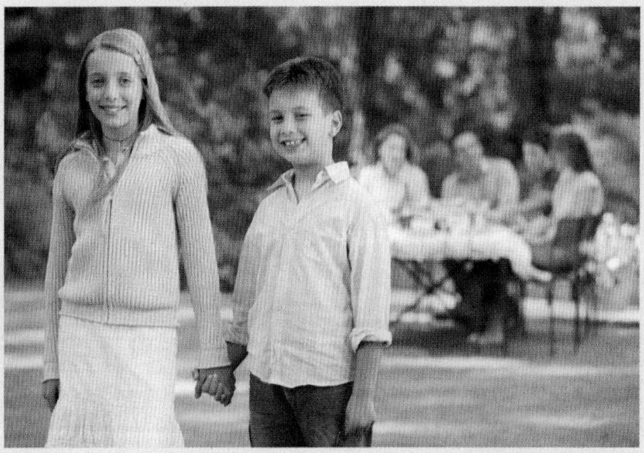

Although the benefits of hormone therapy, such as GH, are well documented for children with a medical need, some situations are quite controversial. One of the more commonly known practices is a parent wishing to add inches to a normally developing child so her or his will hopefully have a better chance of success in sports, that is, without full consideration of possible detrimental long-term effects. However, one of the more unknown practices was recently brought to our attention—hormone therapy to stunt the growth of young girls projected to be (too) tall. A young girl's mother, whom was tall, remembered being teased and embarrassed about her own height at school. Apparently, the social culture in 1950s and 1960s did not appreciate tall females. Girls wanted to remain below 5′6″ so that they could, for example, be a ballerina, become airline stewardess, or improve their chances of finding a husband. Not wanting this for her daughter, she asked a specialist to stunt her child's growth (height). The pediatrician, affiliated with a prestigious U.S. academic medical center, confidently prescribed synthetic estrogen in doses 100 times greater than the estrogen found in today's high-dose oral contraceptives. Apparently, this practice was performed on several females during the 1970s. A follow-up of these cases when the ladies were adults found that several experienced reproductive problems (miscarriage and difficulty conceiving). In the case of the young lady described, doctors also diagnosed her with a condition that put her at risk of breast cancer.

Although this information does not represent scientific study of true cause, this case brings to light the need for parental education and stronger ethical restrictions for the use of hormone therapy with children and adolescents.

Source:
Cohen, S., & Cosgrove, S. (2010). Too tall, too small? The temptation to tinker with a child's height. *The Lancet*, *375*(9713), 454–455.

Thyroid Gland

The thyroid gland is second only to the pituitary in terms of influence on human growth and development. This gland produces **thyroxine**, which is important to cell multiplication and growth in the fetus and young child. In contrast to GH, thyroxine is essential to CNS development. Its presence is so important that regardless of other hormones, its absence would result in retarded and abnormal growth. Thyroxine is vital to the production of all forms of RNA, and its presence stimulates ribosome production and protein synthesis. Other functions include metabolizing fats and carbohydrates, stimulating the cell's use of oxygen, and, along with sex hormones, facilitating skeletal development through calcium and phosphate absorption. GH is relatively ineffective without thyroxine. In contrast to GH, which has little if any effect on fetal and early infant growth, thyroxine is very influential. Children who have too little thyroxine grow at a below-average rate but with prompt treatment typically catch up to normal size.

As people age, the cells within the thyroid gland undergo several structural changes and collagen fibers appear. With increasing age, the blood levels of thyroxine do not drop although the thyroid itself produces fewer hormones. The thyroid gland continues to function normally in healthy adults throughout the life span.

The pancreas, which is well developed by the end of prenatal development, secretes a powerful anabolic hormone called *insulin*. Insulin functions primarily to metabolize sugars in the diet and increase the transport of glucose (blood sugar) and amino acids across the plasma membrane. Insulin also enhances protein synthesis, although tissue hypertrophy can occur in its absence, and appears to increase the synthesis of DNA and RNA in muscle and bone tissues. The commonly known disorder of diabetes is a result of an abnormality in the body's ability to metabolize blood sugar. With increasing age, many people experience longer and higher levels of blood sugar as a result of the aging cell's tendency to absorb less blood sugar and decrease its active insulin secretion.

Adrenal Glands

Of the several groups of hormones the adrenal glands produce, androgens are the most important to a discussion of factors influencing growth and development. Although androgens are secreted by the adrenal cortex in both sexes, they also are produced by the testes in the male; their release is triggered by actions originating from the pituitary gonadotropins.

Chapter 3 discussed the importance of adrenal hormones to the development of muscle tissue and skeletal growth. Other functions include causing the release of epinephrine and norepinephrine to mediate the response to stress, mediating the kidney's absorption of sodium and chloride, and metabolizing fat and carbohydrates. Although a major portion of the adrenal cortex is developed and differentiated by the third fetal month, it does not reach its adult character until about the third postnatal year.

As the system ages, the production of some adrenal hormones, including androgens, declines. The hormone secretions that regulate fat and carbohydrate metabolism do not decline with aging, although individuals will require more time to complete this metabolic process as they age. Hormones affecting fluid balance in kidney function remain relatively stable well into old age.

Other Glandular Functions

Closely associated with sex differentiation, physical growth, and sex hormones are the functions of the *gonads* (the testes and ovaries). Adrenal and gonadal tissues originate from similar cells; both are known as *steroid-producing glands*. Exposure of the brain to sex hormones during early fetal development is associated with future reproductive physiology and sex-oriented behavioral characteristics. For example, during the early stages of fetal development, androgens interact with the immature CNS to imprint future male characteristics. Ovarian estrogens in females, like testosterone in males, normally are not secreted in physiologically effective quantities until shortly before puberty. Similar to GH in men, declining testosterone levels occur with advancing years. The loss of testosterone has been linked to significant changes in body composition (decreased lean body mass and increased fat mass). For females, the loss of estrogen and its effect on bone loss is well documented.

Hormones secreted by the *parathyroid glands* also play a major role in normal growth and development. At birth, the parathyroid glands are similar morphologically to those of the adult. These hormones are responsible for normal skeletal development by regulating calcium and phosphorus metabolism. In addition to its function in skeletal development, these hormones also enhance calcium absorption in the presence of vitamin D. The parathyroid glands, located at the base of the throat, grow heavier until males turn 30 years and females reach 50 years of age. After these peaks, their size and rate of hormone production remain stable.

Most experts agree that physical activity probably influences many of the relationships among hormonal activity, growth, and behavioral characteristics. Although exercise of varying levels and types has been shown to affect specific hormone concentrations, the consensus is that it does not significantly influence physical growth beyond that which would occur naturally.

Summary

Several factors may affect the normal course of growth and development throughout the life span. A number of maternal and external factors can have a profound effect on development of the unborn infant. Among the potentially harmful maternal factors are age of the mother, nutrition, genetic abnormalities, and the mother's emotional state.

Although the fetus appears safe in its protective membrane, the fetus can still be affected by external environmental factors through the placenta. Broadly, external factors can include anything the expectant mother breathes, drinks, eats, or smokes or the disease-producing bacteria with which she comes in contact. Exposure to harmful agents (teratogens) can cause negative reactions in the form of birth defects and behavioral dysfunctions. Teratogens include infectious diseases, tobacco, alcohol, and drugs.

The intake of essential nutrients and water are vital to growth and development throughout the life span. In general, infants with malnourished diets (especially diets low in protein and total calories) show below-average physical growth by early childhood. However, the primary concern for children in the United States appears to be the overconsumption of fat, refined sugar, and salt rather than a deficiency of protein and calories.

Although the literature is unclear regarding what level of physical activity is beneficial or harmful to physical growth and development, its effects on specific characteristics have been documented. In general, habitual physical activity has been shown to have a positive influence on body weight, lean body mass, skeletal mineralization and density, muscular development and strength, and cardiorespiratory development. Most of the literature, however, does not claim that habitual physical activity has any significant influence on stature, skeletal maturity, or any long-term effect on body proportion and physique. Some research has suggested that intense exercise may be a factor in delayed menarche, but there is no evidence that physical activity has a positive influence on sexual maturation. For the typical young competitive athlete, training does not appear to adversely affect pubertal growth.

One of the most influential factors in physical growth and development throughout the life span is hormonal activity. Hormones, in general, are highly interactive and are affected by numerous factors, many of which are unknown.

think about it

1. What does research tell us about exercising while pregnant? Are there any possible effects on the fetus?
2. Consider how maternal factors affect postnatal motor development.
3. Advances in science are telling us more and more about what affects prenatal development. Are you suspicious of any other (than the already described) agents that might affect prenatal development? Explain.
4. What do you think is the greatest problem with children's health: lack of exercise or poor diet?
5. What activities (not specific exercises) would you recommend for stimulating bone health, and why?
6. This discussion noted the effects of normal habitual physical activity on development. What is your reaction to Olympic-style programs (e.g., 3 to 5 hours daily of swimming and gymnastics) for children?

■ LEARNING ACTIVITIES:

Objective: To compare physical activity recommendations. Using the Web, compare the physical activity recommendations set by ShapeAmerica, CDC, and ACSM. How are they similar and how are they different? Anything to add?

Objective: To create a program for bone health? In reference to the *Think About It* question regarding bone health, what specific activities would you recommend for a young child (3 to 5 years) and an older person (65 years and older)?

part three

Perception and Information Processing

part three takes a developmental perspective to focus on the way people perceive and act on sensory information from the external and internal environments. This general process is called *information processing*. From a motor behavior perspective, information processing involves both *perception* (monitoring and interpreting sensory information) and *motor response* (deciding on and organizing response activity). Figure 6.1 illustrates the information-processing, or *perceptual-motor process*, model. The model contains four primary components: sensory input, reception of information, interpretation of information and decision making (planning), and overt motor response. From a more simplified perspective, consider the workings of a computer, *input*, *processing*, and *output*.

The processing stage is studied in two separate chapters. Chapter 6 focuses on the developmental aspects of the perceptual systems with regard to receiving, monitoring, and interpreting sensory data. Chapter 7 covers the developmental aspects involved in processing and acting on the information. It gives special emphasis to attention, memory, processing speed, motor programming, and theories of motor control. Chapters 6 and 7 together provide a framework for studying the complex processes involved in the central issue of the text understanding.

Perception → Action
(motor response)

Chapter 6

Perceptual Development

OBJECTIVES

Upon completion of this chapter, you should be able to

6.1 Diagram the information-processing model (perceptual-motor process) and briefly explain the four primary components.

6.2 Briefly describe the basic visual process and structural changes that occur over the life span.

6.3 List and describe basic functional aspects of the visual modality and the changes associated with visual development.

6.4 Describe the basic function and structure of kinesthetic perception.

6.5 List the five components of basic movement awareness associated with the kinesthetic modality and describe how they function and change over time.

6.6 Discuss the developmental characteristics of auditory perception.

6.7 Describe tactile perception and identify the significant events that take place in its development.

6.8 Provide a general definition of perceptual integration and discuss the specific visual-auditory, visual-kinesthetic, and auditory-kinesthetic intermodal relationships.

6.9 Describe the major changes that occur in perception with advanced aging.

6.10 Discuss *Gibson's ecological perspective* and its role in understanding perception to action.

6.11 Describe the merits and limitations of perceptual-motor training programs.

KEY TERMS

- perception
- information processing
- visual acuity
- object permanence
- A-not-B error
- perceptual constancy
- spatial orientation
- spatial awareness
- directional awareness
- vestibular awareness
- rhythmic awareness
- perceptual integration
- figure-ground perception
- depth perception
- field of vision
- visual-motor coordination
- coincident timing
- kinesthesis
- body awareness
- intermodal perception
- Gibson's ecological perspective
- affordances
- ecological fit
- embodiment

Objective 6.1

focus on change

Change in information-processing ability drives *changes* in motor planning and performance.

The essence of human behavior and motor performance is based on the ability to receive and interpret sensory information. Human beings live in a vast sea of sensory information, yet they thrive rather than drown because of an elaborate network of perceptual systems. The human perceptual system, in fact, has a constant need to receive sensory input from the external world and from its own internal environment. When sensory input is reduced or eliminated, the system reacts negatively. This same negative reaction also can occur when the system is overloaded by too much sensory input. This happens when you try to carry on a telephone conversation while reading a paper, or when a beginner in dance class tries to stay in step with the teacher's instructions during a fast-paced song.

Perception refers to the processes used to gather and interpret sensory information from the external and internal environment. The two related processes of sensation and perception enable the body to receive stimulation and organize it for further processing.

Sensation refers to the stimulation of sensory receptors (Fig. 6.1) by physical energy received from the internal and external environments. The retina of the eye, for example, reacts to light rays (sensory input) and translates the message into nerve impulses (reception). The nerve impulses then are transmitted via the

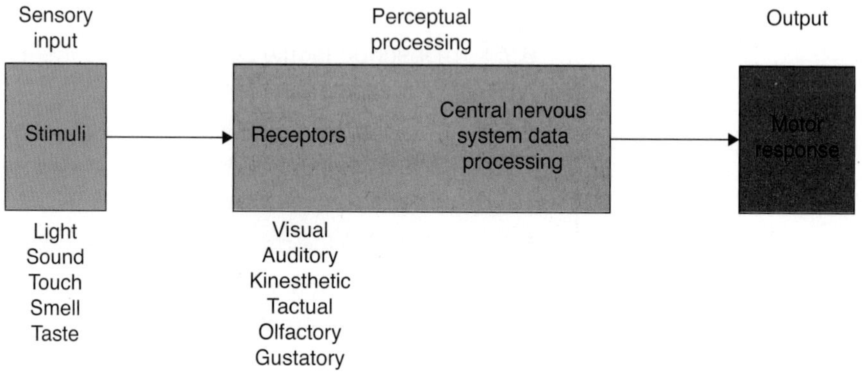

Figure 6.1 The general information-processing (perceptual-motor) model.

perceptual modality to the brain, which reacts to the stimulation in various ways. At this point, perception occurs. Basically, perception involves the monitoring (reception) and interpretation of sensory information. The interpretation given to the information is based on past experience (memory) and cognitive analysis (judgment) of the information. Intertwined with interpretation is the ability to discriminate among various types of sensory stimuli with varying degrees of precision—the similarities or differences, arrangements, and organization.

Another complex function of the brain in this process is to integrate information coming from different perceptual modalities. This information provides the basis for formulating a motor response, which completes the information-processing cycle. This sequence may be thought of as the information-gathering segment of the general **information-processing** model.

Of the six perceptual modalities, perhaps *the two that provide the most relevance to the study of motor behavior are vision and kinesthesis.* This is not to minimize the importance of audition and tactile information; these modalities are discussed briefly along with system integration. However, human movement is universally described in terms of its spatial-temporal characteristics—the spatial coordinates and timing of the body with moving stimuli as well as internal rhythmic awareness. Although individuals can move in the environment without visual information (as the blind do), this modality is crucial in determining reference points and judging the movement of objects. The visual modality provides spatial-temporal information about the external environment, and the kinesthetic system may be described as the body-knowledge network that provides information about the body's movements without reference to auditory or visual cues.

VISUAL PERCEPTION

Objective 6.2

In many ways, vision is the dominant perceptual modality. For human beings, the visual world is the richest source of information about the external environment. Experts estimate that approximately 80% of all sensory information derived outside the body is channeled through the visual system. In terms of movement, visual input provides a primary source of information from which motor behavior is organized and carried out. Visual information is used to formulate a motor program, monitor movement activity, and provide the feedback that allows for immediate correction. Visual input is such a dominant source of information that people tend to rely on it although other sensory information may be more useful.

Most of the available data on this subject focus on infants and children during the growing years. Until about 25 years ago, it was believed the newborn infant was incapable of processing information meaningfully. Today, most experts agree that the visual system of the newborn is relatively well developed at birth and that the neonate demonstrates considerable visual ability. On the other end of the lifelong developmental continuum, several deficits attributed to aging have been documented, although the information on perceptual changes during adulthood and old age is sparse.

The Visual Process

Three basic functions occur in the course of visual perception. First, the eyes receive light and generate messages through nerve impulses about that light.

Second, visual pathways transmit those messages through the optic tract from the eye to the visual centers of the brain. Finally, the visual centers interpret those messages.

Light enters the eye through the pupil, passes through the lens and chambers, and terminates in the retina. The retina is a complex structure consisting of numerous photosensitive receptors and other cells that assist in optic transmission of visual nerve impulses. After nerve impulses are transduced from light energy in the retina, they are transmitted over the optic nerve. The optic nerve from each eye resembles a cable that contains approximately 1 million wires and acts as a huge communication line. The optic nerves must input all of the visual information that comes into the brain for neural processing. Optic nerves from the two eyes pass backward to unite at the optic chiasma and from there, project posteriorly even further as the optic tracts. Fibers from these tracts make synaptic connections with several subcortical structures in the brain. Signals then enter the visual projection areas located in the occipital lobes, at which point impulses are dispersed in various directions to the association areas where interpretation, or perception, takes place.

Developmental Change in Visual Structures

Every structure in the visual system undergoes some early postnatal change. Although all of the visual structures are intact at birth, several are immature in terms of myelinization and synaptic potential. There is also great variability in the growth rate of different parts of the eye. The size of the eye approximately doubles between birth and maturity.

The newborn retina, the part of the eye that turns light into nerve signals to the brain, is similar in structure to that of the adult but is thicker and has no distinct fovea. The fovea is the area in which central visual images are formed. Without this structure, the processing of spatial resolution is poor in the central retina; thus, the ability to see images clearly is relatively weak in comparison to the mature structure. Development proceeds rapidly. By the end of the first year, the major structures of the retina are like those of the adult.

The part of the nervous system that relays visual impressions between the retina and the cortex of the brain also develops quickly and reaches a large part of its ultimate efficiency during the first 11 to 12 months. In the visual cortex, dendritic development at the ends of the nerve cells forms more branches, and by 4 to 5 months of age, the myelinization process is almost complete. At about 2 months, the infant's visual cortex begins to process visual stimuli.

Compared to that of the adult, the newborn's eyeball is short, and the distance between the retina and the lens is reduced. This results in a temporary form of farsightedness. Many infants also will have astigmatism (difficulty in focusing) during the first year because their cornea is not yet symmetrical. Another developmental difference between the neonate and the adult is in the strength and control of eye muscles. Because of weak ciliary muscles attached to the lens, few newborns can change the shape of the lens to accommodate the shifting plane of focus for visual targets, as occurs in the adult eye. Until the end of the first month, infants can adjust their focus only for targets between 5 and 10 inches away. By 4 months of age, infants can accommodate to shifting planes of focus as well as adults. Figure 6.2 illustrates a comparison of the adult and newborn eye.

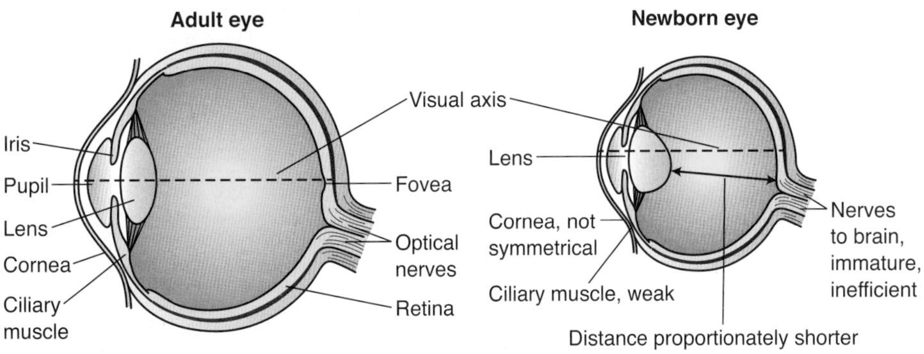

Figure 6.2 A comparison of an adult and newborn eye that indicates limitations of the infant's visual system.

Developmental Change in Visual Functions

Objective 6.3

Visual Acuity. **Visual acuity** refers to clearness of vision and the capacity to detect both small stimuli and small details of large visual patterns. From a motor behavior perspective, visual acuity often is classified as static or dynamic. *Static visual acuity*, the most common form of assessment, is concerned with the ability to detect detail in a stationary object. *Dynamic visual acuity* refers to the ability to perceive detail in a moving object.

At birth, the neonate can see; however, it is not known with what degree of clarity. It was once assumed that the newborn could not see more than a blur until 3 or 4 weeks of age. Researchers now know that soon after birth, a baby can focus on a near object and respond visually to a moving light. By 3 months, a baby can focus quite well but not with good clarity. Using Snellen values as a reference, a newborn's acuity has been estimated between 20/200 and 20/600. This means an individual sees an object 20 feet away as if it were 600 feet away. The 20/600 value is about 30 times lower than adult visual acuity (20/20). By the end of the first year, the baby sees about as well as an adult.

Although these comparative figures might lead one to speculate that a young infant cannot see well, it can detect the contours of many common objects. For example, young infants can see the contrast between hair and skin on a parent's face and can detect large objects at close range. Figure 6.3 illustrates the visual acuity of a newborn compared to that of an adult.

The perceptual component of dynamic visual acuity reflects the ability of the central nervous system (CNS) to estimate the direction and velocity of an object and the ability of the ocular-motor system to catch and hold the object's image on the fovea long enough to permit resolution of its detail. Different estimates of age-related acuity levels have been reported. It is quite evident, however, that static visual acuity matures before dynamic acuity and that the ability to focus on a moving object is a function of the speed at which the object is moving (i.e., efficiency decreases as speed increases). Dynamic acuity increases gradually, with efficiency remaining relatively stable from 12 years of age to the beginning of middle-age adulthood.

As noted earlier, among the primary factors that affect visual acuity are development of the fovea, degree of myelinization, number of neural connections in the visual cortex, shape and structure of the eye, and strength of the ciliary muscles. There is also some indication that the quality of visual acuity coincides with the development of binocular vision (the ability to use both eyes together and fixate on an object), which is evident by 2 months of age.

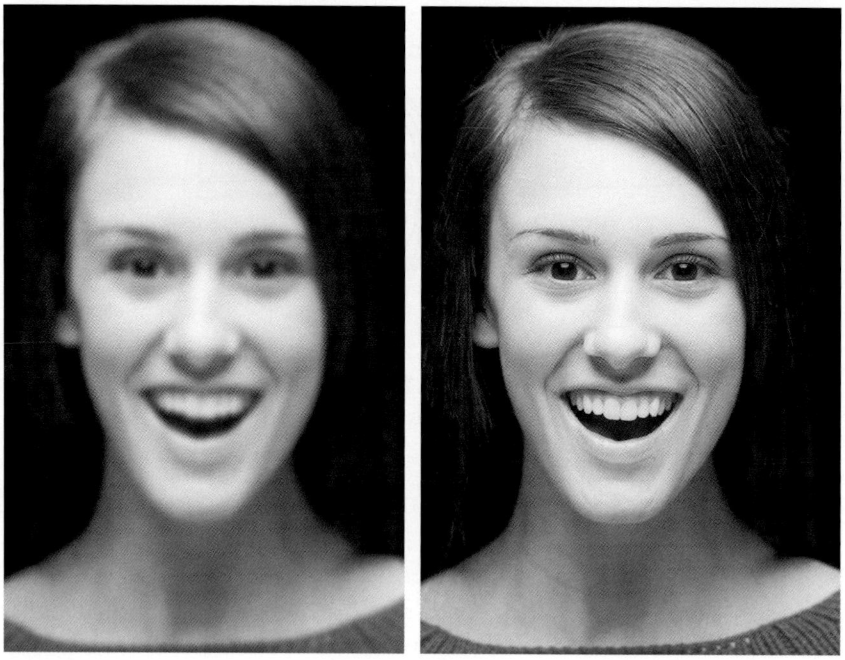

Newborn view Adult view

Figure 6.3 To the newborn (about 2 months), the image appears fuzzy and has far less detail.

OBJECT PERMANENCE

The realization that objects continue to exist when they are no longer in view is **object permanence**. This ability is considered one of the more notable achievements in sensorimotor development. Young infants typically rely heavily on vision and movement to derive information about an object. When an attractive (distinctive) object is shown, then hidden from view, babies (from 1 to 4 months) typically lose interest, as though the object did not exist (Fig. 6.4). This observation was noted frequently in Piaget's (1952) early work. Between the ages of 4 and 8 months, when infants can successfully reach for objects, they continue to be disinterested unless the object is partially visible. Between the ages of 8 and

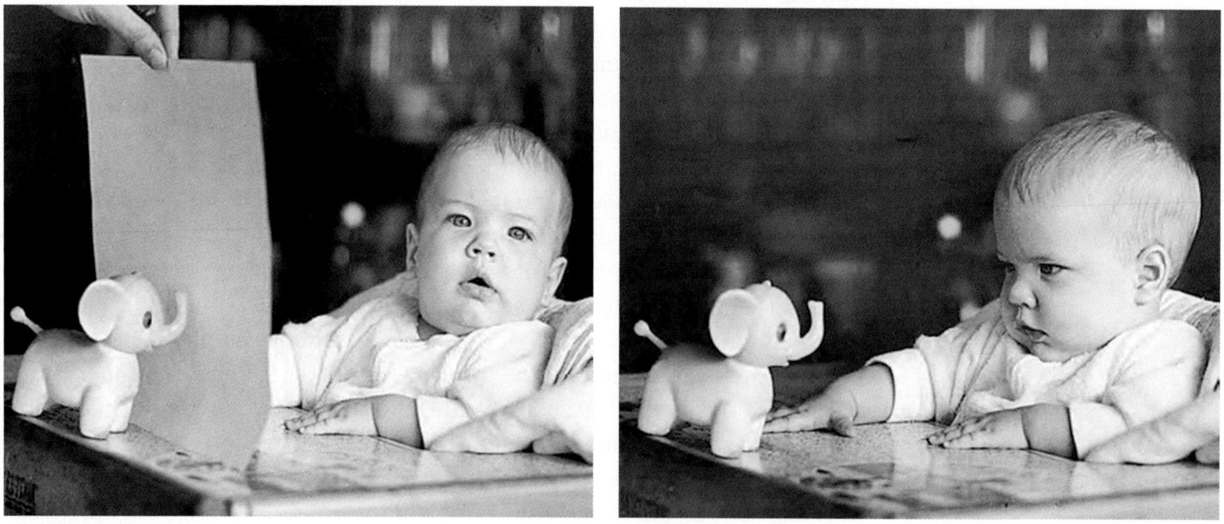

Figure 6.4 A baby shows no sign that she knows the toy is still there.

12 months, signs of object permanence begin to emerge. However, at this stage, infants will typically search for a hidden object *where they first found it* rather than where they saw it last (when the location is switched) (Fig. 6.5). This phenomenon is known as the **A-not-B error**, a classic (hide-and-seek) experimental design introduced by Piaget and used with variations in contemporary research. Between the ages of 12 and 18 months, this ability improves significantly; infants search for the object *where they last saw it*. However, infants still have difficulty perceiving invisible displacement and programming a reach response. Between the ages of 18 months and 2 years, infants are capable of making this integration. It appears that developmentally, infants have difficulty integrating knowledge (perceptual information about an object) with action, which requires a certain level of cortex maturation that may not be present until after the first year.

WebLink

http://www.youtube.com/, or other site; see *Piaget—The A not B Error*.

Ruffman and colleagues (2005) reviewed the research on this topic and found that the explanations for the A-not-B error focused primarily on deficits in *attention*, *inhibition*, and *memory*, or that the infants might genuinely believe the object is in A (a conceptual deficit). The inhibition hypothesis, which is associated with memory, suggests that infants do not have the ability to inhibit previously successful searches at A. The memory explanation contends that infants have the tendency to repeat previous (motor) actions, thereby not searching B. In regard to the attention hypothesis, some researchers believe that the difference is in the extent to which the B location captured attention. In their conclusions, Ruffman et al. agreed with most theorists that there may be more than one cause of A-not-B errors, including the belief that the object is in A. In their series of experiments, even when conditions were equated for infants' attention, inhibitory ability, and motor memories, infants were more likely to make A-not-B errors when they had seen an object placed in A previously.

think about it

Consider child's play. How is it related to embodiment?

The phenomenon of the A-not-B error continues to be a highly studied and debated issue in child development. In fact, the basic concept provides a key experimental vehicle by which contemporary researchers are studying the notion of *embodiment* (also known as *embodied cognition*), that is, the role of motor behavior in higher cognition such as memory and decision making. The underlying hypothesis is that perceptual and motor abilities are inseparably linked and together form the basis for cognition, emotion, and language. Supporters point out that in order to successfully complete the reaching task in the A-not-B setup, the infant must

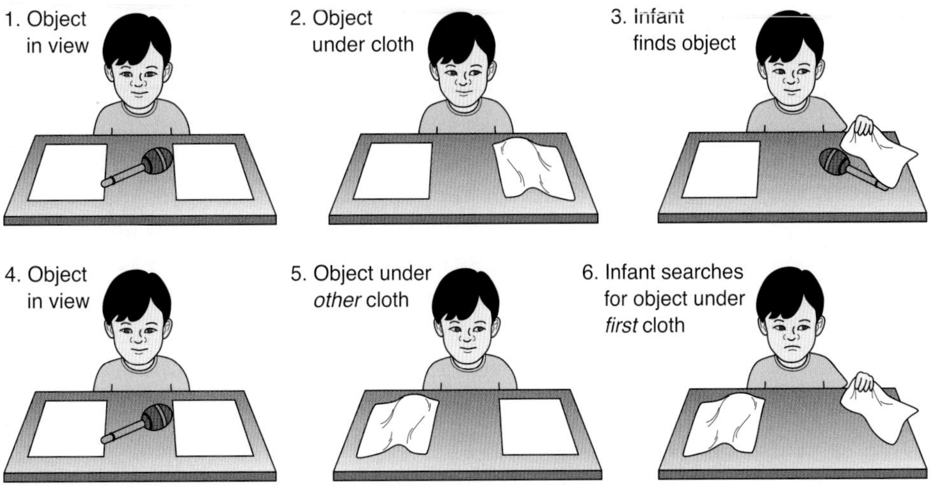

Figure 6.5 Illustration of A-not-B error phenomenon.

perceive, remember, create a plan of action, and reach. Embodiment is discussed further in a subsequent section of this chapter.

PERCEPTUAL CONSTANCY

Of the various aspects of **perceptual constancy**, the one most closely related to the study of motor behavior is the perception of size constancy. Other constancies include shape and color. When an object becomes known to an infant, it becomes recognizable as that specific object regardless of the angle or distance from which it is observed. The object has constancy because it remains the same form, although the retinal image changes. Hence, the ability to perceive constant size is referred to as perceptual constancy.

Another way of describing constancy is the notion that the perceived size is scaled. That is, one unit of measurement is converted, or scaled, into another (perceived size). Road maps, for example, typically include scales that transform inches into miles; theoretically, the visual system contains a mechanism that scales an image into object size.

An example of constancy is perceiving that the airplane on the ground before takeoff is the same object that, minutes later, is several thousand feet in the air. The importance of constancy is that it represents perceptual stability and underlies the ability to interpret the environment consistently and accurately.

In the past, researchers thought this ability did not appear until 4 to 5 months of age, but it seems that even newborns know something about an object's size (Slater et al., 1990). Important stimuli for perception appear to be kinetic cues noted as an object approaches and recedes. This ability steadily improves; maturity is typically reached by 11 years of age. As noted earlier, the ability to understand the constancy of objects is essential to motor development, especially when the infant explores *affordances* in the environment.

SPATIAL ORIENTATION

Perception of **spatial orientation** refers to the ability to recognize an object's orientation or position in three-dimensional space. Closely associated with this visual ability is a component of kinesthetic perception known as *spatial awareness*. This is the internal awareness of the position (orientation) of objects and of the body in three-dimensional space. This discussion concentrates primarily on the visual perception of objects rather than on aspects of internal awareness of spatial orientation and movement in the external environment.

It is important to recognize the differences in spatial orientation of objects. Most older children and adults have the ability to immediately notice these differences, whereas young children do not have this facility. Young children first must learn to recognize the spatial characteristics of objects before they can ignore irrelevant information. In some everyday tasks and motor skill activities, it is important to recognize an object even if it is upside down, rotated, or angled to one side. In the case of recognizing letters such as *d* and *b*, and *p* and *q*, proper identification of spatial orientation is critical. Successfully performing certain target-projecting tasks, gymnastic events, and game activities by recognizing boundary lines and designated spaces also necessitates the accurate perception of spatial orientation.

By 3 to 4 years of age, children are aware of most basic spatial dualisms such as over/under, high/low, front/back, in/out, top/bottom, and vertical/horizontal. However, until these characteristics become commonplace and perceptually refined in their spatial worlds, children are likely to get things reversed, inverted, and confused. It also has been observed that children appear to master spatial dimensions in a fairly, orderly sequence—vertical to horizontal and then to diagonal or oblique. Although 3- and 4-year-olds have some ability to distinguish vertical from horizontal, they still lack the ability to effectively perceive mirror images (left-right reversals) and oblique lines and diagonals. By 8 years of age, most children can perceive the spatial orientation of objects, although some individuals continue to have problems with right-left or mirror-image reversals.

FIGURE-GROUND PERCEPTION

Figure-ground perception refers to the ability to distinguish an object from its surrounding background. This ability, as with most meaningful motor behavior tasks, requires an individual to concentrate on and give selective attention to a visual stimulus. Examples of figure-ground perception include the ability to track and/or intercept objects in sports such as softball, golf, soccer, and ice hockey. To catch a softball hit into the sky, the outfielder must first focus on and track the ball (figure) against the backdrop (ground) of white sky or lights (if at night). Figure-ground perception appears to improve steadily between the ages of 4 and 12 years. Individuals at all ages are more proficient at identifying familiar figures embedded in distracting backgrounds than they are at perceiving unfamiliar figures from similar backgrounds.

DEPTH PERCEPTION

Depth perception is the ability to judge the distance of an object from the self. This automatic occurrence takes place every time an individual judges the distance to other vehicles when driving or attempts to shoot a basketball. Reacting quickly to such tasks requires the individual to know where the object is located in three-dimensional space.

Depth perception is referred to in absolute distance and relative distance. Absolute distance refers to a precise judgment of the space from the person to an object. For example, a short stop attempting to throw out a runner at first base must judge the distance between himself and the base. An infant attempting to place a cap on a bottle and an adult reaching for a cup of coffee are other examples of judging absolute distance.

Relative distance refers to the estimation of distance between one object and another or between different parts of a single object. Examples include discriminating the distance between two rattles or determining whether an opponent or partner is closer to the goalpost. The ability to judge relative distance is much more precise than the detection of absolute distance.

The perceptual system uses two types of cues to detect depth: oculomotor cues and visual cues. The development of each is tied to independent perceptual systems (i.e., visual and kinesthetic). Oculomotor cues are kinesthetic in nature, which means cues are derived from the kinesthetic receptors located in the muscles and joints. An example of this is evident in the absolute distance task of using the arm and hand to reach for a glass of water. Visual cues, in contrast, provide good relative depth information but also might offer additional information about absolute distance. Information is gathered through visual perception with either binocular cues (using both eyes), which appears at about 2 months, or monocular cues (using one eye). The independent development of kinesthesis (kinesthetic sense), monocular vision, and binocular vision all have developmental implications for the individual's ability to judge distances.

think about it

In what ways can you modify the visual cliff experiment to study other aspects of depth perception?

WebLink

http://www.youtube.com/; see *Visual Cliff Experiment*.

It is generally agreed that depth perception is absent at birth. *Most sources indicate that by the age of 6 months, children are capable of judging depth with fair accuracy.* A simple observation of 4-month-old infants grasping objects reveals they have some degree of depth perception. When an object is placed within grasping range, most infants will attempt to grasp it; when the item is placed out of reach, infants rarely grab for it.

The classic study of depth perception in children involved the use of a visual cliff (Gibson & Walk, 1960). The apparatus consisted of a table several feet high covered with a heavy sheet of glass. On one side of the table (runway), a checkerboard pattern was fixed just beneath the surface of the glass. On the other side, the same checkerboard pattern was set 3½ feet below the surface of the glass, thus creating a visual cliff. Infants were placed on the shallow side and beckoned by their mothers to cross the glass over the cliff. The investigators found that infants as young as 6 months of age clearly paid attention to depth cues and would not crawl to their mothers over the deep end, even when coaxed (Fig. 6.6). Refinement (especially of absolute distance) continues until approximately age 12 years.

FIELD OF VISION

Also known as *peripheral vision*, **field of vision** refers to the entire extent of the environment that can be seen without changing the fixation of the eye. References to peripheral vision frequently are described in terms of lateral and vertical capabilities. According to Blake and Sekuler (2005), normal adult lateral peripheral vision is approximately 90 degrees from straight ahead, which creates a visual field of about 180 degrees. In contrast, vertical peripheral vision in adults is approximately 47 degrees above and 65 degrees below the visual midline.

Information on the development of peripheral vision, especially the vertical aspects, is quite limited. At 7 weeks, lateral peripheral vision is about 35 degrees, roughly 40% of adult capability. According to a review by Cummings et al. (1988), most sources indicate that by the end of the first postnatal year, visual field

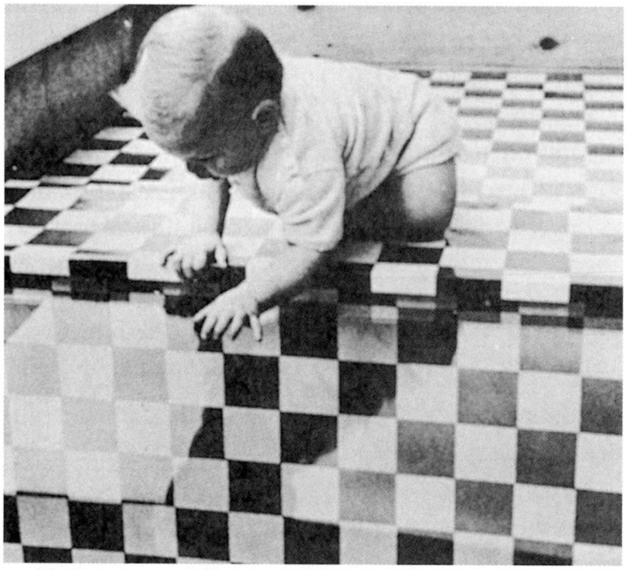

Figure 6.6 Confronting the visual cliff.

extension is still immature. Only after age 5 years, visual fields are equivalent to those of adults. Although the role of peripheral vision in children's motor performance is not clear, its importance in sports at the adult level is evident. In activities that involve quick responses and numerous visual cues (e.g., basketball, tennis, hockey, and soccer), central and lateral peripheral vision are essential for spatial orientation.

PERCEPTION OF MOVEMENT AND VISUAL-MOTOR COORDINATION

One of the most important and complex perceptual abilities related to motor behavior is the detection, tracking, and interception of moving objects. Many more demands are placed on the perceptual system when objects begin to move in space and individuals are confronted with dynamic rather than static conditions. Just a few of the difficulties are evident when one considers the differences between static (stationary) objects and dynamic visual acuity, and the perception of depth in reference to moving (dynamic) objects in comparison to stationary objects.

In addition to the functional aspects of these perceptual abilities, the developmental dynamics of eye movement changes are also factors that influence the ability to perceive moving objects. *Saccadic eye movements* are rapid movements between one point of visual fixation (i.e., focusing one's gaze on something) and another. These movements are slower and more numerous in young infants than in older children and adults. At maturity (approximately 12 years), a saccade moves the eye about 90% of the distance to the visual target, but in infants, several saccades are required to reach their visual target. An infant's eyes also move less smoothly in tracking a moving object and tend to refixate frequently, or focus first on one spot and then another. It is difficult for the newborn to focus both eyes on the same point (convergence) and thus to see only one stimulus.

By 48 hours after birth, most infants can track a slow-moving object. This response is uneven, however, and focus is easily lost. Smoother, more accurate tracking is evident by 2 months. By 4 months, the more complex task of tracking and predicting the path of a slow-moving object is within most infants' capabilities. Around the same time, the infant has reached an unrefined visual-motor stage and exhibits approaching movements with the upper body as if attempting to receive the object.

The ability to coordinate visual abilities with movements of the body is **visual-motor coordination**. This aspect of movement combines both visual and kinesthetic perceptions with the ability to make controlled and coordinated bodily movements that usually involve eye–hand or eye–foot integration. Development of these actions generally follows the proximodistal (midline to periphery), cephalocaudal (head to toes), and gross-to-fine motor order. Much of the contemporary research on this topic involves reaching, which is discussed in greater detail in Chapter 8. Briefly, eye–hand coordination emerges during the first 6 months of life, as evidenced by reaching to objects reasonably well by 4 months. By 7 months of age, the trajectory of most reaches is more adultlike, due in large part to better use of visual information. At approximately 14 months, the infant's form for reaching and grasping is more adultlike. In fine motor tasks such as lacing shoes or writing, the small muscles of the hand or foot are synchronized and, in turn, are coordinated with vision. Table 6.1 presents a selection of fine visual-motor behaviors characteristically exhibited by children during the developmental period of

TABLE 6.1 Selected Fine Visual-Motor Characteristics of Children 3 to 8 Years Old

Age (Year)					
3	4	5	6	7	8
Uses hand constructively to direct visual responses	Makes visual manipulation; does not need support of hands	Understands horizontal and vertical concepts	Easily performs copying tasks	Prefers pencil over crayons	Copies a diamond shape
Makes skillful manipulations	Makes discoveries in depth perception	Copies squares and triangles	Prints fairly well	Makes uniform size letters, numbers, etc.	Attempts cursive writing
Draws lines with more control	Laces shoes	Increases fine finger control		Draws a person more accurately	Aligns letters uniformly
Copies circles and crosses	Buttons large buttons	Colors within the lines			
Stacks 1-inch cubes	Orients movements from center of periphery	Cuts fairly accurately			
Handles utensils like adults do	Draws a recognizable picture with some detail	Draws a recognizable person			
Strings beads					
Cuts with scissors					

think about it

What are the constraints to effective coincident timing in young children (e.g., 5- to 7-year-olds)?

3 to 8 years of age. The development of gross motor abilities that require visual-motor coordination is discussed in subsequent sections.

Coincident timing, another aspect of tracking and intercepting objects, also appears to improve with age. Coincident timing tasks are commonly used in sport activities that involve the ability to coordinate visual and motor behavior to a single coincident point (interception) such as in catching a ball, kicking a moving ball, and passing a ball to a running player. An important determinant in coincident timing performance is the relative direction of the moving object. And, as might be expected, accuracy tends to decrease as velocity increases.

Other than the fact that coincident timing abilities seem to improve through adolescence, with significant change from about age 6 to 12 years, the specific developmental mechanisms involved are not well understood. A longitudinal study that tracked the coincident timing abilities from ages 6 to 12 years noted an interesting finding (Kuhlman & Beitel, 1997). For both sexes, the amount of time spent playing sports (e.g., soccer and softball) and video games was a better indicator of ability than age was. This ability is an excellent example of complete information processing; much more is involved than the simple perception of moving stimuli. Coincident timing involves a complex interplay between visual-perception proficiency and motor control. The discussion of motor performance provides a more complete treatment of visual-motor abilities. Table 6.2 summarizes visual perception milestones.

Focus on Application
Can You Pitch a Ball Too Slow to Young Children?

In an effort to make the much-loved sport of baseball more developmentally appropriate for young children, activities such as t-ball, machine pitch, and coach pitch have been good lead-ups to the regular game. One of the problems that younger children have is the ability to judge fast-moving objects and time their actions for contact (coincident timing ability). With some practice, by approximately 8 to 9 years of age, most children experience some success with such activities.

Aside from t-ball, in which the ball is stationary—a good thing for beginners—what is the optimal pitching speed for children? Obviously, too fast is not good, but how slow should pitching be? Interestingly, recent evidence suggests that young children (5 years of age) may have more difficulty hitting very-slow-moving balls. Apparently, it is more difficult because their brains are not wired to handle slow-motion information. This explains in part why a young child holding a bat or a catcher's mitt often will not react to a thrown ball, which in many instances prompts the parent or coach to continue throwing the ball at an even slower speed.

By adding a little speed to the pitch, children may be able to judge speed more accurately. Furthermore, it appears that even adults are worse at slow speeds than they are at faster speeds. Apparently, the human brain possesses fewer neurons for interpreting slow motion than it does for detecting faster motion. The immature neurons in a child's brain make a child especially poor at judging slow speeds. Once the brain develops to maturity, it becomes more adept at handling slower speeds.

Source:
Ahmed, I. J., Lewis, T. L., Ellemberg, D., & Maurer, D. (2005). Discrimination of speed in 5-year-olds and adults: Are children up to speed? *Vision Research*, *45*(16), 2129–2135.

TABLE 6.2 **Summary of Visual Milestones**

Aspect	Basic Function	Adultlike
Visual acuity (static)	3 mo can focus	12 mo
	6 mo 20/100	
Object permanence	8–12 mo	2 y
Field of vision	12 mo	5 y
Spatial orientation	3–4 y	8 y
Perceptual constancy	4–5 mo	11 y
Depth perception	6 mo	12 y
Visual-motor coordination	(highly dependent on task)	
(reaching and grasping)	4 mo	14 mo
(fine motor)	3–8 y	
(interception)	4 mo	12 y
Figure-ground	<4 y	12 y

KINESTHETIC PERCEPTION

Objective 6.4

Often referred to as the sixth sense, kinesthetic perception is a comprehensive term that encompasses the awareness of movement and body position. The word **kinesthesis** derives from two Greek words meaning "to move" and "sensation." It involves the ability to discriminate positions and movements of body parts based on information that derives from the individual's internal environment. Unlike the visual, auditory, and tactile perceptual modalities that receive sensations from outside the body, the kinesthetic system receives sensory input from receptors located in muscles, tendons, joints, and the vestibular (balance) system. Although kinesthetic information is not the exclusive determinant of the way movement patterns are organized, it provides body and movement knowledge without reference to visual and verbal cues. This modality is basic to all movement and, along with the visual modality, dominates the learning and acquisition of motor skills.

think about it

What motor skill activities require a high degree of kinesthetic ability?

Structure and Function of the Kinesthetic System

In spite of several years of inquiry on the subject, kinesthesis is not fully understood either physiologically or psychologically. Its complexity is due, in part, to the fact that kinesthetic perception is not a single sensory system. Rather, the kinesthetic system consists of several different sensory receptors.

The group of kinesthetic receptors is associated with the *somatosensory system* that handles sensations from the body. Somatic receptors are located in the skin, muscles, joints, and vestibular apparatus of the inner ear. Somatic receptors may be further subgrouped into cutaneous receptors and *proprioceptors*. Cutaneous receptors are located near the skin and perceive touch, pressure, temperature, and pain. The sensations these receptors pick up come primarily from outside the body and do not appear to play a primary role in motor behavior. However, because there is such a strong relationship between the two perceptions, they often are referred to as *tactile-kinesthetic perception*. Collectively, the proprioceptors of the muscles (spindle receptors), joints, tendons (Golgi), and inner ear (vestibular apparatus) form the perceptions known as kinesthesis (kinesthetic perception). All are sensitive to stimuli arising from movement.

As noted in Chapter 2, spinal tracts are the major pathways for transmitting signals from these receptors via the periphery to the specific brain interpretation centers. Spinal tracts are located alongside the vertebrae that make up the spinal column. Input to the CNS, except for kinesthetic input from the structures in the head (vestibular apparatus), comes through roots (nerve bundles) that collect and guide the input to the spinal cord at each segment, which serves a specific region of the body. One of the most important concepts concerning kinesthesis is the understanding that any one of the kinesthetic receptors in isolation from the others is generally ineffective in signaling information about the movements of the body. The various receptors are often sensitive to a variety of aspects of body motion at the same time.

Development of Kinesthetic Perception

The developmental aspects of kinesthetic perception may be measured and described in terms of their basic physiological qualities and in their applied context involving knowledge of the body and movement awareness.

The two basic physiological aspects of kinesthetic perception are kinesthetic acuity and kinesthetic memory. *Kinesthetic (discrimination) acuity* refers to the ability to proprioceptively detect differences or match quantities such as location, distance, weight, force, speed, and acceleration. Examples include the ability to discriminate the difference between two objects of slightly different weights when placed in the hands while blindfolded (weight discrimination) and the ability to detect when blindfolded which arm has been raised slightly higher than the other (location).

If the stimulus is removed after presentation, then *kinesthetic memory* is involved. Tests of kinesthetic memory usually involve a reproduction of movements. For example, a blindfolded individual is asked to move one hand to a distance of choice or at a measured speed and, after a pause, to reproduce the movement. In another passive variation, the experimenter moves the subject's limb and then asks the subject to reproduce the movement. The subject has less motor information in the passive situation.

A review of the studies on this topic suggests that kinesthetic acuity improves faster and earlier than kinesthetic memory. The ability to discriminate kinesthetic information approaches adult levels by age 8 years, *whereas the mature stage of kinesthetic memory generally is not reached until after 12 years of age*. Although very little information is available on young children, research findings note substantial yearly decreases in performance errors after age 5 years.

Basic Movement Awarenesses

Objective 6.5

Several different descriptors may be found in the literature concerning the more applied developmental aspects of kinesthetic perception. Some sources use single descriptors, such as body knowledge, body awareness, or spatial awareness, whereas other sources have identified several subcategories. All of these terms have been used to identify movement awareness (both cognitive and motor) abilities theoretically associated with kinesthesis and one's internal awareness of various movement parameters. The following basic movement awareness components are related to kinesthetic perception: body awareness, spatial awareness, directional awareness, vestibular awareness, and rhythmic (temporal) awareness. These awarenesses are closely interrelated and are inseparable in most movement conditions. The components have been identified to aid in categorizing the various kinesthetic abilities based on the notion that presenting the parts to such a complex process will produce a better understanding of the whole.

BODY AWARENESS

Sometimes referred to as body concept, body knowledge, or body schema, **body awareness** involves an awareness of body parts by name and location, their relationship to each other, and their capabilities and limitations. As children age, they become increasingly more aware of their body parts in reference to the aspects described. With this basic movement knowledge, they gradually improve their ability to perform desired movements efficiently.

The knowledge of body parts and their functions is one of the most basic aspects of kinesthesis and one of the more researched topics. At birth, the newborn is not capable of true conscious body awareness. However, during the first month, a relatively crude awareness appears to emerge that the body is distinct from the surroundings. With growth, the infant then becomes increasingly aware of the capabilities of various body parts in moving the eyes, head, trunk, arms, and legs. By the end of the first year or so, correct reactions to verbalizations of body parts become more evident. Although infants at this age cannot identify specific parts verbally, they are capable of indicating a few body parts (tummy, nose, ears, eyes, and feet) correctly when given verbal cues. They can do this first on their own bodies and then later on other people. As their body-part vocabulary increases, so does their accuracy at physically touching and verbally identifying specific body parts. By age 6 years, the majority of children can accurately identify the major parts. Shortly after, the ability to distinguish the minor parts (ring finger, wrists, heels, ankle, and elbows) also has been mastered.

The ability to identify various body parts depends heavily on both conceptual and language abilities as well as other sensory perceptions. For example, a response to "Where is your left ankle?" involves both auditory memory and the ability to plan a motor response. If a series of responses to commands such as "Touch your right elbow to your left knee" is required, the demands of the situation are increased significantly. It is reasonable to assume that children who have been tutored in body-part identification will show superior abilities in comparison to the norm described.

SPATIAL AWARENESS

As noted earlier, the spatial awareness aspect of kinesthetic perception interplays with the visual perception of spatial orientation. Both perceptions involve the ability to recognize objects in three-dimensional space. The two differ in that **spatial awareness** involves the ability to draw inferences in relationship to self-space or position as well as object recognition. In essence, it is the sense of the location of one's body in space in relationship to the environment. This aspect of kinesthesis also has been viewed in the developmental psychology literature as the general sense of direction required for spatial mobility.

Spatial awareness may be described in terms of *egocentric localization* and *allocentric (object) localization*. These terms are also synonymous with *egocentric* and *allocentric frames of reference*. Egocentric localization refers to the ability to locate objects in space in reference to the self, which is characteristic of younger children. Allocentric localization generally follows egocentric perception; it is the ability to locate objects using something other than the self as a reference. Such behavior is exhibited by older individuals who can locate an object relative to its nearness to other objects. Knowledge of the spatial environment and of the body is necessary for an individual to formulate a motor program (plan) and project the body effectively.

Before individuals can effectively project their bodies into space, they must have a sense of where objects are located. For example, an individual might perceive or learn the location of an object relative to himself or herself (e.g., second base is directly in front of me when I am batting) to demonstrate the use of an egocentric frame of reference. If an allocentric frame of reference is in use, the individual might learn the location of second base relative to various landmarks in the area (e.g., second base is between first and third, or second base is next to the shortstop). The strategy used in allocentric localization is quite similar to that required in map reading and orienteering.

Typically, adults have the ability to use and exercise both egocentric and allocentric frames of reference. For example, an adult may learn a new pathway through a mountain bike course in an egocentric way ("Go to the first sign and turn right, then go straight ahead until you get to the fork and turn left, etc."). In other situations, however, the cyclist may use allocentric localization in checking out the possibility of a shortcut on the second run or in looking at a map and then using his or her sense of direction to proceed. Apparently, young infants under 12 months of age do not have the ability to use allocentric frames of reference and are restricted to egocentric orientation. Allocentric localization appears sometime between the ages of 12 and 16 months and seemingly is used with increasing frequency through childhood. Use of both frames of reference are important in action processing such as in reaching and throwing; more on action processing is discussed in Chapters 7 and 8.

DIRECTIONAL AWARENESS

In theoretical terms, **directional awareness** is that aspect of kinesthetic perception assumed to be an extension of body and spatial awareness. Directional awareness refers to the conscious internal awareness of two sides of the body (*laterality*) and the ability to identify various dimensions of external space and project the body within those dimensions (*directionality*). The term *lateral preference*, which involves hemispheric control and preferential use of one eye, hand, or foot over the other, also is associated with directional awareness and is discussed in Chapters 8 and 9 in reference to asymmetries.

Briefly, the internal awareness that the body has two sides (laterality) and that those sides can be differentiated as right or left improves steadily until approximately 5 years of age, when the understanding that the body has two distinct sides is well developed. Around this same time, a more advanced form of laterality begins to emerge—the ability to label specific body parts as right or left (i.e., left-right discrimination). As this aspect of laterality develops, the child clearly moves from the perceptual-motor phase of development to the conceptual-cognitive phase. Children at this age may realize that right and left are opposite sides of the body. But they may not perceive which is which, or they will oftentimes reverse the two. By the age of 8 years, most children can respond accurately to questions regarding the left-right discrimination of specific body parts.

> **think about it**
>
> What physical activities and sports require a high level of directional awareness?

Directionality is the motoric expression of laterality and the perception of spatial orientation. Along with the understanding that the body has two distinct sides that work independently and in unison, the identification of the dimensions of external space is prerequisite to purposeful movement in the environment. By 4 years of age, as discussed earlier, children are aware of the most basic spatial dualisms such as over/under, high/low, front/back, in/out, top/bottom, and vertical/horizontal. As mentioned earlier, children appear to master spatial dimensions in a fairly, orderly sequence: from the vertical to the horizontal, to the diagonal or oblique. Although most children by age 8 years have the basic ability to effectively perceive the spatial orientation of objects, some individuals continue to have problems with right-left or mirror-image reversals.

Refinement of directionality continues to about age 12 years, when this aspect of kinesthetic perception approximates adult behavior.

VESTIBULAR AWARENESS

The successful performance of virtually all motor skills depends on the individual's ability to establish and maintain *equilibrium* (balance). The general description for this component is **vestibular awareness**. The newborn must establish equilibrium before achieving any of the early developmental milestones of maintaining head position, sitting, and standing. Remember, the vestibular apparatus is the part of the kinesthetic modality that provides the individual with information about the body's relationship to gravity and its head position. In a general sense, balance, which depends primarily on information from the vestibular apparatus, refers to the ability to maintain equilibrium in relation to the force of gravity. Regardless of how the term is defined, it is clear that balance involves the successful integration of several anatomical and neurological functions (e.g., the skeletal, muscular, sensory, and motor systems) (Fig. 6.7).

Typically, balance is subdivided into three types: postural, static, and dynamic. *Postural balance* refers to the relatively unconscious level of basic reflex functioning that enables one to maintain upright posture, hold the head erect, sit, and stand (to be discussed in greater detail in Chapter 8). *Static balance* is the ability to maintain a desired body posture when the body is relatively stationary. Common testing procedures include standing on one foot and balancing on a stabilometer or balance board. *Dynamic balance* refers to the body's ability to maintain and control posture while in motion. This type of equilibrium is used in numerous motor skill activities; it usually is evaluated based on the ability to walk on balance beams of different widths and heights. Although these definitions may appear somewhat simple and relatively clear, balance tasks are complex. The assessment of balance at any age is related to the specific task used to measure it. Thus, balance is better described as a set of specific characteristics or components that describe the task to be performed, rather than as a single, unitary ability.

Specificity of the task appears to be a major determinant in the exact pattern of change. For example, improvement for a group of children on some tasks may be significant and steady over a number of years; performance on other tasks may change very little, change not at all, or decline. Table 6.3 shows selected balance abilities of young children in approximate developmental order.

In addition to the relatively simple balance tests such as standing on one foot and walking across a beam, researchers now use an array of sophisticated measurement techniques to better determine the specific mechanisms involved. Typically, these techniques involve a moving surface to momentarily destabilize the person, with focus given to postural sway and/or specific muscle group activation (electromyography responses). Although refinement with specific tasks may continue

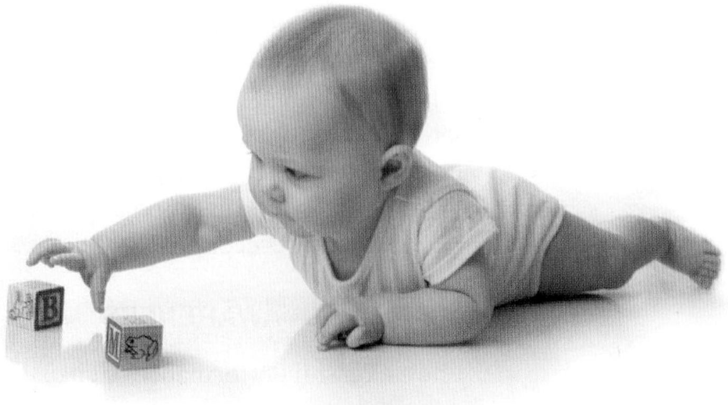

Figure 6.7 Postural control underscores virtually all motor skill proficiency.

TABLE 6.3 Selected Balance Abilities

Type of Balance	Task	Approximate Age (Year)
Static	Balances on one foot (3–4 s)	3
	Balances on one foot (10 s)	4
	Supports body in basic inverted position	6
Dynamic	Walks on straight line (1-in. line)	3
	Walks on beam using alternating steps (4 in. wide)	3
	Walks on circular pattern (1-in. line)	4
	Walks on beam using alternating steps (2–3-in. wide)	4½
	Hops proficiently (traveling)	6

across the life span, Peterson and colleagues (2006) observed evidence that children do not demonstrate adultlike balance prior to 12 years of age. Their assessment included the use of sensory information in maintaining stability; therefore, it also assessed sensory integration. Postural responses are similar to those of adults. From a dynamic systems perspective, as with other motor skills, success with balance is based on the individual's ability to adapt (self-organize) his or her motor abilities to the characteristics of the changing environment, that is, to integrate at times very complex, perceptual information with the motor system.

The ability to maintain and control equilibrium is widely acknowledged as a fundamental motor component. It is included in almost all motor assessment batteries, especially those that focus on the abilities of young children. As one might expect, balance ability is a good predictor of overall fundamental gross motor skill performance in children 3 to 5 years of age. Further discussion of balance ability is presented in Chapter 8 (rudimentary behavior) and Chapter 11 on adult motor performance.

RHYTHMIC (TEMPORAL) AWARENESS

All motor activities consist of spatial-temporal characteristics (i.e., movement takes place in both space and time). Coincident timing, one aspect of temporal awareness that already has been discussed, involves the ability to gauge one's position relative to the changing position of an object or another person. Another aspect of the internal awareness of time is rhythmic awareness. As with other kinesthetic perceptions, considerable interplay exists among the various aspects of temporal awareness.

think about it

Is there any practical application of the information on movement awarenesses?

Rhythmic awareness refers to creating or maintaining a temporal pattern within a set of movements. The temporal pattern may be initiated from within by the individual or may be matched with some external pattern. Even young infants seem to be born with the tendency to make rhythmic movements with parts of their bodies. These movements appear within a predictable time during the first year and seem to be triggered by an internal awareness (i.e., an internal drummer) rather than in reaction to any observable external stimulation. Examples of rhythmic awareness are found in such activities as keeping time to music, tapping the hands or feet to stay in rhythm with a sound or light, reproducing a pattern from memory, and creating a rhythmic beat or pattern without external stimulation. Two major differences between this aspect of temporal awareness and coincident timing are evident. Coincident timing occurs primarily in unpredictable situations (i.e., with moving stimuli) and requires visual information for effective completion.

Little information is currently available on the individual's ability to initiate rhythmic movements without an external stimulus. The absence of criteria by which to make judgments and the strong possibility that most rhythmic responses are not original but are derived from past experiences or memory make this a difficult question to answer experimentally. However, there have been reports related to *keeping time*. One (classic) study observed the ability of children (from 2 to 5 years) and adults to keep time to piano music played at several different tempos when walking and beating time with their hands (Jersild & Bienstock, 1935). The accuracy rate of the 5-year-olds about doubled that of the 2-year-olds, and the adults' values were almost double those of the 5-year-olds. These data suggest that children between 2 and 5 years of age improve considerably in their ability to keep time to a rhythmical stimulus and that periods of improvement continue to adulthood. Another interesting note is that better accuracy scores were recorded at faster rather than slower tempos. This type of behavior also has been observed in coincident timing tasks. One could speculate from these observations that the body's rhythmic mechanism responds more effectively to an external stimulus in which the tempo falls within a range of quite fast and quite slow.

AUDITORY PERCEPTION

Objective 6.6

The importance of auditory cues is obvious, although they generally are not as vital to motor behavior as visual and kinesthetic information. Very few sport activities are learned or carried out without auditory information and verbal cues. As with all the perceptual modalities, auditory perception derives from a complex system that involves the ability to detect, discriminate, associate, and interpret auditory stimuli. Commonly addressed aspects of auditory perception include auditory localization, auditory discrimination, and auditory figure-ground perception.

An infant's sense of hearing is functional prior to birth. Immediately following birth, however, hearing usually is impaired because the auditory canals are filled with fluid. Normal hearing function usually is restored within a few days, and hearing improves rapidly. Young infants have been observed at birth to turn their eyes in the direction of the source of sound, although they seem unable to locate the exact position from where the stimulus originated. Although the ability is unrefined, newborns are able to make crude discriminations among different pitches. It appears that low-pitch sounds have a calming effect on newborns, whereas high pitches tend to elicit stress reactions. Shortly after birth, the neonate can differentiate sounds of different duration, which is critical to processing spoken language. After 4 months, most new sounds (as opposed to ambient sounds) stimulate searching activities in the infant, an aspect of auditory localization. These activities may include head turning, reaching, and movement toward the sound. Some evidence also suggests that by 6 months of age, infants are almost as sensitive to sounds as adults are. The ability to localize distant auditory stimuli occurs around 12 months and continues to improve. By age 3 years, children can localize, or determine, the general direction of sounds quite effectively. The ability to discriminate auditory sounds also continues into childhood. There is significant improvement that extends to at least the early teens. Little information is available on the developmental characteristics of auditory figure-ground perception, other than the observation that some children have more difficulty than others separating irrelevant stimuli (background) from the primary task (figure). As with the other aspects of auditory perception, auditory figure-ground perception is closely associated with the ability to selectively attend to the stimuli in the environment.

In summary, although mastery of basic auditory skills is evident by the age of 3 years, refinement continues steadily until approximately 13 years of age, when near adult levels are reached.

TACTILE PERCEPTION

Objective 6.7

Tactile perception (touch) refers to the ability to detect and interpret sensory information cutaneously (of or on the skin). Most textbooks give little if any attention to tactile perception, perhaps because relatively little information is available on its developmental characteristics and because most aspects of this ability are not closely related to the study of motor behavior. Most information on tactile perception discusses the individual's ability to perceive pain, light, and temperature differences. However, from a motor behavior perspective, several considerations warrant a brief treatment. As we learned in an earlier section, the first phase of motor behavior is the reflexive phase. Several of these initial movements (e.g., grasping, rooting, and Babinski reflexes) are elicited through touch stimulation and are dependent on the infant's ability to detect tactile sensations. In conjunction with kinesthetic perception, often referred to as the *tactile-kinesthetic system*, the individual receives vital information in a movement context with regard to the position of the body in space. For example, a competitive gymnast walking across a balance beam relies primarily on tactile input through the feet and depends relatively little on visual or auditory information. Individuals who are blind depend heavily on tactile input to get feedback for organizing their movements.

Tactile sensations are picked up by numerous receptors and are transmitted to different areas of the brain for interpretation. With growth, increasing numbers of receptors are found in the skin over a wider area and in closer proximity.

The first responses to touch are elicited in the facial area of the fetus, specifically the lips. The general trend of sensitivity to tactile stimulation during the prenatal stage follows a cephalocaudal progression (i.e., head, trunk, and limb). The first prenatal reflex, elicited by tactile stimulation around the mouth, is opposite-side neck flexion at about 7½ weeks after conception.

The available information suggests that the development of touch discrimination and localization, as determined by a one-point tactile stimulus, is well developed by 5 years of age. By 8 years of age, children consistently are able to reproduce designs that have been drawn on one of their body parts such as the back of their hand. Interestingly, evidence also suggests that infant and adult females tend to be more sensitive to touch than males are.

One of the most researched aspects of tactile perception is the ability to recognize objects (e.g., letters and shapes) through tactile manipulation. Observations indicate that young children generally go from tactile to visual recognition of objects, which suggests that tactile perception may develop before the ability to visually identify objects does. In the context of learning, this type of behavior is quite evident in infants and their first responses to something hot, cold, or sharp.

The infant learns by touch, places this in memory, and from that time is able to recognize the characteristics of similar items by sight (e.g., fire or a red stove burner). After the age of 4 years, however, visual recognition of objects is consistently superior to the use of tactile manipulation.

PERCEPTUAL INTEGRATION

Objective 6.8

The discussion thus far has focused on the perceptual modalities as independent systems. The description of developmental characteristics and improvements within individual sensory systems is referred to as *intrasensory development*. The perceptual and perceptual-motor processes, however, frequently involve the simultaneous use of more than one system (i.e., *intersensory*). This process is known as **perceptual integration**. This type of functioning is commonplace in motor skill settings. For example, a skill such as hitting a baseball requires the interaction of visual, tactile, and kinesthetic information. The normal academic task of learning to read aloud requires vision and auditory integration. As the dynamic system develops and the individual experiences the environment with various affordances, this ability increases uniquely to the individual.

Closely associated with this ability and one of the most studied aspects of perception is **intermodal perception**, the ability to translate (perceive) information from one sensory modality to another. It is generally acknowledged that intermodal perception is partially functional at birth and improves with increasing age beyond the childhood years. The basic level involves the recognition of a specific stimulus or the features of a stimulus as the same or equivalent (match) when they are presented to two different perceptual modalities. For example, after being allowed to manipulate an object tactually (without use of vision), a child can recognize the object as the same item when permitted to use the visual modality.

One of the difficulties in interpreting any improvements in intersensory development is isolating improvements in intrasensory functioning, which may help improve perceptual integration. Researchers also have found it very difficult to explain how intersensory functioning affects the development of motor behavior. Despite these and other related problems, perceptual integration generally appears to increase with age through childhood as the person gains valuable experience. In subsequent pages, we discuss the effect of experience (i.e., the environment) on perceptual development as viewed by prominent theories, namely, Gibson's ecological perspective. The following briefly describes the development of intermodal perception.

Visual-Kinesthetic Integration

Visual and kinesthetic (VK) perceptual modalities appear to have some integrative characteristics in the very early stages of infancy. In fact, the abilities associated with VK integration seem to become refined before those of visual-auditory integration. Information on this topic usually includes mention of tactile integration due to its interrelation with kinesthetic awareness.

The research findings on this aspect of intermodal perception are relatively consistent; most sources note an improvement with increasing age through childhood, up to about 11 years of age. Some of the first indications of VK integration

think about it

Describe a few examples of sport activities that have a high degree of perceptual integration.

have been observed in children as young as 2 to 3 weeks of age. For example, babies at this age are able to imitate the mouth and tongue movements of adults. This is quite impressive considering that they cannot see (and probably never had) their own matched movement. Gibson and Walker (1984) reported that babies only 1 month old could recognize by sight (match) objects they had sucked previously. In these instances, the infants translated visual input into an equivalent body movement, thus exhibiting kinesthesis.

By 6 months of age, there are numerous studies indicating that children who explore an object with their hands alone can recognize it by sight alone. This type of intermodal perception appears to be nearly mature by the age of 5 years, with slight improvement until about 8 years (Williams, 1983). Evidence also suggests that, among the visual, tactile, and kinesthetic types of perception, VK integration abilities are the most advanced in 5-year-olds. Hence, the refinement of VK integration appears, in general, to lag behind visual-tactile integration. The interweaving process that occurs between the VK modalities is still somewhat of a mystery, as is the way in which intersensory integration affects the development of motor behavior. How experience affects the total process is perhaps as intriguing.

Visual-Auditory Integration

Although unrefined, visual and auditory (VA) perceptual abilities also appear to be integrated at birth. A common observation on which many research studies have been developed is that infants will orient their eyes in the direction from which sounds originate. For example, newborns turn their eyes and head toward the sound of a voice or rattle. By 4 months, infants can link VA information in a relatively coordinated manner. When shown a film of a bouncing toy monkey on one screen and a bouncing kangaroo on another screen, infants preferred to observe the film of the animal that bounced in rhythm with the sound track (Spelke, 1987). Thus, they apparently were able to identify the way in which the visual information matched the auditory stimuli. In a somewhat more sophisticated study (Wagner et al., 1981), the researchers found what has been suggested are quite remarkable abilities for young children 9 to 13 months of age. The children were presented with pairs of VA stimuli that matched each other abstractly. For example, a visual pair of a broken line and a continuous line was matched with an auditory pair of a pulsing tone and a continuous tone. The researchers determined that the infants were able to perceive similarity (i.e., match) in three of the eight stimuli sets. This was considered quite remarkable because infants typically are not exposed to these kinds of events.

In general, VA integration abilities are quite functional by 4 months and continue to improve markedly up to approximately 12 years.

Auditory-Kinesthetic Integration

Information on auditory-kinesthetic integration is limited. However, the available information suggests there is a natural compatibility between the auditory and kinesthetic modalities. In a frequently used testing procedure, the tester tells the child the name of an object or shape. The child then is asked to select the item tactually from a number of items to create an auditory-tactile/kinesthetic match. Consistent development differences have been reported between individuals 5 and

8 years old. The evidence also suggests that older children are markedly less variable as a group than younger children. Therefore, although only scant information on a small age range is available, evidence indicates that auditory-kinesthetic/tactile integration improves during childhood. Although intermodal perception is basically functional by the end of childhood, other forms of perception integration continue to improve throughout adolescence, with experience a significant influence.

CHANGES WITH ADVANCED AGING

Objective 6.9

As most people begin their middle-age years, the perceptual systems generally become less responsive to stimulation. However, most of these changes do not significantly interfere with everyday functions until the later adult years. Aside from the basic performance decrements associated with the VA perceptual modalities, little is known or understood about the effects of aging on the perceptual processes. This is especially evident with the various aspects of kinesthetic perception.

Visual Perception

A loss of visual abilities is one of the most noticeable changes in perceptual functioning as the body passes its peak performance level. Most people begin to notice changes in visual acuity between 40 and 50 years of age. Although individuals in their 70s and 80s have 20/20 acuity, only about 25% of 70-year-olds and 10% of 80-year-olds exhibit this level of clarity. The loss of acuity is especially severe at low levels of illumination and for moving objects.

focus on change

Change in perceptual abilities with advancing age can influence (constrain) daily living activities.

Closely related to loss of acuity with age is the condition known as *presbyopia*. This is the reduction in the elasticity of the lens of the eye to the point where the lens can no longer change its curvature sufficiently to allow accommodation for nearsightedness (close vision). By age 60 years, this condition can greatly affect the eye's ability to focus on objects at close distance. As the eye ages, the lens also becomes thicker and less transparent, thus reducing the transmission of light through the lens.

Sensitivity to light is important to optical functioning; it is a major consideration with the elderly. As a result of increased density and yellowing of the lens, the amount of light that enters the eye is reduced; thus, older adults are less able to see in low levels of illumination. Closely associated with this is the ability of the eyes to adapt to dim light; this is particularly evident after age 60 years. Another form of light sensitivity that appears to affect older individuals, especially after age 60 years, is glare. This also is attributed in part to age changes in the lens that affect the scattering of light over the retinal surface. This, along with problems related to deteriorating acuity, has some practical implications for older individuals who attempt to function in reduced light conditions. One obvious suggestion for minimizing the effects of these changes is to increase the light levels in environments where older adults live and participate in leisure activities.

The information related to aging and its effects on depth perception suggests little or no change up to 60 years. However, in late adulthood, this aspect of perception declines, making it difficult for the person to determine how close, how far away, how high, or how low something is. Lateral field of vision reaches a peak at approximately 35 years of age and gradually decreases until about 60 years of age, when the decline continues at a much more rapid rate. In addition to associative changes within the visual modality, age-related changes in facial structure (i.e., upper eyelid and orbital eye sockets) also have been linked to the decrease in field of vision.

Auditory Perception

With aging comes a gradual loss of hearing that begins around the mid-30s and continues to progress at least into the 80s. The most common type of age-related hearing loss is associated with the gradual deterioration and hardening of the auditory nerve cells. As a result of this condition, the sensitivity to high-frequency tones is impaired earlier and more severely than the sensitivity to low-frequency tones is. The term used to describe this kind of hearing loss is *presbycusis*.

Beginning at about age 40 years, there are marked sex differences in auditory perception. There is some suggestion that hearing loss is due in part to environmental noise stress, especially in male-dominated occupations. Hearing loss at higher frequencies becomes more apparent after age 50 years, especially in males. For age groups older than 60 years, hearing loss progresses to affect the lower frequencies, so that hearing in the elderly is generally impaired for a wide range of tones.

Kinesthetic Perception

Most of the research on kinesthetic perception is grouped under the heading of somesthetic senses. Recall that the word *somatosensory* refers to sensations from the body, which in this context also includes tactile perception. Except for functioning of the vestibular system (balance) and tactile perception, little is actually known about the effects of aging on the kinesthetic receptors and the individual's sense of body position. As with the other perceptual modalities, it might be expected that people approaching middle age would have diminished somesthetic function that would result in a reduced awareness of bodily orientation, movement, and touch. However, research findings on age differences in somesthetic sensitivity have not provided clear-cut evidence of this parallel. Although structural and functional age effects have been found, no overall deterioration across modalities in the somatic domain is evident. This should be considered a preliminary evaluation of the somesthetic domain, however, because documentation of many of these areas is sparse or absent.

Perhaps the most abundant information available about age effects on somesthetic sensitivity is in tactile perception. Some evidence suggests that elderly persons frequently suffer a loss in sensitivity to touch; however, the degree of loss varies widely among individuals and differs for various parts of the body. For example, with advancing age, touch sensitivity of the lower extremities is typically more impaired than that of the upper body. Caution should be taken in interpreting results such as these, for impairments observed might be related to factors other than age, such as disease, injuries, or circulatory problems. The primary age-related factors responsible for diminished touch sensitivity have been fairly well established. For example, there are cross-sectional age reductions in the number of touch receptors (i.e., Pacinian corpuscles and Meissner's corpuscles) in the skin.

Malfunctioning of the vestibular system, as evidenced by decreased performance on balance tasks, dizziness, and vertigo, is a common characteristic among

TABLE 6.4 Summary of Selected Perceptual Changes with Advanced Aging

Perceptual Characteristic		
Visual Perception	**Auditory Perception**	**Kinesthetic Perception (Somesthetic)**
Acuity (decreases)	Sensitivity to high and low frequencies (decreases)	Touch sensitivity (decreases)
Sensitivity to light (decreases)		Sense of body position and movement (no major change)
Depth perception (little change <60 and then declines)		Weight discrimination (decreases)
Visual information processing (decreases)		Balance (decreases)
Perception of movement (decreases)		

older adults. From approximately 40 years of age, a gradual deterioration of vestibular nerve cells takes place. Sensory cell loss may begin as early as the fifth decade in the semicircular canals. It may be quite marked in the saccule and utricle as well after the age of 70 years. As in the case of the cochlear nerve fibers, evidence suggests that the loss of fibers is due to the accumulation of bony material around the opening through which the nerve fibers pass. Apparently, as the holes become smaller, the nerve fibers compress and gradually degenerate. Although decreasing balance performance points to vestibular malfunction in older adults (as one factor), the underlying mechanisms responsible for this response have not been defined clearly. Chapter 11 discusses balance in greater detail.

As noted earlier, currently, little is known about sense of body position (kinesthesis) in the elderly. Although older persons generally show a decrease in the ability to discriminate weight (e.g., held in hands while blindfolded), there are some indications that no major changes occur in active joint-movement (body positioning) sensation. For example, Meeuwsen and colleagues (1992) reported no significant differences in young and older adults in their ability to blindly compare upper limb body position by location and extent (degree of change). More important, however, the researchers suggest that age-related declines in the elderly cannot be generalized to all perceptual systems.

Table 6.4 summarizes selected perceptual changes due to advanced aging.

think about it

Describe the impact of regression of perceptual abilities on daily living activities in the elderly. Consider the impact on playing a simple game of softball.

GIBSON'S ECOLOGICAL PERSPECTIVE

Objective 6.10

Although the role of biology/environment in children's perceptual development represents one of the classic debates in developmental psychology, most contemporary theorists view the process from an interactive perspective. That is, they believe changes in the ways human beings perceive the world reflect a fundamental interplay between nature (maturation) and nurture (experience and learning within their cultural context). Thelen and Smith (1994) introduced the importance of this body of information profoundly by suggesting that "movement as perception,

focus on change

Ecological context is a strong determinant in developmental *change*.

is the critical role of movement in development" (p. 193). More recently, Adolph and Robinson (2015) stated that "children learn to choose appropriate (motor) actions by perceiving and generalizing affordances for action" (p. 115).

The perceptual theory that has had the greatest impact on our understanding of how infants perceive and act on that information in the form of movement is **Gibson's ecological perspective**, proposed by Eleanor Gibson (2001) and James Gibson (1979, 2014). An important characteristic of this theory is the assumption that infants can directly perceive information that exists in the environment. Perception is an active cognitive process in which each individual selectively interacts with a richly varied field of perceptual possibilities. This ties in with our earlier discussion of intermodal perception. According to this perspective, infants actively explore for *invariant features* of the environment—that is, features that remain stable in a constantly changing perceptual world. They search for features that stand out and then they explore their internal characteristics. In this exploration, over time, the infant makes finer and finer distinctions about the feature. This process is *differentiation* (hence, another name for this perspective is *differentiation theory*). This perspective is in contrast to the traditional (constructivist) view that, rather than being able to directly perceive information in the environment, individuals have to make a construction based on sensory input and past experience. In other words, the environment has no meaning without experience. With ecological theory, perceiving is experiencing. The child is an active explorer in the process, where perception and action are coupled.

think about it

In the perception → action model, where and how does Gibson's ecological perspective fit?

Movement plays a critical role in this perspective because it provides the infant with means of exploration and a diverse sampling of environmental stimuli. Central to this notion is the observation that infants constantly explore ways in the environment that afford opportunities for action. The environment provides *affordances* that invite and challenge the infant to perceive and act on information (invariant features). **Affordances** are opportunities for action that objects, events, or places in the environment provide (e.g., toys, stairs, and dance class). This is a major concept in the study of motor skill development today. How the infant acts on the affordance depends on the infant's

1. Developmental level
2. Past experiences
3. Present need
4. Cognitive awareness of what the object might be used for

focus on change

Environmental affordances promote developmental *change*.

The notion of affordances emphasizes there is an **ecological fit** between the individual and the situation. The following examples apply to our study of motor development.

First is the concept of graspability, that is, whether an object is the appropriate size and shape and within reach. By exploring the object, the infant learns a great deal. A considerable body of research suggests that infants as young as 3 months actually perceive graspability before they are capable of successfully performing the action. That is, after viewing objects that are and are not graspable, they show indications of reaching for those that are the appropriate size and distance for grasping, and simply track the others (Bower, 1989).

In what is arguably a classic study, Adolph and colleagues (1993) observed two groups of infants, 14-month-old walkers and 8½-month-old crawlers, as they moved up and down ramps sloped at varied degrees (Fig. 6.8). The researchers predicted that older infants would react more carefully to the inclines due to prior

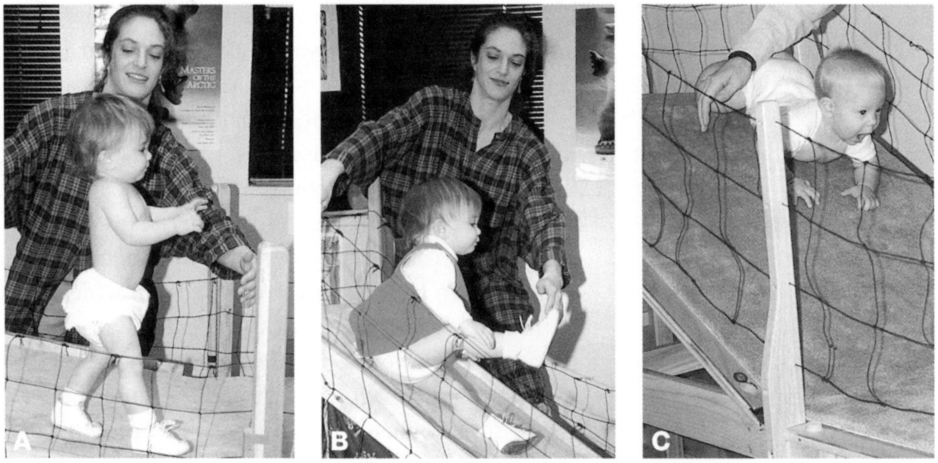

Figure 6.8 Like the other 14-month-olds in Karen Adolph's study, Lauren perceives that a gently sloping ramp **(A)** affords walking and confidently descends the ramp. When later confronted with a steep slope, **(B)** Lauren, like the other experienced walkers in the study, perceives the affordance of falling, and consequently slides down the slope. **(C)** This is in marked contrast to the inexperienced 8-month-olds, who, like Jack, try to descend every slope, no matter how steep it is, by crawling, and sometimes end up in a nose dive.

think about it

Identify some typical affordances in the environment that challenge the prewalking infant. What motor skills do they trigger?

experience with walking; that is, they would perceive the affordance of falling. Their prediction was correct. Older infants confidently walked down gentle slopes and negotiated steeper inclines by sliding down (some went down backward). In comparison, the young group of infants, regardless of slope difficulty, tried to crawl down (mothers were there to catch them) and never attempted alternative ways of descent. In essence, the older group, due to experience and perceptual ability, found a fit between their abilities and the environment (slopes).

More recently, using a wider developmental scope, Ishak and colleagues (2014) examined the development of affordance perception for reaching through openings of various sizes. The study involved five age groups of children 16 months to 7 years and young adults. The researchers examined the *affordance function* of participant's actual ability to fit the hand through openings, and the *decision function* of attempts to reach. In some cases, the openings were not feasible. The study determined that compared to adults, decisions were less accurate in children and they were more likely to attempt impossible openings and to touch openings prior to refusing. That suggested a slow developmental trend in learning to perceive such affordances. Interestingly, although not as accurate, the youngest participants were equally consistent in their decision making as the oldest ones and that every age group showed sensitivity to changes in the environment by scaling their attempts to opening size. Why the difference between children and adults? The first possibility is that affordance perception does not approach adultlike accuracy until later in childhood. Also, errors stem from a liberal response criterion—meaning, young children may consider more options and not consider errors a problem. Third, young children are driven to explore new affordances, and fourth, the immaturity of executive function in young children. In summary, young children were more exploratory. Although accuracy improves with age, young children are no less consistent or sensitive to affordances compared with adults.

Overall, the ecological perspective provides us with one idea of how perception → action works, perhaps the most relevant question in the study of motor development. See Adolph and Robinson (2015) for an excellent summary of affordance research with young children.

EMBODIMENT

The idea drives **embodiment**, also known as *embodied cognition*, is that *cognitive processes, including thinking, are deeply grounded in our bodily interactions* with the environment (e.g., Barsalou, 2008; Glenberg, 2015; Sadeghipour & Kopp, 2012). That is, cognitive representations and actions are inextricably linked—actions are central to the development of new representations. One of the major propositions of this general body of work is the notion that the motor system contributes to higher level cognitive processing. One of the first tactics used to study embodied cognition was the classic A-not-B error paradigm described earlier. In most of those studies, associations between attention, reaching (bodily action), and memory were explored; for more contemporary uses of the paradigm, see Marcovitch et al. (2015) and Zmyj et al. (2015).

More recently, several innovative approaches have been used to study the connection between bodily actions and cognition (Fig. 6.9). For example, research with school children shows that using physical activity and gestures that align with scientific concepts, math, reading, and foreign language improves learning (e.g., Mavilidi et al., 2015; McClelland et al., 2015; Toumpaniari et al., 2015).

Another interesting line of interesting inquiry has emerged. These studies have examined the interactions between the motor system and the processing of numbers (e.g., Lindemann & Fischer, 2015; Noël, 2005). The implications are that the representation of numbers and finger movements in the adult brain maybe linked to finger-counting strategies used in childhood. Noël's (2005) data supported this idea in part when the research reported that finger differentiation ability in Grade 1, predicted numerical ability at the end of Grade 2. A follow-up study by Gracia-Bafalluy and Noël (2008) reported that finger differentiation training in young children improved the learning of numerical skills. In summary, the studies mentioned support the notion of a bodily foundation and role in cognitive development.

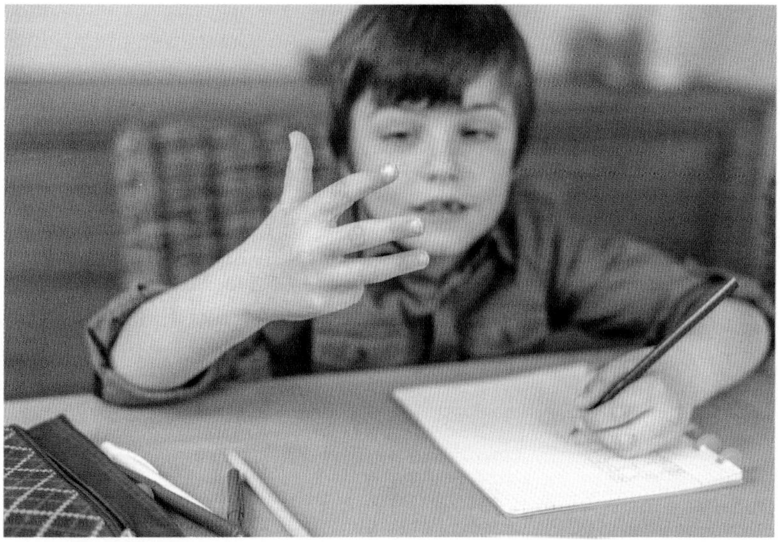

Figure 6.9 Research indicates that finger counting is an embodied process associated with analytical (numerical) skills.

PERCEPTUAL-MOTOR TRAINING PROGRAMS

Objective 6.11

Several perceptual-motor programs introduced during the 1950s and into the early 1970s received considerable attention in the educational and research communities (e.g., Delacato, 1966; Kephart, 1971). It should be noted that with the current push and pressure on education to demonstrate student achievement, similar programs have emerged. Underlying most of these earlier theories was the assumption of a strong direct link between perceptual-motor functioning and cognitive functioning. Deficiencies in cognitive performance, such as reading and spelling, were attributed primarily to poor sensory integration. Perceptual shortcomings were seen to be remediable through perceptual-motor training activities requiring those perceptual judgments. For example, some theorists believed that participation in activities involving eye–hand coordination, laterality, directionality, and balance could enhance cognitive and academic abilities.

Although some proponents of these theories still exist and such programs are available, little general support from the scientific community can be found. Convincing evidence of a true link between perceptual-motor skills and cognition has not been presented. Most studies have reported little or no relationship among perceptual-motor development, perception, and academic performance. Kavale and Mattson (1983) conducted a sophisticated study of 180 scientific reports designed to research the efficacy of perceptual-motor programs. The researchers concluded that perceptual-motor intervention appears to be ineffective and noted that, compared with other forms of educational intervention, the effects of such programs are negligible. Furthermore, Salvia and Ysseldyke (1991) state, "There is a tremendous lack of empirical evidence to support the claim that specific perceptual-motor training facilitates the acquisition of academic skills or improves the chances of academic success. Perceptual-motor training will improve perceptual-motor functioning" (p. 322). This in itself is a reasonable goal in motor development programming, especially during the childhood years.

think about it

How would you present the position that movement-based activities are important to child development?

It is interesting to note that with the recent findings in early brain research and the effects of stimulation on development (Chapter 2), dramatic claims for training effects have emerged. Claims are being made, for example, that music and movement activities for infants and young children enhance intellectual abilities. For example, the Mozart effect theory suggests that exposing young children to classical music may boost their brainpower. It was reported in a major national newsmagazine in 2001 that balancing activities improve learning of math. One trademarked national program currently active claims that "specific exercises . . . improve reading, writing, and overall academic achievement."

First of all, as discussed in Chapter 2, there is little doubt that early stimulation positively affects brain development. However, there is little evidence to suggest that structural change relates to change or improvement in specific functional behavior. Bigger is not necessarily better.

As a final word at this time, the National Academies convened a group of the top developmentalists to address this issue. In the final report *From Neurons to Neighborhoods: The Science of Early Childhood Development* (Shonkoff & Phillips, 2000), it was noted that although early stimulation and relationships are critical to development, "there are no special programs that are guaranteed to accelerate early learning during infancy. Despite the proliferation of materials that claim to raise babies' IQs, there is lack of hard scientific evidence on how enrichment activities affect early brain development. For example, the so called Mozart effect has never been studied in young children."

Summary

Both perception and the perceptual-motor process are related to information processing, which involves monitoring and interpreting sensory information, and deciding on and organizing a motor response. Of the six perceptual modalities, the two that provide the most relevance to the study of motor behavior are vision and kinesthesis.

Visual perception, considered to be the dominant modality, undergoes several structural and functional changes across the life span. Significant structural differences between the newborn and adult are accompanied by functional changes associated with motor behavior.

Kinesthetic perception, often referred to as the sixth sense, encompasses the awareness of movement and body position. It involves the ability to discriminate positions and movements of the body based on information derived from sensory receptors in the body. The various aspects of kinesthetic perception may be described with regard to their physiological and more applied characteristics (movement awarenesses).

Although they are generally not considered as vital to motor behavior as VK perception, the auditory and tactile modalities provide important cues to successful movement responses.

Although discussions of perceptual development usually focus on the various modalities as independent systems (denoting intrasensory change), the actual perceptual-motor process frequently involves the simultaneous use of more than one system (perceptual integration). A much studied aspect of this ability is intermodal perception that is partially functional at birth and improves with increasing age beyond the childhood years.

Although most people experience some form of regression in perceptual function beginning in middle age, most changes do not significantly affect everyday activities until old age. Most noted among the forms of regression are losses in visual acuity, sensitivity to light, hearing, and a loss of balance.

Gibson's ecological perspective provides insight into our understanding of how infants perceive and act on information in the environment. Embodied cognition is based on the idea that cognition is largely influenced by bodily (sensorimotor) actions. In the past and even today, there have been claims that specific movement-based perceptual-motor programs directly affect academic skills. But they have received little support from the scientific community.

think about it

1. **Consider child's play. How is it related to embodiment?**
2. **In what ways can you modify the visual cliff experiment to study other aspects of depth perception?**
3. **What are the constraints to effective coincident timing in young children (e.g., 5- to 7-year-olds)?**
4. **What motor skill activities require a high degree of kinesthetic ability?**
5. **What physical activities and sports require a high level of directional awareness?**

6. **Is there any practical application of the information on movement awarenesses?**
7. **Describe a few examples of sport activities that have a high degree of perceptual integration.**
8. **Describe the impact of regression of perceptual abilities on daily living activities in the elderly. Consider the impact on playing a simple game of softball.**
9. **In the perception → action model, where and how does Gibson's ecological perspective fit?**
10. **Identify some typical affordances in the environment that challenge the prewalking infant. What motor skills do they trigger?**
11. **How would you present the position that movement-based activities are important to child development?**

LEARNING ACTIVITIES

Objective: To explore A-not-B error and object permanence. View research via the Web to find two contemporary (not older than 3 years old) scientific journal articles that expand the A-not-B error idea. Write a brief one-page summary of each describing the researcher(s) intent, method, results/discussion, and how the experiment is relevant to earlier work.

Objective: To assess the home environment for motor affordances. Using one of the Affordances in the Home Environment for Motor Development (AHEMD) (Chapter 13) assessment tools, evaluate the home of a baby or young child. With the assessment results, provide recommendations for improvement of the environment.

Objective: To assess a perceptual-motor (movement) program advertised on the Web. Briefly describe the program, its goals, and claims (if given). Then, provide a critique of the program.

Suggested Readings

Goldstein, B. E. (2014). *Sensation and perception* (9th ed.). Wadsworth, OH: Cengage Learning.

Spirduso, W. W., Francis, K. L., & MacRae, P. G. (2005). *Physical dimensions of aging* (2nd ed.). Champaign, IL: Human Kinetics.

Chapter 7

Information Processing and Motor Control

■ OBJECTIVES

Upon completion of this chapter, you should be able to

7.1 Discuss the roots of information-processing theory.

7.2 Diagram the information-processing model and describe its four basic components.

7.3 Describe the functional and developmental aspects associated with attention.

7.4 Discuss memory with regard to definition, structures, processing strategies, and changes across the life span.

7.5 Discuss the various processes and developmental characteristics associated with information-processing speed and movement time.

7.6 Define *programming* and explain its relationship to motor planning.

7.7 Discuss the three developmental theories and approaches to the study of motor control.

7.8 Describe the theory and application of the constraints model.

7.9 Briefly describe the possible effects of advanced aging on the various aspects of information processing.

KEY TERMS

- divided attention
- selective attention
- recognition memory
- recall memory
- working memory
- contextual learning
- processing speed
- reaction time (RT)
- programming
- motor program
- coordinative structures
- dynamic systems
- rate controller
- self-organizing properties
- subsystems
- neuronal group selection theory (NGST)
- developmental cognitive neuroscience (DCN)
- constraints model
- constraint

Information processing is involved in virtually all forms of human behavior. Whether from the perspective of cognitive psychology or the acquisition and performance of a motor skill, the ability to process information is a major contemporary issue in human development.

Chapters 6 and 7 provide a general framework for studying the complex processes involved in perception → action. Chapter 6 focused on the developmental aspects of the perceptional systems and provided insight into how individuals act on information in the environment (ecological perspective). Chapter 7 extends our quest to understand the issue by underscoring two critical factors in the perception-to-action process: *programming* a motor plan and *theories and approaches to the study of motor control* (i.e., executing the plan via the motor system). In addition, the constraints model is provided as an excellent applied approach to the study of motor behavior. The topics of attention, memory, and processing speed also are covered, given their developmental significance in the formulation and execution of a motor plan.

focus on change

Change in information-processing ability represents the core element in movement and sport performance.

Objective 7.1

Information processing is an approach to understanding human development and behavior that became established during the 1970s with the mass popularity of computers. The roots of the information-processing approach are in the fields of computer science (manipulation of symbols), communications theory (information coding and channel capacity), and linguistics (language). As long ago as 1949, psychologists compared human processing to basic computer functions in which information is encoded, stored, transformed, retrieved, and acted on. During these early stages of information theory, mathematical models were developed to make quantitative predictions about human behavior. Of the numerous traditional and contemporary theories of human development, information processing now dominates the field of cognitive psychology.

think about it

Reflecting back on Chapter 6, how does the information presented here fit the general information-processing model (Fig. 6.1 on page 150)?

Objective 7.2

One of the popular approaches to studying the execution of a motor response has been to conceptualize the process in terms of an information-processing model. Motor developmentalists are concerned with the way individuals use information in perceiving, making decisions, and organizing activity in relationship to the demands the environment places on them. Four basic components have been

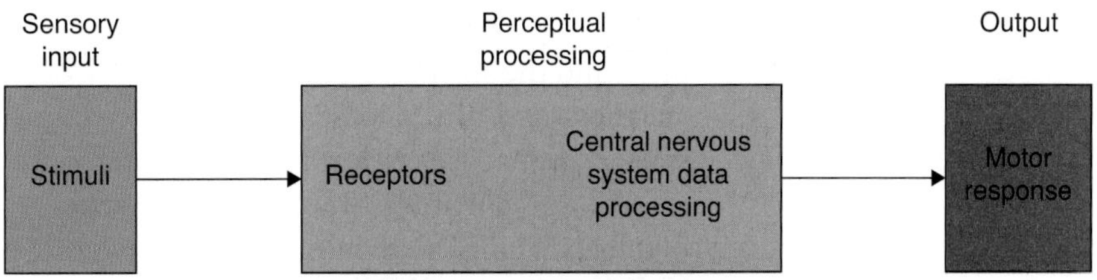

Figure 7.1 The basic information-processing model.

identified in the simplified model of information processing in Figure 7.1: sensory (afferent) input, reception of information through the various perceptual modalities, interpretation and decision making (processing), and an overt motor (efferent) response.

As individuals progress toward adulthood, they are able to process more information in a shorter period of time. This concept is relatively simple. Yet, the structural and functional aspects of information processing to which it refers are complex and, in several instances, remain in the little black box of the unknown or highly theoretical.

ATTENTION

Objective 7.3

Attention usually is considered the core of information-processing models. And there is convincing evidence this aspect of information processing changes across the life span. More than a century ago, William James, one of the earliest and most renowned experimental psychologists, described *attention* as "focalization, concentration, and of consciousness" (James, 1950). Although several definitions have been proposed since James's work, two features inherent in his statement are still prominent today. First is the notion that attention is *limited* (an individual capacity exists) so that an individual can attend to only one thing at a time, or think only one thought at a time. From a motor behavior perspective, this statement suggests an individual's capacity could be exceeded if too much activity were attempted. Second, attention is apparently performed in a *serial manner*, which suggests that individuals attend to one thing and then another and that it is difficult (sometimes impossible) to combine certain activities.

Although attention is a key component in information-processing models, it is also a strong factor in the successful performance of a motor task. Three basic concepts associated with attention and motor behavior have been identified: (a) Attention involves alertness and preparation of the motor system to produce a response; (b) attention is related to individuals' limited capacity to process information; and (c) the successful performance of a motor task requires selective attention, the ability to select and attend to meaningful information. The following pages discuss the functional and developmental aspects associated with these concepts and give particular emphasis to capacity and selective attention. For detailed discussions of attention theory as it relates to motor behavior, see Magill and Anderson (2013) and Schmidt and Lee (2014).

Alertness

Alertness and preparation of the perceptual-motor system prior to any initiated motor task are vital aspects of attention and successful movement response.

These conditions are evident in the softball batter preparing for the incoming pitch and the sprinter in the starting block before the gun. The levels of perceptual alertness and physiological preparation immediately preceding the pitch or the starter's signal are critical to the outcome of these events.

A large portion of the research on this aspect of attention has dealt with individuals' ability to exhibit alertness and response preparation by assessing their ability to detect a visual or auditory signal in a predetermined fashion. Researchers have typically used *reaction time* (RT) experiments to test these abilities. RT is the interval of time between the onset of a stimulus and the initiation of a response. This topic is discussed in greater detail in a subsequent section. However, an example of alertness is relevant.

In the case of the sprinter, RT is the period of time from the moment the auditory stimulus (gunshot) was received by the auditory receptors to the point just prior to the first motor response. The RT phase includes attention (alertness) to the stimulus, motor system preparation (body position and muscle tension), reception and transmission of the stimulus, interpretation of the information, and organization of a motor program with which to execute the response. Numerous sophisticated functional characteristics are performed within the general alertness and preparation stages. Successful athletes, such as the softball batter, learn to anticipate upcoming conditions by being alert.

Divided Attention

Another aspect of attention that has strong implications for motor performance is the concept of limitations in the capacity to handle information from the environment. This aspect of attention represents the concept of **divided attention**. This term refers to concentrating on more than one activity at the same time, in essence, dividing your attention. Because capacity is believed to be limited, *interference* will occur if another activity requires the same resources. Interference could result in the following: (a) a loss of speed or quality in the performance of one of the activities, (b) both activities could be affected, or (c) the second activity could be ignored.

The operational definition of attention generally includes the notion of interference. However, it is possible to perform two tasks simultaneously as long as the total amount of processing capacity is not exceeded. The amount of the capacity resources required for any task or tasks depends on the activity and the individual. Examples of divided attention are abundant in everyday life as individuals try to handle several cognitive tasks at once, sometimes unsuccessfully. The act of driving a car while conducting a conversation may not be difficult if both conditions are relatively light and undemanding. However, if the road conditions deteriorate or the conversation turns to something complex or emotional, processing capacity may become overloaded and performances may suffer.

Numerous studies of the processing capacity of attention have used the dual-task paradigm in which subjects are observed as they perform two tasks simultaneously. Typically, under this method, individuals are presented a primary task and secondary task separately and then are asked to perform the tasks simultaneously. Presumably when the tasks are executed simultaneously, any differences between the events indicate where and how individuals allocate their capacity resources. Younger children most often allocate their available attention somewhat equally between two tasks, whereas older children appear to recognize the significance of the primary task, attend to it, and perform better on it.

Focus on Application
Texting and Driving

Virtually, everyone agrees that texting and reading text while driving is dangerous, but how much does it impair the driver? Caird and colleagues (2014) did an analysis of "scientific" studies completed up to that year. The researchers concluded that texting (typing) and reading text messages while driving adversely affected several abilities important to safe driving; for example, eye movements, reaction time, lane positioning, speed, and maintaining the correct headway (lane).

Rumschlag et al. (2015) examined the influence of driver age (18 to 59 years old) and other factors on the disruptive effects of texting on simulated driving behavior. While driving, the participants were engaged in a series of brief text conversations with a member of the research team. Their primary aim was to examine texting effect on *land excursions*, defined as any time the vehicle moved outside the directed driving lane. Excursions were not observed when not texting, *but 66% of subjects overall exhibited excursions while texting*. Text task duration was significantly correlated with the number of excursions, and texting skill level and driver age were significantly correlated with the percentage of excursions (see figure). Gender of the driver was not an influence. Interestingly, among "highly skilled" (versus less skilled) texters, driver age was significantly correlated with the number of excursions. For those self-identified as not highly skilled texters, text task "duration" was a factor in the number of excursions.

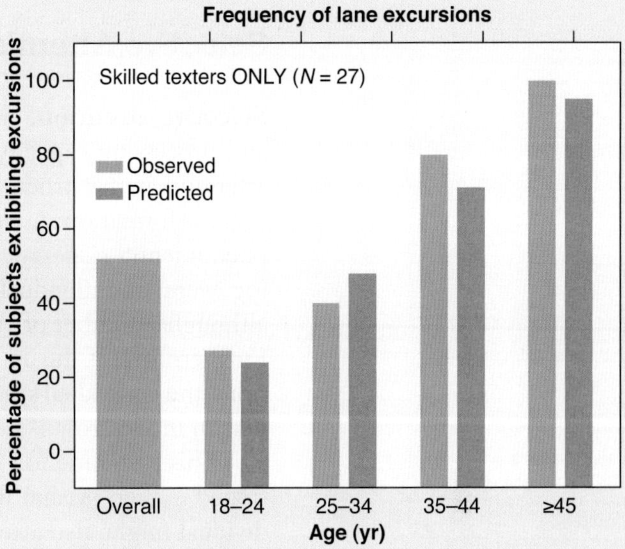

As the researchers and others studying this topic have concluded, the best practice is "no texting while driving."

Sources:

Caird, J. K., Johnston, K. A., Willness, C. R., Asbridge, M., & Steel, P. (2014). A meta-analysis of the effects of texting on driving. *Accident Analysis & Prevention*, *71*, 311–318.

Rumschlag, G., Palumbo, T., Martin, A., Head, D., George, R., & Commissaris, R. L. (2015). The effects of texting on driving performance in a driving simulator: the influence of driver age. *Accident Analysis & Prevention*, *74*, 145–149.

Capacity allocation (time-sharing efficiency) improves with age, and developmental differences in attending to dual tasks primarily are due to automation and attention deployment skills. *Automation* is a possible source of age-related improvement in which the performance on one task remains the same with less attention used, thus freeing up processing resources for performing a concurrent task. For example, because driving a car requires more attention for the novice, interference while talking to another person is much more likely than with an experienced driver. For many of us, driving in normal conditions is relatively automatic. The underlying notion is that the cognitive processes involved in a task compete for limited central-processing capacity. Therefore, as children grow older, they become more adept at controlling the allocation of their attention (through the use of strategies) and require less of the capacity resources.

A much-debated issue on the topic of processing ability is whether improvements are due primarily to structural increases (actual capacity) or control operations (e.g., the use of strategies). However, it is quite likely that change is a result of structural changes in the central nervous system (CNS) as well as qualitative alterations due to experience.

Selective Attention

Selective attention, although closely related to alertness, response preparation, and processing capacity, is a distinguishable characteristic of attention. Selective attention is the processing of relevant information and nonprocessing of irrelevant information. A frequently used generalization is the "classic" cocktail party phenomenon (Cherry, 1953). During a large gathering such as a party or sporting event, an individual can attend selectively to a conversation with one person, although a number of other conversations and noise are taking place around them. Furthermore, if during that personal conversation someone in the crowd mentions the individual's name, his or her attention is immediately diverted to that person in the crowd.

This phenomenon is related closely to another perceptual characteristic mentioned earlier—visual figure-ground perception. Under these conditions, the individual might also attend selectively (visually) to the relevant information in the environment (the figure) and set it apart from its background. Selective attention, however, may involve more than one sense; for example, an individual catching a fly ball must separate relevant information (the ball) from an environment that may be filled with trees, clouds, and crowd noise.

Evidence suggests that children as young as 4 months of age have impressive selective attention abilities; however, refinement appears to continue during the childhood years. In general, older children show better control of selective attention by processing more stimulus features relevant to a particular task and by not processing those that are irrelevant. In contrast, younger children tend to select features of a task that stand out or are salient. And, as noted in the dual-task paradigm studies, older children are more organized and strategic in their processing abilities.

As a general observation, older (school-age) children can concentrate longer than younger children can and can focus on the information they need while screening out irrelevant information. For example, young children (2 to 5 years) most often pay exclusive attention to one event. Observations of younger children also suggest they are more easily distracted than older children. For example, while watching television, they are more likely to play with toys, look around, and talk with other people during the viewing. The ability to concentrate and filter out distracting information steadily improves until early adolescence, around age 12 years (Tabibi & Pfeffer, 2007).

As with the other aspects of attention, age differences in selective attention abilities are attributed primarily to experience and the refinement of operational functions (i.e., the use of strategies). Through experience, adolescents and adults learn which stimuli are relevant to a particular situation and which are not relevant. They then adopt a strategy to address the situation. For example, the experienced softball batter knows from past events at what approximate point in the pitcher's delivery the ball will be released. The batter selectively attends to the point of release and follows the ball exclusively to the anticipated point of contact. In contrast, the young, inexperienced batter's attention may be diverted to crowd noise, words from opposing players, and unfamiliar actions of the pitcher. Because the past experiences of younger children likely will be limited, the use of selective attention strategies likely will be restricted. Several studies have noted that children can be taught to resist irrelevant cues and acquire selective attention strategies.

MEMORY

Objective 7.4

The study of *memory* and its various systems is vital to understanding information processing and motor performance. Up to this point in the text, various discussions have focused on the developmental aspects of the way information is selected and perceived by the CNS in preparation for a meaningful motor response. However, at some point in information processing, data entering the system must be retained or stored for future use. There have been numerous structural and operational definitions proposed for the term memory. In a broad sense, *memory refers to the retention and subsequent retrieval of information*. Some operational definitions also use the term synonymously with *remembering*. In a more global treatment, Tulving (1985) describes memory as the "capacity that permits organisms to benefit from their past experiences" (p. 385). Relevant to our discussion of memory from a developmental perspective are the two primary types: recognition and recall memory. **Recognition memory** involves noticing whether a stimulus is identical or similar to one previously experienced. In contrast, **recall memory**, the more advanced form of memory, involves remembering a stimulus that is not present.

think about it

Do you perceive general memory and the ability to recall movements (motor memory) as different from each other?

Most evidence suggests that developmental differences in memory system effectiveness derive primarily from functional refinement (*control-processing strategies*) rather than structural (capacity) increases. A basic knowledge of the various memory structures and their capacities is important to a more detailed understanding of developmental differences.

Memory Structures

To use a contemporary analogy, the operational relationship between the structural and functional components of memory is like that of a computer; the structure is similar to computer hardware, whereas control processes (strategies) are similar to software. Although numerous computerlike schematics and models have been developed and a vast array of terminology used to explain the concept of memory and its elements, the two-component model is mentioned most often in contemporary literature (e.g., Baddeley, 2012). According to this view, memory consists of two components: *working memory* and *long-term memory*. A theoretical representation of these systems and their relationship to a motor response is shown in Figure 7.2.

WORKING MEMORY

Working memory is the concept of short-term memory as a place for mental work—that is, a workbench that allows individuals to manipulate and assemble information. This component incorporates characteristics and functions traditionally associated with sensory, perceptual, attentional, and short-term memory processes involved in processing information. It also serves as a processing center to transfer information to long-term memory. This system has a small and limited capacity with a storage duration of generally not more than 30 seconds. Evidence of the way this workspace and moment of attentional focus come into play appears in numerous everyday situations. For example, an individual looks up a telephone number, closes the phone

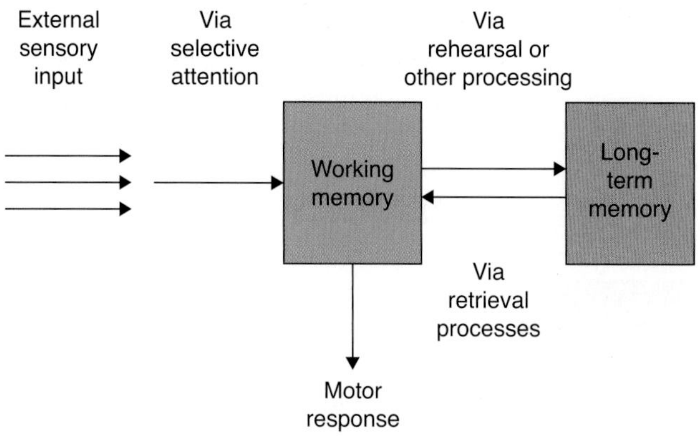

Figure 7.2 Memory systems and their relationship to motor response.

book, and by the time he finds the change for the call, forgets the number. Or, picture being introduced to three or four people at a meeting. You could remember the names immediately after introductions were made. But if you conversed for a minute or two and could not rehearse the names, you easily may have lost them.

The working memory system has a capacity of only about five to nine items (7+ or −2). For experimental purposes, the term *item* also has been used to designate the capacity of the system to hold single words or digits. Grouping separate items in some way to make larger collections is a process known as *chunking*. This technique, along with *rehearsal* (repeating the information one is trying to retain), significantly increases the number of items that can be retained; however, without practice or rehearsal, the capacity limit is about five to nine items.

The capacity of working memory is commonly determined using the memory span technique, in which an individual is presented with a list of digits or words at a given rate (usually one item per second) and asked to repeat the list. The number of items in the list is increased after each perfect recall. Memory studies using this technique are described in subsequent pages. The question of whether verbal and motor working memory are separate features of the memory system is yet to be resolved. Speculation suggests, however, there is one memory system that adapts to the unique requirements of verbal and motor skills.

LONG-TERM MEMORY

When items are rehearsed, they are transferred in some manner from short-term memory storage to long-term storage, where they can be held on a more permanent basis. Both the storage duration and capacity of *long-term memory* are seemingly unlimited. Storage can span hours, days, and, with several items, years. Perhaps the most often cited examples of long-term motor memory are the abilities to ride a bicycle and to swim after several years without any intervening practice. One thing that is clear is that long-term memory depends on what control processes and strategies people use when they are learning and remembering information such as rehearsal, coding, decisions, and retrieval strategies.

The following brief overview discusses the development of memory abilities most relevant to the study of motor development.

EARLY PROCESSING ABILITIES

The identification and extent of processing strategies and abilities infants use are difficult to determine. However, there are indications that primitive forms of recognition memory are present shortly after birth. Evidence of this phenomenon has been gathered primarily through observing *habituation*. A stimulus is presented to an infant and its responsiveness is monitored (e.g., time and quality of gaze). If the stimulus is repeated, reaction declines (reduced attention) and habituation is said to have occurred; but if a different stimulus is substituted, responsiveness generally increases. Theoretically, the renewed responsiveness to a new stimulus (referred to as *dishabituation*) can be viewed as evidence for recognition memory. Given adequate familiarization and relatively simple stimuli, memory in the form of dishabituation has been reported in numerous studies of newborns. For this type of behavior to occur, it appears that even newborns actively attend to the environment and encode information from it. Habituation improves dramatically throughout the first year, with 5- to 12-month-olds exhibiting the ability quite well. For an excellent review of habituation, see Aslin (2007).

WebLink

http://www.youtube.com/; see *Infant Looking Time Habituation.*

In general, the available evidence suggests that adultlike conscious recall memory emerges in the second 6 months of life, with this form of memory more evident by age 2 years, as exhibited in imitation and on memory span tests (Bauer, 2009). With imitation (nonverbal), infants are typically shown an action or action sequence and then allowed to imitate it. However, in a remarkable set of experiments conducted by Rovee-Collier and Barr (2001) with infants 3 and 6 months of age, cued recall (long-term) memory has been shown, that is, a recollection prompted by a cue associated with the setting (context) in which the recalled memory originally occurred. This phenomenon also is associated with **contextual learning**, a much-studied topic in memory today. Perhaps most intriguing about these studies is the experimental setup, which is presented in a motor domain. Infants are placed on their backs in a baby crib, with one of their ankles attached by a ribbon to an overhead mobile (Fig. 7.3). The infants learn within a few minutes that by kicking their leg, the mobile moves; the faster and harder they kick, the more the mobile jiggles

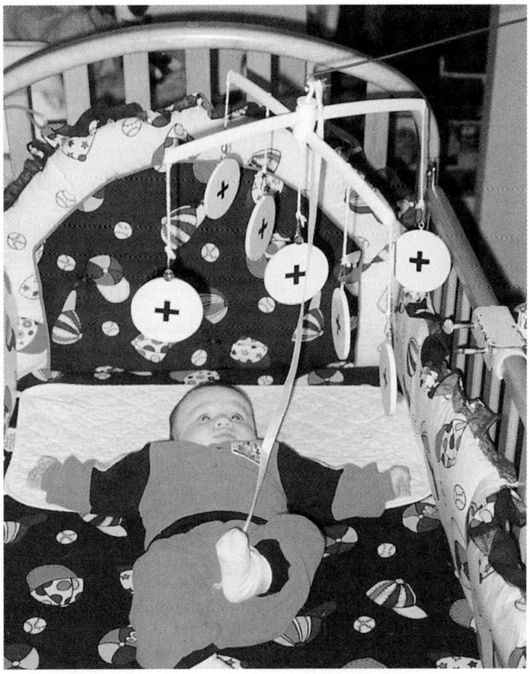

Figure 7.3 The technique used in Rovee-Collier's (2001) investigation of infant memory. The mobile is connected to the infant's ankle by the ribbon and moves in direct proportion to the frequency and vigor of the infant's kicks.

WebLink

http://www.jove.com/; see *Quantifying Learning in Young Infants: Tracking Leg Actions During a Discovery-learning Task*

think about it

Can you think of any application of contextual learning to sports?

and fascinates them with sights and sounds—a spectacle they truly enjoy. Before each training (learning) session begins, the number of kicks is recorded with the ribbon not attached (the infant simply views the interesting mobile). These data are used as the baseline for comparison with learned (attached) behavior in various conditions. Three-month-old infants typically double or triple their rate of kicks with a few minutes of training. After the ribbon is detached, the number of kicks decreases to baseline level. Then, as a test of immediate recognition, the ribbon is again attached and the rate of kicks compared to the previous attached behavior. Delayed retention (cued recall) of up to 42 days was measured by comparing original kick rate with the same or a novel mobile (ribbon attached). The prediction was that kick rate would be immediately similar within the same context and significantly less when compared to the novel condition.

The findings? Three-month-old infants exhibit near perfect retention 3 to 4 days after the training session, convincing evidence for (cued) long-term memory. At 6 months, another very interesting phenomenon occurs—the infants can discriminate with detail differences between the training mobile and the novel task for up to 2 weeks. In the training session for the older infants, the lining of the crib had a distinctive bumper pattern, which they apparently remembered, as evidenced by a significantly lower kick rate in a novel (different pattern) context. Several researchers consider this evidence for contextual learning and suggest that a unique and distinctive context serves as an effective retrieval cue. Researchers once thought infants were not capable of encoding information about where events occur; however, these results suggest otherwise. It also is suggested that this type of information is picked up and encoded in 3-month-old infants.

WORKING (SHORT-TERM) MEMORY ABILITIES

Evidence of working (recall) memory ability as shown by memory span research suggests that it improves markedly up to early adolescence. Memory span increases from about two digits in 2- and 3-year-olds to about five digits in 7-year-olds. And interestingly, from age 7 years to adulthood, the increase is only about two and a half digits (to a maximum of seven and a half digits).

A common method for testing short-term memory within a motor context is the use of an arm-positioning task in which the subject is asked to reproduce the location and distance of a movement. The general findings suggest that individuals are most successful in recalling location and that, in comparison, distance information seems to decay rather quickly.

An interesting study (Thomas et al., 1983) produced similar results in a field environment. The working memory of children (from age 4 to 12 years) was studied by asking them to reproduce location and distance after jogging through a predesigned course. The researchers suggested that all the children encoded location before distance information. They also found that the ability to recall distance improves with age, as does the apparent use of processing strategies such as rehearsal.

Overall, working memory increases with age. Children and older adults experience more difficulty with working memory than young adults. One of the explanations often cited is that as individuals age, they become *more efficient information processors*. With increasing age, they are quicker to recognize relevant information and more skilled at performing cognitive operations that tie to motor acts. As a result of practice or experience, children become more efficient at using their working memory space (Bjorklund, 2004). Another explanation that has gained attention is the *general capacity hypothesis*, which suggests that age-related changes primarily (but not exclusively) are related to processing capacity (e.g., Cowan et al., 2015).

Swanson et al. (1999) drew this conclusion after comparing a large sample of nine age groups, from ages 6 to 76 years. Subjects performed a series of verbal and visuospatial working memory tasks. Results indicated that young children and older adults experience a generalized lower level of performance due primarily to processing capacity constraints. Perhaps most important, age-related differences were not isolated to specific processes or strategies.

It appears the question remains: Are age-related differences due to process capacity or to efficiency? The extent of each is perhaps in need of continued debate, but there is no doubt that optimal performance is dependent on both.

LONG-TERM MEMORY ABILITIES

By age 2 years, children can recall interesting events that happened months ago and even relate them in the form of a story. However, their ability to do this is far from that of older children. Limitations are primarily in control processes and strategies related to coding, elaboration, rehearsal, decision making, and retrieval of information.

As children become older, they begin to engage in more formal memory strategies, such as *rehearsal.* Although evidence suggests that children as young as 5 years of age are able to rehearse and memorize information successfully if they are aided, they generally do not begin to independently rehearse on memory tasks efficiently until approximately 10 years of age (Flavell et al., 1993). Children around this same age group information rather well, but younger children are still relatively weak in their use of this strategy. However, evidence also suggests that compared to fourth graders (9 and 10 years old), adults tend to organize information in ways that make retrieval much easier.

Retrieval processes pertain to finding information located in long-term storage. The process requires the ability to both search the memory and decide the appropriate information has been retrieved. Differences between children and adults are evident in the retrieval process. The developmental pattern for retrieving ability is similar to that of rehearsal; that is, 10- and 11-year-old children are likely to use *elaboration strategies* (engaging in more extensive processing) to retrieve information from long-term storage, but 5- and 6-year-old children are not. Apparently, older children are better at conducting a thorough and systematic search of the memory store and selecting appropriate material.

With regard to general long-term memory performance and effective use of the control processes, most development appears to occur between the ages of 5 and 12 years. Younger children exhibit more deficiencies than older children.

Due perhaps to methodological problems associated with studies of memory over long periods of time, little information about long-term motor memory, particularly in children, is available. However, as evidenced by the Rovee-Collier and Barr (2001) (contextual learning) studies, memory for perceptual-motor actions can be substantial. General observations suggest that for well-learned continuous motor skills (i.e., skills with no distinct beginning or end), such as riding a bike and swimming, long-term motor memory loss is minimal.

With regard to discrete motor tasks (i.e., skills with a distinct beginning and ending) such as kicking and throwing, however, evidence suggests that forgetting can be considerable. For example, Schmidt and Lee (2014) suggest that discrete skills generally have more verbal-cognitive components, and these characteristics are more quickly forgotten than motor components are. In a review of discrete tasks that are highly motor in nature, Schmidt and Lee suggests that there is more to the difference than the motorness of the task.

think about it

Why can we recall how to ride a bicycle (and do it) after years of not practicing but forget what we wore to class last week?

TABLE 7.1 **Summary of Selected Memory Abilities**

Recognition	Recall
Habituation (newborn)	Higher level
cued recall (3 mo)	
contextual learning (6 mo)	
(6 mo) *short-term* emerges	
2 y evident	12 y
long-term 2 y	12 y
<8y weak encode/elaboration	

Not a great deal is known about how individuals code information for long-term storage so it might be retrieved several years later (e.g., how to ride a bicycle or swim). One possible explanation from a motor behavior perspective is that the specific patterns of a movement are not stored but rather a generalized motor program is formulated and placed in long-term storage. Motor programs are discussed later in this chapter.

KNOWLEDGE

It is a widely accepted notion that the knowledge an individual possesses probably contributes to memory abilities. In an interesting study that compared adults and children on memory for chessboard displays, it was found that children had significantly better recall than adults did (Chi, 1978). Initially, this result seems unusual, but the children were skilled chess players, whereas the adults were novices. It is suggested that due to the children's advanced knowledge base, they used chunking strategy to be more proficient at grouping items of information. It also could be assumed that because of their familiarity with the game, their processing was more efficient. Evidence such as this provides strong confirmation of the power of the effects of knowledge on long-term memory. More contemporary research supports this general observation (Staszewski, 2013).

Table 7.1 provides a summary of selected memory abilities.

PROCESSING SPEED AND MOVEMENT TIME

Objective 7.5

Processing speed is the rate of speed at which information is processed. Although not all cognitive or motor tasks require information to be processed at a fast rate, processing speed may account for many performance differences between children and adults. In a movement setting, there are numerous instances when the ability to recognize a stimulus and process information quickly is critical to an effective motor response (e.g., catching a ball or playing table tennis or badminton). Successful motor performance is based on a combination of perceptual recognition (attention), speed of memory functions, and neuromuscular response time.

Reaction time (RT) is the basic measure of processing speed. It refers to the interval of time between the onset of a stimulus (e.g., light, buzzer, or shock) and the initiation of a motor response (e.g., lifting a finger off a button). When the individual being tested is asked to respond to only one stimulus, the task is referred to as *simple reaction time*. *Choice RT* tasks are more complex and involve a greater information load because more than one signal requires discrimination in a more unpredictable setting. For example, a red light may mean move one way, blue another, and yellow another. A well-known concept related to processing speed, information load, and complexity is *Hick's law*: RT increases linearly as information load increases. That is, as the complexity of the processing task increases, so does the time it takes to process that information.

think about it

As future teachers and coaches, is there any practical value to this information: We (as adults) are about twice as fast with processing and reaction as a 5-year-old?

The time required to complete a motor response is referred to as *movement time*. Movement time combined with the RT is known as *response time*. RT usually is calculated as the amount of information (or bits) processed per second.

Comprehensive reviews about age differences in information-processing rates and performance on speeded tasks suggest that differences are large and remarkably consistent speed of processing, as determined by reaction time, improves with age up to the early adult years and then remains stable until about age 60 years (Salthouse, 2007). The period of greatest improvement appears to occur between the ages of 6 and 15 years (Fig. 7.4).

As a general observation, it takes a 5-year-old nearly two to three times as long as a 17-year-old to process one bit of information. This estimate was based on differences between simple and choice RTs. It has been suggested that the slower processing speed of children is due primarily to central processing factors, such as attention and speed of memory processes.

It was alluded to in the earlier discussion of memory storage that children and adults differ in their ability to process information into memory. It is also apparent there is a difference in the speed with which these memory functions are performed. Along with the greater difficulty they have in searching for and retrieving information, children appear to take longer than older individuals to encode information into memory.

Most discussions of RT also include movement time, particularly within the context of motor behavior. The close or, in most conditions, inseparable association between the two phases of a movement response time has been discussed (see Fig. 7.4).

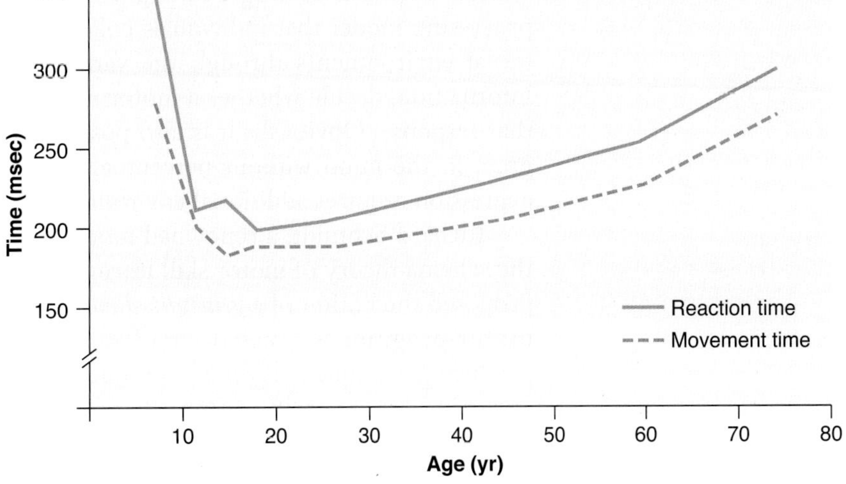

Figure 7.4 RT and movement time as functions of age.

A well-known law of motor behavior closely associated with movement is *Fitts's law* (Fitts, 1954). This law also is referred to as the *speed-accuracy tradeoff*, which means that when performers attempt to do something more quickly, they typically do it less accurately. That is, under most movement conditions, as speed increases, accuracy decreases. Exceptions are those conditions in which moving too slowly is not conducive to motor efficiency that can affect accuracy (e.g., striking a fast-moving object).

Other factors such as task complexity and movement distance also affect an individual's movement time. Movement time often is described as the capacity of the motor system to use an amount of information per second. Within this definition, capacity is expressed as the index of difficulty divided by the movement time; it is evidenced when movement times become faster (lower) for a specific information load.

Using a life-span approach to the study of rapid aiming arm movements, Yan and colleagues (2000) report data relevant to the concepts of processing speed and Fitts's law. The researchers examined four age groups of 6-, 9-, 24-, and 73-year-olds. As you would predict, young children and older adults were slower, more variant, and less smooth in their movements than the other groups were. Much of the difference was related to task characteristics involving movement accuracy demands and response uncertainty. In general, the younger and older groups performed in a similar manner. However, the younger group's performance is improving over time (a finding supported by Lambert & Bard, 2005), whereas the older adults' performance is regressing. The researchers concluded that the lower performances for the two groups were due in large part to their making more on-line movement adjustments, as opposed to movement under central (programming) control.

PROGRAMMING

Objective 7.6

Perhaps the most sophisticated mental operation is **programming**. In a broad sense, programming is cognitive processing that results in the formulation of a thought, cognitive expression, or motor program. Depending on the task, several factors are involved in these functional operations. For example, attention, perceptual awareness, and information stored in the working and long-term memory systems all influence programming. You may recall from the general information-processing model that individuals collect information from the external and internal environments through the various perceptual modalities, interpret that information, decide whether a motor response is appropriate, and, if so, generate that response. Obviously, it is also possible to generate a thought or motor program in the mind without perceptual information. But in most cases, an overt expression requires additional environmental information.

Richard Schmidt, a renowned motor behavior scientist and the originator of the schema theory of motor skill learning (Schmidt, 1975; Schmidt & Lee, 2014), proposed the notion of a *generalized motor program* (GMP). Schmidt describes the **motor program** as a memory representation of a class of actions responsible for producing a unique pattern of motor activity if the program is executed. For a person to produce a specific action, the person must retrieve the appropriate program from memory and then add movement-specific parameters such as force, duration, and movement pattern that must be used to perform the skill. The emphasis and application of the motor program concept are the core of schema theory.

Schema Theory (Generalized Motor Program)

Briefly, *schema theory* offers an explanation of the way individuals learn and perform a seemingly endless variety of movements. The theory suggests that the motor programs stored in memory are not specific records of the movements to be performed; rather, they are a set of general rules, concepts, and relationships (schemas) to guide performance in keeping with the concept of a GMP. Basically, individuals store past movement experiences in memory. Storage of movement elements and the relationship of these elements to each other are called *movement schema*. Individuals call up the schema for programming or, in a sense, they piece together desired movements.

An example of the theory in practice is the performance of an individual playing shortstop in baseball or guard in basketball. The shortstop can field a ball from numerous positions, many of which are unpracticed, and still get the ball to first base, just as the basketball player can shoot successfully from almost any position on the court.

There are two control components: the GMP and the motor response schema responsible for dictating the specific rules governing an action. Thus, the motor response schema provides parameters to the GMP. The motor schema (concept) for a general skill area (e.g., throwing and jumping) is bounded by dimensions related to space, time, and force. Each dimension represents a continuum that, depending on experience, may be limited or diverse. Theoretically, the greater the variety of experiences produced by the individual, the more diverse the schema becomes and the greater the capacity to move. The motor schema enables the individual to select the appropriate level from each dimension to program a task that may be known or novel. In shooting a basketball, for example, the child calls on a program consisting of a relationship among the distance the ball has to travel, required muscular force, arm speed, and angle release—all of which may change from one attempt to the next.

A major prediction of schema theory is that increasing *variability in practice* on a given task will result in increased transfer to a novel task of the same movement class. The strength of the schema is a positive function of the amount and variability of practice of responses within a movement class. Studies have tested these predictions by manipulating the variability of practice factor. It is predicted that subjects exposed to a high variability of practice regime but who never experience the test condition will perform as well or better than subjects who practice only on the test condition relevant to a final observation on that test condition. In addition, it is predicted that the high-variability group will outperform the specificity group on transfer to novel tasks.

Variability in practice is predictably more effective for children, especially young children, than it is for adults simply because young individuals have considerably more to learn. Generally, schema theory supports variability in practice and problem solving (within the same class of movements and rules) during early years rather than instruction in specific sport skills. For a review of research using variability of practice, see Boyce et al. (2006). Since its introduction more than 40 years ago, schema theory has generated numerous lines of inquiry. Although critiques now suggest that the motor learning process is more sophisticated than a GMP, a review indicates that the theoretical existence of a motor program is generally accepted by the research community (Summers & Anson, 2009), and new theories should be built on the foundation and evidence laid by schema theory.

think about it

As a physical education teacher for children, how would you use this information for teaching, for example, the manipulative skill of throwing?

Developmental Theories and Approaches to the Study of Motor Control

Objective 7.7

Although it is generally accepted that the control of motor behavior is under the direction of some type of motor program, what the program actually controls and how control develops have been two of the most active issues in contemporary motor development research. Under the heading of developmental biodynamics, this general approach to the study of perception and action is based on the general hypothesis that *change* in motor coordination and control emerges from continual and intimate interactions between the nervous system and the periphery, the limbs and body segments (in essence, the brain and body). From this multifaceted approach, three theories continue to have exciting implications for better understanding the processes and mechanisms involved in motor development (perception → action): *coordinative structures*, *dynamic systems*, and *neuronal group selection*. Obviously, some scientific approaches incorporate more than one of these ideas into the same study. With advances in brain imaging and muscle activation measurement, such approaches will become more commonplace. And, as noted in Chapter 1, these approaches are often associated with the emerging and dynamic scientific field of *developmental cognitive neuroscience*.

COORDINATIVE STRUCTURES

The general consensus in past years was that the individual muscles were given instructions by the commands produced in the motor program. Bernstein (1967) challenged this notion. He argued there are too many independent operations for the motor program to control them all simultaneously. In more recent years, numerous researchers have supported Bernstein's initial concern. They find it difficult to consider that the nearly 600 muscles and 100 mobile joints of the body are under the control of the CNS in all the possible *degrees of freedom* (i.e., controlled action of an independent joint movement). Bernstein suggested that motor programs control groupings of muscles instead of individual muscles. These groupings of muscles with associated joints have been termed **coordinative structures**, dynamic structures, and *synergies*. The commands generated by the motor program are said to be directed toward the specific coordinative structure that is constrained to act as a single functional unit. For a simplified analogy, consider the actions of a puppeteer who controls several degrees of freedom (e.g., the action of the whole arm of the puppet) with a single finger (Fig. 7.5). From this general notion, a new definition of the term *coordination* has been proposed. It is the process by which an individual constrains, or condenses, the available degrees of freedom into the smallest number necessary to achieve a goal (Rose & Christina, 2006).

The idea of coordinative structures has stimulated considerable inquiry in developmental research, much of which has been associated with the dynamic systems perspective. A common technique with this type of research is use of electromyography to determine the creation and use of synergies in learning and executing various motor actions (e.g., reaching/grasping, postural responses, and locomotion). For a more detailed description of coordinative structures, refer to Magill and Anderson (2013) and Latash (2008).

DYNAMIC SYSTEMS

In Chapter 1, we saw that the **dynamic systems** perspective seeks to provide an understanding of how movement and control emerge or unfold developmentally.

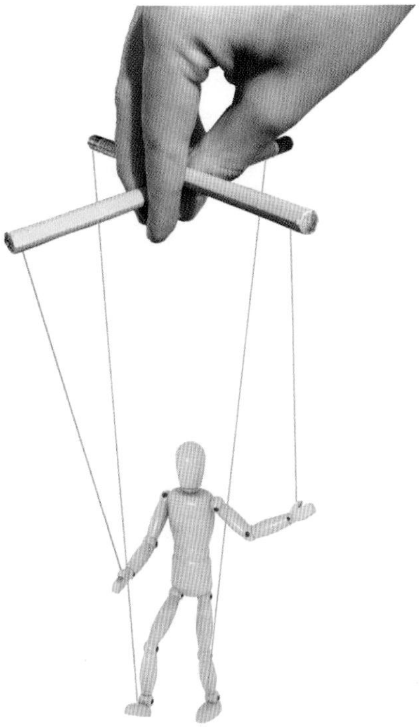

Figure 7.5 The brain's control of synergies is much like the puppeteer controlling several actions with only a few movements.

Based on highly complex principles from theoretical physics, theoretical mathematics, and ecological psychology, this theory proposes that qualitative changes in motor behavior emerge out of the naturally developing dynamic properties of the motor system and coordinative structures (Kugler et al., 1982).

The following features of dynamic systems should be noted (as interpreted from Thelen, 2005; Thelen & Smith, 1998):

1. The first assumption of the dynamic systems approach is that developing organisms are complex systems that consist of many individual elements that are embedded within and are open to a complex environment. In essence, this relates to the developmental systems perspective.
2. Movement emerges from **self-organizing properties** *of the body*. Individuals are composed of several complex and cooperative **subsystems** (e.g., perceptual, postural, muscular, and skeletal), with each system developing at developmental different rates, thus resulting in the intricacy of coordinated movement. Even the simplest skill requires a cooperative effort, with each system providing critical input. For example, muscular strength of the legs and postural control are critical controllers for walking.

   Figure 7.6 illustrates the subsystem idea in regard to skill function. Subsystems may also be thought of as a form of "constraint" (see "Constraints Model"). The "other constraints" in the figure are, for example, flexibility, body fat, speed, etc. Supposedly, there is a **rate controller** for each skill that organizes the system or subsystems needed to execute the task. Rate controllers may be influenced by, for example, maturity, disease, and neurological impairment.

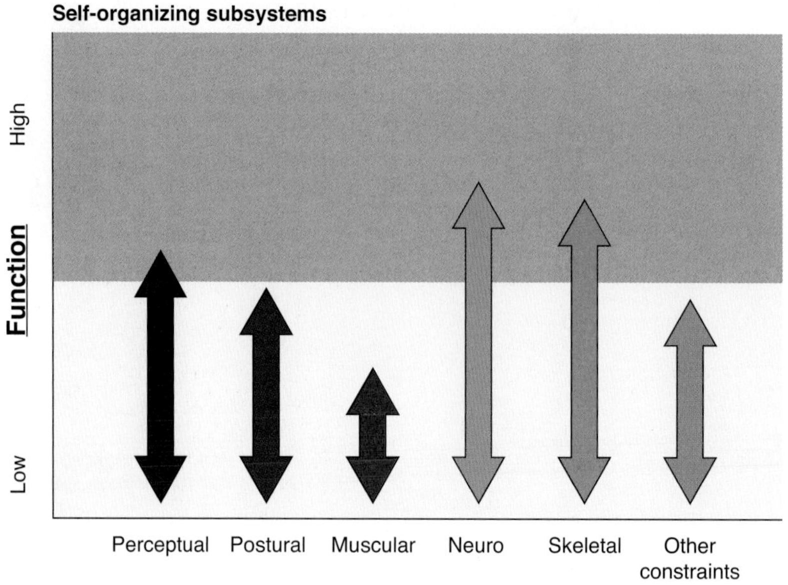

Figure 7.6 Illustrating the idea of self-organizing subsystems and level of function.

3. Another assumption is that movement is determined not only by muscular forces but also by mechanical interactions (e.g., body segments and joint reaction forces). The contribution of these forces may be influenced by speed of movement, body position, length and mass of body segments, and the intentions of the movement. Research in this area seeks to examine the developmental characteristics associated with the generation and apportionment of forces and the timing-based control system.
4. With regard to the question of continuity, the dynamic systems perspective suggests that in the transition from old movement patterns to new ones, referred to as a *phase shift*, disruptions (discontinuities) occur in performance. The major challenge is to account for these characteristics from processes that are inherently continuous.

Using the dynamic systems perspective in motor behavior are unfolding the developmental picture of how interlimb coordination emerges. Specifics from some of these studies are described in Chapter 8, with the discussion of early movement behaviors (e.g., stepping, cruising, reaching, and walking).

This line of developmental research has accomplished much toward our understanding of motor control and performance across the life span, including the identification of factors that both facilitate and constrain development. It is hoped that future studies will complete the picture of lifelong development by observing the effects of advanced aging on the coordinative structures of older adults. Because the presence of dedifferentiation and other neurological losses are assumed sometime during late adulthood, there is likely some accompanying effect on the coordinative structures.

NEURONAL GROUP SELECTION

The dynamic systems perspective provides a glimpse into self-organizing properties of developing and mature motor systems, but it does not identify specific underlying neural mechanisms. The **neuronal group selection theory (NGST)** (Edelman, 1989, 1992) holds such promise and is tied to the theory that the emergence of coordinated movement is tied closely to the growth of the musculoskeletal system and development of the brain. A key issue is how changes in brain circuitry-controlling synergies (coordinative structures) become matched to developmental changes in the musculoskeletal system and the environment of the organism.

According to Sporns and Edelman (1993), during the early stages of development, neuronal circuits are not precisely wired to execute specific skills. Instead, the brain contains variant circuits (structural variability) that have dynamic properties. That is, those circuits selectively form *neuronal groups*, localized collections of hundreds to thousands of interconnected neurons. Neuronal groups are arranged in the brain in neural maps that represent the body surface. Although they are separated in regions of the cortex, they are linked anatomically through long-range neural connections and thus allow for global mapping. Theoretically, these selected neuronal groups temporarily share functional properties to accommodate the desired task.

In essence, NGST accounts for the brain's organization of synergies as functional units of motor control (coordinative structures). One of its merits is that it accounts for the spontaneous adaptability of coordinative structure in response to biomechanical and environmental changes. Therefore, as with the dynamic systems perspective, NGST supports the contextualist approach to the study of motor development. Refer to Hadders-Algra (2010) for additional information on this attractive theory. And, for a life-span perspective, see Leversen et al. (2012).

DEVELOPMENTAL COGNITIVE NEUROSCIENCE

As mentioned in Chapter 1, **developmental cognitive neuroscience (DCN)** is a rapidly growing field that examines the relationships between the developing brain and cognitive ability, in the context of this text–action processing. DCN is an interdisciplinary scientific field that is situated at the intersection of neuroscience, cognitive science, genetics, psychology, and movement sciences. One of the common research tools used in this field is brain imaging (see Chapter 1). With recent and frequent technological advances, we have a new generation of "functional" maps of brain activity based on either changes in cerebral metabolism, blood flow, or electrical activity. These tools allow observation of changes that are linked to the developing brain and changes in human behavior (Fig. 7.7). Another methodological advance is related to the emergence of techniques for formal computational modelling of neural networks. Such models allow us to begin to bridge data on developmental neuroanatomy to data on behavioral changes associated with development.

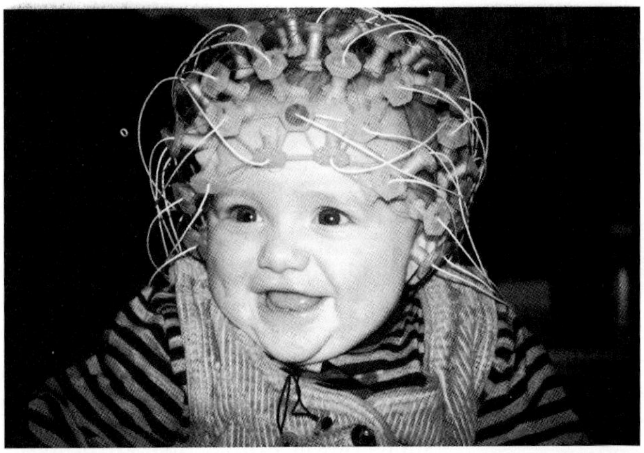

Figure 7.7 Researchers, from a DCN perspective, are using EEG to study perception in infants.

think about it

Summarize the issue of prewired versus self-organized motor development.

Underlying much of this work is the goal of understanding the link between the developing brain and changes in behavior—in our case, motor behavior. Studies range with identifying the brain structures and function involved in coordinating infant reach movements to understanding brain deficits associated with motor behavior in special populations. A prominent research noted, "Accordingly, the field appears to be moving in a direction that recognizes age-related changes in brain morphology as well as age-related changes in behavior" (Luciana, 2010, p. 3).

A commonality among all the theoretical notions and Gibson's ecological perspective is the suggestion that the brain and body are not prewired for skilled movements; rather, they have amazing adaptable *self-organizing properties* that adjust for biological and environmental contexts. In this dynamic process, exploration and selection are critical factors. To illustrate this observation, the following dynamic events explain how infants acquire new movement skills.

Foremost, there is a coupling of perception and action. This notion suggests perception and movement continually interact in learning. As described earlier in reference to Gibson's ecological theory (Chapter 6) and the concept of environmental affordances, infants coordinate their movements with concurrent perceptual information. The infant derives meaning from the environment through a continuous input of multisensory information. Change is driven primarily by the infant's need and desire to *select* and *explore* specific features of the environmental context. In many situation, these processes are stimulated by environmental *affordances* and the desire to act.

think about it

Using the theories and discussion from Chapters 6 and 7, how would you tell the story of perception → action?

With exploration of the environment, there is development of *adaptable and functional movement synergies*. Basically, motor control progresses from movements of great variability to more restrictive functional motor synergies. Complementing our previous discussions of neuronal and muscle group selection, this idea suggests the basic units of motor behavior are functional synergies or coordinative structures rather than the actions of specific muscles. These synergies are highly adaptable to meeting the demands of the infant's changing movement patterns to complement the challenges of the environment.

And, as the infant progresses from one level of skill to the next, *there are phase shifts in which new movement patterns are explored and selected*. During this transition, movement is typically quite variable and performance unstable. The infant may experiment with a wide variety of movement patterns that are driven primarily by exploration and the need to find a solution(s) to the new task. This phase of development has been described as beginning with an assembly of early movements, followed by a tuning to establish the more desired stable pattern (Goldfield, 1995). All of this illustrates the adaptive and self-organizing properties of the dynamic system.

WebLink

www.youtube.com; see Abigail and Brittany as they age into adulthood.

A truly remarkable example that helps summarize this concept and section on the development of motor control is the phenomenon of *conjoined twins*. Extremely rare, these identical twins have separate necks, heads, and hearts, and their nervous systems are distinct. They are joined together at the chest. Perhaps most remarkable, they share one set of upper and lower limbs. In the case reviewed, 6-year-olds share motor acts; one controls the right side and the other controls the left side (Fig. 7.8). Although coordination does not come easy, these are among their amazing feats: They learned to walk at 15 months and now can swim and ride a bicycle. How can two separate brains coordinate such complex functions? Although researchers contend that specific answers are out of reach presently, one could speculate that the self-organizing dynamics of

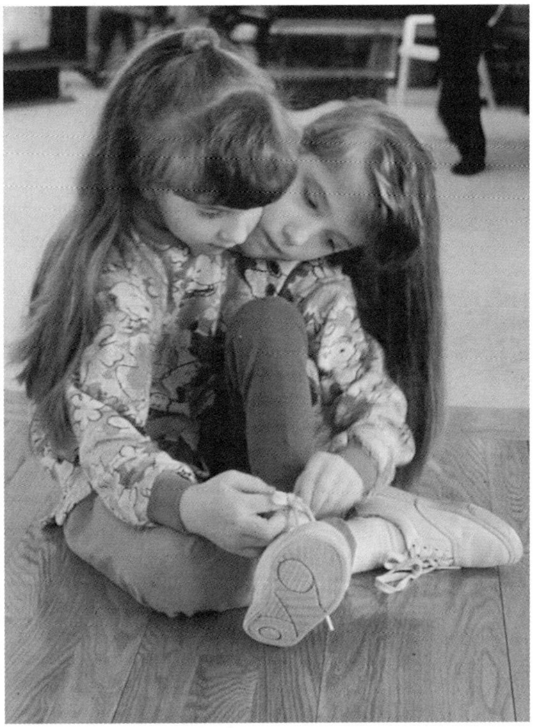

Figure 7.8 Tied together: Abigail controls the right hand; Brittany controls the left hand.

think about it

What explanation is there for how conjoined twins learned to swim?

control are truly at work. Today, the twins are in their 20s and each has a driving license.

Constraints Model

Objective 7.8

As mentioned in Chapter 1, the **constraints model** (Newell, 1986) offers an excellent framework for the observation and assessment of lifelong motor development. Arguably, its greatest value is its application for use by teachers and clinicians. It combines both the biological and ecological systems perspectives. This is applied by describing the constraints to behavior in reference to the individual, to the task to be performed, and to the environment in which it is to be executed (Fig. 7.9). In this context, the term **constraint** refers to factors that either facilitate or restrict development. Underscoring this view is the perspective that new motor behaviors emerge as a result of changing individual (organismic), environmental, and task constraints. In essence, this model supports the developmental systems perspective.

Individual constraints, originally referred to as *organismic factors*, can be divided into two categories: structural and functional constraints. For example, weight, height, and reach may be structural constraints, whereas speed, coordination, postural stability, and strength are considered functional constraints. It is not difficult to understand that, depending on the task, we could be limited to some extent by strength, flexibility, and balance.

Environmental constraints can be related to the physical environment or sociocultural factors (see Chapter 14). This may include gravity, terrain, surface, space, temperature, and characteristics of the home. For example, the space and terrain that an infant has available for movement are constraints on the development of locomotion.

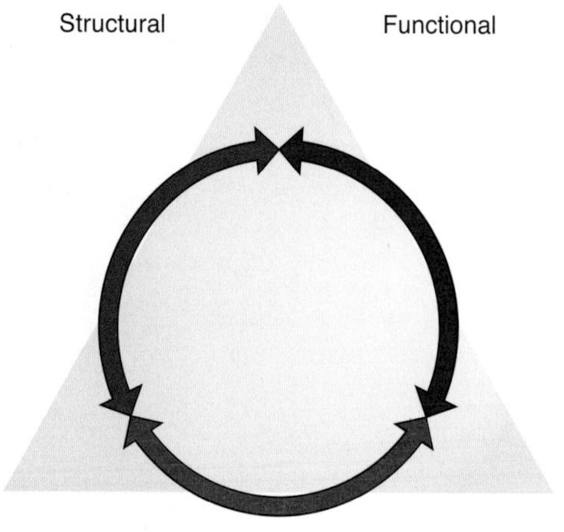

Figure 7.9 Constraints model. A version of the triangle (performer-task-environment) was first published in a textbook by Keogh and Sugden (1985, p. 15).

WebLink

http://www.vimeo.com/; see *Constraints in Motor Development*.

Task constraints are broadly grouped into categories of task goal, task rules, and equipment/materials used with the task. Closely associated with the first two constraints (task goal and task rules) are the cognitive demands of the activity. In regard to equipment, a young child may not be successful with a normal-sized bat or racquet, but after modification, more success or a better movement pattern may emerge. In regard to object size, the same concept applies to the infant learning to reach and grasp.

Obviously, there are more specific constraints than those mentioned. Let's consider an example using all three constraints: a young child (a typical 5-year-old) learning to strike a ball with a bat. The individual constraints may be coincidence timing ability, power, and selective attention. Environmental factors may include lighting, temperature (too hot or too cold), and audience (at practice or the game). In regard to task constraints, there is understanding of the goal, ball and bat size, and speed of the ball (also considered an environmental factor). No wonder that most 5-year-olds play T-ball.

Certainly, one can think of numerous situations across all age groups. That is the merit of the constraints model. It can be used for evaluating performance and can influence the type of instructional strategies used. The goal of the professional physical educator or physical therapist, for example, is to assess individual level of performance (individual constraints) and prescribe developmentally appropriate instructional strategies, which require changing environmental or task constraints to fit the individual.

Given the instructional and clinical merits of the model, elements are incorporated into the *Think About It* and *Learning Activities* in chapters describing motor behaviors (Chapters 8 to 12).

CHANGES WITH ADVANCED AGING

Objective 7.9

The discussion of the effects of aging on brain structures (Chapter 2) noted that not only does a significant loss of neurons occur but also other possibly debilitating changes occur within neurons themselves (e.g., senile plaques, vacuoles, and tangles). However, even with these conditions, it is believed that the brain may lose only a small portion of its ability to function.

Attention

focus on change

The rate of negative *change* with advanced aging is highly influenced by individual difference and environmental factors.

As a general observation, as long as the two competing tasks (divided attention) are relatively easy, younger and older adults perform in a similar manner. However, as task difficulty increases, younger persons do better. Explanations focus on reduced amounts of processing capacity and the notion that the total amount of capacity stays constant across age, but that older persons require more capacity to perform elementary functions. Thus, less space would be available for higher level processing operations. Although these views are somewhat different, both suggest that capacity (i.e., total or space capacity) is affected by older age.

With regard to selective attention, older adults generally are less adept than younger adults. However, when appropriate environmental supports are available (e.g., distinctive features), differences are less evident in filtering out irrelevant stimuli. However, *if speed is a requirement*, older adults are slower than young persons.

Working (Short-Term) Memory

think about it

What are the everyday implications for a decline in working memory with advanced age?

In general, working memory declines during the late adulthood years. A study by Botwinick and Storandt (1974) found that memory span remained relatively constant from the 20s through the 50s and then dropped only about one item following those years. However, greater comparative deficits between young and older adults have been found on other tasks, such as math problems and the linear ordering of items. Once again, is the age difference due to processing efficiency or capacity (refer back to the discussion regarding children on pages 187–191)?

One explanation for any age difference is that, compared with young adults, older persons are slower in searching or scanning short-term memory. From another perspective, the difference is a result of information-processing abilities growing less flexible with age, a loss of information during reorganization (encoding), or a diminished ability to process the encoded information. In addition to this processing deficit explanation, the hypothesis that older adults have a storage capacity deficit compared to young persons also has been supported by research (Cowan et al., 2015). In short, it appears that the deficit with age is both a hardware and a software problem.

Long-Term Memory

Older adults often exhibit significant deficiencies on memory tasks that involve the transfer of information between short- and long-term stores. In general, older adults are less able to recall details of past events (e.g., Friedman, 2013; Ward et al., 2013). This deficiency likely is due to the difficulty that elderly people have with both encoding and retrieving information from long-term storage. Older adults, like young children, apparently do not engage as frequently as young adults in deep elaborate encoding strategies. However, wide individual differences are normal. Long-term memory in older adults has been shown to improve with instructions to use imagery and when plenty of time is provided for the task.

Knowledge

A number of studies suggest that past experience and knowledge of specific content positively can affect age differences in children, it also can override age differences in adults.

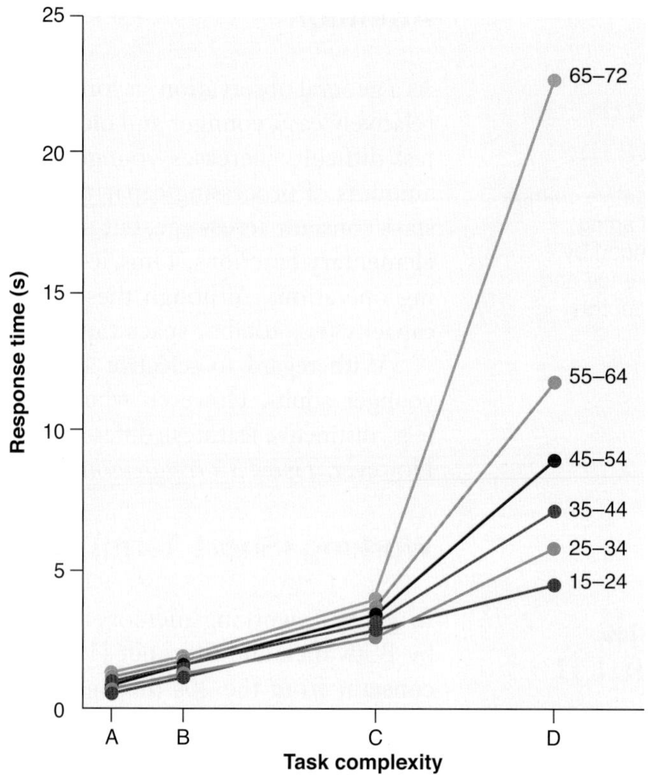

Figure 7.10 Age-related increase in processing speed (response time) with increase in complexity.

Processing Speed and Movement Time

A consistent finding in the study of aging is a decline in processing speed as measured by RT and other speeded manipulative tasks. Overall, processing speed of many types reaches a peak in young adulthood (20s) and declines slowly thereafter (Salthouse, 2009). If it takes a 20-year-old 200 milliseconds to perform an RT task, the same task will take a 60-year-old about 250 milliseconds and an 80-year-old over 300 milliseconds (see Fig. 7.4 on page 193). In contrast, a 6-year-old typically performs the task in just less than 350 milliseconds. Figure 7.10 shows response time changes with task complexity (demonstrating Hick's law) by age.

Apparently, with advancing age, there is little change in the speeded performance of single, discrete arm/hand actions and simple repetitive tasks that can be programmed in advance. However, much greater decrements among older persons have been found on timed (speed) tasks that involve decision making based on perceptual information and the programming of movement sequences. This is partially evidenced by large performance decreases on complex sequential tasks that require a series of different movements, particularly when speed is a critical factor. Overall, older adults are capable of demonstrating accurate motor performance on well-rehearsed tasks when speed is not a critical factor.

think about it

Do you suppose the rate of psychomotor slowing in the elderly can be controlled? If so, how?

The general slowing of the body with advanced aging constitutes a universal phenomenon referred to as *psychomotor slowing*. Although the mechanisms responsible for this condition remain unexplained, it appears that slowing is attributed to numerous factors associated with advanced aging (e.g., neuron loss, synaptic delay, decrease in excitability, and decrease in nerve conduction velocity), which causes disruptions of connections within the neural network. Supposedly, each disruption increases the time to process information. Other researchers also agree that, although neuromuscular factors contribute to slowing with age, most of the decrement can be attributed to central mechanisms (i.e., CNS). The topic of psychomotor slowing is discussed in greater detail with performance examples in Chapter 11.

Programming

Recall from the discussion of processing speed and Fitts's law, while studying life-span differences in rapid arm movements, researchers noted that older adults were slower, more variant, and less smooth than young adults were. Much of the difference was attributed to the older group making more on-line movement adjustments as opposed to movement under central (programming) control, especially when confronted with accuracy demands and response uncertainty. In essence, it was speculated that older adults lacked programming control. However, when accuracy was not critical and practical trials were provided, older adults performed much better. More recent studies also demonstrate that older adults can learn (program) new skills with practice, but they are slower than younger persons are. This conclusion applies to relatively simple and more complex tasks (e.g., Onushko et al., 2014; Seidler, 2007).

think about it

In regard to driving a car, which of the factors listed in Table 7.2 could be a constraint in the elderly? How so?

A summary list of selected information-processing changes with aging is presented in Table 7.2. A general observation is that young children and older adults have several characteristics in common.

TABLE 7.2 Summary of Selected Information-Processing Changes with Advanced Aging

Information-Processing Characteristic	
Attention	Declines
Working memory	Declines
Encoding and retrieval abilities	Decline
Long-term memory	Declines
Metamemory and knowledge	No apparent change
Processing speed	Slows
Movement time	Slows slightly
Response time	Slows on tasks requiring that movement sequences be performed quickly
Programming	Ability to learn new motor tasks and program movement sequences (little change, but slower)

Summary

The four basic components of the information-processing model are sensory input, reception through the various perceptual modalities, interpretation and decision making (programming), and overt motor response. Although much about information processing is unknown, it generally has been observed that as individuals progress toward early adulthood, they are able to process more information in a shorter period of time.

The core of most information processing is attention. The primary importance of attention to motor behavior involves alertness and the ability to select and attend to meaningful information. Age differences in this aspect of information processing are attributed primarily to experience and the refinement of strategies.

The two primary types of memory are recognition and recall.

Evidence that primitive forms of recognition memory are present in the newborn is found in the observation of habituation. There are also indications that young babies learn to remember (cued recall memory) using contextual information. Most evidence suggests that developmental differences in memory derive from functional abilities (strategies) rather than structural abilities (capacity) increases.

The rate at which information is processed, as reflected by an individual's reaction time, improves with age up to the early adult years, and then remains relatively stable until later adulthood. Although not all motor tasks require information to be processed at a fast rate, processing speed may account for many age-related performance differences. This appears to be especially evident when comparing young adults to young children and the aged.

Programming is considered one of the most sophisticated operations in information processing. With regard to the development of a theoretical base for motor programming, the concept of a schema has received considerable attention as a result of the schema theory of motor skill learning.

The notion of some form of motor program generally has been accepted but does not explain the link between brain and body (motor control). Three aspects of the developmental biodynamics perspective offer some insight: coordinative structures, dynamic systems, and neuronal group selection. A promising field that utilizes one or more of these approaches is developmental cognitive neuroscience. A commonality among these ideas is the suggestion that the brain and body are not prewired for skilled movements; rather, they have adaptable self-organizing properties that adjust for biological and environmental contexts. The constraints model provides a good framework for the study of motor behavior across the life span. There are several special populations that have common motor disorders that affect motor performance.

It is fairly well accepted that changes in the brain structure with advancing age produce some degree of regression in information-processing abilities. A general observation is that the abilities of the old approximate those of children; both perform below the level of the young adult.

think about it

1. **Reflecting back on Chapter 6, how does the information presented here fit the general information-processing model (Fig. 6.1 on page 150)?**
2. **Do you perceive general memory and the ability to recall movements (motor memory) as different from each other?**
3. **Can you think of any application of contextual learning to sports?**
4. **Why can we recall how to ride a bicycle (and do it) after years of not practicing but forget what we wore to class last week?**
5. **As future teachers and coaches, is there any practical value to this information: We (as adults) are about twice as fast with processing and reaction as a 5-year-old?**
6. **As a physical education teacher for children, how would you use this information for teaching, for example, the manipulative skill of throwing?**
7. **Summarize the issue of prewired versus self-organized motor development.**
8. **Using the theories and discussion from Chapters 6 and 7, how would you tell the story of perception → action?**
9. **What explanation is there for how conjoined twins learned to swim?**
10. **What are the everyday implications for a decline in working memory with advanced age?**
11. **Do you suppose the rate of psychomotor slowing in the elderly can be controlled? If so, how?**
12. **In regard to driving a car, which of the factors listed in Table 7.2 could be a constraint in the elderly? How so?**

LEARNING ACTIVITIES

Objective: To identify selective attention needs in sport. Name at least three sport activities that require considerable selection attention. Rank them in order by complexity and explain why you ranked them as you did.

Objective: To personalize the "constraints" concept. Consider the questions "What constraints influence my physical activity and daily life. Is there one or more that currently impedes my optimal performance?" Also, think of one of your parents or grandparents and how constraints affects them.

Suggested Readings

Adolph, K. E., & Robinson, S. R. (2015). Motor development. In L. Liben & U. Müller (Eds.), *Handbook of child psychology and developmental science: Cognitive processes* (7th ed., Vol. 2, pp. 114–157). Hoboken, NJ: Wiley.

Shumway-Cook, A., & Wollacott, M. H. (2012). *Motor control: Translating research into clinical practice* (4th ed.). Baltimore, MD: Wolters Kluwer.

Spencer, J. P., Samuelson, L. K., Blumberg, M. S., McMurrary, B., Robinson, S. R., & Tomblin, J. B. (2009). Seeing the world through a third eye: Developmental systems theory looks beyond the Nativist-Empiricist debate. *Child Development Perspectives*, 3(2), 103–105.

part four

Motor Behavior Across the Life Span

part four In the study of motor behavior, researchers gather information related to *growth*, *development*, and *motor performance* across the life span. The text up to this point has addressed the growth and development of the various dynamic systems of the human body and the factors that can affect them. Part Four builds on this foundation by documenting observable movement characteristics that typically occur within the phases of motor behavior.

In essence, motor behavior is the movement expression of the human body with regard to its physical size, neurological and physiology functioning, information processing abilities, and *self-organizing properties*.

The information provided so far serves as the basis for understanding characteristic movement abilities within each phase and what factors of change are responsible for the transition across phases. For example, what factors are responsible for the regression of motor performance? What factors account for the transition from reflexive behavior to voluntary movement? These questions are the foundation of motor development inquiry.

Part Four is divided into four chapters. Chapter 8 describes the reflexive, stereotypic, and rudimentary behaviors that span the prenatal stage through infancy (2 years of age). Chapter 9 documents the development of fundamental movement patterns and manipulative behaviors characteristic of the early childhood years (approximately ages 2 through 6 years). Chapter 10 presents information related to motor behavior during later childhood and the adolescent years (ages 7 to 18 years), in which individuals generally exhibit sport skill abilities and rapid periods of physical growth and development. Chapter 11 deals with the characteristic behaviors of the adult years, which normally feature peak motor performance and the inevitable course of regression. And finally, Chapter 12 describes selected behaviors associated with special populations.

Accompanying each chapter are "constraint" applications (*Think About It* questions and *Learning Activities*) that ask you to consider the constraints model in real-world situations.

Chapter 8

Early Movement Behavior

OBJECTIVES

Upon completion of this chapter, you should be able to

8.1 Discuss reflexes with regard to definition, control, relevance, and developmental characteristics.

8.2 Identify the three general types of reflexes and provide examples of each.

8.3 Explain the various theoretical views of reflex behavior.

8.4 Describe the developmental characteristics of spontaneous movements (stereotypies).

8.5 Provide a brief overview of the rudimentary phase of motor behavior.

8.6 Outline the developmental milestones associated with basic postural control and rudimentary locomotion.

8.7 Describe the developmental characteristics involved in manual control during the first 2 years of life.

8.8 Discuss the theoretical views associated with motor asymmetries.

KEY TERMS

- reflexes
- primitive reflexes
- postural reflexes
- locomotor reflexes
- spontaneous movements
- rudimentary behavior
- developmental cascade
- crawling
- creeping
- walking
- prehension
- manipulation
- manual control
- motor asymmetries

The Developmental Continuum

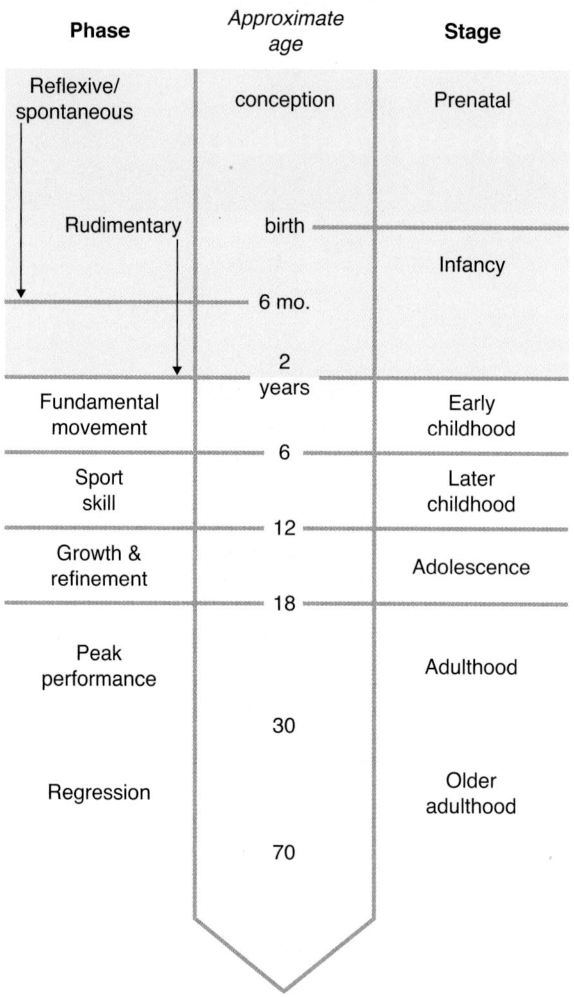

focus on change

The body's self-organizing properties and the environment promote *change* in motor behavior.

The beginnings of human movement are those characteristic behaviors that appear during the prenatal and infancy stages of development. Coinciding with these stages that cover the first 2 years of life are the reflexive/spontaneous and rudimentary phases of motor behavior. This chapter describes and explains the importance of reflexive and stereotypic (spontaneous) behaviors. It also documents the development of early voluntary movement with regard to postural control, locomotion, and manual control. Evidence of early motor asymmetries and theoretical views on this topic also is discussed.

REFLEXIVE BEHAVIOR

Objective 8.1

It already has been established that motor development has its origins in the prenatal period. Reflexes can be elicited in the fetus as early as the second or third month after conception, and most are present by the time of birth. In fact, many of the superficial, cutaneous reflexes are present by the fifth or sixth fetal month. **Reflexes** are involuntary movement reactions elicited by such forms of sensory stimuli as sound, light, touch, or body position. They are controlled primarily by the subcortical areas (lower brain centers), which are also responsible for numerous involuntary, life-sustaining processes such as breathing and heart rate.

The body's initial movement responses are controlled in the subcortical areas due to the maturational stage of the central nervous system (CNS). As the nervous system matures, reflexes come under the command of the brain stem and midbrain rather than remaining solely under spinal cord control. Finally, as the cerebral cortex (higher brain center) matures, most of these transient reflexes gradually become inhibited and voluntary motor behavior eventually takes over. The motor area of the cerebral cortex generally is considered to be minimally functional in the developing fetus and newborn infant; thus, most movement behavior is thought to be primarily involuntary. The human organism in the first 6 months to 1 year is essentially a reflex machine that undergoes a continuous process of neuromuscular functional maturation. Of the estimated 27 major infant reflexes, most are suppressed (disappear) by 6 months of age in the typical developing child, and few are observable after the first year. However, some reflexes, such as coughing, blinking, and sneezing, persist throughout life. There are also indications that specific reflexes reemerge due to neurological trauma or insult.

Importance of Reflexes in Infant Development

The importance of reflex behavior primarily is associated with its role in stimulating the CNS and muscles, in infant survival, and in its use as a diagnostic tool for assessing neurological maturity. Until the information-processing mechanisms become mature enough to consciously formulate motor programs and execute movement responses, *reflexes are a primary mode of stimulating the CNS and muscles*. However, the role of reflexes in the development of voluntary movement is controversial. That is, is there a direct or indirect link between specific reflexes and later voluntary movements? Theoretical views on this topic are discussed later in this chapter.

The presence of some reflexes offers infants certain survival advantages with regard to seeking nourishment and, perhaps to a lesser degree, protection. Two prime examples of these *primitive reflexes* are the *rooting reflex* and the *sucking reflex*. The rooting (search) reflex is exhibited when newborns automatically turn their mouths toward the mother's nipple (or bottle) when it touches their cheek or lips. In the sucking reflex, newborns reflexively suck on anything that touches their lips. Interestingly, the neonate is not born with the voluntary capacity to ingest food. Thus, the sucking reflex enables the newborn to feed by involuntary means.

Although perhaps not as critical to survival as the reflexes related to feeding, certain involuntary responses also have been described as *protection mechanisms*. One example of this type of survival response is the Moro reflex. When a newborn is startled or begins to fall, the arms and legs fling outward, the hands open, and the fingers spread. As the reflexive action for protection continues, the arms draw close to the body, the fists clench, the eyes open, and the infant lets out a loud wail.

Reflexes not only are important to the survival of infants but also serve as an indicator of general neurological status. The genesis of reflex behavior is well documented with regard to onset, persistence, and disappearance. Because infant reflexes occur within predictable age ranges, pediatricians have used these behaviors extensively as diagnostic tools for assessing neurological maturity. The failure of reflexes to appear, their prolonged continuation, or their uneven strength characteristics may cause the physician to suspect neurological impairment. Two universal assessments of neonatal behavior (described in Chapter 13) are the *Apgar scale* and the *Brazelton scale*; both include reflex measures as indicators of neurological adequacy. The Moro, Babinski, and asymmetrical tonic neck reflexes commonly are used with infant assessment scales and during normal physical examinations. These measurements can provide highly critical information. For example, if the asymmetrical tonic neck reflex or certain postural reflexes persevere past the time it normally disappears, it is an indication that cerebral palsy or other neurological impairment may be present (Lorton & Lorton, 1984).

Although most measures of reflex behavior indicate generalized neurological status, they may be used in a selective way by specialists to determine the presence of localized neurological defects of such areas as the cranial nerves, spinal roots, and spinal cord (e.g., spina bifida).

Types of Reflexes

Objective 8.2

Although it may not be possible to precisely and systematically classify reflexes into neat categories, they generally may be grouped under the descriptors of primitive, postural, and locomotor.

Primitive reflexes primarily are associated with the infant's instinct for survival and protection. Upon stimulation, the infant reflexively seeks nourishment with the rooting and sucking responses and shows indications of protecting itself with the Moro and grasping reflexes. The term *primitive* may be appropriate in view of the infant's ultimate potential; however, the term also may be associated with the level of neurological control. Because most of these reflexes are mediated by the lower brain centers (e.g., spinal cord and lower brain stem) as opposed to the higher centers of control (e.g., midbrain and cerebral cortex), use of the word *primitive* in this context also seems to be appropriate. Compared with the other types of reflexes, most of the primitive responses are functional prenatally and can be elicited in utero. As the cerebral cortex matures and gains control of lower brain functions (around 3 to 4 postnatal months), many of the primitive reflexes are suppressed.

As the higher brain centers begin to function and suppress the lower control centers, postural reactions enter the infant's repertoire. **Postural reflexes** provide the infant with the ability to react to gravitational forces and changes in equilibrium. These involuntary reactions are the mechanisms by which the infant is able to maintain an appropriate posture with a changing environment. General functions of these reflexes include coordinating movements of the head, trunk, and limbs to keep the head upright; maintaining equilibrium; rolling over; and attaining vertical postures. There is also a protective response with postural control, as evidenced with the parachute reflex. When infants are tilted forward (face down) from an upright position, they reflexively extend their arms as a protective mechanism to brace against the forward displacement.

It is not unusual to find classification methods that use only the primitive and postural categories. However, another group of reflexes has enough common characteristics to justify including a third category. **Locomotor reflexes** are unique in that they resemble later voluntary locomotor movements. Involuntary responses such as the reflexes associated with climbing, walking (stepping), and swimming have been described as precursors of the voluntary movements of the same name. Although these reflexes normally are suppressed by the fifth or sixth month, their voluntary counterparts do not appear until months later. Consequently, there has been much debate concerning their possible linkage. This issue arises again in the discussion of the various theoretical views concerning the role of reflexes in motor development.

A fourth group of involuntary responses, known as *tendon reflexes*, should be noted with regard to their initial appearance. These reflexes are used throughout the life span to evaluate neuromuscular response (primarily contraction) and are present in standard sites of the jaw, biceps, knee, and ankle by the second day of postnatal life.

WebLink
http://www.teachertube.com/; http://www.youtube.com/; see *Infant Reflexes*

The following section does not attempt to describe all infant reflexes. Rather, its purpose is to discuss those involuntary responses considered most appropriate to the study of motor development. For a more detailed description of specific reflexes, refer to the work of Fiorentino (1981) and Kliegman et al. (2015). Table 8.1 summarizes the approximate timetables for appearance, persistence, and disappearance of selected reflexes.

TABLE 8.1 Approximate Timetable of Selected Reflexes

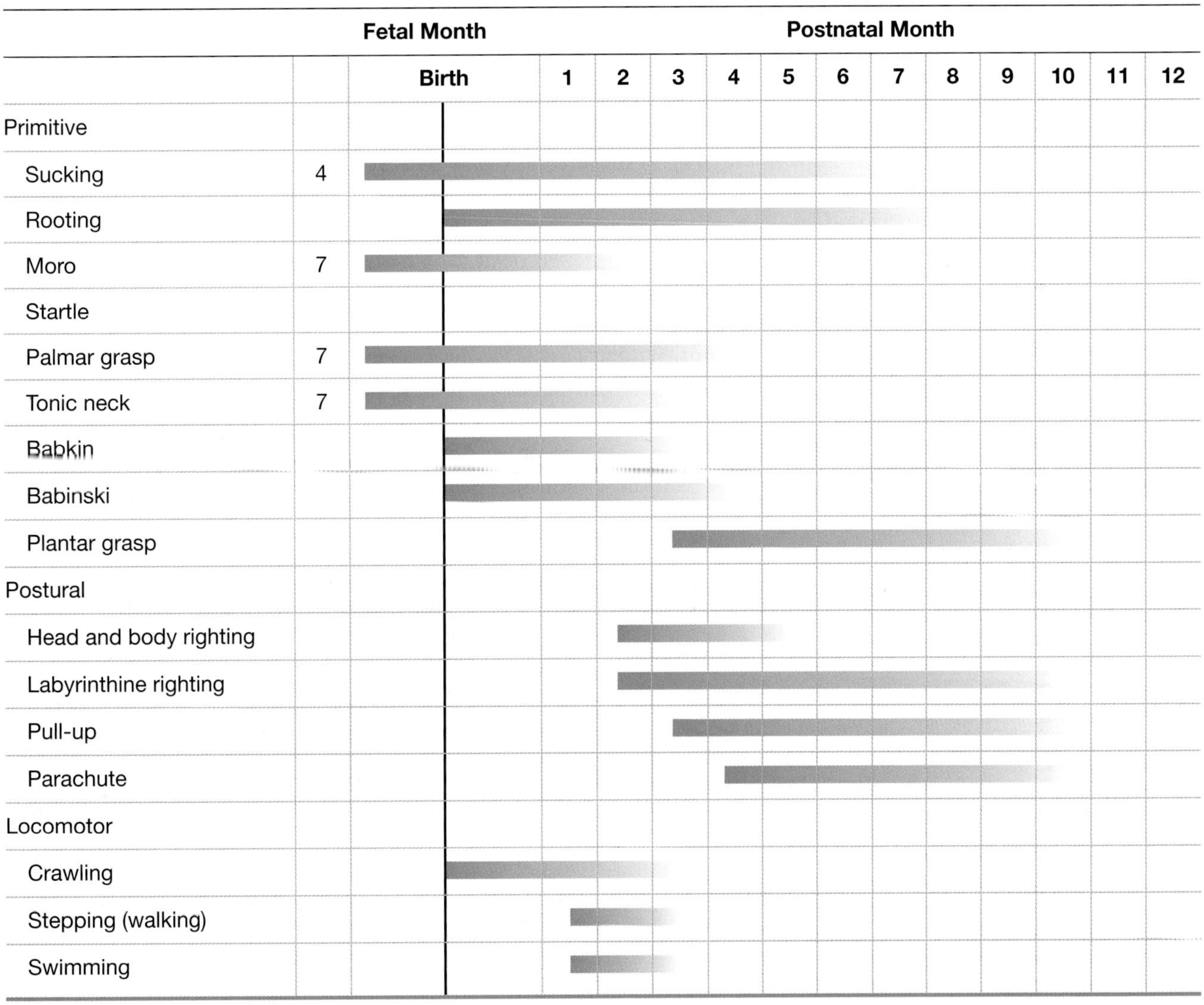

SOURCE: Data from Forfar, J. O., & Arneil, G. C. (Eds.). (2003). *Textbook of pediatrics* (6th ed.). London, United Kingdom: Churchill Livingstone.

PRIMITIVE REFLEXES

One of the earliest involuntary responses to appear is the sucking reflex. This response is evident in the 4-month-old fetus as it protrudes its lips in unmistakable preparation for sucking. Some babies have sucking blisters at birth caused by this sucking action during the prenatal state. In newborns, the sucking reflex is elicited by anything that touches its lips.

In conjunction with the sucking response, the tongue and pharynx adequately adapt to swallowing so the newborn can feed. Newborns can suck and inhale simultaneously and swallow between breaths about 3 times faster than adults can. After a couple of weeks, most newborns have mastered the complex function of synchronized sucking, swallowing, and breathing.

The reflexive behavior of sucking for nourishment is joined with the instinctive response to seek food using the *rooting reflex*. This response is activated by a light touch on the cheek, which causes the newborn to turn its head toward the stimulus in search of nourishment. This response also is referred to as the *search reflex*. Although the sucking response appears to be voluntary around the third month of infancy, characteristics of the reflex are still evident until 6 to 9 months of age, when feeding is totally under voluntary control. The rooting reflex follows a similar timetable; it persists until approximately the ninth month.

When the newborn is startled or begins to fall, its arms and legs extend outward, its hands open, and its fingers spread in the instinctive protective response called the *Moro reflex* (see Fig. 8.1). As noted earlier, the Moro reflex commonly is used for assessing generalized neurological status. The response can be elicited in several ways. One way is abruptly to remove support from the newborn's head by allowing it to drop sharply backward a short distance and then catching it with the hand. Another way to produce the reflex is to make a loud noise by clapping or slapping a table. After the arms and legs extend in response to the stimulus, the limbs return to a normal flexed position against the body. The Moro reflex crystallizes in the seventh fetal month and normally disappears by the third month of postnatal life.

Although quite similar to the Moro response, the startle reflex may not appear until months after the Moro reflex has disappeared (at about 7 months). When startled, the infant initially flexes its arms and legs rather than extending them as in the Moro reflex. The startle response normally is suppressed by the end of the first year; however, less intense indications of it may persist throughout the life span.

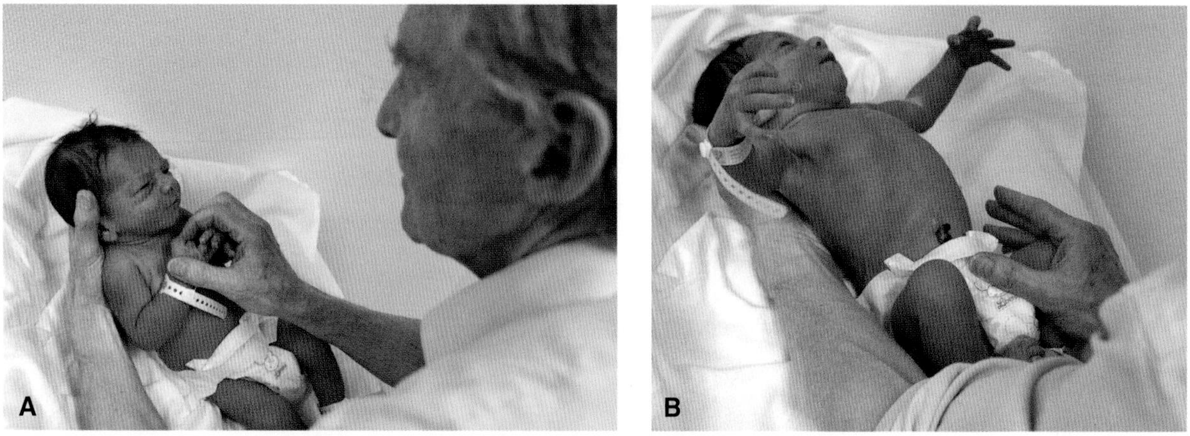

Figure 8.1 Moro reflex: **(A)** position of rest and **(B)** extension of limbs.

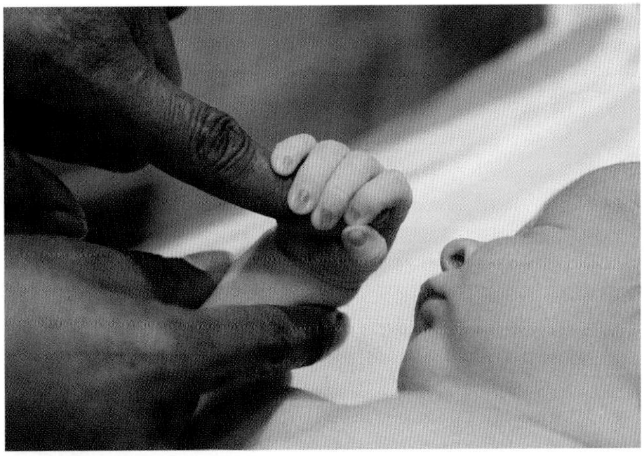

Figure 8.2 The grasping reflex.

Grasping reflex behavior is one of the most well-known and interesting responses in the infant's involuntary movement repertoire. This reflex is evident when a small rod or someone's finger touches the newborn's palm. The fingers (excluding the thumb) fold tightly around the object with a grasping action. The reflex is present by the seventh fetal month, although in a weaker form, and gradually grows stronger for several weeks after birth. The reflex then weakens and is suppressed entirely by the time the infant is about 4 months old. Around this time, the involuntary response is replaced by the initial stages of voluntary grasping, or manual control. This association is described later with regard to the developmental progression of manual control.

Another interesting facet of involuntary grasping behavior is its strength characteristics (Fig. 8.2). When pulled toward suspension while involuntarily clinging to a rod with both hands, infants typically are able to support more than 70% of their body weight (Eckert, 1987). In a classic study of the grasping reflex, Richter (1934) recorded the suspension time of 37 newborns, 1 to 23 days old, who grasped with both hands. Large individual differences were evident, but only one infant failed to hang for any length of time. The longest suspension of 128 seconds equals that found among the better efforts of adults. It also has been noted that strength of the reflex is greater about 2 weeks after birth.

Two forms of the *tonic neck reflex* have been identified: asymmetric and symmetric. Both responses appear at about 7 fetal months of age and disappear by approximately 5 months of age. The asymmetric tonic neck reflex can be elicited by placing the infant in a supine position (on its back, face upward) and turning the neck so the head faces either side. In response to the stretch of the neck muscles as the neck turns, an increase of tonus in the limbs is triggered. The infant exhibits a fencer's on guard position (Fig. 8.3A) as the limbs extend on the side of the body in which the head is facing and flex on the opposite side.

Right-side limbs respond differently than the left-side limbs in the asymmetric pattern. In the symmetric tonic neck reflex, the limbs move symmetrically, a response that can be elicited by placing the infant in a supported semistanding position and tipping the neck forward or backward. If tipped backward, which causes the neck to extend, the infant's arms will extend reflexively and the legs will flex (Fig. 8.3B). If tipped forward, which causes flexion of the neck, the infant's arms also will flex and the legs will extend (Fig. 8.3C).

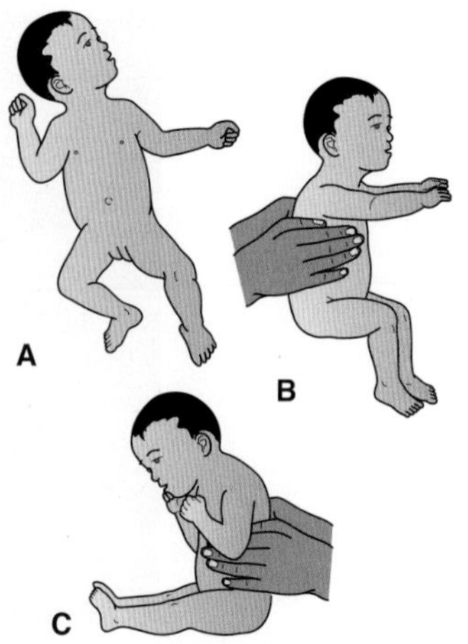

Figure 8.3 Tonic neck reflexes: **(A)** asymmetric, **(B)** symmetric when tipped backward, and **(C)** symmetric when tipped forward.

One unusual infant reflex is the *Babkin reflex*, also known as the *palmar mandibular reflex*. This response can be elicited by providing pressure simultaneously to both palms, which causes the infant to exhibit one or all of the following behaviors: mouth opens, eyes close, neck flexes, and head tilts forward. The Babkin reflex can be elicited at birth and normally disappears by the third month.

The *Babinski* and *plantar grasp* reflexes are involuntary responses to stroke stimulation along the sole of the infant's foot. In the Babinski reflex, which is present at birth, pressure applied to the sole of the foot causes the infant to reflexively fan out and extend its toes (Fig. 8.4). This reflex normally is suppressed by the fourth month. Around this same period in the infant's life, stroking the sole will induce the plantar grasp reflex in which the toes contract or flex as if attempting to grasp the object. The plantar grasp reflex may persist through the first year of life.

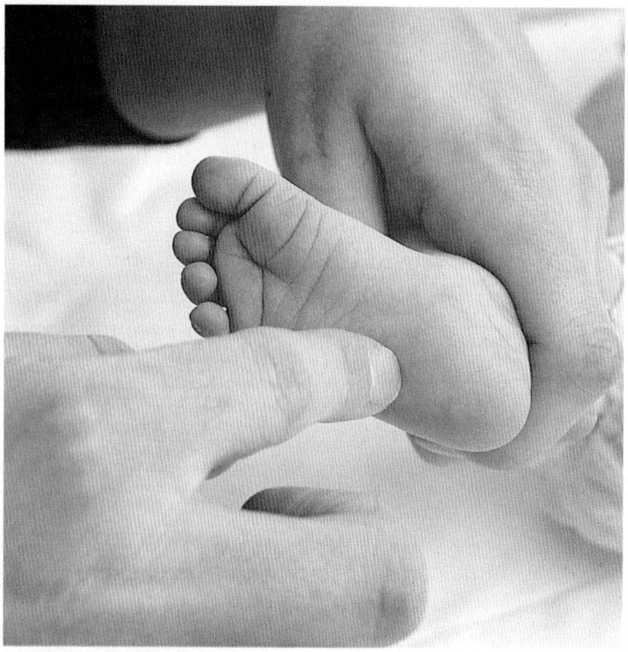

Figure 8.4 The Babinski reflex.

POSTURAL REFLEXES

Head and *body righting* are reflex behaviors believed to form the basis for future voluntary rolling movements. Both involuntary responses appear around the second month and persist until about 6 months of age. The head (and neck) righting reflex can be elicited by gently turning the infant's body in either direction while in the supine position (on its back). The infant will respond reflexively by righting, or turning, its head in the same direction. In contrast, the body-righting reflex is elicited by turning the head in one direction while the infant is in a supine position. The body will reflexively right itself by turning in the same direction—first the hips and legs and then the trunk.

The *labyrinthine righting reflex* characteristically involves both righting and gravity reactions. This reflex enables the infant to maintain an upright body posture; it is believed to contribute to the ability to move in a forward direction. The first evidence of this reflex is seen around 2 months when the infant, while lying on its stomach, attempts to orient its head to gravity and look up. It is this upright head position while the infant is on its hands and knees at around 6 months that establishes the posture for forward locomotion.

The labyrinthine righting reflex can be elicited by holding the infant in an upright position and tilting its body forward, backward, or to the side. In response, the infant will reflexively attempt to maintain an upright posture of the head by moving it in the direction opposite that in which the trunk was moved (Fig. 8.5). The head tends to maintain the original upright posture with relation to gravity. This response also detects functioning of the otolith organs housed in the labyrinth of the inner ear. The labyrinthine righting reflex generally appears around the second month of life, becomes stronger during the middle of the first year, and normally disappears by 12 months.

The *pull-up reflex* is an involuntary attempt to maintain an upright position. The response is elicited by placing the infant in an upright sitting position while holding its hands and carefully tipping it backward or forward. In response, the infant will flex or extend its arms in an apparent effort to maintain the upright posture (Fig. 8.6). This reflex usually appears around the third month and disappears by the end of the first year. It has been suggested this involuntary response is related to the attainment of voluntary upright posture.

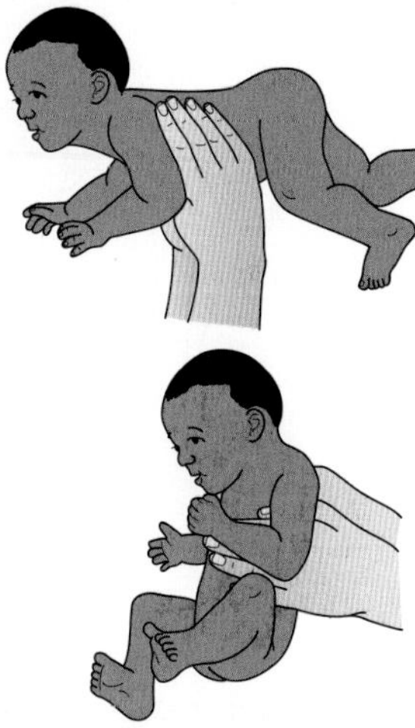

Figure 8.5 The labyrinthine righting reflex.

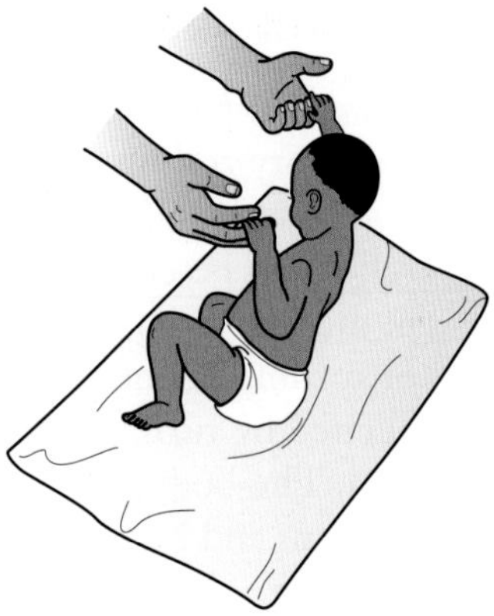

Figure 8.6 The pull-up reflex.

Also referred to as propping reflexes, the *parachute reflexes* serve as protective and supportive movements for the infant. Protective responses are evident when the infant is tipped off balance in any direction. Forward and downward parachute reflexes are present around the fourth month. The forward response is elicited by holding the infant in an upright position and tilting it toward the ground. In response, the infant reflexively extends its arms in a protective movement to break the fall (Fig. 8.7A). The downward response is observed when the infant suddenly is lowered downward (from an upright position) a distance of about 3 feet. The infant's legs will extend and spread, and the feet will rotate outward.

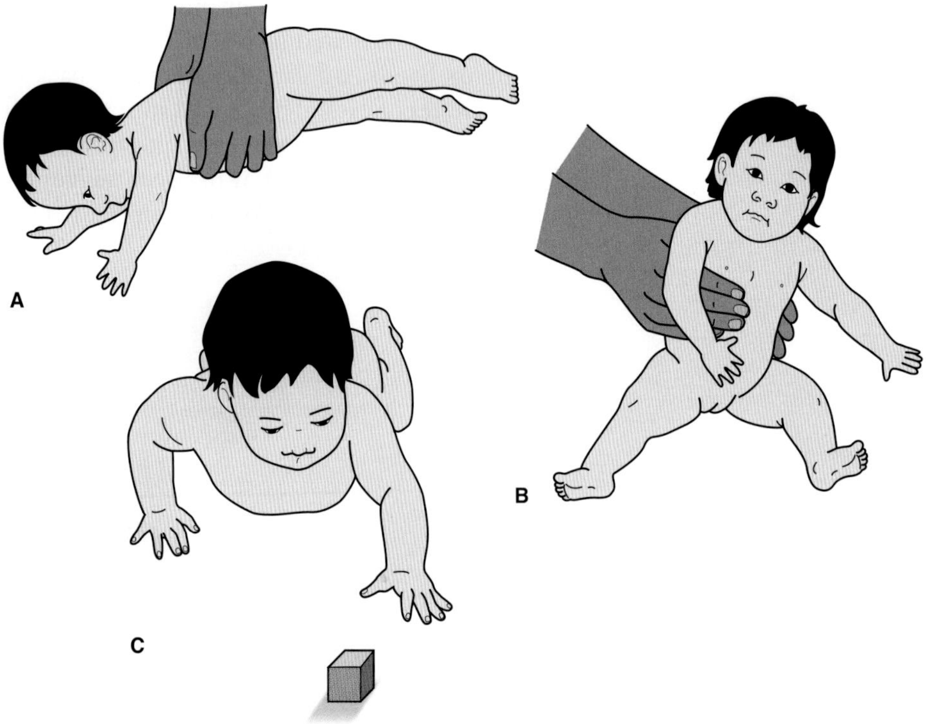

Figure 8.7 Parachute reflexes: **(A)** protective reaction to sudden downward movement, **(B)** protective reaction to being tilted from a balanced position, and **(C)** propping reaction using one arm for support in reaching for a toy.

These reflexes also are seen when the infant is tilted off balance in either direction from a sitting position (Fig. 8.7B). The sideward propping movement usually is not observable until around the sixth month. The backward response usually is not observable until sometime between 10 and 12 months. In response to being tilted backward, the infant also may rotate the body to avoid falling in that direction. Until these reflexes are present, infants will make no attempt to brace or catch themselves when falling. It is not unusual for these protective responses to persist beyond the first year.

Parachute reflexes are supportive as well as protective movements. The supportive response is observable when the infant (voluntarily) extends an arm for support while reaching with the other hand (Fig. 8.7C). It may be assumed this supporting (propping) action enables the infant to attain a better visual perspective of the surroundings and perform other tasks such as reaching, grasping, and crawling.

LOCOMOTOR REFLEXES

The *crawling reflex* can be observed from birth and, as noted earlier, there is a definite similarity of movements between this response and the voluntary pattern that appears months later. If the infant is placed in a prone position (on the stomach) and pressure is applied to the sole of one foot or both feet alternately, the infant will reflexively crawl using its arms and legs (Fig. 8.8). There is some speculation that this reflex (and others in this category) is a precursor to the voluntary crawling pattern, although there is a distinct time lag between the disappearance of this reflex and the appearance of the voluntary pattern. Although the crawling reflex normally disappears by the fourth month, voluntary crawling generally is not observed until around the sixth or seventh month. The crawling reflex is important for the development of sufficient muscle tone for voluntary crawling.

The *stepping reflex* is one of the most debated involuntary responses in the infant's repertoire. The primary point of contention is its assumed link with voluntary walking behavior. Normally present by the end of the first week after birth, this reflex can be elicited by holding the infant upright with the feet touching a flat supporting surface. Pressure on the bottom of the infant's feet will cause it to reflexively respond with crude but characteristic walking movements. The reflex will consist of a distinct knee lift but will not involve an arm swing or hip motions. A variation of the stepping response is the *placing reflex*. This reflex is similar in kinetics to the stepping reflex but is elicited by bringing the front of the infant's foot lightly in contact with the edge of a table. The infant responds by appearing to place the foot on the table (Fig. 8.9). It also may appear as though the infant is lifting its foot over an object. Interestingly, after testing infants at 2, 4, and 6 weeks, Thelen et al. (2002) found that at each age, overall arousal was the best predictor of number of steps. In addition, those infants who were "chubby" stepped less often. One of the implications of this research is that reflex behavior is influenced by factors other than the CNS (maturation). The stepping reflex normally persists to the fourth month.

think about it

Of the types of reflexes, how would you rank their importance?

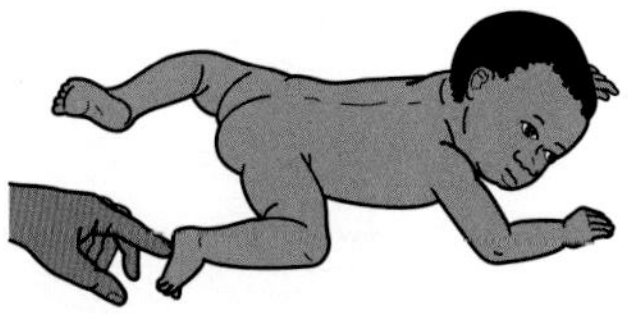

Figure 8.8 The crawling reflex.

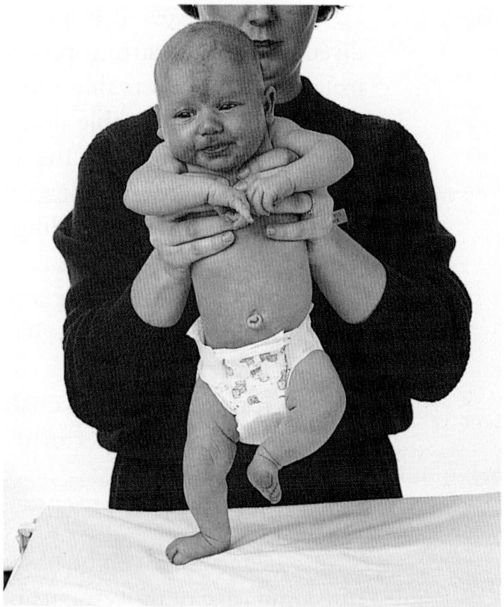

Figure 8.9 The stepping reflex.

The *swimming reflex* is one of the most interesting involuntary responses seen in infants and can be elicited during the second week after birth by holding the infant horizontally in the water with its head up or over the surface of the water. The infant responds by moving the arms and legs rhythmically in a swimming movement pattern (Fig. 8.10). Researchers also have noted that a breath-holding reflex is elicited in the newborn when its face is placed in the water. However, a month or so later, an infant may experience severe anxiety when its head is submerged. This involuntary response usually disappears by about the fourth month.

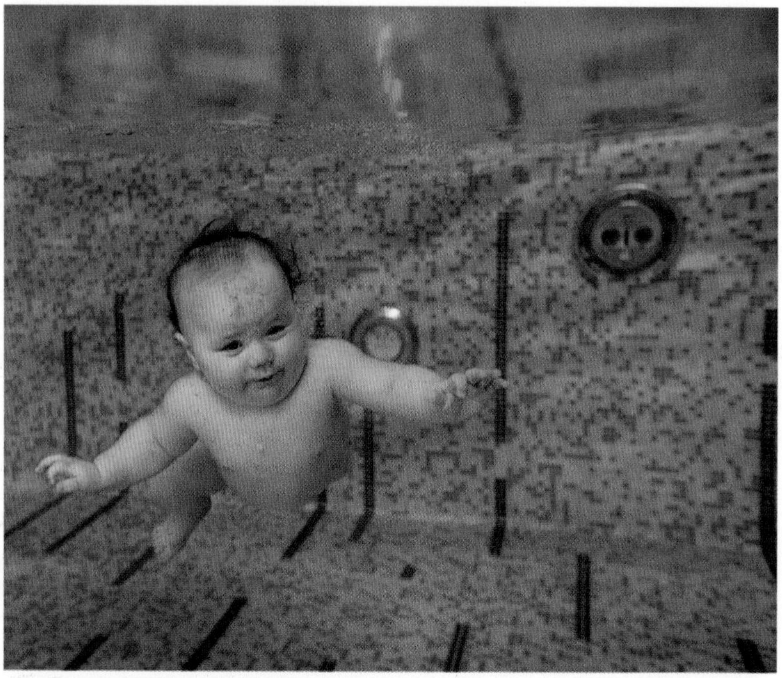

Figure 8.10 The swimming reflex.

Theoretical Views of Reflex Behavior and Voluntary Movement

Objective 8.3

The developmental evolution of reflexive behavior followed by voluntary motor control can be described generally. However, an explanation of how and why these changes occur has been debated from several differing viewpoints. The primary issue from a motor behavior context has been related to the possible connections between involuntary responses and voluntary movement. This has been especially true of the reflexes that resemble voluntary movements, such as grasping, crawling, stepping (walking), and swimming. The question is, is there a direct or indirect relationship?

Most contemporary viewpoints support the general notion that reflex and spontaneous behavior, to some degree, forms the basis for later voluntary movement. Furthermore, reflexes do not actually disappear but, rather, are suppressed and integrated into the hierarchy of controlled behavior. Tied to the theoretical view of a *direct relationship* is the notion that stimulation of the reflex will positively affect later voluntary control. This point of view has been supported by research on the effects of stimulation on stepping and reaching reflexes. Researches in one well-known series of studies (review by Zelazo et al., 1993) had infants "practice walking" by stimulating their stepping reflex. They then compared the results with various control groups. In general, results indicated that infants whose stepping reflex was stimulated began to walk voluntarily at an earlier age than did the infants who had not practiced walking. One noted limitation of this research is that it is not known when the infants would have begun walking without stimulation. Bower (1976), who subjected infants to practice reaching movements during the involuntary phase, obtained similar results; the emergence of voluntary reaching was accelerated and, in some cases, children (presumably) experienced no disappearance phase. Results such as these have led some researchers to speculate that there a direct link between specific involuntary reflexes and later voluntary control.

Dynamic systems research (e.g., Adolph & Robinson, 2015; Thelen et al., 2002) generally supports the notion of *continuity* between specific reflexive movements and voluntary control. This view differs somewhat from Zelazo's theory that a reflex is transformed to a voluntary action by practice. Rather, it is suggested that, for example, increased stepping frequency and the earlier onset of independent walking may be the result of strengthening the infant's musculature. In one set of studies, Thelen and Fisher (1982) found that kicking and stepping reflexes involve the same neuromuscular functioning and suggest the reflex disappears because muscle growth does not keep up with leg growth. That is, the muscle is not strong enough to lift the leg mass in the upright position. In the horizontal position, the pull of gravity is less, so kicking can occur. Therefore, the researchers suggest the stepping reflex actually is linked (but not directly related) to later walking through spontaneous kicking. Underlying both reflexes and voluntary action are common motor *primitives*, such as for neural and muscular synergies (Dominici et al., 2011).

The role of reflexive behavior in the later development of voluntary movement remains unclear. Available evidence seems to suggest that *specific reflexes play at least an indirect role in preparing the infant for later voluntary movement*. Partial justification for this assertion is based on the fact that reflexes play a significant role in the regulation, strength, and distribution of infant muscularity. Most developmentalists determine this supportive element to be vital to the attainment of voluntary movements. This same line of reasoning may be used with other readiness elements, such as postural control and balance, for which specific reflexes can provide practice. It should be noted that most of the same may be said for this next class of involuntary movements—spontaneous movements.

SPONTANEOUS MOVEMENTS (STEREOTYPIES)

Objective 8.4

In contrast to reflex behavior, **spontaneous movements**, or stereotypies, are stereotypic repetitive motions that appear in the absence of any known stimuli. Compared to rudimentary behaviors, stereotypies cannot be characterized as voluntary, goal-oriented motor behaviors. Infant stereotypies may also be viewed as *transitional behaviors* because they are performed when some level of control over body parts is involved but intentional, goal-oriented action is not yet possible. Spontaneous movements create sensory experiences that elicit neural activity that in turn assists in shaping neural development (Hepper, 2003). These early patterns of coordinated movement occur in isolation (e.g., single kick) and in bouts of rhythmic limb flexion and extension. Spontaneous movements occur with increasing frequency and peak between 6 and 10 months of age. Stereotypic behavior such as persistent rocking, waving, and other nonpurposeful spontaneous movements are considered abnormal in older children and adults.

WebLink

http://www.vimeo.com/; see *Reflexes and Spontaneous*. http://www.youtube.com/; see *Spontaneous Movements*.

Researchers have identified 67 forms of spontaneous movements (Piek & Carman, 1994; Thelen, 1979). Of the different forms, most common and first noticed is rhythmical leg kicking (single leg, two legs, and alternate leg), at about the 10th fetal week; shown in Figures 8.11 and 8.12. Other commonly found stereotypies are arm waving, arm waving with an object, arm banging against a surface (with or without an object), and finger flexion. Researchers have noted and found that these early movements are subject to several sets of organizing constraints. That is, although appearing to be random, they actually have an underlying temporal (timing) structure (von Hofsten & Rönnqvist, 1993). Once again, this adds credence to the underlying dynamic properties of the human body (see Fig. 8.11).

Other characteristic stereotypies include arching the back and rocking when on hands and knees, rocking and bouncing when sitting, and bouncing while standing with support. These movements typically reach their peak later than the

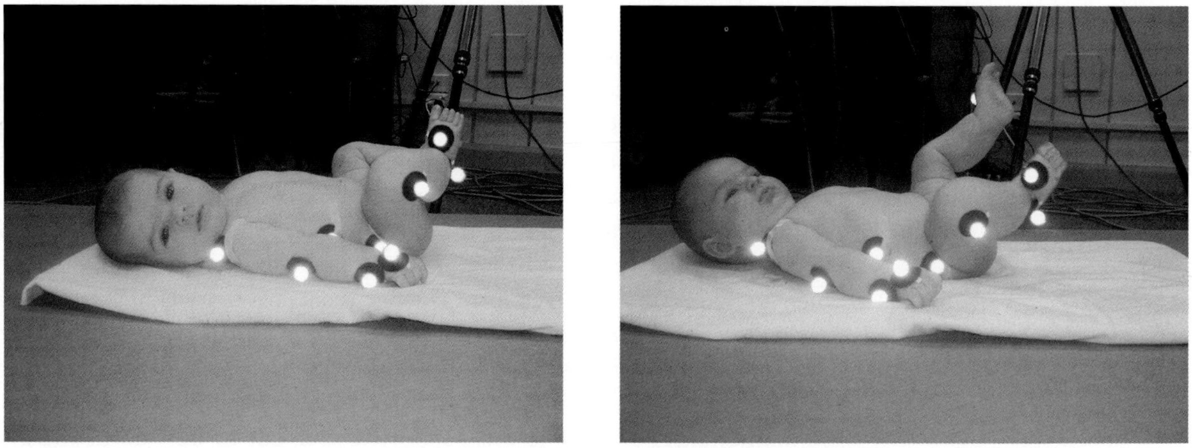

Figure 8.11 Motion analysis has been used to investigate interlimb coordination in rhythmic kicking.

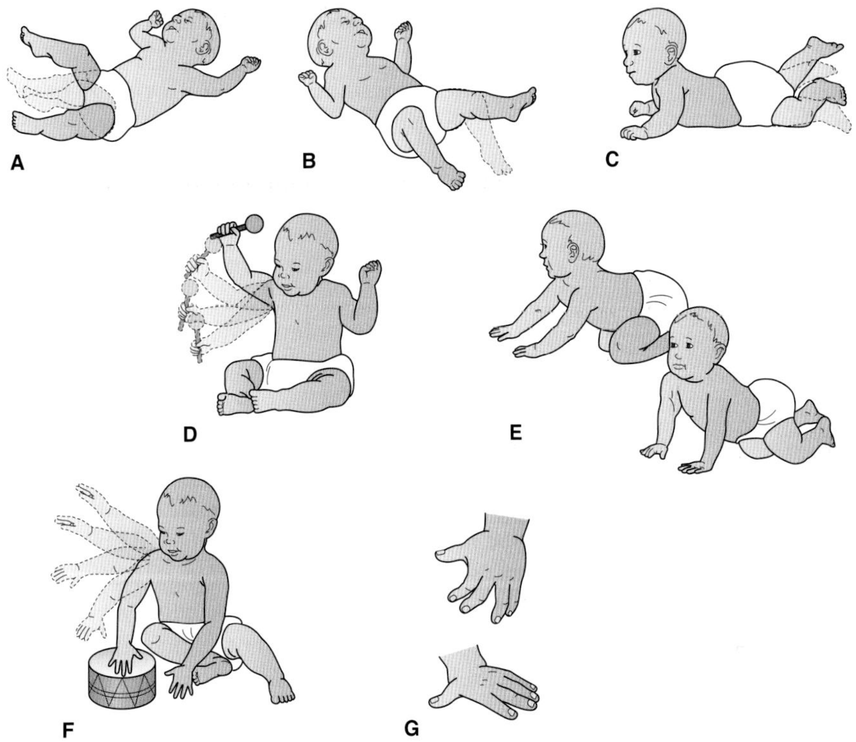

Figure 8.12 Common stereotypies: **(A)** alternate leg kicking, **(B)** single leg kicking, **(C)** kicking with both legs together, **(D)** arm waving with object, **(E)** rocking on hands and knees, **(F)** arm banging against a surface, and **(G)** finger flex.

other stereotypies. An interesting observation by Piek and Carman (1994) is that posture has a significant influence not only on the type of movement but also on movement frequency. They found that the greatest frequency was produced in the supine position (on the back). And, as infants moved to a prone position (sitting and upright), the frequency lessened. This observation underscores the postural constraint factor in this type of movement.

> **think about it**
>
> How can we be sure stereotypies are not purposeful and goal-oriented?

Although these movements do not appear to be goal-oriented and the purpose of the movements is not evident, it is apparent that their appearance is relatively predictable and orderly, and, more important, of developmental significance. Spontaneous movements provide (ensure) practice for future goal-directed actions (Adolph & Robinson, 2015). For example, stereotypic kicking characteristically precedes and accompanies voluntary control of the legs, spontaneous finger flexion normally precedes voluntary grasping attempts, and rocking on the hands and knees precedes creeping. This typical order of normal maturation prepares the infant for more complex use of the neural pathways that complement skilled motor actions.

Although stereotypies have not been determined clearly to be precursors of voluntary motor behavior, the fact that newborn infants can exhibit this degree of neuromuscular coordination with relatively little CNS activity has been a revelation. Figure 8.12 shows seven of the more common stereotypic behaviors. Refer to Piek (2006) for more information. For assessment of these movements, refer to Prechtl's method (Einspieler et al., 2008) and Karch et al. (2012). Also note that assessment of spontaneous movements is a common practice with suspected and diagnosed atypical populations (Chapter 12).

RUDIMENTARY BEHAVIOR

Objective 8.5

Rudimentary behavior typically occurs in that phase of motor development that spans the period from birth to approximately 2 years of age. As the infant's nervous system matures, a gradual increase in basic voluntary motor behavior occurs. During the first 6 to 10 months of the infant's life, these *initial voluntary movement responses* coexist with various reflexes and stereotypies. As more voluntary behavior is achieved, the infant develops a basic level of postural control, locomotion, and manual control. The acquisition of these basic abilities, in turn, provides the foundation for fundamental movement skill abilities.

The development of rudimentary movements, *although based in part to maturation, are highly influenced by the environment* (e.g., stimulation and affordances). The order of motor control generally develops in a cephalocaudal-proximodistal direction and in a relatively predictable sequence. That is, functions appear and develop earliest in the infant's head and neck, then in the shoulders and upper trunk, and later in the lower trunk and legs. The order also proceeds proximodistally from the shoulders, to the elbows, and then to control of the fingers. Progression also is characterized by the performance of gross motor before fine motor acts. This is evident in the development of manual control when, for example, infants initially use their whole arm to corral a toy before they are able to grasp it securely with a hand.

think about it

What are the implications of the exception to the cephalocaudal pattern reported by Galloway and Thelen (2004)?

However, one should keep in mind that, as noted in Chapter 1, there are exceptions to the general cephalocaudal pattern as reported by Galloway and Thelen (2004). In this study, infants (2 to 4 months old) were observed from the beginning of toy interest and provided equal opportunity to reach with either their feet or hands while seated upright off the ground. In this situation, the infants reached with their feet weeks before using their hands. These results add to an increasing body of evidence suggesting that purposeful behavior is driven by factors other than maturation.

The remainder of this chapter describes the general sequence of early voluntary movement behavior with regard to the achievement of postural control, rudimentary locomotion, and manual control. When viewing the developmental milestone charts for these actions, it is important to keep in mind that the timing of the events may vary by 2 to 4 months, and experience can modify the onset. Also, some infants may not follow the sequence described. For example, some infants may never crawl (on their belly) or creep (Adolph & Robinson, 2013).

Postural Control

Objective 8.6

The ability to maintain body posture and to move the body voluntarily into a desired position underlies all motor behavior. Postural control requires a dynamic interaction of neural and musculoskeletal systems. The infant must be able to perceive and assess sensory information and generate forces to make adjustments in body position. In general, the development of these rudimentary abilities begins with control of the head and neck muscles and proceeds in a cephalocaudal direction until the infant is able to stand alone, a course of rapid development during the first year of postnatal life. However, before the infant can stand without support and progress to the landmark achievement of upright locomotion, a number of developmental milestones must be reached. Figure 8.13 depicts the well-documented general sequence of postural control and approximate age at which

Head and upper trunk	**Approximate age (mo)**
Holds head erect voluntarily	1
Holds head and chin up	2
Holds chest up with arm support (prone)	3
Elevates head when supine	4–5
Rolls (turns)	
Side to back	2
Back to side/stomach to side	3–4
Back to stomach	5–6
Stomach to back	8
Sits	
With support	3–4
Alone	$5^1/_2$–$6^1/_2$
Gets into sitting position	8
Sits down	9
Stands	
Holding on	6–8
Pulls self to stand	$7^1/_2$–$9^1/_2$
Alone	11–13

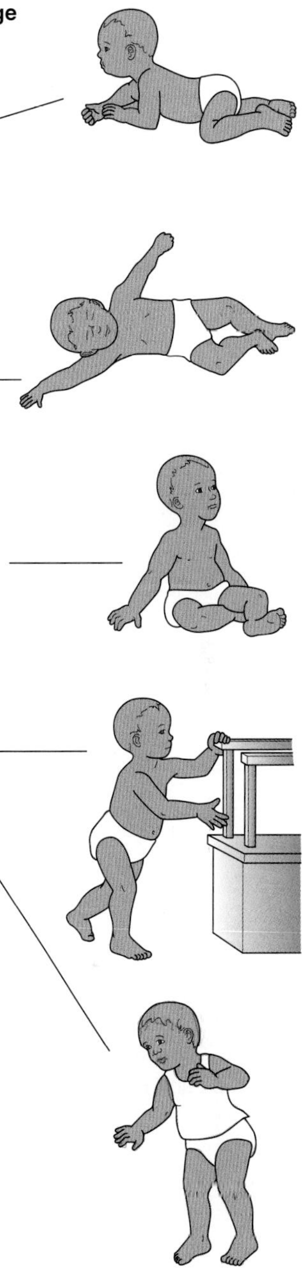

Figure 8.13 Typical sequence of rudimentary postural control.

50% to 75% of infants achieve these milestones (e.g., Bayley-3 Scales [Bayley, 2006]). However, keep in mind that with virtually all of the behaviors described in this chapter, there is considerable variability and individual difference.

HEAD AND UPPER TRUNK

Although some involuntary behavior may be evident at birth, the newborn has minimal voluntary control over the head, neck, and upper trunk. At about 1 month, the infant gains enough control of its head to hold it erect momentarily when supported at the base of the neck. When prone, the infant can hold its head up only for seconds; the movement is unsteady and the angle of vision is quite low.

focus on change

Change in postural control underscores virtually all *change* in motor skill.

By the second month, the infant is able to hold its head and chin steadily off a supporting surface while in the prone position. The head can be lifted as much as 30 degrees above the horizontal plane, thus allowing for greater visual field. At 3 months, the cephalocaudal progression is even more evident in that the infant is able to hold its head and chest up off the surface using arm support. By the fifth month, the infant can accomplish the more difficult task of lifting the head off the surface when on its back.

ROLLING (TURNING)

Rolling the body requires a certain level of control over the head, neck, and trunk. The first signs of voluntary rolling appear at about 2 months with the infant turning from its side to its back. By approximately 4 months, the infant can roll from a supine position to the side and from the prone position to the side. As the infant matures and gains greater control of the hips and shoulders, more advanced abilities, such as rolling from the supine to prone position at around 6 months, become evident. The most difficult task, rolling from the prone to the supine position, normally is achieved by 8 months.

SITTING

think about it

What are the constraints on the infant to sit and reach for an object?

By approximately 3 to 4 months, infants, while being supported, can sit with their heads relatively steady. The first attempts at sitting without support (after being placed into position) are characterized by an extreme forward lean, which may be an attempt to gain control of the lumbar region. By 6 months, the infant is able to remain in the sitting position for a short time without additional support. However, before the infant can independently position itself into a sitting posture, it must have some basic body rolling ability (indicating some control of the upper body) and possess various support reactions (e.g., parachute reflex). By 8 months, infants generally can position themselves from a prone or supine position into a sitting posture and remain there without support.

A rather important early achievement is the ability to sit down from a crouched or standing position. This task requires additional postural control and flexibility, especially if the infant is attempting to position itself in a chair. The ability to sit down with reasonable control normally is achieved around 9 months of age.

STANDING

The achievement of upright posture while standing is a major milestone in the infant's first year of development. With the ability to gain control over gravity and remain upright, the infant is ready to proceed with efforts to achieve upright locomotion (walking), perhaps the most monumental landmark in development. The first attempts to stand may occur early when the infant is held under the armpits by a parent and brought into contact with a surface. The ability to remain in the standing position while holding on to something usually occurs by the seventh or eighth month. By about 9 months of age, the infant becomes capable of pushing or pulling itself to a standing position. Typically, the infant can stand unassisted by the end of the first year. The infant does this by first getting to its knees, pushing itself upward using the power of the legs, and pulling downward with extended arms.

RESEARCH IN POSTURAL CONTROL

One of the questions explored in postural control is whether infants depend on the same stimuli for balance as adults do. A primary factor is vision, coupled with kinesthetic perception (vestibular and somatosensory). It is generally thought that in adults, visual information plays a primary role, as evidenced by sway when standing with the eyes closed. One of the more innovative ways that researchers have examined this question is by use of the moving room—a room in which the floor and participant are stable, but the walls move forward and backward (see Bertenthal et al., 1997). This setup presents a conflict of visual cues and kinesthetic information; the body is not actually moving, but it appears to be doing so. The evidence suggests that in this context, infants use visual information in a manner similar to adults (Barela et al., 2000; Bertenthal et al., 2000). However, as one might predict, infants are slower and may rely on visual information to make needed postural adjustments even more than adults do. With increasing age and experience, such as in sitting and standing, infants respond sooner. That is, they learn to couple visual cues with kinesthetic perception to make postural adjustments. See the chapter on postural control in Shumway-Cook and Woollacott (2012).

focus on change

"*Changes* in bodies, skills, and environments are especially dramatic during infancy" (Adolph, 2008, p. 27).

Rudimentary Locomotion

Generally, it is acknowledged that the two most basic motor skills in the human repertoire are the maintenance of upright posture and bipedal locomotion. Within roughly the first 6 months of life, the infant develops postural control, the ability to detect changes in the body's center of gravity in relation to the base of support. For contemporary views on the development of early locomotion, refer to Adolph and Berger (2015).

Before infants will attempt the complex task of forward upright locomotion (walking), they will move about their surroundings in a variety of ways. As early as the third month, infants have been observed to scoot along in a sitting position, using one leg to push the body along. However, basic forward locomotion normally begins during the second 6 months after birth. Although virtually all infants will develop through the orderly progression of moving forward in a prone position with crawling and creeping movement patterns, some also will use more unorthodox methods such as edging sideways like a crab and walking on all fours.

After they are able to pull up to an upright standing position at around 8 months old, some infants may be observed to cruise around by moving unsteadily from spot to spot while holding on to furniture or similar supports. This form of walking with support usually is done with sideways motion, which enables the infant to use the arms for support and control. Cruising is an important behavior because it provides opportunities to improve strength and postural control and to learn to adjust with the flow of perceptual information (see Haehl et al., 2000 for an in-depth analysis of cruising). By the age of 13 months, most infants will have achieved the single most important milestone in motor development: independent walking.

Although walking is considered a fundamental motor skill, which is the topic of the next chapter, much of the development and refinement of walking occurs before the rudimentary phase of motor behavior and infancy is over (Fig. 8.14).

Another interesting developmental observation has been noted by Adolph and Robinson (2015) using a constraints view. Within such locomotor actions as crawling, cruising, and walking, experienced infants adapt their responses to the current biomechanical constraints on movement. That is, they self-organize movements to fit the environmental challenge. For example, when infants are present with a

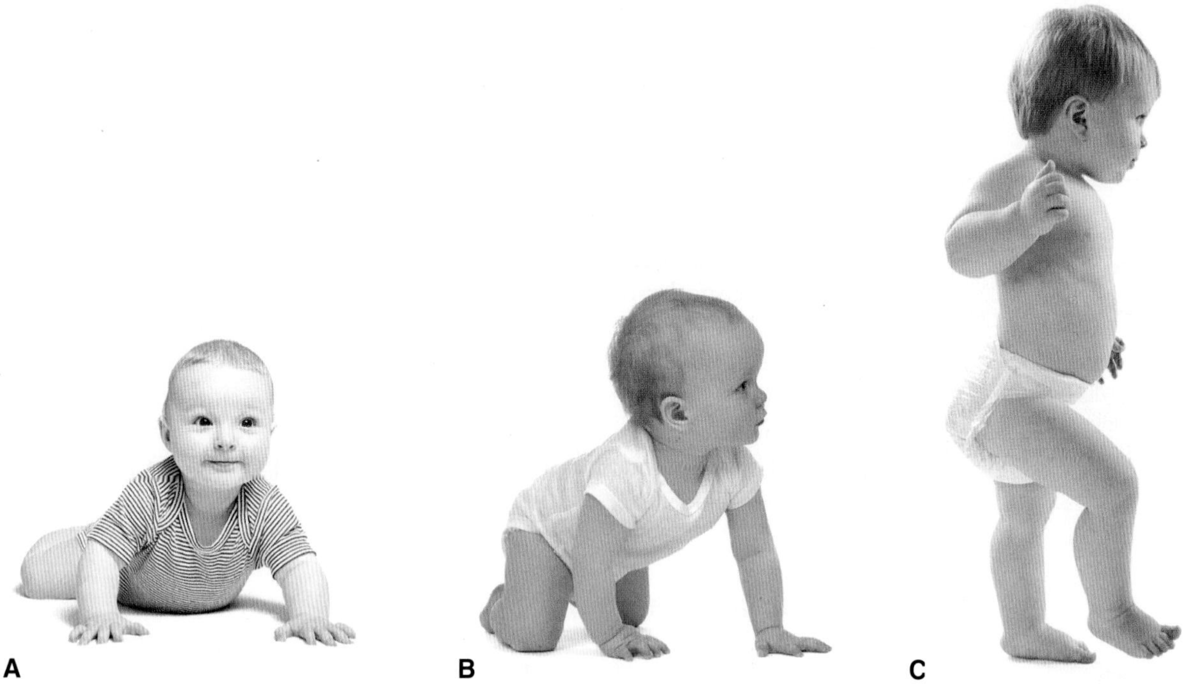

Figure 8.14 Typical sequence of rudimentary locomotor abilities.

new challenge such as crawling over objects, walking downstairs, or down a slope, infants must continually assess (update) their physical capabilities with the current task. With this experience, *infants are learning to move as they move*. Furthermore, *infants are learning as they move*. This idea supports the embodied cognition notion described earlier. Adding to that is growing evidence that early movement behavior can "instigate a **developmental cascade** of events that extend beyond mere movement of the body, effecting changes in perceptual, cognitive, and social development" (Adolph & Robinson, 2015, p. 115). That is, with newly acquired motor skills, infants explore and solve novel problems in the environment—problems that require perceptual and cognitive awareness. For example, sitting facilitates reach behavior, object awareness, and manual skill. Crawling and walking lead to more contact and interaction with the surroundings. Evidence does exist indicating that such behaviors can be a catalyst for future academic achievement (Bornstein et al., 2013).

CRAWLING AND CREEPING

Both *crawling* and *creeping* are well-known terms, but they sometimes are used in the developmental literature in ways that cause confusion. Some popular infant assessment batteries describe creeping as a precursor to crawling, whereas others note creeping as the advanced form of prone locomotion. By dictionary definition, crawling is the slow movement by dragging the prone body along the ground; creeping is the act of moving the body along slowly and close to the ground on the hands and knees. Although their differences are evident, both are slow, deliberate forms of progress. Many individuals tend to perceive creeping as a slower (thus less mature) form of locomotion. However, most contemporary references to motor development and this text use crawling to designate the movement that precedes creeping.

Focus on Application
Heavy Babies Move Less—and Later

Babies that are chubby are viewed as cute; however, new research indicates that many of those infants, compared to thinner babies, will exhibit delayed development in locomotor skills such as crawling and walking. The study examined 217 African American babies from 3 to 18 months of age. Overweight infants were about twice as likely (1.8 times) as nonoverweight infants to have a low score on the Psychomotor Development Index test, reflecting delayed motor development. Infants with high subcutaneous fat (rolls of fat under their skin) were more than twice as likely (2.32 times) as babies without fat rolls to have a low score. The primary concern is that potentially, children with delayed motor skills are less likely to be physically active.

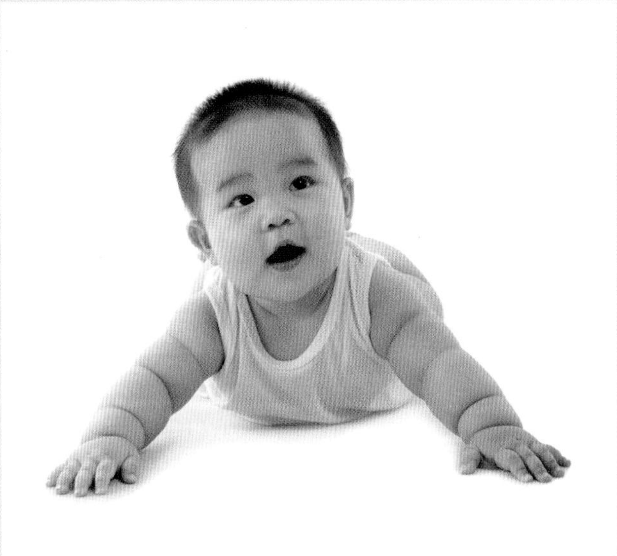

Source:
Slining, M., Adair, L. S., Goldman, B. D., Borja, J. B., & Bentley, M. (2010). Infant overweight is associated with delayed motor development. *Journal of Pediatrics*, *157*(1), 20.e1–25.e1.

Crawling represents the infant's first purposeful efforts at prone locomotion, which normally occurs between the ages of 6 and 8 months. Infants crawl using their arms and legs to drag the body along a surface. An important characteristic of this ability is that the abdomen remains in contact with the surface. Infants may use only their arms and legs, or a variety of arm–leg combinations, to achieve forward progress. Important prerequisites to crawling are control of the muscles of the head, neck, and upper trunk. It may be speculated that for crawling and creeping, certain reflex movements (e.g., asymmetrical tonic neck, labyrinthine, body righting, and crawling) provide some of the stimulus for neural and muscular development.

Creeping occurs approximately 2 months (between 8 and 10 months of age) after the appearance of crawling. In contrast to crawling, creeping movements involve moving in a prone position on hands and knees with the abdomen clear of the surface. Initial efforts are characterized by minimal elevation off the supporting surface and a *homolateral pattern of movement*; that is, the leg and arm of one side move together, alternating with the limbs of the opposite side. Shortly after sufficient strength has developed to support the abdomen above the surface, the infant's elevation increases, as do the flexion and extension of the limbs. These factors support the more efficient *contralateral pattern* of movement in which the right leg and left arm are used together, alternating with the left leg and right arm. Creeping appears to be an enjoyable mode of locomotion for the infant. In fact, infants who have become independent walkers at times revert to creeping as the desired form of speedy travel. By the end of the first year, most infants have become very efficient creepers and use this pattern to move up and down stairs. For excellent reviews of crawling and creeping behavior, refer to Adolph et al. (1998) and Freedland and Bertenthal (1994).

Walking

Walking is the movement by means of shifting weight from one foot to the other, with at least one foot contacting the surface at all times. Walking is perhaps the single most significant milestone in motor development, and its characteristics have probably been researched more than any other motor skill. Although some infants may be observed taking their first independent steps at 8 or 9 months, most children will not walk independently with any degree of efficiency until approximately 13 months of age. Children usually will not achieve the mature walking pattern until the age of 5 years. Before these efforts can be attempted, the infant must possess a certain level of upright postural control as evidenced by the ability to pull up to a standing position (achieved around 8 months) or stand without assistance (achieved around 12 months). With at least some control of upright posture, infants will begin walking with the support of a parent holding their hands, or by cruising, usually laterally, from point to point while holding on to furniture or other supports (achieved around 8 to 10 months).

think about it

If all physical properties were equal in two infants, why is it likely that one will walk before the other does?

Movement Pattern Descriptions. Even when the infant walks independently, the movement pattern is usually immature (Fig. 8.15). Balance is easily lost, and falls are frequent in initial walking efforts. To compensate for the general sense of instability, the infant uses a relatively wide base of support and takes short steps. The leg action is inefficient, as demonstrated by the short steps with limited leg and hip extension. Little, if any, trunk rotation is evident. Contact with the ground is flat-footed with one knee locked and the other knee bent. Out-toeing is also present with minimal ankle movement and a slight pelvic tilt. Arm action is characterized by a high guard position in which the limbs are fixed and do not swing on each stride.

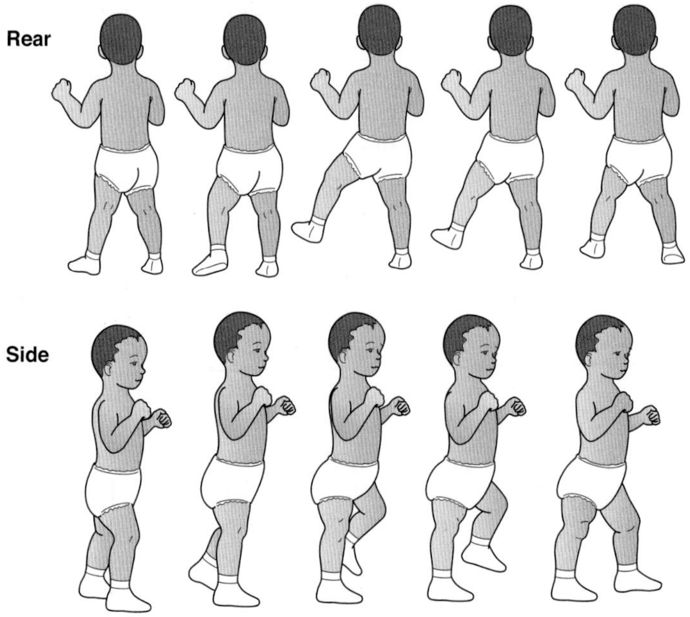

Figure 8.15 Initial (immature) walking pattern: rear and side views.

SOURCE: From Wickstrom, R. L. (1983). *Fundamental motor patterns* (3rd ed.). Philadelphia, PA: Lea & Febiger.

think about it

Also referring to Chapter 11 (older persons), compare typical walking movements of the very young (beginner) and elderly person?

With the mature walking pattern, each leg alternates between a supporting phase and a swinging phase. The heel strikes the surface first as the back leg pushes off, which shifts the weight to the front leg. The body leans forward slightly after the lead foot contacts the surface. The weight then is transferred from the heel to the outside of the foot, ball of the foot, and toes. The base of support is approximately shoulder-width, and the feet are parallel to each other with toes pointed forward. The arms swing rhythmically in opposition to the legs; the right arm swings forward with the left leg, and the left arm moves forward with the right leg.

Infants also exhibit some characteristic patterns while walking up and down stairs. This skill is sometimes referred to as *climbing stairs*, although in the truest sense, climbing involves use of the upper body. Initial efforts of walking up stairs are characterized by *marking time*. With this pattern, the infant places one foot forward to the next step and then follows with the other foot to the same step. This pattern is repeated with each succeeding step. Marking time without the support of a handrail or another person's hand generally occurs between the ages of 24 and 28 months.

By the age of about 3 years, the child will progress to the more advanced *alternate stepping* movement pattern (without support). With this pattern, the first foot moves to the first step, the other foot is placed on the second step, and the cycle is repeated. Descending stairs by marking time occurs just a few months after the child learns to walk up the stairs. However, the ability to descend using the alternating step without support does not occur until around 5 years of age, about a year (12 to 15 months) after the child learns to ascend the stairs without support.

Developmental Characteristics. The walking pattern improves gradually from initial independent walking (around 13 months) to maturity at about 5 years of age. According to Shumway-Cook and Woollacott (2012), there are three requirements for successful locomotion that apply to walking: a rhythmic step pattern, control of stability, and the ability to modify gait to changes in the environment. The following general developmental trends parallel the transition from initial to mature walking:

1. The *base of support* (dynamic base) narrows to within the approximate lateral dimensions of the trunk (Fig. 8.16). This normally occurs by 4½ months after the onset of independent walking. In general, *maturation of the equilibrium system* is critical to independent walking.

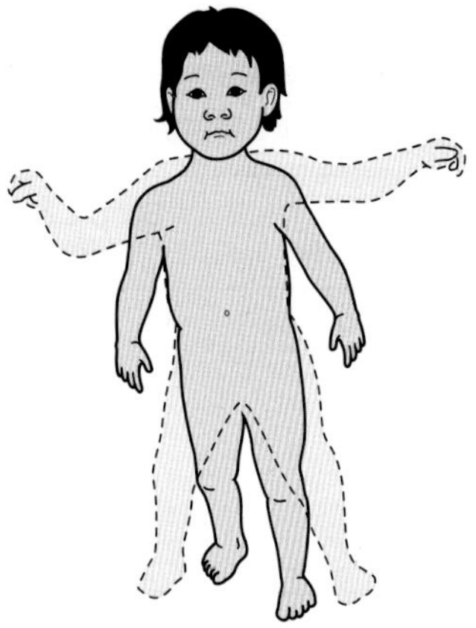

Figure 8.16 Change in arm position as base of support narrows.

2. *Foot contact* changes from flat-footed to the heel-toe pattern. The appearance of heel striking commonly is achieved by the age of 19 months. Toe stepping is common in novice walkers who have not yet reached the more advanced pattern.
3. *Foot angle* changes show a decrease in the degree of toeing out. In-toeing is usually rare and considered abnormal.
4. The single knee-lock pattern is abandoned for the more mature *double knee-lock variation*. This pattern involves heel strike with knee extension, followed by slight knee flexion as the body moves forward over the supporting leg, then extension once again at the push-off phase. This action creates a greater range of leg motion.
5. *Pelvic rotation* increases to allow full leg motion and oppositional movement of the upper and lower body segments. This action normally is observed in infants by 14 months of age.
6. The *high guard arm position* (elbows flexed and abducted) is gradually lowered and oppositional arm swinging starts. The infant's first efforts at arm swing are frequently not equal and regular; both hands might swing forward in unison. A mature arm action involves movement of the opposite arm and leg together with slight movement at both the shoulder and elbow of each arm. The change in arm position usually parallels a narrowing base of support and is achieved at approximately 18 months (see Fig. 8.16).
7. *Step and stride length increase*, which reflects greater application of force and greater leg extension at push-off. Step and stride length nearly double between 1 and 7 years of age and then increase by approximately 50% by adulthood (Table 8.2). In general, step and stride length increase linearly with increasing leg length. With this, there is a decrease in *double-support*, that is, time when both feet are in contact with the ground.
8. *Walking speed* increases and *step frequency* (steps per minute) decreases during the development of walking (see Table 8.2). Sutherland (1984) notes that younger people normally must take more steps per unit of time to increase walking speed, which is due primarily to lack of neuromuscular control.

focus on change

In regard to walking activity (steps), Adolph and colleagues (2012) reported that toddlers will accumulate more than 14,000 steps covering the length of 45 football fields in a day!

Research in Walking. Along with basic infant reaching, one of the most active lines of developmental biodynamics research has been conducted on walking using the dynamic systems approach. What follows is a glimpse of selected pioneering achievements.

TABLE 8.2 Developmental Characteristics of Gait Length and Speed

Age (y)	Step Length (cm)	Stride Length (cm)	Steps/Minute	Walking Speed (cm/s)
1	21.6	43.0	175.7	63.7
2	27.5	54.9	155.8	71.8
3	32.9	67.7	153.5	85.5
7	47.9	96.5	143.5	114.3

SOURCE: Data from Sutherland, D. H. (1984). *Gait disorders in childhood and adolescence*. Baltimore, MD: Wolters Kluwer.

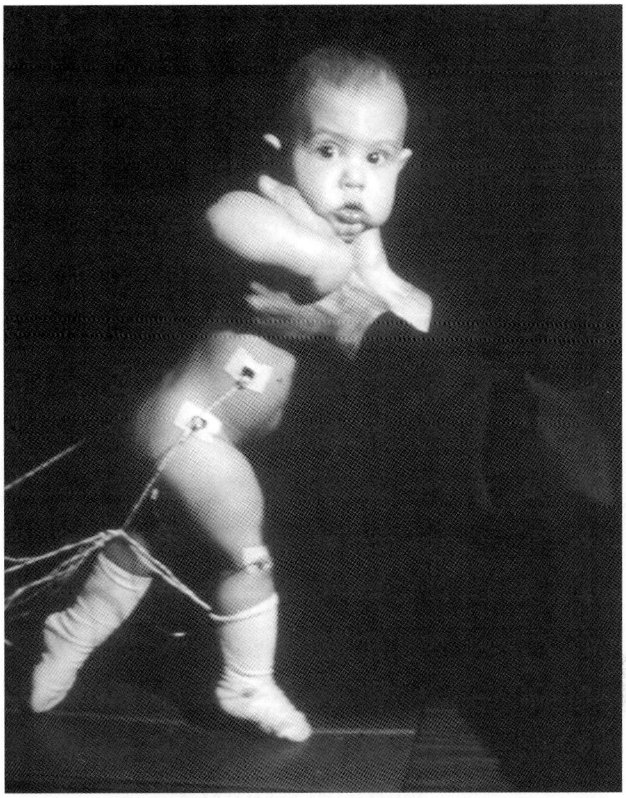

Figure 8.17 Experimental setup Thelen and her colleagues used to study dynamic components of upright locomotion.

As noted earlier (review Chapters 1 and 7), the dynamic systems approach seeks to identify and explain the *processes* associated with motor control and of change. For example, experiments by Thelen et al. (1991) have noted that some infants as young as 3 months exhibit well-coordinated, alternating stepping movements typically not common until several months later. In the experiment, infants were held by an adult over a motorized treadmill to facilitate the *stepping action* (Fig. 8.17), not a stepping reflex. By holding the infant upright, balance and leg strength (subsystems), critical *rate controllers* in independent walking, were supported, therefore allowing the apparently more mature neuromuscular component to emerge. This study supports the general dynamic systems hypothesis that the development of motor control is an *emergent* rather than a prescribed (preset) process turned on in the brain. Walking emerges as a consequence of sufficient development and cooperation of contributing subsystems that are quite adaptive for use in other contexts as well. As you may recall, this *functional adaptability* also was noted as a characteristic of neuronal group selection. Other constraints, such as environmental contexts (walking surface, slope, etc.), also contribute to behavior. An example of this was described in Chapter 6 with Karen Adolph's slopes experiment.

Clark and Phillips (1993) added to the dynamic systems literature by studying the dynamic properties of intralimb coordination in infants over the course of their first 12 months of walking. The researchers note that others have suggested that such components as body mass, limb length, and strength contribute to the dynamic system. Clark and Phillips observed that two additional control parameters, force production and balance, also play integral roles in independent walking.

think about it

What are the developmental constraints in learning to walk?

It is noted that the propulsive forces needed in coordinated walking are potentially destabilizing, but the infant's *self-organizing* system appears to compensate by spending more time with both feet on the ground than the more forceful adult does. The novice walker begins quite slowly but after a few months produces gait parameters that are much more adultlike. The researchers suggest that perhaps to compensate, the infant's control parameters are being scaled to contribute to stability and coordination.

While studying arm posture during early acquisition of walking, from high guard to coordinated alternating arm swing, Ledebt (2000) concluded (confirmed) that efficient walking is not a prewired synergy or pure reflection of neural maturation. Rather, it is a motor behavior that must be learned. Infants in this study self-organized their movements to adapt the most efficient means to overcome the problem of destabilization while shifting their weight and moving forward. This same example of *self-organization* seems to apply with learning to ski, roller-blade, or walk on ice.

As you will recall from previous discussions, one of the main principles of dynamic systems research is that behaviors emerge from the constraints that surround them, such as the organism, environment, and specific task. These findings present us with examples of how the environment influences the developmental dynamics of motor behavior.

Clearly, future research of this type will add significantly to our understanding of the mechanisms and processes that govern the development of motor behavior.

Manual Control

Objective 8.7

In addition to the attainment of basic postural control and upright locomotion, the first 2 years are characterized by several developmental milestones that involve manual coordination. Three terms commonly are used to describe this area of motor development: *prehension*, *manipulation*, and *manual control*. **Prehension** is the initial voluntary use of the hands as characterized by basic seizing or grasping. In contrast, **manipulation** refers to skillful use of the hands, such as in stringing beads or threading a needle. Skillful manipulative behaviors usually are not observed until the middle childhood years (ages 5 to 8 years), although they are a basic part of the early childhood curriculum. The term **manual control** encompasses both descriptors by referring to the developmental characteristics of hand movements. The three basic components of manual control are reaching, grasping, and releasing. Table 8.3 shows the general phases of manual control across the life span. This chapter focuses on the involuntary and prehension phases.

think about it

Cite specific examples of affordances that could stimulate the development of early manual control.

NON–GOAL-DIRECTED BEHAVIOR

The first reaching and grasping movements appear as reflexes and spontaneous movements. Involuntary grasping usually appears in the seventh fetal month and disappears by 4 months of age. Spontaneous arm and hand (flexion and grasping) movements also have been observed prior to and during voluntary manual behavior (e.g., von Hofsten & Rönnqvist, 1993; Prechtl & Hopkins, 1986). Spontaneous prereaching (arm) and finger movements may appear as early as newborn to 3 months, whereas stereotypic hand movements are generally observed between 3½ and 5½ months. These seemingly nonpurposeful stereotypic behaviors normally parallel voluntary efforts and reach their peak between 6 and 12 months of age. Refer back to Figure 8.12 on page 225 for illustrations of spontaneous (stereotypic) behaviors involving arms, hands, and fingers.

Focus on Application

Diapers Influence Infant Walking

Many parents, due to cost and what they believe feels better, prefer to provide their babies with cloth diapers. Some are bulkier and deliver a non–form-fitting shape. Obviously, some disposable diapers have the same problems. With that said, you could ask the question, "Do diapers hinder infant walking?"

According to a study published in *Developmental Science* in 2012 entitled, "Go Naked: Diapers Affect Infant Walking," the answer is yes and that relates to cloth and disposables. The study involved 30 walking babies aged 13 months and 30 aged 19 months. Each baby's walking pattern was measured while wearing disposables, old-fashioned cloth diapers, and while naked. Results for the younger group indicated that wearing diapers had an adverse effect on quality of gait. That is, babies stumbled many times more with diapers on, especially the cloth type, than when naked. The babies were tested again at 19 months of age, but it was still an issue but only with the cloth diapers and not with disposables.

Source:
Cole, W. G., Lingeman, J. M., & Adolph, K. E. (2012). Go naked: Diapers affect infant walking. *Developmental Science*, *15*(6), 783–790.

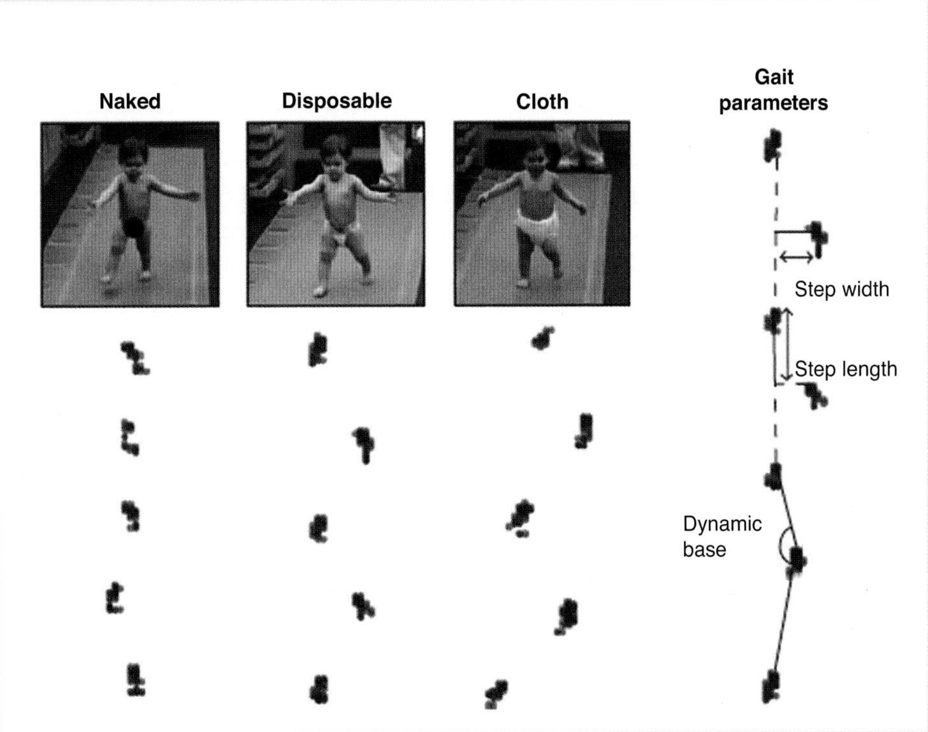

GOAL-DIRECTED BEHAVIOR

By 4 to 5 months, most infants make their initial goal-oriented efforts in reaching and grasping. With regard to the reaching segment, researchers use a dynamic system's perspective report that initial movements (trajectories) are jerky and do not follow a straight-line path (Konczak et al., 1997). However, within a few months of experience, infants make remarkable progress, and their reaches become smoother and much straighter over the first year. By age 7 months, the ability to make corrections based on visual information is quite functional.

TABLE 8.3 General Phases of Manual Control

Phase	Approximate Age	Characteristics
Involuntary	Newborn	Reflexive and spontaneous reaching and grasping
Prehension	4 mo	Initial voluntary efforts
		Corralling (both limbs)
		Palmar grasp
	5–6 mo	Smooth arm and hand action
		One-hand/pseudothumb opposition
	8 mo	Accepts two objects
	9–10 mo	Pincer grasp (thumb opposition)
	14 mo	Adultlike reaching and grasping
	18 mo	Effective release
Manipulation	5–8 y	Skillful behavior (Chapter 9)
Regression	>50 y	Fine motor control declines (Chapter 11)

Interestingly, Konczak et al. (1997) also noted that some of the basic patterns of coordination found in these infants were observed in early spontaneous movements, which provide evidence for continuity of developmental behaviors. It also has been suggested that, although young infants lack the fine motor control of adults, they learn to adjust their trajectories as a consequence of previous experience that they match with their current level of control. Learning to stabilize the body in a reaching posture and control movement speed are important factors in the early development of goal-oriented reaching and subsequent grasping. Dynamic systems research with young infants provides convincing data that support the general claim that *virtually every movement is nested into a postural set* (Reed, 1989). This suggests a functional relationship between manipulative behavior and level of postural control. This assumption has some anecdotal support as derived from laboratory studies of infants' reaching and grasping behavior. For example, van der Fits et al. (1999), while studying postural adjustments during spontaneous and goal-directed reaching in the first 6 months of postnatal life, observed that even before the onset of successful reaching (around 4 to 5 months), arm movements were accompanied by a high amount of postural activity. More specifically, early reaching success required the need for head stabilization, which the authors believed facilitates the processing of visual information. With increasing age and reaching success, the amount of postural activity decreased. In essence, this and other research indicates that the quality of reaching movements improve when infants master postural skills such as sitting without support.

In a more recent review of the history and developmental theories used to explain reaching, Williams et al. (2015) mention that, particularly, dynamic systems theory, next generation sequencing theory, and approximate optimal control theory (Barto, 2003; Berthier et al., 2005) provide a fruitful way to examine how *movement exploration* (through repeated cycles of perception and action) can lead to the *selection* and *emergence* of infant reaching. Although not described in this text, approximate optimal control theory uses modeling technology to extend and specify the notion of "value" in relation to neural mechanisms and the emergence of reaching. One of their conclusions, one that fits the developmental systems perspective used in this text, was that contemporary developmentalists believe that "the emergence and development of reaching can only be understood by considering the *continuous interactions among all levels of the developing system.* Factors such as genetics, neural maturation, anatomical structure, developmental history, current movement preferences, sensory-motor experiences, and task demands, just to name a few, continuously interact and cooperate to impact the development of behavior" (p. 7).

Grasping. The first efforts with grasping usually are characterized by a corralling action in which both arms and hands work together to pull in the object. At this point, the infant picks up the object by using the immature palmar grasp. With this form of manual control, the infant grasps the object without thumb opposition and instead uses the thumb and fingers as a unit to hold the object against the palm of the hand. Evidence indicates that young infants successfully alter grip size based on orientation and size of the object (Berthier & Carrico, 2010; Corbetta et al., 2000). That is, children learn to integrate (self-organize) perceptual information characteristics of the task and environment with their developing motor system.

During the fifth to sixth month, development normally reaches the level of reaching and grasping with one hand using *pseudothumb opposition.* Here, the thumb opposes the fingers (but not the fingertip as in true opposition) to pick up an object; there is minimal contact of the object with the palm. Infants also may transfer an object from one hand to the other during this period. By 8 months, infants normally exhibit the ability to receive two objects (holding one object in the opposite hand).

A major developmental milestone that usually occurs between 9 and 10 months is the ability to grasp small objects using true opposition of the thumb with one finger. Often referred to as the *pincer grasp,* this advanced form of manual control progresses to the level of fine motor coordination using the thumb and forefinger to manipulate objects.

think about it

What task constraints can affect grasping in young infants and the elderly?

With regard to learning to grasp large objects with two hands, Fagard and Jacquet (1996) note a few interesting observations. First, infants younger than 11 months did not perceive the need to use both hands to grasp a large object as well as older infants (12 to 13 months of age) did. Younger infants tended to activate their second hand only after the first one completed its trajectory, whereas older infants displayed more bimanual flexibility. The researchers concluded that a critical factor in development appears to be visuomanual experience.

To summarize, the sequence of manual control moves from no thumb opposition, to pseudo-opposition, to true opposition. This developmental pattern also involves a shift in the positioning of the grasped object from the little finger side (ulnar) to the thumb side (radial). During the course of development, grasped objects are positioned to occupy a more radial and distal position next to the thumb and index forefinger rather than in the palm. Figure 8.18 illustrates the basic grasping techniques and changes in object positioning. By the time the infant is 14 months old, reaching and grasping have evolved into a smooth, coordinated, adultlike action.

Unquestionably, *releasing is a difficult component of manual control.* The ability to control and relax the muscles in the arms and hands to provide a well-coordinated and accurate release is one of the final acquisitions in the development of manual

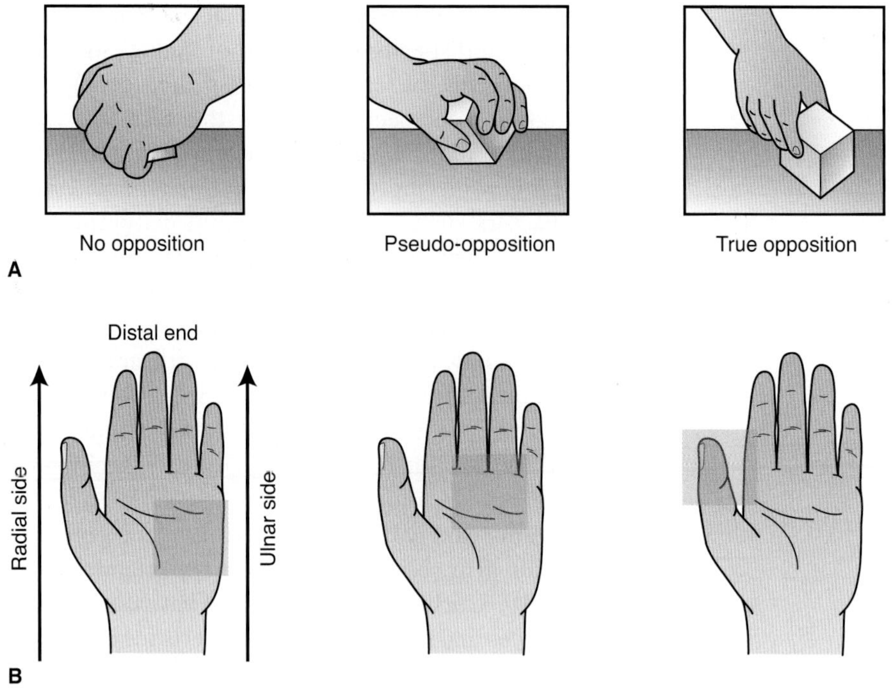

Figure 8.18 **A.** Basic grasping techniques. **B.** Changes in object positioning.

control. Although a crude form of object release may be observed as early as 8 months, when the infant opens its hand and simply allows the object to drop, accuracy of release normally is not achieved until 18 months of age.

Related to the ability to grasp and accurately release objects is the infant's perception of object weight and ability to control the amount of applied force. Prior to about 9 months of age, the application of force with the grasp appears to be unrelated to the weight of the object. Regardless of object weight, infants apply a similar force in the arm and grasping movements. By 9 months, the infant normally can adjust the force used to grasp objects of varying weights but only *after* the initial grasp of the object (Palmer, 1989). Not until approximately 18 months of age can the infant anticipate the weight of objects (after repeated presentations) and apply the appropriate amount of force. By this age, most infants apparently acquire the perception that similar objects weigh more or less based on their length. Therefore, by approximately 18 months of age, infants have acquired the general ability to reach, grasp, and release objects in a relatively well-coordinated manner.

USE OF VISUAL INFORMATION

Obviously, the perception and use of visual information are critical to the development of manual control via reaching. To succeed at reaching, infants must integrate visual and kinesthetic input and accommodate their movements to the constraints of the task. Several weeks prior to goal-oriented (voluntary) successful grasping at around 4 months, the infant projects arm and hand movements in the presence of visible objects. In a very clever setup, known as the "sticky mittens" experiment, Needham and colleagues (2002) provided nonreaching (grasping) infants with Velcro mittens that attached to objects on contact. The infants were trained at home by parents to use the mittens. Compared to age-matched controls, the sticky mitten group performed significantly more intentional attempts via visual contact with the object (toy). Several variations of this experiment have

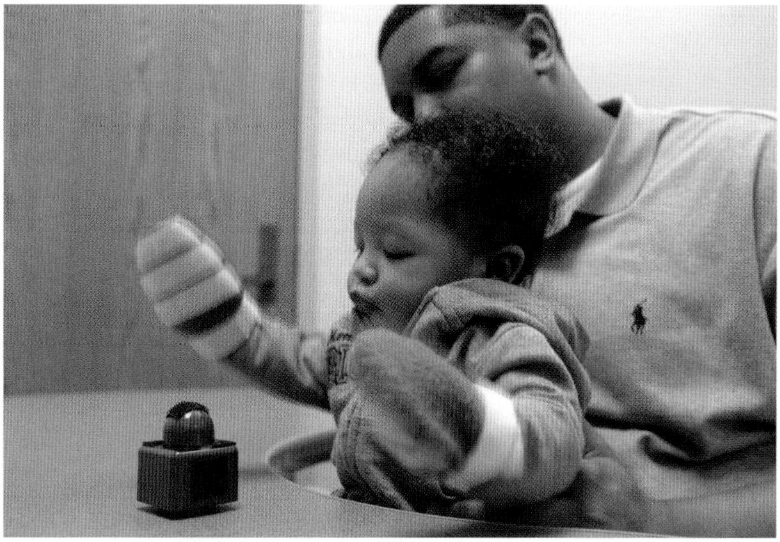

Figure 8.19 Needham and colleagues exploring infant reach via "sticky mittens."

followed using younger infants and showing similar results (e.g., Williams et al., 2015). Figure 8.19 illustrates the general experimental setup used to study reaching in infants using sticky mittens.

With the onset of goal-oriented behavior, the use of visual stimuli in reaching movements can be described as visually guided and visually elicited. The first stage, *visually guided*, describes the infant as learning to grasp by bringing both hand and object into view, thus guiding the hand toward the object. *Visually elicited* behavior begins around 6 to 7 months of age (Clifton et al., 1993; Robin et al., 1996). That is, the infant visually sights the object and follows with a trajectory, without need for sight of the hand. A common experimental setup is to have infants reach for a moving object in the light and then reach for a glowing object in the dark so they cannot see their hands. In essence, infants at this stage of development can grasp a moving object successfully without sight of their reaching hand. This behavior adds to the weight of evidence that emphasizes the importance of proprioceptive (kinesthetic) control of reaching. However, the use of visual information, whether visually guided or elicited, does play a vital role in reaching behavior. By about 9 months, reaching becomes less dependent on visual feedback and more ballistic, with corrections made toward the end of, instead of during, the movement.

For an excellent review of reach and grasp in infants, see Williams et al. (2015).

Motor Asymmetries

Objective 8.8

Some of the most evident behavioral manifestations of brain lateralization are **motor asymmetries**. That is, although the human body (and brain hemispheres) is symmetrical in general appearance, the paired limbs (hands, feet) and sensory organs (eyes, ears) are used in an asymmetric manner. Complementing this phenomenon is the fact that the cortex of the right hemisphere controls muscular activity in and receives sensory input from the left half of the body; the left hemisphere has a complementary role in conscious movement on the right side of the body (Chapter 2). Other terms often used interchangeably with motor (and functional) asymmetries are *lateral preference* and *lateral (hemispheric) dominance*.

Lateral dominance generally means that one side of the brain has developed to the point of establishing dominance for motor control; therefore, the individual has an internalized lateral preference for use of one side with a specific action or task. Although *lateral preference* most often is identified as *right-sided* or *left-sided*, there are individuals who do not consistently favor the use of one limb or the other on a specific task; these individuals are identified as *mixed-sided*.

THEORETICAL VIEWS

Perhaps the most evident and intriguing manifestation of motor behavior is that the vast majority of people are right-sided. Complementing this phenomenon is the much-debated issue of whether motor asymmetries stem from innate biological factors inherited from parents or are learned behaviors influenced by environmental contexts. In other words, is handedness (or footedness) learned, or is it primarily genetically based (inherited)? Despite volumes of literature dating back over a century (e.g., Broca, 1865; Brown-Séquard, 1877), no single theory that explains the nature and developmental characteristics of this phenomenon has been widely accepted. However, most reviews on the subject conclude there is an underlying biologically based explanation. For example, van Strien (2000) states in sum that handedness appears to be determined by genetic, intrauterine, and perinatal factors (p. 58).

One of the most widely accepted theoretical positions is the genetic model proposed by Annett (1985, 1996). According to the general tenets of Annett's right-shift theory, although the majority of the population has a strong right-shift genetic factor underlying cerebral asymmetry, the remaining portion of individuals may not express a dominant limb due to a weaker right-shift gene or lack of this inheritance (no right-shift factor). This suggests that environmental factors could influence the distribution of limb preference (right, left, or mixed) in this portion of the population. Arguments by Corballis and Morgan (1978; see also Corballis, 1983) also suggest that limb preference is specified innately, but they contend that in most of the population, there is a *left-right maturational gradient* programming the left hemisphere to mature more rapidly than the right hemisphere, thus providing the bias toward right-sidedness in limb preference.

In essence, although functional asymmetries may have origins in genetic makeup and possess maturational characteristics, few theorists would deny that specific behaviors maybe modified by cultural/environmental factors (i.e., experience). More specifically, *while direction (right, left, or mixed) of limb preference may be more fixed to biological foundations, the degree of preference could vary considerably depending on the environment* (e.g., experience, culture, manipulatives). Thus, the environment may account for developing a strong or weak phenotype (functional asymmetry).

Although there have been some exceptions, research in general has supported the variant developmental trend for handedness and footedness. This has been evidenced by a general shift toward right-sidedness with increasing age (from early childhood) for hand preference (e.g., Dargent-Paré et al., 1992; McManus et al., 1988) and foot preference behavior (as reported in a review of the literature by Gabbard & Iteya, 1996).

EARLY INFANT MOTOR ASYMMETRIES

Well before children are capable of understanding and responding reliably to conventional preference inventories, evidence of asymmetric bias may be observed. Remarkably, indications of handedness have been observed before birth.

Using ultrasound observations of fetuses during the last two trimesters, Hepper et al. (1998) and Hepper et al. (1991) noted a marked bias for arm movements and thumb sucking of the right side. The conclusion of two reviews on early infant asymmetries found the majority of newborns and young infants exhibit reflexes and spontaneous movements that are stronger and more coordinated on the "right side of the body" (Grattan et al., 1992; Provins, 1992). Types of responses favoring the right side include spontaneous head turning, spontaneous fisting, rooting reflex, asymmetric tonic neck response, right foot lead in walking reflex, and the plantar and palmar grasps. Also worthy of note is that the asymmetry described was found only in the motor (efferent) parameters (strength and coordination) and not the sensory (afferent) parameters. This may be indicative of the developmental state of the population observed (primarily neonates). As mentioned earlier, although the relationship appears complementary, the question of whether right-biased involuntary movement behaviors in infants are the basis for right-sided voluntary responses in older persons still is debated.

In regard to voluntary unimanual hand preferences in infants, evidence also shows a right-side lateral bias; a trend that increases over time (e.g., Domellöf et al., 2015). In the beginning, many infants prefer to reach with either hand toward an object, something that may persist up to 14 months of age (Campbell et al., 2015). Another interesting note, when objects are presented on the ipsilateral (same) side, older infants are more likely to reach with the same side hand, as opposed to reaching across with the "dominant" limb (Domellöf et al., 2015; Fagard et al., 2009).

think about it

Which functional asymmetry, handedness or footedness, do you think is more affected by the environment and why?

Complementing the development of motor control during childhood is a stronger emergence of *functional asymmetries* such as handedness, footedness, and eye preference. The development of these behaviors is most evident during the early childhood years and is discussed in the next chapter.

Summary

Early movement behavior is categorized by movements associated with reflexes, spontaneous actions, and rudimentary behavior. Reflexes are involuntary movements controlled by the subcortical areas of the brain. They primarily are associated with the stimulation of the CNS and muscles, infant survival, and their usefulness as a diagnostic tool for assessing neurological maturity. Theoretical viewpoints concerning the relationship between reflex behavior and voluntary movement focus on whether the link is direct (continuity view) or more indirect (reflexes must disappear before voluntary actions emerge). Most are suppressed by 6 months of age, and only a few are observable after the first year.

Spontaneous movements are stereotypic, rhythmic patterns of motion that appear in the absence of any known stimuli and do not appear to serve any apparent purpose. Some of the more frequently observed stereotypies include kicking, waving, rocking, and bouncing. Stereotypies are observable early in fetal life and reach a general peak between 6 and 10 months of age. Because their appearance is predictable and orderly, it has been suggested they are of developmental significance.

The first 2 years of life are characterized by the development of several rudimentary behaviors that follow the general trend of cephalocaudal-proximodistal growth and motor control. In general, the development of postural control begins with control of the head and neck muscles and proceeds in a cephalocaudal direction until the infant is able to stand alone. Forms of early locomotion that precede independent walking are scooting, cruising, crawling, creeping, and walking with support. Like other voluntary movements, the theory that walking is an emergent rather than prescribed (preset) process has been confirmed by research. Independent locomotion emerges as a consequence of sufficient development, cooperation of several contributing subsystems, and experience.

The first signs of hand use in the form of reaching and grasping appear as reflexes and spontaneous movements during the prenatal stage. Rudimentary (initial) voluntary manual control, referred to as *prehension*, develops rapidly during the first 2 years in the form of reaching, grasping, and releasing abilities.

Several motor asymmetries (linked to brain lateralization) are evident during the first 2 years of life. With regard to its origin, the primary debate focuses on to what extent these behaviors stem from biological factors or the environment (learning).

think about it

1. **Of the types of reflexes, how would you rank their importance?**
2. **How can we be sure stereotypies are not purposeful and goal-oriented?**
3. **What are the implications of the exception to the cephalocaudal pattern reported by Galloway and Thelen (2004)?**
4. **What are the constraints on the infant to sit and reach for an object?**
5. **If all physical properties were equal in two infants, why is it likely that one will walk before the other does?**
6. **Also referring to Chapter 11 (older persons), compare typical walking movements of the very young (beginner) and elderly person?**
7. **What are the developmental constraints in learning to walk?**
8. **Cite specific examples of affordances that could stimulate the development of early manual control.**
9. **What task constraints can affect grasping in young infants and the elderly?**
10. **Which functional asymmetry, handedness or footedness, do you think is more affected by the environment and why?**

■ LEARNING ACTIVITIES

Objective: To find a contemporary paper that describes infant (or elderly) brain activity during walking. Find a scientific paper (not older than 3 years old) that describes brain activity during walking. Summarize the paper in one or two pages in reference to aim, method (type of brain imaging), results, and your thoughts.

Objective: To create a program for assisting infants in learning a locomotor skill. After reviewing the information on rate controllers and constraints, consider how you might help an infant acquire a locomotor skill through manipulation of environmental and/or task constraints. Identify the skill, approximate age of the child, and create a lesson progression (from beginner to skilled) that systematically changes constraints to encourage emergence of the motor skill.

Suggested Reading

Marcdante, K., Kliegman, R. M., Behrman, R. E., & Jenson, H. B. (2010). *Nelson essentials of pediatrics* (6th ed.). Philadelphia, PA: Saunders.

Chapter 9

Motor Behavior During Early Childhood

OBJECTIVES

Upon completion of this chapter, you should be able to

9.1 Provide a brief overview of the fundamental movement phase of motor behavior.

9.2 List and describe basic terminology associated with fundamental movement behavior.

9.3 Discuss the methods used to study movement pattern development and the type of questions that each method attempts to answer.

9.4 Compare the composite and component approaches to describing movement pattern characteristics.

9.5 Identify key descriptive and developmental characteristics associated with fundamental locomotor and manipulative motor skills.

9.6 Describe the key developmental characteristics of manual manipulation.

9.7 Identify the basic developmental aspects of functional asymmetries.

■ KEY TERMS

- locomotor skills
- nonlocomotor (stability) skills
- manipulative skills
- fundamental movement skill
- movement pattern
- process characteristics
- product values
- composite approach
- component approach
- running
- jumping
- leap
- vertical jump
- standing long jump
- hopping
- galloping
- sliding
- skipping
- throwing
- catching
- striking
- kicking
- ball bouncing
- climbing
- manipulation
- bimanual control
- functional asymmetries

The Developmental Continuum

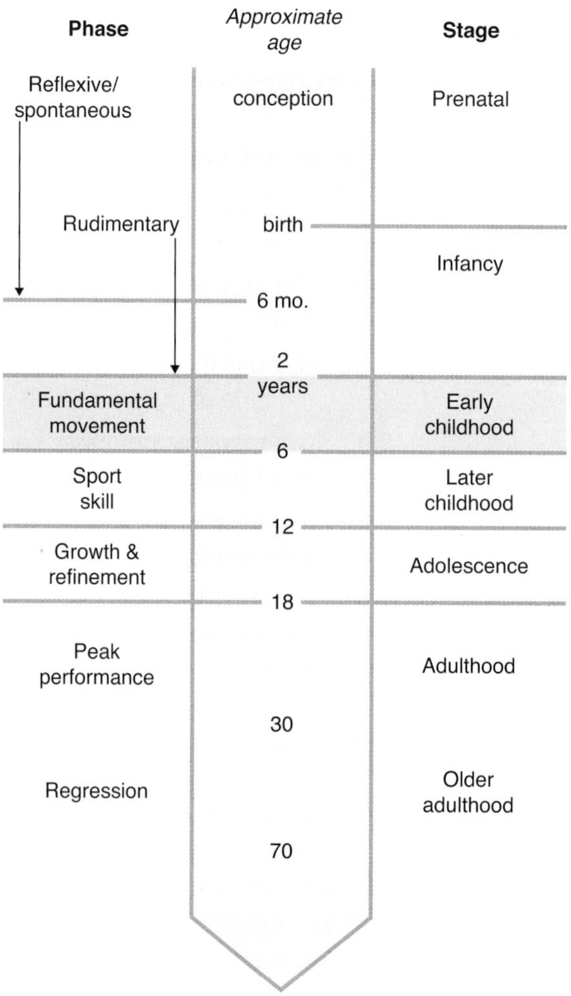

Objective 9.1

After the acquisition of rudimentary motor abilities, the individual's movement repertoire expands to include fundamental movement behaviors. The period during which these behaviors emerge normally spans the early childhood years (from approximately ages 2 to 6 or 7 years), a period of landmark significance for motor development. This phase of motor behavior sometimes is referred to as the *movement foundation*. This is based on the notion that the elements of movement behavior that develop and emerge during this period provide a substantial part of the motor skill foundation on which more complex motor programs are formed. Keep in mind that although individuals will display at least some of these behaviors, attainment is strongly influenced by *experience*, *sociocultural factors*, and *one's self-organizing properties*.

focus on change

Change in fundamental movement behavior is highly dependent on environmental as well as biological factors.

Fundamental movement behaviors may be classified into three general motor skill groups: locomotor, nonlocomotor, and manipulative. **Locomotor skills** are movements that transport an individual through space from one place to another; examples are walking, running, and skipping. **Nonlocomotor (stability) skills** involve axial movements and movements of balance executed with minimal or no movement of the base of support; examples are bending, twisting, and swaying. **Manipulative skills** include fine motor manual movements and gross motor skills that involve the control of objects primarily with the hands and feet; examples are throwing, catching, kicking, and striking. From this foundation, children begin to perform movement activities that include more advanced combinations of skills and specificity and require greater temporal and spatial accuracy.

This chapter focuses on fundamental motor skill development and places specific emphasis on those skills in which developmental motor patterns have been established. Complementing this material are descriptions of process-oriented assessment tools (tests) in Chapter 13.

FUNDAMENTAL MOTOR SKILL DEVELOPMENT

Basic Terminology

Objective 9.2

The development of fundamental motor skills is perhaps the most extensively researched area of motor development because the study of basic developmental movement patterns is considered by many to form the core of the field. As early as the 1930s, researchers sought to identify the sequence and primary developmental components of basic movement patterns. In recent years, this area of inquiry has continued to be active through the efforts of several established and promising researchers.

The terminology associated with fundamental movement skills is a vocabulary that has developed over the years of research in that field of scientific inquiry.

focus on change

"Movement forms and outcomes are determined by goals, context, and individual constraints that continually *change*" (Davis & Broadhead, 2007).

FUNDAMENTAL MOVEMENT SKILL

Also referred to as a *basic motor skill*, a **fundamental movement skill** is a common motor activity (e.g., walk, run, jump, and throw) that has specific movement patterns. It also is believed that these basic skills are general—they form the foundation for more advanced and specific movement activities.

MOVEMENT PATTERNS

Often used interchangeably with the term *motor pattern*, a **movement pattern** is the basic functional structure of a fundamental motor skill. The primary description involves a series of movements organized in a particular time–space sequence. The term also is used in reference to common elements observable in more than one motor skill. For example, several throwing and striking skills share common movement pattern elements in terms of arm, trunk, and leg action. Another term frequently associated with the identification of movement elements is *movement form*. This term also is used to describe the process rather than the product (performance) characteristics of movement.

Proficiency in fundamental movement pattern execution has been described using terms ranging from *initial* to *mature*. Each term identifies the developmental movement pattern characteristics of children in the approximate age range of 2 to 7 years. *Initial* descriptors generally depict the minimal standard of a movement pattern characteristic of children 2 to 3 years of age.

With sufficient practice, by 7 years, most children acquire at least some features of the *mature movement pattern*. This pattern represents the composite of the common elements that skilled performers used. Mature pattern performance is *skill-related* rather than age-related. That is, with practice and maturity, most children will acquire some, or perhaps all, mature pattern characteristics; however, others may not achieve a mature level until years later, if ever. This appears to be especially true of the overhand throwing pattern and standing long jump (with the two-foot takeoff and landing).

Mature fundamental movement patterns that have been adapted to the special requirements of a particular advanced movement activity such as pitching in baseball (from basic throwing) and running hurdles (from basic leaping) are known as *sport skill movement patterns*. These advanced skill movements retain most of the characteristics found in fundamental patterns and generally emerge during later childhood and adolescence.

Methods for Studying Change

Objective 9.3

Several perspectives may be taken when observing and analyzing motor pattern development. Tools of assessment range from simple observation, using the human eye, to sophisticated three-dimensional cinematography, using computers, to calculate and analyze even slight movement changes; changes that can may be viewed on your PC and smartphone. Much of the available literature on movement pattern development is based on descriptive analysis that uses relatively subjective interpretation. Over the years, however, an increasing number of researchers have deemed it more appropriate to use a biomechanical approach in analyzing movement changes.

This trend has become evident in recent research activity that studies coordinative structures (dynamic systems theory). *Biomechanics* is the physics of human motion, a study of the forces produced by and acting on the body. Two associated terms are kinematics and kinetics. *Kinematics* refers to the temporal and spatial characteristics of motion, whereas *kinetics* is concerned with the forces that act upon (i.e., cause, modify, facilitate, or inhibit) motion. The term *kinesiology* literally means the *science of motion*.

think about it

Describe what a comprehensive study of walking skills could involve.

The study of movement pattern change generally includes collection of the following types of specific information: descriptive characteristics of the movements in a pattern, range of motion at each joint, muscle action, angular velocities accompanying segmental movement, timing of the movement sequences, time devoted to each phase of a pattern, and projection angles and velocities. For a more detailed discussion of the analysis of human movement, refer to Hall (2014).

Much of the literature related to the development of fundamental movement patterns is based on qualitative descriptions. That is, the focus is on changes in "form" (**process characteristics**) rather than "performance" (**product values**). Product values are quantifiable measures of performance, such as the number of yards a ball is thrown, running velocity in seconds, and the height of a jump in feet and inches.

Objective 9.4

Researchers have used various approaches to describe and interpret *observable* movement changes using qualitative information. Currently, two practical yet scientific approaches have drawn considerable attention: the **composite approach** and the component approach. To some degree, both are *stage-oriented* and employed primarily to identify movement pattern changes across time and to describe developmental trends. The composite approach (Painter, 1994) describes motor pattern changes through a series of discrete steps (or stages) in the developmental process. Characteristic of this approach is the attempt to break down movement pattern changes into a *sequence of stages* that covers all parts of the body; hence, it is also known as the *total (whole) body approach*. Identified for each stage (e.g., step 1, step 2, and so on) are the actions of various primary body parts (e.g., for the skill of throwing, the arm action, trunk action, and leg action). The number of stages inevitably varies from skill to skill.

The **component approach** (e.g., Langendorfer & Roberton, 2002) proposes that movement pattern changes must be divided into substages to gain more accurate developmental information. Under this approach, each body component (rather than the general pattern) is followed through the development process. For example, if the stage theory uses the general description of stages 1, 2, and 3 in the development of the throwing pattern, the component approach might identify five arm action stages but only three marked changes for the legs. Obviously, for research purposes, this approach provides more precise scientific information relative to studying changes. On the other hand, the composite approach may be quite useful as a practical assessment for teachers and coaches.

The desired outcome of any hypothesized developmental sequence is that it is a valid representation of most children. As mentioned in Chapter 1, one of the best methods of developmental research is the longitudinal design. In this context, the first step is to hypothesize a developmental sequence as a result of numerous observations for children of different ages and experience. Then data would be collected from an appropriate number and age range of subjects. Subjects' performances are evaluated and compared with the hypothesized longitudinal model. The desired outcome is that the youngest (and less experienced) subjects exhibit the less proficient motor pattern characteristics, whereas the older subjects perform advanced (mature) patterns. To establish validity over time, subjects are retested periodically (e.g., yearly) to determine whether, for example, a child who originally was identified at step 1 fits the model for step 2.

To determine that they depict distinct developmental throwing changes, validation of the hypothesized sequences typically involves biomechanical (quantitative) analysis; that is, analysis of the time and spatial characteristics of particular movements. For example, a study of throwing would involve observing changes in stride length, pelvis rotational velocity, and greater trunk tilt, to name a few variables. To date, only a few of the proposed sequences have been validated to that extent; one such study is described in the section on throwing.

Why Are Fundamental Motor Skills Important?

In addition to acquiring movement proficiency with the goal of performing at a higher level either for personal enjoyment or sport, fundamental motor skills are viewed as an important vehicle for physical activity. As noted in Chapter 5, associated with the overweight and obesity problem are lower physical activity levels. The study of such has been given much attention in recent years. Research indicates, for example, that childhood motor skill proficiency predicts adolescent physical activity—children who are more proficient are more likely to become active and more physically fit adolescents (Barnett et al., 2009; Jaakkola et al., 2015). Studies of children (preschoolers and preadolescents) reveal that if they are more proficient with fundamental motor skills, less time is spent being sedentary (Hume et al., 2008; Williams et al., 2008). A similar finding has been reported with young adults (Stodden et al., 2009). In essence, children and adults that are relatively skillful tend to use those skills in an active lifestyle.

think about it

What is the role of biology/environment in the development of fundamental movement patterns during early childhood? Consider information from previous chapters to support biological change.

The following section discusses the process characteristics associated with key fundamental movement patterns that emerge during early childhood. In addition to a summary of movement pattern and developmental characteristics for each skill, examples of component and composite sequence models are included. For instructional (teaching) purposes, focusing on the mature pattern should be helpful. Also, see Graham et al. (2013) for excellent strategies in analyzing and teaching fundamental motor skills. Much of the following discussion was derived from the seminal works of Wickstrom (1983).

INFLUENCING FACTORS

As noted earlier, the attainment of fundamental movement skill proficiency is influenced by several factors. Among those, as with virtually all voluntary movements, are biology (maturation, self-organizing properties) and the environment (experience and sociocultural) factors. Two related influences that have garnered the attention of researchers are body composition and perceived motor competence.

Body composition, more specific body fat, and its relationship with motor behavior was mentioned in Chapter 3. In summary, being too small or being overweight may hinder motor performance. In this section, we focus on gross motor activities requiring motor coordination. In studies involving children 6 to 14 years old, the evidence is clear that there is a negative association between, for example, body mass index (BMI) and motor coordination (Cliff et al., 2012; D'Hondt et al., 2013; Lopes et al., 2012). That is, those with high BMI performed at a lower level than those within the normal range. Those studies compared normal-weight individuals and those who were overweight/obese on an array of fundamental movement skills.

The other influencing factor is *perceived motor competence*—an individual's awareness and belief of their capability to perform motor tasks. This is in contrast to *motor competence*, defined as a person's "actual" ability to execute different motor acts. It appears and evidence shows that the two are closely related. Perceived motor competence is typically measured using a questionnaire consisting of "confidence level" items. In studies of children, the findings suggest that motor competence is associated with perceived competence (e.g., Barnett et al., 2015; LeGear et al., 2012; Robinson, 2011). These studies examined an array of locomotor and object-control fundamental movement skills. In one study that examined the association with physical activity (Barnett et al., 2015), neither perceived nor actual motor competence was associated with physical activity. However, there does appear to be a positive association between perceived competence and adolescent physical activity (Biddle et al., 2005; Sallis et al., 2000). This is a finding that aligns well with the idea that being competent and having confidence in one's movement skill ability could be a significant factor in lifelong physical activity.

WebLink

http://www.youtube.com; see thePoint FMS collection, YouTube, or other sites for specific fundamental movement skill videos.

The next section describes a variety of common fundamental movement behaviors. For video observation and analysis, see the WebLinks provided, links that may also be used for learning activities and assignments.

MOVEMENT PATTERNS (PROCESS CHARACTERISTICS)

Running

Objective 9.5

Running is a natural extension of walking and is characterized by activity in which the body is propelled into flight with no base of support from either leg. This is in contrast to walking, in which one foot is always in contact with the surface. Because it contains a nonsupport phase, running is less stable than walking and therefore demands more bodily control. Most children take their first running steps at about 18 months and exhibit a true flight phase (minimum standard) between 2 and 3 years of age. By the age of 5 years, most children attain a reasonably skillful running form, and speed becomes a primary stimulus for performance. The general development of a skillful running pattern usually occurs without need for specific help or instruction. However, depending on the nature of the running task (e.g., sprints and long-distance running), education usually is needed to attain mastery.

Movement Pattern Descriptions. The description of the developmental pattern for running has been established primarily on running performance at maximum velocity (short sprints of 30 to 50 yards). Sprint-action analysis is used because it yields relatively constant performance, and the high degree of effort required produces maximum movement and acceptable reliability. During the initial (immature) stages of running, there is no observation flight phase and the base of support is relatively wide (Fig. 9.1). The stride is short, with the feet rotated outwardly and laterally. The center of gravity is forward and foot-to-surface contact is usually flat-footed, with some children exhibiting a tiptoe style. Arm swing is relatively rigid and more lateral and horizontal than vertical.

In the mature stage, the arms are bent at the elbows in approximate right angles and are swung vertically in a large arc in opposition to the legs. The recovery knee is raised high and swung forward quickly, whereas the support leg bends slightly at contact and then extends completely and quickly through the hip, knee, and ankle. Stride length and duration of the flight phase are at their maximum. There is little rotary movement of the recovery knee or foot as stride length

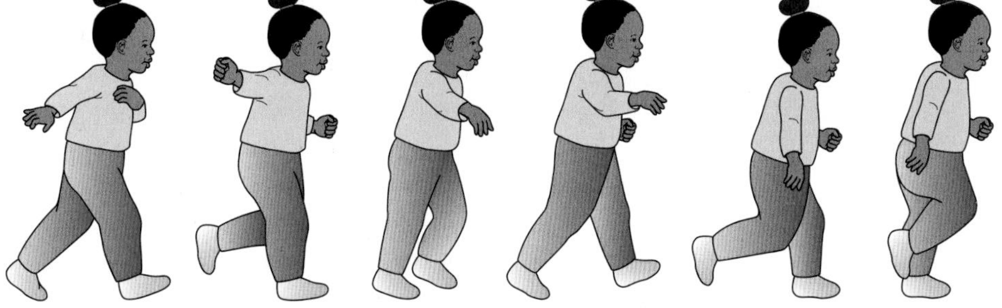

Figure 9.1 Initial running attempts of a 15-month-old.

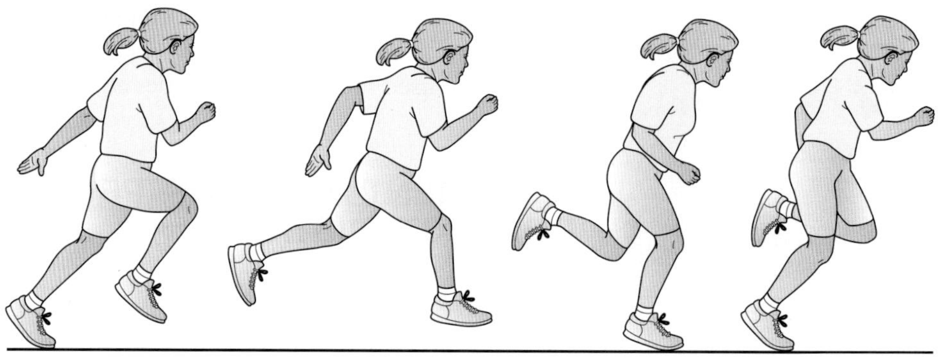

Figure 9.2 The mature running pattern.

increases. Figure 9.2 shows characteristics of the mature pattern in a young girl. The essential characteristics of the mature running pattern are as follows:

1. The trunk maintains a slight forward lean throughout the stride pattern.
2. Both arms swing through a large arc in a vertical plane and in synchronized opposition to the leg action.
3. The support foot contacts the ground approximately flat and nearly under the center of gravity.
4. The knee of the support leg bends slightly after the foot has made contact with the ground.
5. Extension of the support leg at the hip, knee, and ankle propels the body forward and upward into the nonsupport phase (*flight phase*).
6. The recovery knee swings forward quickly to a high knee raise and there is simultaneous flexion of the lower leg, which brings the heel close to the buttock.

Unfortunately, little developmental information is available on the long-distance running pattern, although it is considered a fundamental skill. Because all national physical fitness assessments include tests of distance running (rather than sprints), it is anticipated that more research in this area will follow. There are postural similarities between sprinting action and long-distance patterns, but many mechanical differences are evident. Proper mechanics and speed are primary factors in sprinting, but efficiency, pace, and endurance are paramount to the distance runner. Due to the sprinter's need for maximum forward propulsion, knee lift and rear kickup of the recovery leg are higher and the sprinter's arms move more vigorously. In contrast, the distance runner normally displays less knee flexion, uses less arm motion, contacts the ground with more of a heel-to-toe action, and displays more vertical movement. The sprinter normally relies on a combination of long stride and high frequency, whereas the distance runner exhibits a relatively short stride with low frequency and pace to conserve energy. Although the concept of pace is generally difficult for young children, the long-distance running pattern is acquired by 5 years of age.

think about it

What are the individual *constraints* driving efficient running for speed?

Developmental Characteristics. Among the numerous developmental studies of the running (for speed) movement pattern, the following major trends are frequently noted:

1. Length of stride increases. This developmental trend coincides with the age-related increase in running speed.
2. Base of support narrows.

3. Relative amount of vertical movement decreases so there is greater horizontal displacement of the center of gravity.
4. Relative distance of the support foot from the center of gravity at contact decreases.
5. Hip, knee, and ankle extension during the takeoff increases.
6. Duration of the nonsupport (flight) phase increases.
7. Support knee flexion on contact increases.
8. Knee flexion in the recovery leg increases, as exhibited by the closeness of the heel to the buttock on the forward swing.
9. Height of the swing of the forward knee (recovery leg thigh) increases.
10. Lateral leg movements and out-toeing are eliminated.
11. Arm action evolves from the immature high and middle guard positions (rigid and held laterally) to elbows flexed at approximate right angles that move in opposition to the legs.

Table 9.1 presents Roberton and Halverson's (1984) component view of the running pattern.

TABLE 9.1 Developmental Sequence (Components) for Running

Leg Action Component	
Step 1	The run is flat-footed and has minimal flight. The swing leg is slightly abducted as it comes forward. When seen from overhead, the path of the swing leg curves out to the side during its movement forward. Foot eversion gives a toeing-out appearance to the swinging leg. The angle of the knee of the swing leg is greater than 90 degrees during forward motion.
Step 2	The swing thigh moves forward with greater acceleration, which causes 90 degrees of maximal flexion in the knee. From the rear, the foot is no longer toed-out and the thigh is not abducted. The sideward swing of the thigh continues, however, which causes the foot to cross the body midline when viewed from the rear. Flight time increases. After contact, which may still be flat-footed, the support knee flexes more as the child's weight rides over the foot.
Step 3	Foot contact is with the heel or the ball of the foot. The forward movement of the swing leg is primarily in the sagittal plane. Flexion of the thigh at the hip carries the knee higher at the end of the forward swing. The support leg moves from flexion to complete extension by takeoff.
Arm Action Component	
Step 1	The arms do not participate in the running action. They sometimes are held in high guard or, more frequently, middle-guard position. In high guard, the hands are held about shoulder high. Sometimes, they ride even higher if the laterally rotated arms are abducted at the shoulder and the elbows flexed. In middle guard, the lateral rotation decreases, which allows the hands to be held waist high. They remain motionless except in reaction to shifts in equilibrium.
Step 2	Spinal rotation swings the arms bilaterally to counterbalance rotation of the pelvis and swing leg. The frequently oblique plane of motion plus continual balancing adjustments gives a flailing appearance to the arm action.
Step 3	Spinal rotation continues to be the prime mover of the arms. Now the elbow of the arm swinging forward begins to flex and then extends during the backward swing. The combination of rotation and elbow flexion causes the arm rotating forward to cross the body midline and the arm rotating back to abduct and swing obliquely outward from the body.
Step 4	The humerus (upper arm) begins to drive forward and back in the sagittal plane independent of spinal rotation. The movement is in opposition to the other arm and to the leg on the same side. Elbow flexion is maintained; the elbow oscillates at about a 90-degree angle during the forward and backward arm swings.

SOURCE: Data from Roberton, M. A., & Halverson, L. E. (1984). *Developing children—Their changing movement*. Philadelphia, PA: Lea & Febiger.

Jumping

Jumping is a motor skill in which the body is projected into the air by a force generated by one or both legs and then lands on one or both feet. One of the most diverse and fundamental of all motor skills, jumping patterns range from simple leaping (a one-foot takeoff and opposite-foot landing) to hopping (jumping from one foot to the same foot rhythmically).

For the young child, the primary challenges of jumping are sufficient leg strength to propel the body off the ground (for a longer period than required in running) and the ability to maintain postural control in the air and on landing. For these reasons, most jumping patterns are considered more difficult than walking or normal running.

Some sources document the first stage of jumping as an exaggerated step down from a higher level (stairs or box) at about 18 months. But it is generally agreed that the first true jumping movements do not occur until the child is able to project the body off the ground into flight. This form of jumping, described as a **leap**, is normally evident by approximately 2 years, when the child propels himself or herself forward and upward into flight with one foot and lands on the other foot. Although simple leaping is achieved by the age of 2 years, maximum height and distance (flight) are not accomplished until approximately age 5 years.

Table 9.2 shows the sequence of general jumping patterns and approximate age of skillful achievement. It should be emphasized that achievement levels are for the basic patterns of jumping and that these movements provide the elements for more advanced jumping variations (sport skills) commonly displayed by older children (e.g., running long jump, triple jump, and high jump).

Of the several jumping variations, the patterns that have received the most attention in the developmental literature are the vertical jump, the standing long jump, and the hop.

Both the vertical jump (for height) and the standing long jump (for distance) involve a two-foot takeoff and landing as well as distinctive preparatory, takeoff, flight, and landing phases. In the mature form of both skills, the jumper must (a) initiate a preparatory crouch; (b) vigorously swing the arms forward and upward to initiate the action; (c) extend the legs rapidly to propel the body from the ground; (d) extend the entire body during flight; and (e) flex the hips, knees, and ankles to absorb shock upon landing.

TABLE 9.2 General Sequence for Jumping Patterns

Movement	Approximate Age of Skillful Achievement (y)
One-foot takeoff and opposite-foot landing (simple leap)	2–2½
One-foot takeoff and two-foot landing	
Two-foot takeoff and one-foot landing	5
Two-foot takeoff and landing (vertical jump, standing long jump)	5–6
One-foot takeoff and same-foot landing (hop)	5–6

The standing long jump pattern is slightly more difficult than the vertical style due primarily to the angle of projection and the coordination of arm action with the leg movements required. The long jump requires the body to be propelled forward and upward. This necessitates the center of gravity to be slightly ahead of the base of support at takeoff, which may create difficulty in maintaining forward balance; there is a strong tendency for the novice to step out with one foot to avoid falling. At this angle (about 45 degrees), the jumper also must swing the legs forward under the trunk in preparation for landing, whereas in the vertical jump the legs and trunk remain relatively vertical throughout execution.

Although rhythmical hopping (one foot to the same foot repeatedly) does not require maximum effort, it is the most difficult and complex of the three forms noted. The difficulty lies primarily in the requirement of greater leg strength and better balance as well as the ability to perform controlled, rhythmical movement. All three of the jumping patterns, however, exhibit common developmental changes in relation to increased depth of preparatory crouch and increased use and effectiveness of arm action. With few exceptions, initial jumping patterns lack effective arm action. As a general rule, leg action is considerably more advanced than arm movements in the early stages of jumping. With maturity, arm movements are used effectively to aid in takeoff propulsion and in maintaining stability through flight and on landing.

think about it

What forms of jumping do we typically use in everyday life? What do young and older persons use?

VERTICAL JUMP

The **vertical jump** movement pattern involves a two-foot takeoff and landing with the primary purpose of achieving maximum height. Assessment of pattern characteristics usually is conducted by observing the skill while the individual reaches for an overhead target that elicits maximum reach. This form of vertical jumping often is described as the jump-and-reach version. If the jumping task does not include purposeful reaching (to a target) by the arms, less mature pattern characteristics usually are displayed. Although mature process characteristics of the vertical jump have been observed in children as young as 2 years old, most children do not achieve mastery until approximately age 5 years.

Movement Pattern Descriptions. In the performance of skillful vertical jumping, the knees are bent in a preparatory crouch and the arms are lowered with the elbows slightly flexed. As the knees straighten, the arms swing upward. The body stretches and extends as far as possible into vertical flight. The landing should be on the balls of the feet, with knees flexed to absorb the force of impact. However, the novice jumper frequently displays the following immature characteristics: (a) minimal preliminary crouch, (b) arms fixed at the middle- or high-guard position, (c) slight forward lean at takeoff, and (d) quick flexion at hips and knees following takeoff. An important factor in accomplishing maximum reach is the position of the shoulders and nonreaching arm at peak height. Figure 9.3 on page 258 illustrates three arm positions commonly observed in novice jumpers when reaching for an overhead target.

In the mature vertical jump pattern, the preparatory phase is characterized by flexion at the hips, knees, and ankles. A vigorous forward and upward lift by the arms initiates the jump, and thrust is continued by forceful extension at the hips, knees, and ankles. Just prior to the peak of the jump, the nonreaching arm is pushed downward. This movement tilts the shoulder girdle laterally and raises the

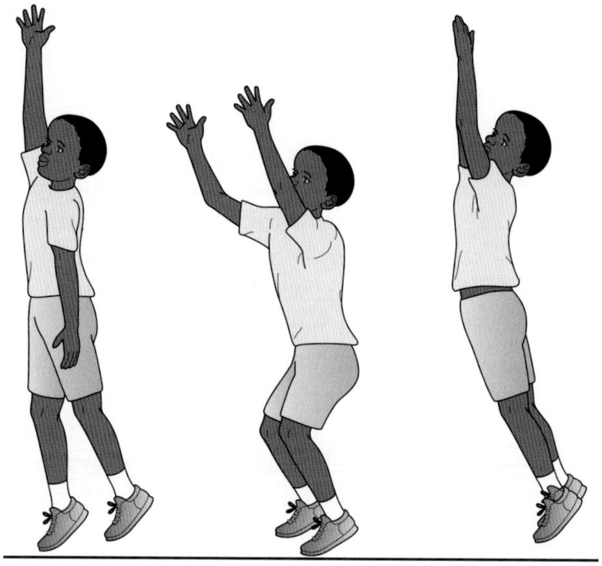

Figure 9.3 Arm positions in novice jumpers. The arm position of the child on the left is the most effective of the three arm positions shown for attaining maximum reach.

hand of the reaching arm higher. Upon landing, the ankles, knees, and hips flex to absorb the shock (Fig. 9.4).

Developmental Characteristics. The following general developmental trends have been noted in the vertical jump pattern:

1. A gradual increase in preparatory crouch
2. Increased effectiveness of arm opposition
3. Improved extension at takeoff and in flight
4. Change from a forward flexion of the head throughout the jump to deep dorsiflexion (backward) during the entire sequence
5. Greater extension of the trunk at the crest of the reach

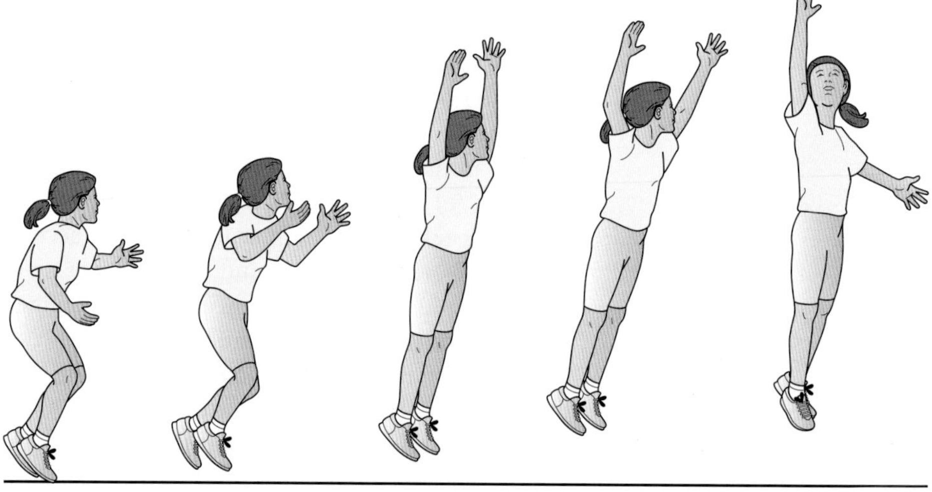

Figure 9.4 Mature vertical jumping pattern.

STANDING LONG JUMP

The **standing long jump** (two-foot takeoff and landing) for maximum horizontal distance may be considered the standard fundamental jumping skill. This form of jumping has been included in numerous motor and physical fitness assessment batteries over the years to determine jumping ability in relation to maximum distance (product). Research on the early childhood years, however, has brought focus to the development of process characteristics. These components form the basis for several advanced jumping variations older children use in a sports setting. As noted earlier, the standing long jump pattern is slightly more difficult than the jump-and-reach pattern is due primarily to the angle at which the body is projected. Although most children achieve a relatively high degree of vertical jump proficiency by age 5 years, mastery of the standing long jump usually is not observed until age 6 years.

Movement Pattern Descriptions. Skillful execution of the standing long jump requires, in general, a deep preparatory crouch and forward lean of the body that is counterbalanced by swinging the arms backward and then forcefully forward. Both feet leave the ground together with the angle of takeoff at approximately 45 degrees. The body achieves extension during flight, and the landing is on both feet. However, arm, leg, and trunk action in the initial (immature) stages of jumping are quite limited. The jumping action is not initiated effectively by the arms because of their limited swing. Several ineffective arm positions may be observed in the novice jumper. Two of the most common are arms held rigidly at the side with elbows flexed and a winging position. At takeoff, which is usually at an angle of less than 30 degrees from vertical, the trunk is propelled in more of a vertical direction with little emphasis on the length of the jump. The preparatory crouch is limited and generally inconsistent with regard to the degree of leg flexion. Extension of the hips, legs, and ankles is incomplete at takeoff, and one leg frequently precedes the other upon takeoff and upon landing. Figure 9.5A shows two immature movement patterns for the standing long jump. In Figure 9.5B, the child displays the characteristic winging arm position.

With maturity and practice, greater coordination of arm and leg movements is achieved to result in a mature movement pattern. The mature pattern is

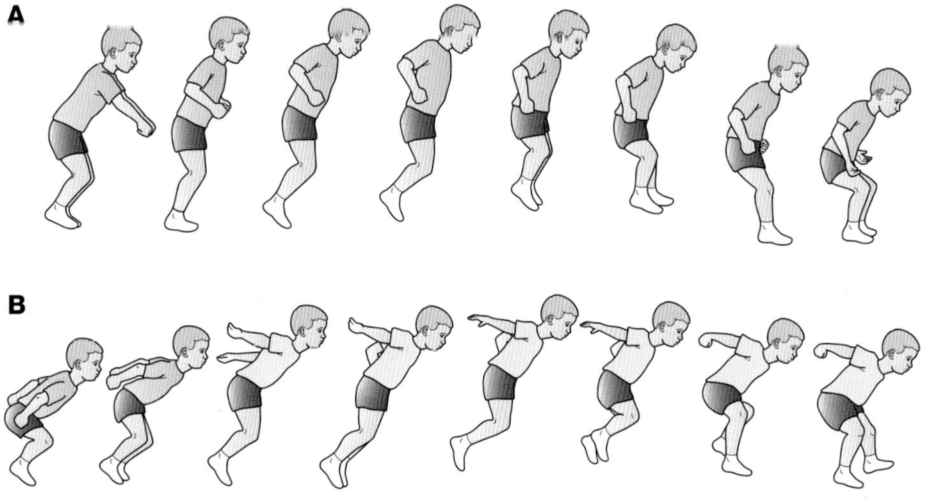

Figure 9.5 Initial patterns of the two-foot takeoff. **A.** Arms are held rigid at the sides with elbows flexed. **B.** Arms are held in a winging position.

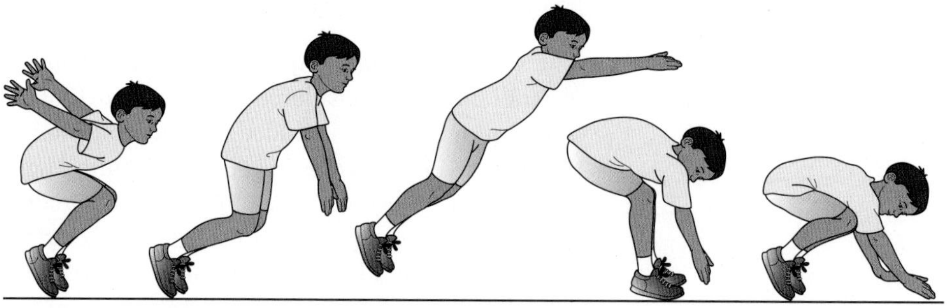

Figure 9.6 Mature stages of the horizontal jumping pattern.

characterized by a relatively deep preparatory crouch while the arms swing backward and upward (Fig. 9.6). At takeoff, both feet leave the ground together, with the thrust initiated in a horizontal direction at an angle of approximately 45 degrees. As the body moves forward, the hips, legs, and ankles extend in succession. During flight, the hips flex, which brings the thighs to a position nearly horizontal to the surface. The lower legs extend prior to landing. When the body lands on both feet, the knees bend and the body weight continues forward and downward. The arms reach forward to keep the center of gravity moving in the direction of the flight.

Developmental Characteristics. General developmental trends in the standing long jump movement pattern are similar to the developmental characteristics described for the vertical jump-and-reach:

1. An increase in the preparatory crouch
2. Greater efficiency in use of the arms as displayed by an increase in the forward swing in the anteroposterior plane
3. A decrease in the takeoff angle; theoretically, a projectile angle of 45 degrees is ideal.
4. An increase in total body extension at takeoff
5. Greater thigh flexion during flight
6. A decrease in the angle of the leg at the instant of landing

Hopping

Hopping is a coordinated one-foot takeoff and landing on the same foot repeatedly. It is considered the most difficult form of basic jumping because hopping requires greater leg strength and better balance as well as the ability to perform controlled, rhythmical movement compared to other jumping patterns. Prerequisite to hopping is the ability to balance on one foot momentarily (static balance), a skill not acquired until approximately 2½ years of age.

Because hopping is a dynamic (moving) skill, repeated steps generally are not observed until after the age of 3 years. By 3½ years of age, most children can hop one to three steps; by the age of 5 years, the ability to hop 10 consecutive times is commonly seen. However, in a study of the process components of children ages 3, 4, and 5 years, Halverson and Williams (1985) found few children who displayed advanced levels of hopping and therefore concluded the development of this skill may not reach the mature stage until the age of 6 years or older. The researchers also concluded that females are developmentally more advanced than the males are. This finding appears consistently in the literature.

Movement Pattern Descriptions. The early attempts at hopping are performed primarily in place with little forward movement. The general pattern is usually jerky with little extension and flexion of the support leg. As a result, the hop has minimal elevation and landings are flat-footed. As one would expect, arm opposition is ineffective (held in the high-guard position and to the side for balance) and the nonsupport (swing) leg often is lifted high and held awkwardly to the side or in front of the body.

As the child's balance, leg strength, and coordination improve, arm and leg actions gradually transform into a smooth rhythmical mature movement pattern. Mature hopping is characterized by arm opposition that moves forward and upward in synchrony with the swing leg. The other arm moves in direct opposition to the action of the swing leg.

Longitudinal data reported by Roberton (1990) suggest that advanced, smoothly timed arm opposition is the last component of hopping to develop and sometimes takes more than 10 years to achieve. Prior to takeoff, the weight of the child is transferred along the foot to the ball before the knee and ankle extend to takeoff. The support leg reaches maximum extension on takeoff, while the swing leg leads the upward–forward thrust with a pumping action. During this action, the swing leg passes behind the support leg (when viewed from the side). Upon landing, the hip, knee, and ankle joints flex to absorb the shock (Fig. 9.7).

Developmental Characteristics. The following major developmental trends have been observed in hopping behavior:

1. A decrease in the amount of forward body lean
2. An increase in arm action effectiveness from stabilization to efficient arm opposition
3. A change from leg clearance by flexion to clearance as a result of leg thrust
4. Improvement in the use of the nonsupportive (swing) leg, from an inactive forward position to a forward–upward swing connected with takeoff
5. An increase in range and speed of movement at the hip, knee, and ankle of the support leg
6. Change in landing from immediate extension that follows knee and ankle flexion to a delay in extension while the body pivots over the foot

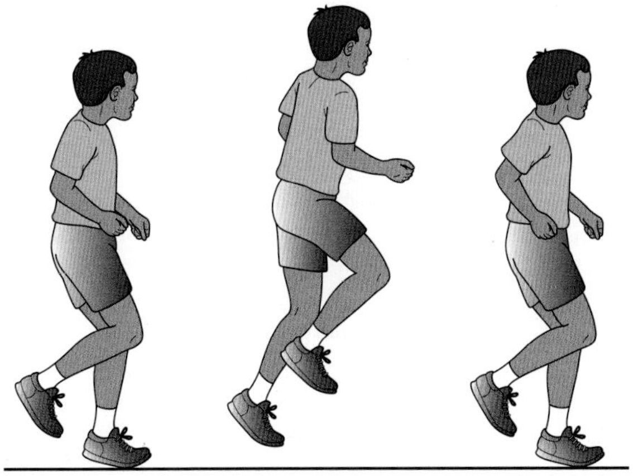

Figure 9.7 Mature hopping pattern.

Galloping, Sliding, and Skipping

Galloping, sliding, and skipping are locomotor skills that consist of a combination of basic movements. Due to their increased complexity, they normally are not mastered until the end of the early childhood years. The relatively late appearance of these skills (around age 4 years) may be expected because they require a certain level of dynamic balancing ability. As children master the ability to propel their body weight onto the forward foot, these patterns begin to appear.

Galloping, which is usually the first of these three skills to emerge, combines the basic patterns of a walking step and the leap; it is an uneven rhythmical pattern. The mature movement pattern is characterized by a slight forward lean and a thrusting forward of the lead leg. The lead foot supports the body weight, whereas the rear foot quickly closes behind the lead foot and takes the weight. During this cycle, there is extension and flexion of both legs with a momentary suspension of both feet in the air. In a series of gallops, the same foot takes the lead and contacts the ground with a heel-toe action. The arms swing freely from the shoulders during execution. In comparison to sliding and skipping, opportunities for galloping and the motivation to gallop as a mature physical activity appear limited.

Sliding is similar to galloping except the direction of movement is sideways. When sliding to the right, the right foot moves sideward and takes the weight, and the left foot follows quickly. As with galloping, the same foot always takes the lead. The first step is usually a slow gliding movement, and the second is a quick closing step. Foot contact is normally on the balls of the feet, with the weight shifted from the lead to the follow-up foot. After the follow-up foot catches the lead foot, a slight jump (momentary suspension) is displayed. At this time, the body is ready for a quick change of direction or continuation in the same pathway. Arms are held in a relaxed position at approximately waist level and to the side (see Fig. 9.8).

Of the three locomotor skills noted, **skipping** is typically the last to be mastered (between the sixth and seventh year). The general pattern involves stepping forward on one foot, quickly hopping on the same foot, duplicating the process on the opposite foot, and so on. Complexity lies in the fact that it consists of a *step-hop pattern* performed in an uneven rhythm. To perform a step-hop on one foot requires additional skill in timing of sequential movements as well as a substantial degree of balance. Another aspect of its complexity is that the step-hop is performed on one foot before the weight is transferred to the other foot.

Characteristic of mature skipping is a well-coordinated and continuous cycle of weight transfer to the opposite foot and the subsequent step-hop. The trunk is held erect with the head focused in a forward direction. The arms swing freely and

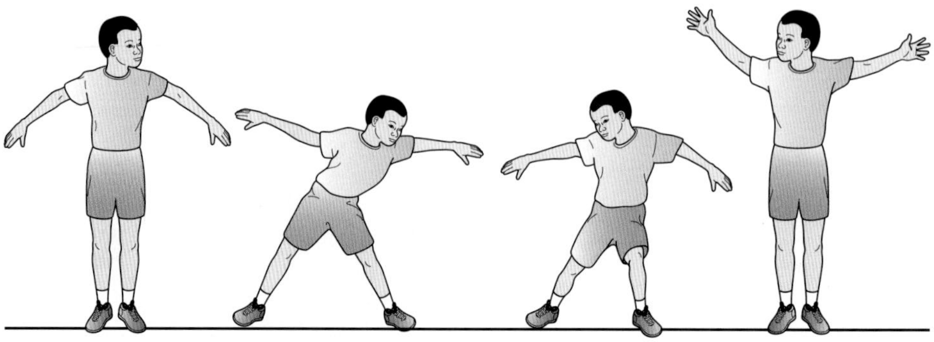

Figure 9.8 Sliding.

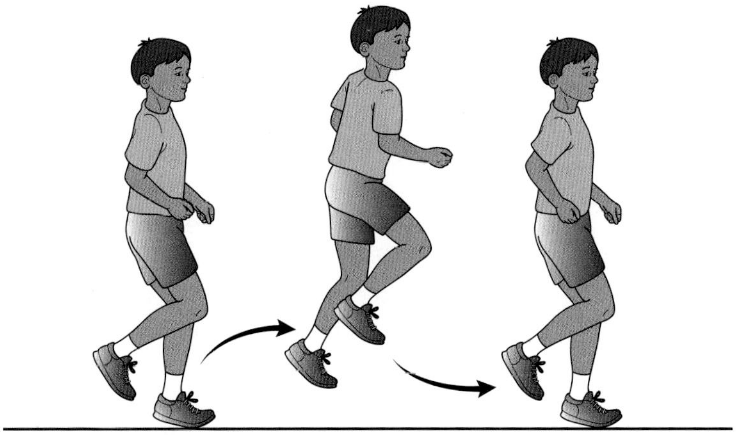

Figure 9.9 Skipping.

in opposition to leg action. The support knee and ankle extend for takeoff (which creates momentary suspension) and flex on landing. The nonsupport leg flexes to aid elevation of the hop. The balls of the feet receive the weight of the body. Figure 9.9 shows the movement pattern in skipping.

Because young females tend to be superior at hopping, it is not surprising the literature shows them to be better skippers also. For example, Haubenstricker and colleagues (1990) found females 2 to 9 years of age were consistently more advanced at skipping than males at all ages were. Males appear to be about 6 months to 1 year behind in the qualitative aspects of skipping in comparison to females. Although it is speculative, this difference could be a result of females' greater interest in and subsequent practice of the skill as well as the fact that females have a slight edge in biological maturity for chronological age.

Throwing

Throwing is a complex manipulative skill in which one or both arms thrust an object away from the body and into space. During the early childhood years, children display many different throwing patterns. There does not appear to be any definite or precise developmental order for the onset of the variations. The pattern a child uses depends on several factors, including size of the child, size of the object, and age. Of the three most common variations (overarm, sidearm, and underhand), the unilateral overarm style is used most commonly and has been studied the most thoroughly.

The first signs of the overarm pattern appear around the age of 6 months, when the child executes a crude throw that involves limited use of the arm while he or she is in a sitting position. Although a wide variation in skill level may be observed at all ages, the majority of children are skillful throwers by age 7 years. As noted, some individuals may never acquire the mature stage of a specific motor skill. The mature overarm throwing pattern is a motor skill that has a relatively high incidence of individuals (especially females) who do not reach mastery.

Data from a longitudinal study that documented pattern changes of kindergarten children to the seventh grade support this finding (Halverson et al., 1982). By the seventh grade, 80% of the males achieved the mature level in upper arm action compared to only 29% of the females. This trend was also evident for actions of the forearm and trunk. The presence of immature throwing patterns among adult females also is not uncommon, which demonstrates not all movement patterns reach the mature level during childhood or even adolescence.

As one might expect, instruction and adequate opportunity for practice are significant factors in the development of throwing technique among children; however, these factors do not appear to affect ball-throwing velocity.

Movement Pattern Descriptions. Although conducted nearly 75 years ago, Wild (1938) is recognized as having directed one of the most definitive studies of developmental form in overarm throwing. Through cinematographic analysis of throwing form in children from ages 2 to 7 years, the researcher identified four developmental stages. Subsequent observations have confirmed much of the characteristics described; as a composite model, they present a good example.

Stage 1 (2 to 3 years) is characterized by minimal trunk rotation and projection of the ball primarily by elbow extension. Virtually all movement is in the anterior–posterior plane. During the entire series of movements, both feet remain stationary and the body faces toward the direction of the throw.

Stage 2 (3½ to 5 years) is distinguished primarily by movements that occur in the horizontal plane. The feet remain stationary, but rotation of the pelvis and spine are evident. Greater projection force also is attained from the forward and downward follow-through.

The most noticeable occurrence at stage 3 (5 to 6 years) is the appearance of a step forward with the delivery. In the preparatory phase, the weight is shifted onto the left (or rear) foot while the body is rotated to the right. The arm is moved obliquely upward and behind (over) the shoulder and set in a flexed position. During delivery, the weight is transferred onto the foot on the same side as the throwing arm (ipsilateral), as the body rotates to the left and the arm projects forward. Upon completion of the follow-through, the body faces partially to the left (for a right-hander), in contrast to facing forward that took place in the preceding stages.

In stage 4 (mature pattern) (by 7 years), the thrower displays proper opposition by transferring weight to the foot opposite the throwing arm (contralateral). This action facilitates greater trunk rotation and, along with the horizontal adduction of the arm during the forward swing, enables the thrower to achieve maximum body leverage. Wickstrom (1983) provides additional clarification (composite) of the mature throwing pattern.

Preparatory phase

1. The body pivots to the right with the weight on the right foot; the throwing arm swings backward and upward.

Execution phase

2. The left foot strides forward in the intended direction of the throw.
3. The hips, and then the spine and shoulders, rotate counterclockwise as the throwing arm is retracted to the final point of its reversal.
4. The upper arm is rotated medially, and the forearm is extended with a whipping action.
5. The ball is released at a point just forward of the head with the arm extended at the elbow.

Follow-through

6. The movement is continued until the momentum generated in the throwing action is dissipated. Figure 9.10 depicts the mature overarm throwing pattern.

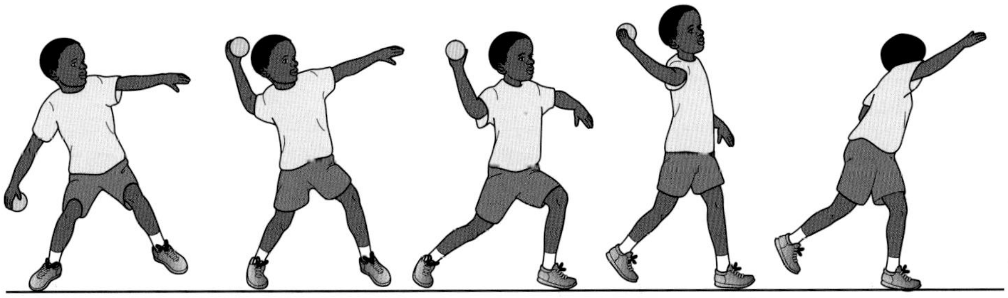

Figure 9.10 Mature overarm throwing pattern.

Roberton and Halverson (1984) (Table 9.3) offer a more precise developmental (component) analysis of the overarm throwing pattern. Research based on this model has verified that development within component parts may proceed at different rates in the same individual or at different rates in different individuals. Perhaps most notably, Stodden and colleagues (2006) determined that the developmental throwing component sequences hypothesized by this model are, with a few exceptions, valid. That is, the component levels are associated with significant differences in kinematic variable changes involving time, space, and the coupling of components. This study also identified the primary constraints (control parameters) in throwing for ball velocity as stepping and trunk actions and humerus and forearm actions. It appears that the differences in kinematics between developmental levels reflect the efficient coupling of these upper and lower extremity components. Highly skilled throwers take advantage of certain mechanical and neuromuscular principles, such as segmental inertial characteristics that promote increased energy generation and transfer to the ball. For example, the researchers note that positional configuration of the upper extremity at stride foot contact is critical to optimizing energy transfer from the lower extremities and to optimizing humerus and forearm segmental interactions during the arm-cocking and arm-acceleration phases of the throw (Fig. 9.11).

Developmental Characteristics. These developmental trends have been noted in relation to the overarm throwing pattern:

think about it

How does Wild's stages (composite of throwing) and Table 9.3 (components for throwing) compare?

1. A gradual shift of movement from a predominantly anterior–posterior plane to a horizontal plane
2. Transition from the use of a stationary base of support to weight transfer on the same side as the throwing arm, followed by functional arm–foot opposition
3. An increase with each successive throwing pattern in effective mechanical projection as evidenced by throwing velocity

Catching

Catching is a fundamental, gross motor, manipulative skill that involves visually tracking an incoming object, stopping its momentum, and gaining control of it with the hands. Receiving objects with the hands is a complex movement pattern for children. This is due primarily to the fact that catching requires coincident timing ability (Chapter 6). Recall that coincident timing is a form of temporal accuracy that involves timing self-movements with an object. Although basic patterns in coincident timing (e.g., catching, kicking, and striking) may emerge during early childhood, considerable improvement occurs

TABLE 9.3 Developmental Sequence (Components) for Overarm Throwing

Trunk Action Component	
Step 1	No trunk action or forward–backward movements. Only the arm is active in force production. Sometimes, the forward thrust of the arm pulls the trunk into a passive left rotation (assuming a right-handed throw), but no twist-up precedes that action. If trunk action occurs, it accompanies the forward thrust of the arm by flexing forward at the hips. Preparatory extension sometimes precedes forward hip flexion.
Step 2	Upper trunk rotation or total trunk block rotation. The spine and pelvis both rotate away from the intended line of flight and then simultaneously begin forward rotation, thus acting as a unit or block. Occasionally, only the upper spine twists away from, and then toward, the direction of force. The pelvis then remains fixed, faces the line of flight, or joins the rotary movement after forward spinal rotation has begun.
Step 3	Differentiated rotation. The pelvis precedes the upper spine in initiating forward rotation. The child twists away from the intended line of ball flight and then begins forward rotation with the pelvis while the upper spine still twists away.
Preparatory Arm Backswing Component	
Step 1	No backswing. The ball in the hand moves directly forward to release from the arm's original position when the hand first grasped the ball.
Step 2	Elbow and humeral flexion. The ball moves away from the intended line of flight to a position behind or alongside the head by upward flexion of the humerus and concomitant elbow flexion.
Step 3	Circular, upward backswing. The ball moves away from the intended line of flight to a position behind the head via a circular overhead movement with elbow extended, an oblique swing back, or a vertical lift from the hip.
Step 4	Circular, downward backswing. The ball moves away from the intended line of flight to a position behind the head via a circular, down, and back motion, which carries the hand below the waist.
Humerus (Upper Arm) Action Component During Forward Swing	
Step 1	Humerus is oblique. The humerus moves forward to ball release in a plane that intersects the trunk obliquely above or below the horizontal line of the shoulders. Occasionally, during the backswing, the humerus is placed at a right angle to the trunk, and the elbow points toward the target. It maintains this fixed position during the throw.
Step 2	Humerus is aligned but independent. The humerus moves forward to ball release in a plane horizontally aligned with the shoulder, which forms a right angle between humerus and trunk. By the time the shoulders (upper spine) reach front facing, the humerus (elbow) has moved independently ahead of the outline of the body (as seen from the side) via horizontal adduction at the shoulder.
Step 3	Humerus lags. The humerus moves forward to ball release horizontally aligned, but at the moment the shoulders (upper spine) reach front facing, the humerus remains within the outline of the body (as seen from the side). No horizontal adduction of the humerus occurs before front facing.
Forearm Action Component During Forward Swing	
Step 1	No forearm lag. The forearm and ball move steadily forward to ball release throughout the throwing action.
Step 2	Forearm lag. The forearm and ball appear to lag, that is, to remain stationary behind the child or to move down or back in relation to the child. The lagging forearm reaches its farthest point back, deepest point down, or last stationary point before the shoulders (upper spine) reach front facing.
Step 3	Delayed forearm lag. The lagging forearm delays reaching its final point of lag until the moment of front facing.
Action of the Feet	
Step 1	No step. The child throws from the initial foot position.
Step 2	Homolateral step. The child steps with the foot on the same side as the throwing hand.
Step 3	Contralateral, short step. The child steps with the foot on the opposite side from the throwing hand.
Step 4	Contralateral, long step. The child steps with the opposite foot a distance of over half the child's standing height.

SOURCE: Data from Roberton, M. A., & Halverson, L. E. (1984). *Developing children—Their changing movement*. Philadelphia, PA: Lea & Febiger.

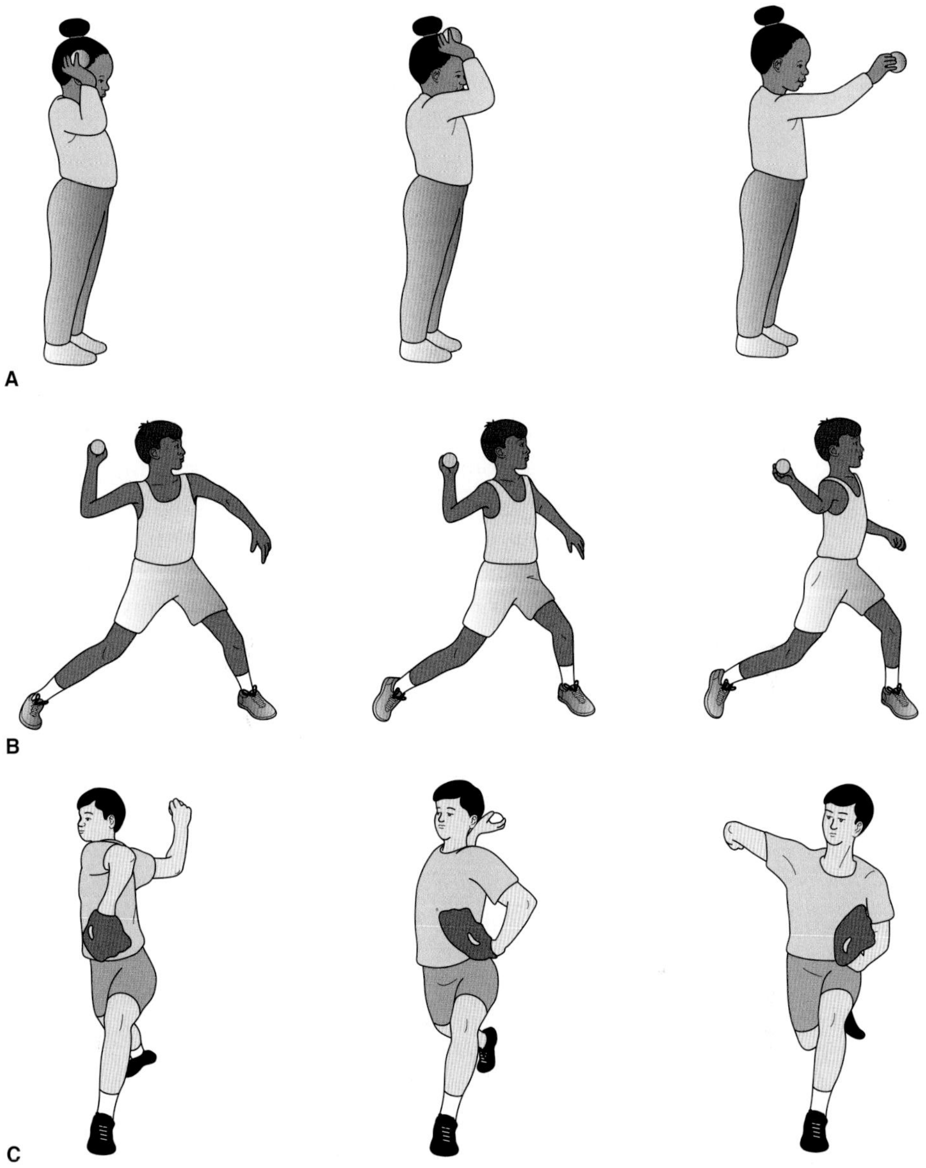

Figure 9.11 Visual description of the transfer of energy while throwing across developmental levels. For the sequence, **(A)** depicts the immature throwing pattern, **(B)** depicts a more advanced throwing pattern, and **(C)** depicts the mature throwing pattern.

from 6 to 12 years and perhaps later. Catching includes a series of complicated perceptual judgments that can vary considerably, depending on catching conditions. In addition, Davids and colleagues (2000) point out from a dynamic systems perspective that postural control may be a significant constraint on successful catching performance. Unfortunately, evidence concerning the emergence of catching skills is insufficient to provide a precise developmental description. Part of the difficulty in studying catching behavior is due to the numerous variables that influence the measurement of performance (e.g., ball size, ball speed and distance traveled, method of ball projection, and angle and level of the receiver). Because of these and other conditions under which catching has been researched, it is difficult to compare and contrast various studies.

think about it

What task *constraints* could you provide to improve catching behavior?

Although throwing and catching have a close functional relationship, catching proficiency normally follows throwing proficiency. A primitive form of catching that involves trapping can be observed in 2- and 3-year-olds, but the reports of children who achieve proficiency at this skill indicate they typically range in age from 6 to 8 years. However, these figures are based on two-handed catching in relatively stable conditions; the ability to catch a ball under more complex conditions continues to develop well into the upper elementary years (from age 10 to 12 years).

Movement Pattern Descriptions. The first attempts to stop and control a moving object occur when a ball is rolled toward a child seated on the floor with legs apart. Initially, the child will stop the ball by corralling and trapping it against the legs. With adequate practice, the child will develop the ability to coordinate arm movements with the velocity of the ball and thus trap it with the hands. As the child rises from the relatively stationary sitting position, he or she develops the ability to chase, stop, and gain control of a moving or bouncing ball. This series of achievements is important in the progression leading to comprehensive catching ability.

The first attempts to catch an aerial ball with two hands are relatively passive. That is, the child simply holds its arms out stiffly in front of the body, regardless of the angle and height of the incoming object. Little or no effort is made to move the body to adjust to the ball's flight. At the point of contact with the ball, the hands exhibit very little give; the momentum is not attenuated. In addition, there is little, if any, flexion at the knees to help absorb the shock of the ball's velocity.

A common observation in novice catchers is a negative reaction to and fear of the ball. These characteristics include turning the head to the side, a slight backward bending of the trunk away from the incoming ball, and closing the eyes. In this stage of development, success in catching is as much (or more) dependent on the accuracy of the throw as it is on the ability of the catcher. Figure 9.12 shows two variations of the immature two-handed catching pattern.

As development approaches mastery, the child displays greater coordination by adjusting the body and the hand and arm positions to accommodate the ball's flight. In addition, the catcher learns to give with the object, thus allowing the body to absorb the momentum of the projectile. The following general characteristics summarize the movements associated with the mature two-handed catching pattern:

1. Body is in alignment with incoming object.
2. Feet are slightly apart and parallel or in forward stride position.
3. Arms are held relaxed at sides (or in front of the body), and elbows are flexed.
4. Hands and fingers are relaxed and slightly cupped (pointing to object).
5. Eyes follow the flight of the object.
6. Hands move forward to meet approaching object.
7. Arms give upon contact to absorb the force and fingers close around the object. Contact and closure are simultaneous with both hands.
8. Body weight is transferred from front to back.

Developmental Characteristics. Because the qualitative evidence concerning the emergence of catching skills is insufficient for a precise developmental description, only generalized observations about developmental trends and characteristics can be made:

1. Catching ability, in general, progresses from trapping (using the arms, body, and hands) to catching an object using the hands exclusively.

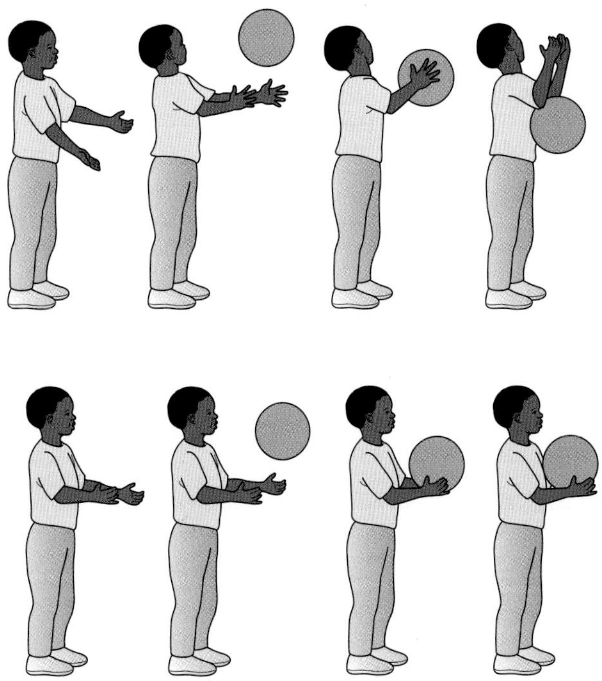

Figure 9.12 Two variations of immature catching pattern. In the upper sequence, the child displays a fear reaction. The child in the lower sequence exhibits urgent actions; the child responds to the ball only after it has touched his or her hands, then traps it against his or her chest.

2. Movement pattern action improves from a relatively passive reception (e.g., simply holding the arms out and trapping after contact) to adjusting the body to the flight of the object.
3. Positioning of the body improves to be in line with the oncoming object.
4. Arm action improves from a stiff outstretched position to a position in which the elbows are flexed and give occurs upon contact to absorb the object's momentum.
5. With practice and a subsequent increase in confidence, fear reactions to catching an aerial ball decrease in most individuals.

Figure 9.13 illustrates the mature two-hand catching pattern (with a small ball). Although no developmental sequence model for two-hand catching has been validated for all components, Table 9.4 presents an update of that endeavor (Strohmeyer et al., 1991).

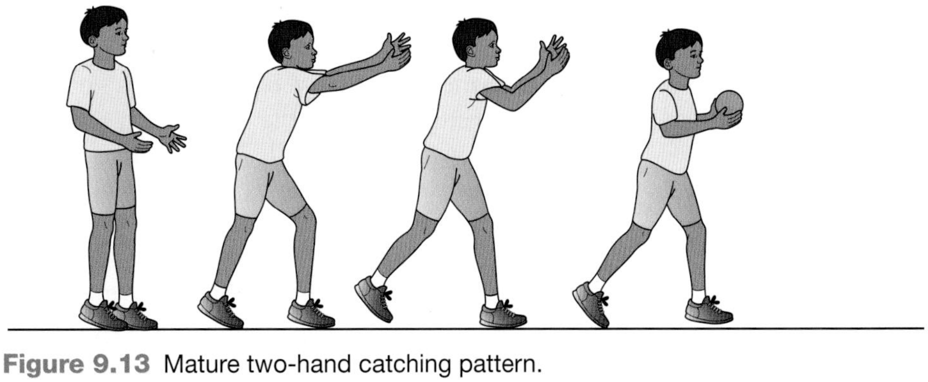

Figure 9.13 Mature two-hand catching pattern.

TABLE 9.4 Developmental Sequence (Components) for Catching

Preparation: Arm Component	
Step 1	The arms are outstretched with elbows extended, awaiting the tossed ball.
Step 2	The arms await the ball toss with some shoulder flexion still apparent, but flexion now appears in the elbows.
Step 3	The arms await the ball in a relaxed posture at the sides of the body or slightly ahead of the body. The elbows may be flexed.
Reception: Arm Component	
Step 1	The arms remain outstretched and the elbows rigid. There is little to no give, so the ball bounces off the arms.
Step 2	The elbows flex to carry the hands upward toward the face. Initially, ball contact is primarily with the arms, and the object is trapped against the body.
Step 3	Initial contact is with the hands. If unsuccessful in using the fingers, the child may still trap the ball against the chest. The hands still move upward toward the face.
Step 4	Ball contact is made with the hands. The elbows still flex but the shoulders extend, which brings the ball down and toward the body rather than up toward the face.
Hand Component	
Step 1	The palms of the hands face upward. (Rolling balls elicit palms down, trapping action.)
Step 2	The palms of the hands face each other.
Step 3	The palms of the hands are adjusted to the flight and size of the oncoming object. Thumbs or little fingers are placed close together, depending on the height of the flight path.
Body Component	
Step 1	No adjustment of the body occurs in response to the flight path of the ball.
Step 2	The arms and trunk begin to move in relation to the ball's flight path, but the head remains erect, which creates an awkward movement to the ball. The catcher seems to be fighting to remain balanced.
Step 3	The feet, trunk, and arms all move to adjust to the path of the oncoming ball.

SOURCE: These sequences were hypothesized by Harper (1979), cited in Roberton, M. A., & Halverson, L. E. (1984). *Developing children—Their changing movement*. Philadelphia, PA: Lea & Febiger.; and updated by Strohmeyer, H. S., Williams, K., & Schaub-George, D. (1991). Developmental sequences for catching a small ball: A prelongitudinal screening. *Research Quarterly for Exercise and Sport*, *62*(3), 257–266.

As noted earlier, the conditions under which catching behavior has been measured vary considerably. Obviously, catching a large ball tossed slowly in front of the body at chest level when stationary is the easier form of catching. Several factors may influence catching performance (e.g., ball velocity, trajectory angle, and ball color), but one of the most consistently noted in the literature is ball size.

As may be expected, catching performance is achieved at a certain level of performance with a large ball before the same level is attained with a smaller ball. Mature catching, using the hands only, seems to appear earlier if the child also practices with a small ball. This practice seems to induce the child to think of using only the hands when catching a small ball rather than using an arm/chest trap. When a larger ball is introduced to children after they have attained some proficiency using a small ball, they seem more likely to resort to the initial pattern. The best catching performance seems to be elicited using a ball that can be cupped in the hands (e.g., tennis ball size) but one that is not so small it requires extraordinary visual-motor control.

Striking

With **striking**, a part of the body or an implement is used to give impetus to an object. Depending on the striking situation, the skill can be executed using a variety of body parts (most commonly a hand, a foot, or the head) and a variety of implements (e.g., a paddle, racquet, or bat). Striking skills also can be performed using various movement patterns; the most common are the overhand, sidearm, and underhand patterns. Kicking, also considered a striking skill, is discussed separately because of its unique pattern characteristics.

Unfortunately, relatively little information is available on the developmental sequence of striking ability. As in the case of catching, a number of factors may affect striking performance, including the size, weight, and length of the implement used; the physical characteristics of the object to be struck; and the speed of the incoming object (whether stationary or moving).

Young children frequently display skillful striking patterns before they gain the ability to contact a moving ball with enough frequency to provide reasonable quantitative measurement. Of the various striking skills, the ones most commonly used are the one- and two-handed sidearm striking pattern in the horizontal plane. A well-defined sidearm pattern may be evident in some children at approximately 3 years of age, but the mature pattern generally is not achieved until age 5 years. The ability to consistently intercept a moving object is more difficult and continues to improve through the late elementary years (from ages 10 to 12 years).

Movement Pattern Descriptions. Striking appears to develop in much the same sequential order as throwing in terms of general age level of performance. In the initial stage, the child uses an overarm chopping action (with or without an implement) in a vertical plane. From that initial stage, the child seems to progress slowly through a downward series of planes that are more horizontal (sidearm) or even underarm.

The position of the object, however, influences the angle of the arm's approach. Most striking skills are performed with a sidearm pattern. One of the techniques most used for eliciting and assessing developmental sidearm striking characteristics is to require the individual to forcefully strike (with a racket or bat) a stationary ball suspended at approximately waist level.

Initial efforts at sidearm striking are similar to immature pattern attempts at overarm throwing. That is, the individual chops at the ball by using an overarm pattern that consists of bending forward slightly, extending at the elbow, and using minimal trunk and leg action. The general striking action is predominantly flexion and extension of the forearm. In addition, the individual usually directly faces the object (instead of standing sideways to it). If a step forward is taken (although none may be evident), it is taken with the foot on the same side as the striking arm (homolateral) (Fig. 9.14). Therefore, as with immature throwing, arm motion occurs primarily in the anteroposterior plane.

With maturity and practice, the individual gradually lowers the striking plane to the horizontal and abandons the arm-dominated movement pattern. Although the one-arm and two-arm variations of the striking skill have their own unique characteristics, each involves the same basic sequence of three movements: the step, the turn, and the swing. Basic actions within this sequence are as follows:

1. In the preparatory phase, the feet are positioned approximately shoulder-width apart.

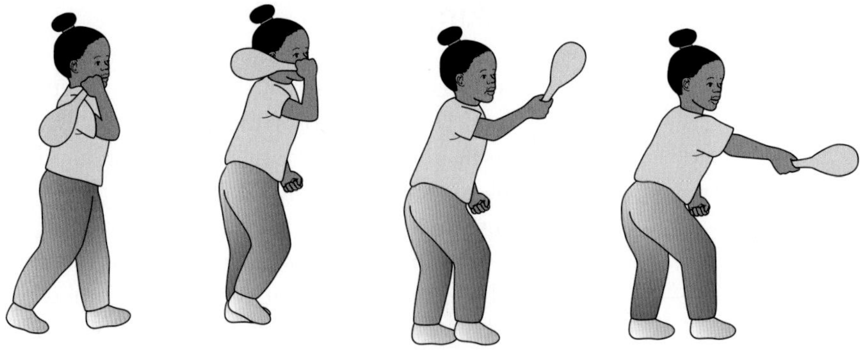

Figure 9.14 Immature one-hand striking pattern.

2. Body weight is shifted initially away from the intended hit, and then in the direction of the strike (sideways to the target), whereas the shoulders and arms are coiled in the opposite direction. That is, for right-handers, the weight is shifted onto the right (rear) foot. The individual steps with the opposite foot into the hit to apply a straight-line direction of force. The length of the step is slightly greater than one-half of the individual's height.
3. Hips and spine are rotated in rapid succession in the same direction as the weight shift.
4. The arm (or arms) swings around and forward (horizontally) in close succession with the other rotary movements. The swing is performed through a full range of motion to apply adequate force.
5. The wrist (or wrists) is cocked in preparation for the strike and uncocked just prior to contact with the object.
6. Eyes follow the flight of the ball until just before contact is made.
7. Follow-through after contact.

Figure 9.15 describes the mature one-arm striking pattern. The only additional basic characteristic unique to the two-arm striking pattern (batting) is the position of the elbow. That is, in the preparatory phase, the lead elbow is held up and out from the body, with the bat held off the shoulder (Fig. 9.16).

Developmental Characteristics. The following developmental trends and characteristics have been noted for the sidearm striking pattern:

1. Increased use of a forward step or a forward weight shift to initiate the pattern
2. Increased range of motion in the various joints during the swing

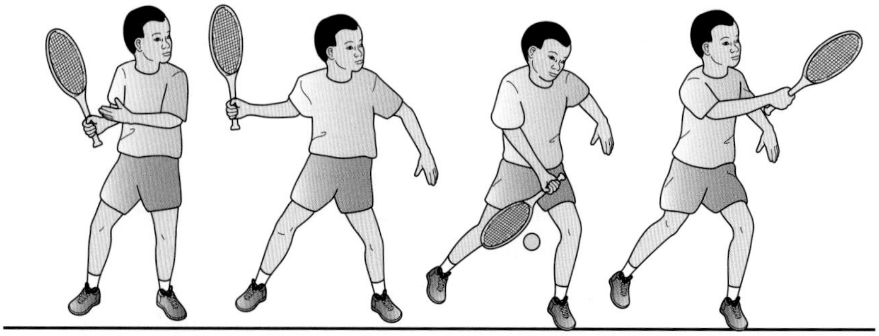

Figure 9.15 Mature one-arm striking pattern.

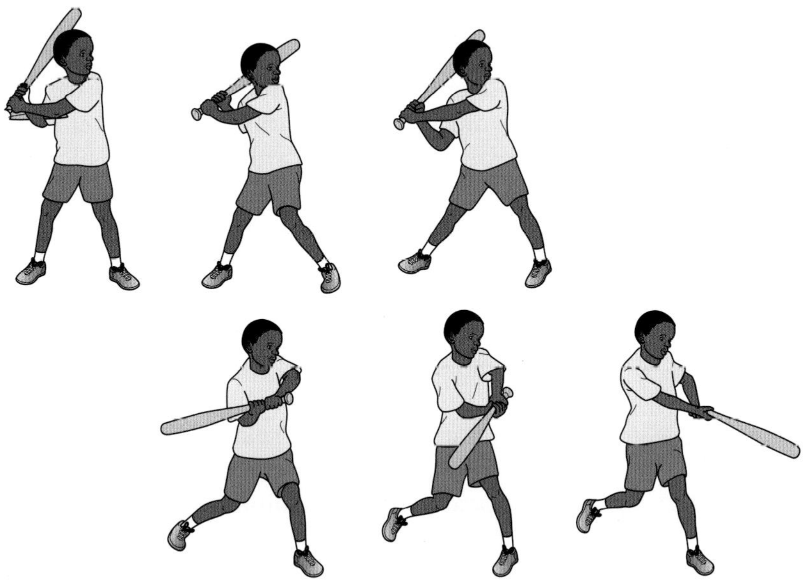

Figure 9.16 Mature two-arm striking pattern.

3. Increased hip and trunk rotation preceding the action of the arm(s) in the swing
4. Change of wrist action from a relatively stiff position to a more distinct cock and uncock action during the swing

Table 9.5 describes a developmental sequence (composite) for striking with a bat.

TABLE 9.5 Developmental Sequence (Composite) for Striking with a Bat

Stage 1	The motion is primarily posterior–anterior in direction. The movement begins with hip extension and slight spinal extension and retraction of the shoulder on the striking side of the body. The elbows flex fully. The feet remain stationary throughout the movement, with the primary force coming from extension of the flexed joints.
Stage 2	The feet remain stationary, or the right or left foot may receive the weight as the body moves toward the approaching ball. The primary pattern is the unitary rotation of the hip–spinal linkage about an imaginary vertical axis. The forward movement of the bat is in a transverse plane.
Stage 3	The shift of weight to the front-supporting foot occurs in an ipsilateral pattern. The trunk rotation–derotation is decreased markedly in comparison to stage 2, and the movement of the bat is in an oblique vertical plane instead of in the transverse path as seen in stage 2.
Stage 4	The transfer of weight in rotation–derotation is in a contralateral pattern. The shift of weight to the forward foot occurs while the bat still is moving backward as the hips, spine, and shoulder girdle assume their force-producing positions. At the initiation of the forward movement, the bat is kept near the body. Elbow extension and the supination–pronation of the hands do not occur until the arms and hands are well forward and ready to extend the lever in preparation to meet the ball. At contact, the weight is on the forward foot.

SOURCE: From Seefeldt, V. & Haubenstricker, J. (1974). *Developmental sequence for striking with a bat* (Unpublished doctoral dissertation). Michigan State University, Michigan. Reprinted with permission of John L. Haubenstricker.

Kicking

Kicking is a fundamental manipulative skill in which the foot strikes an object. Unfortunately, information on developmental kicking behavior has not been extensive. Although the characteristics of mature pattern variations and general trends have been reported, qualitative changes made within the various components are not well documented. Another limitation has been that kicking performance (distance and accuracy) of children younger than 5 years is difficult to measure in quantitative terms. Most research data on the development of fundamental kicking behavior have been collected on pattern characteristics using the placekick with a stationary ball. The placekick is considered the basic foundation on which other skills such as kicking a moving ball, dribbling, and punting are developed. These forms of advanced kicking usually are not achieved until some degree of placekicking skill has been acquired and additional perceptual abilities developed. As with catching and striking, variations in speed and position of the ball in space significantly can alter the level of difficulty.

The ability to kick a stationary ball (with minimal form) appears around the age of 2 years. But the mature pattern is not achieved by most children until 6 years old. It should be noted that proficient kicking, like proficient throwing, may not be achieved through the natural course of childhood development.

Movement Pattern Descriptions. Before an individual can execute a true kicking action, the kicker must be able to maintain an upright posture while balancing momentarily on one foot and imparting force to an object with the other foot. This ability, which is normally present by 2 years, provides the basis for initial kicking behavior.

The initial stage of kicking is characterized by a limited range of action in the propelling leg and minimal backswing and follow-through. There is little movement of the upper body, and the arms are held out from the sides for balance. The kicking leg frequently is deeply flexed while it contacts the ball. General leg movements are described as a "pushing" action and may be displayed with either leg. During the early stages of this skill, the child also may respond to a ball placed in front of the body by running into it.

As the child attempts to kick more forcefully, range of leg motion increases (more backswing and follow-through), forward lean of the trunk increases, and the arms elevate to aid in maintaining balance. Opposition of the arm and foot also begins to develop. The following actions are fundamental to the mature pattern of all basic kicking variations:

1. Preparatory forward step on the support leg to rotate the pelvis backward on the opposite side and to extend the thigh of the kicking leg
2. The support foot is placed to the side and slightly behind the ball.
3. Forward pelvic rotation and swing of the kicking leg, with simultaneous flexion at the hip and at the knees
4. Vigorous extension (whipping) of the lower part of the kicking leg
5. Momentary slowdown or cessation of thigh flexion as the lower leg whips into extension just before the foot makes contact with the ball.
6. Forward swing of the opposite arm in reaction to the vigorous action of the kicking leg (arm/leg opposition)
7. Follow-through is forward and toward the midline.

Figure 9.17 illustrates four typical stages of kicking behavior as described by Deach (1950).

Developmental Characteristics. The following developmental trends and characteristics have been noted for the placekicking movement pattern:

1. An increase in the range of preparatory movement at the hip and the knee of the kicking leg
2. An increase in the range of motion in the kicking leg
3. A tendency to start farther behind the ball and move the total body forward into the kick
4. An increase in compensatory trunk lean and arm opposition

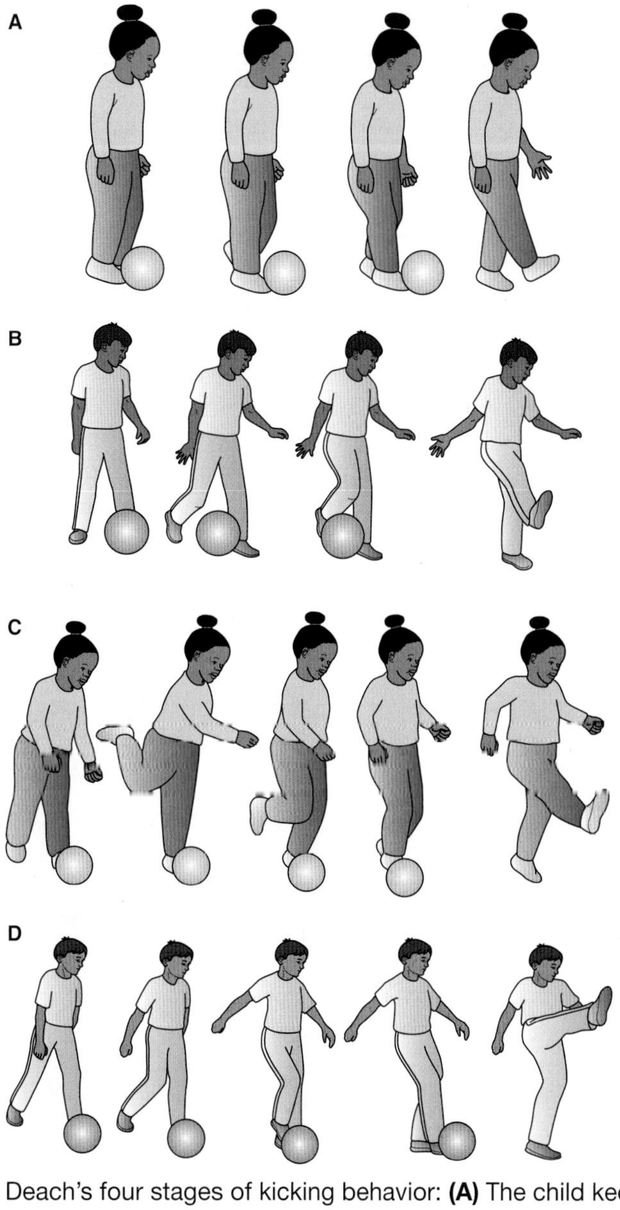

Figure 9.17 Deach's four stages of kicking behavior: **(A)** The child keeps his or her kicking leg nearly straight and exhibits minimal coordination of the rest of the body; **(B)** increased flexion of the kicking leg (precontact) and some arm opposition; **(C)** increased preliminary hip extension, greater range of leg motion, and additional body adjustments; and **(D)** the mature form of kicking behavior.

Ball Bouncing and Dribbling

Ball bouncing and dribbling propel a ball in a downward direction. It has been speculated that the development of bouncing originates as the child drops a ball, causes it to bounce, and attempts to strike the object repeatedly. As the child's control of the ball progresses, the term *dribbling* is used to describe the action; minimal form commonly is determined by the ability to bounce a ball three or four consecutive times.

Although some 2-year-olds may exhibit a minimal degree of skill in two-handed bouncing, the mature pattern of one-handed dribbling in a relatively stationary position is not mastered until approximately 6 years of age. Dribbling proficiency while moving is much more complex than dribbling in a stationary position and is considered a sport skill. The difficulty of this skill is attributed, in part, to the fact that the ball loses forward speed after each bounce and a special push is necessary to maintain the desired forward speed.

Movement Pattern Descriptions. Although a specific developmental sequence has not been validated, the following general progression has been noted:

1. Bouncing and catching
2. Bouncing and slapping on the rebound
3. Dribbling with the ball in control
4. Dribbling with the individual in control
5. Dribbling as a sport skill such as that used in basketball activities

Young children at the lowest skill level typically hold the fingers of the striking hand close together (often hyperextended) and display a distinct slapping motion. Minimal elbow extension follows a quick retraction of the hand after contact (Fig. 9.18). Because of their limited eye–hand coordination, inexperienced dribblers often strike the ball inconsistently. In essence, the ball controls the dribbler.

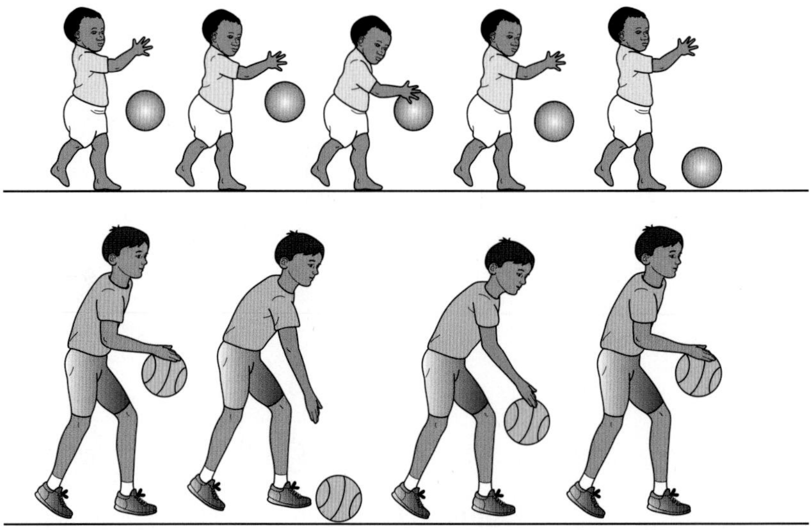

Figure 9.18 Immature and mature dribbling. The upper series demonstrates the slapping motion characteristic of immature dribbling; the lower series shows a mature dribbling action.

Focus on Application

Fundamental Motor Skill Intervention

Although intervention programs for at-risk children are certainly not new to education, thanks in large part to the national focus on physical fitness, such programs are emerging in the field of child motor development. As noted in the text, children who have some proficiency in the basic skills tend to be more physically active—a key component in developing and maintaining physical fitness. Such an intervention program was conducted by Goodway and Branta (2003), with the aim of examining the influence of a 12-week motor skills intervention on the fundamental motor skill development of disadvantaged preschoolers from an urban setting. Underlying the researchers' intent was evidence that some young children who are disadvantaged demonstrate developmental delays in basic skill proficiency.

The researchers administered the Test of Gross Motor Development (TGMD) (see Chapter 13) to both experimental and control groups prior to and following the motor skill intervention. The intervention involved instruction in hopping, galloping, ball bouncing, kicking, catching, and throwing. Overall, the experimental group demonstrated significantly greater improvement when compared to the control group. The 12-week program was described as developmentally appropriate in regard to the tasks presented and level of instruction.

Deli and colleagues (2006) compared three groups of kindergarten children over two 10-week sessions. In addition to a movement program intervention and a music/movement program intervention, the researchers included a free-play group. The researchers focused on seven locomotor skills as assessed by the TGMD. Although the free-play group did show some improvement when compared to the experimental groups, the group's progress was significantly lower on five of the seven skills. What does this type of research tell us? Perhaps foremost is the finding that a developmentally appropriate program can significantly improve the basic skill proficiency of young children. Furthermore, such a program demonstrates better improvement than free-play sessions do. The findings of two systematic reviews indicates that such programs may have sustained outcomes through childhood and adolescence (Holfelder & Schott, 2014; Lai et al., 2014).

Sources:

Deli, E., Bakle, I., & Zachopoulou, E. (2006). Implementing intervention movement programs for kindergarten children. *Journal of Early Childhood Research*, *4*(1), 5–18.

Goodway, J. D., & Branta, C. F. (2003). Influence of a motor skill intervention on fundamental motor skill development of disadvantaged preschool children. *Research Quarterly for Exercise and Sport*, *74*(1), 36–46.

Holfelder, B., & Schott, N. (2014). Relationship of fundamental movement skills and physical activity in children and adolescents: A systematic review. *Psychology of Sport and Exercise*, *15*(4), 382–391.

Lai, S. K., Costigan, S. A., Morgan, P. J., Lubans, D. R., Stodden, D. F., Salmon, J., & Barnett, L. M. (2014). Do school-based interventions focusing on physical activity, fitness, or fundamental movement skill competency produce a sustained impact in these outcomes in children and adolescents? A systematic review of follow-up studies. *Sports Medicine*, *44*(1), 67–79.

Developmental Characteristics. The transition from immature to mature dribbling action is characterized primarily by a progression that moves from slapping to pushing the ball. To achieve the mature form of multiple controlled bounces requires greater consistency in hand position at contact and more continuous contact from the upper part of the rebound through the downward pushing action. Maximum control also necessitates that the proportionate size of the hand and ball allow the dribbler to control the direction of the ball by placing the hands at the center of the ball's mass.

In contrast to the inexperienced dribbler, a pushing action is used to propel the ball with the elbow nearly fully extended. The dribbling arm stays extended with fingers pointed toward the ball and recontacts it after it bounces approximately two-thirds of the way up from the rebound. On contact, the forearm flexes and moves up with the ball; the hand remains in contact with the ball until after the downward push for the subsequent bounce. The fingers stay spread out to conform to the shape of the ball, and the height of the bounce is maintained at approximately waist level (Fig. 9.18).

Climbing

Climbing is a fundamental locomotor skill that involves ascending and descending movement using the hands and feet. The upper limbs usually initiate primary control. Climbing, an outgrowth of creeping, often is performed before walking, especially if the opportunity to practice is made available. Unfortunately, little information is available concerning the developmental process components used in climbing. Depending on the conditions under which climbing takes place (ladders, frames, nets, ropes, or stairs), a number of movement pattern variations may be used. Most information available on climbing patterns (as defined in the context of upper body involvement) has been derived from ladder and stair climbing observations.

Movement Pattern Descriptions. Two basic movement patterns appear to predominate during ladder and stair climbing: the initial pattern of *marking time* and the advanced *cross-lateral pattern*. During the initial stages of climbing, movement is characterized by marking time. That is, the child steps up or down to the appropriate level with the same foot each time. This is followed by movement of the trailing foot to the same level (Fig. 9.19). The dominant arm initiates and guides the action, which is followed by leg movement on the same side. As with the foot action, both arms are placed on the same level before the next cycle begins.

think about it

Of the fundamental skills described in the "Movement Patterns" section, which are culturally gender-biased in children's play and youth sport activities?

With increased maturity and practice, the child progresses to the alternate-foot ascent and descent described as the cross-lateral pattern. That is, rather than placing both feet on the same level, the child alternates sides and places only one foot on each level (Fig. 9.20). Hand placement may vary from positioning both hands on the same level before following with leg action to the more advanced alternating pattern (matching the leg movements). With practice and confidence, the child prefers to reach for the next highest level, therefore, displaying the alternating cross-lateral pattern with the arms as well.

Developmental Characteristics. Although there are wide differences in climbing ability at every age level, children as young as 2 years have been observed to display initial climbing patterns. By 6 years old, the majority of children are reasonably

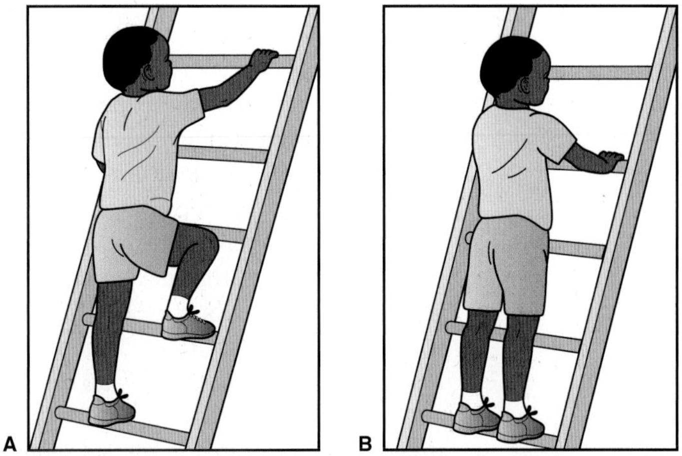

Figure 9.19 Marking time pattern: **(A)** start and **(B)** completion.

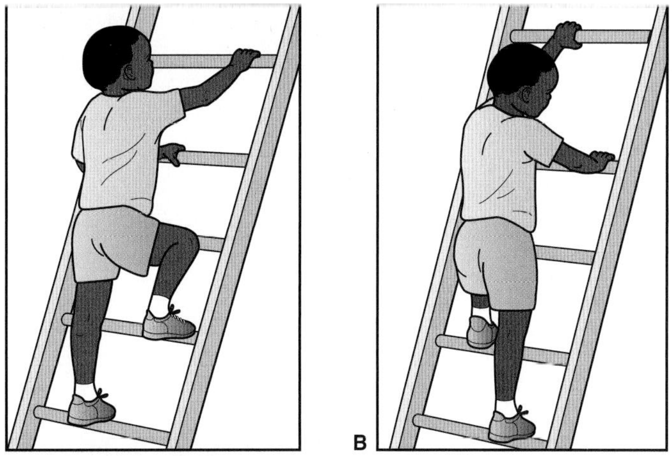

Figure 9.20 Cross-lateral pattern: **(A)** start and **(B)** completion.

proficient climbers and exhibit the mature pattern characteristics. The skill of ascending an apparatus usually is achieved before an individual attempts to descend. Children usually are capable of skillfully descending ladders or stairs by 5 years of age. As one might expect, the physical characteristics of the climbing apparatus markedly may affect climbing performance (e.g., the angle, height, and distance between ladder rungs or step risers). It is not uncommon for children who normally use advanced climbing techniques when operating at low heights to revert to immature and cautious marking time movements when attempting to climb at a significantly greater height.

FINE MOTOR MANIPULATIVE BEHAVIOR

Objective 9.6

think about it

Identify which prenatal factors could affect manipulation.

In the discussion of early movement behavior (Chapter 8), several developmental milestones were noted in relation to manual control. The primitive and rudimentary behaviors of reaching, grasping, and releasing that flourish during the prenatal stage and the first 2 years of life represent three developmental categories: reflexes, rhythmic stereotypies, and prehensile behaviors. The grasping (palmar) reflex appears prenatally and is suppressed by the fourth postnatal month. Rhythmic stereotypies appear in the arms, hands, and fingers shortly after birth and reach their peak during the second half of the first year. The peak of proficient prehensile behavior normally is displayed by 18 months of age. During this period, most children are reasonably proficient in coordinating basic reaching and grasping skills, as evidenced by their ability to use a precision pincer grip and to effectively release objects.

The final stage of manual control, that is, before regression is manipulation. **Manipulation** refers to skillful and refined use of the hands, such as in stringing beads, drawing, and writing. The development of several aspects of manipulation occurs during the early childhood period and shortly after (up to around 8 years of age). With an understanding of the development of manipulation skills and early motor behavior characteristics, a relatively complete picture of manual development is created.

Finger Differentiation

Although most children are capable of displaying a pincer (thumb and forefinger) grip around 10 months, it is several years before they are able to perform precision movements with individual fingers. One task commonly used to evaluate finger differentiation is the test of finger opposition. This task requires the individual to

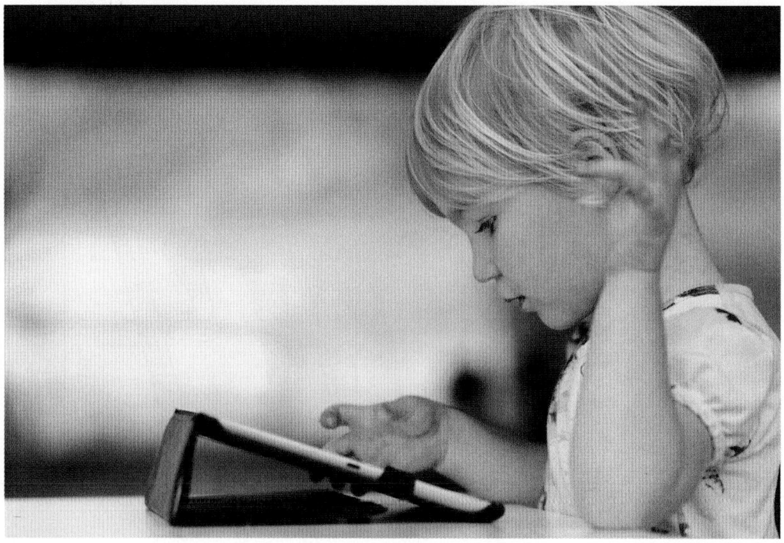

Figure 9.21 Young infant exploring and learning via finger use on an electronic device.

touch each finger, in their order on the hand, to the thumb. Generally, the task is scored under speed stress (e.g., the number of cycles of finger opposition are counted within a given time). This finger opposition test frequently is used by pediatric neurologists to identify possible impairment and by researchers to investigate the developmental characteristics of the hands.

think about it

What do you think is the effect, both short- and long-term, of early use of electronic devices by this generation on finger differentiation?

Early signs of individual finger control (differentiation) appear within the first year of life, as evidenced by the appearance of stereotypic finger flexion, pseudo thumb opposition, and, as noted earlier, true thumb-to-forefinger opposition by 10 months of age. However, the ability to oppose more than one finger to the thumb does not reveal its beginnings until around age 3 years. Initial efforts at this age usually require the tester to provide a slow visual demonstration. Regular improvement continues in finger differentiation until about age 8 years, when performance approximates that of adults (Fig. 9.21).

Other tasks such as stringing beads, moving pegs, and picking up pennies or matchsticks and placing them in a container also are used commonly to determine level of manipulative ability. In general, studies involving these types of tasks have reported similar basic patterns of change. That is, improvement is greater during the early developmental years, with relatively small changes occurring after 8 to 10 years. Figure 9.22 illustrates this trend among individuals from 3 to 15 years of age with the results of a popular test reported by Annett (1970) that measures the speed of moving pegs.

Construction and Self-Help Skills

Widely used developmental scales such as the Peabody Developmental Motor Scales-2 (Folio & Fewell, 2000) and Bayley Scales of Infant and Toddler Development—Third Edition (Bayley-III; Bayley, 2006) typically include several manual construction and self-help tasks. Along with assessing the fine motor abilities used in such tasks as building a block tower, these tasks highlight the importance of manual skills in everyday personal, or self-help, tasks. Such skills as tying one's shoes, buttoning a coat, holding and drinking from a cup, and feeding oneself with a spoon are considered major developmental achievements. Table 9.6 lists

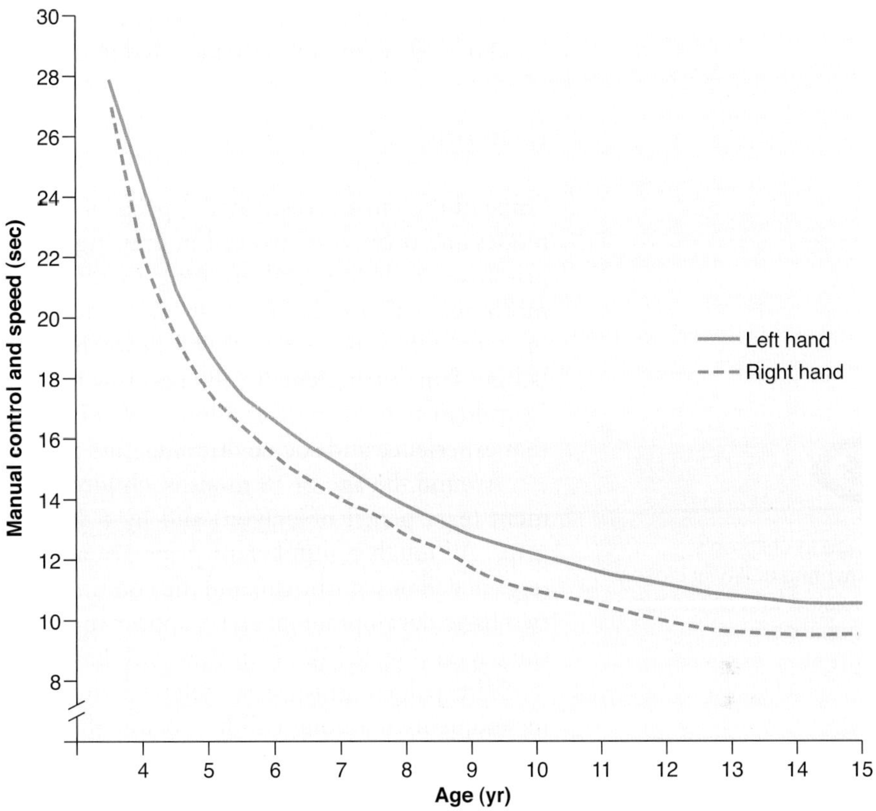

Figure 9.22 Manual control and speed (moving pegs).

TABLE 9.6 Selected Construction and Self-Help Achievements (Ages 1 to 4 Years)

Achievement	Approximate Age (Mo)
Drinks from cup	13
Builds tower of two cubes	14
Uses spoon	15
Builds tower of four cubes	18
Builds tower of eight cubes	24
Puts on shoes	36
Cuts paper	
Buttons up (clothes)	
Feeds self (spills very little)	
Pours well from pitcher	
Laces shoes	48
Brushes teeth	
Cuts paper following line	

SOURCE: Data from Denver II (Frankenburg et al., 1990) and Bayley-III (Bayley, 2006).

selected construction and self-help achievements attained during the early childhood period and commonly included in developmental assessment scales.

Drawing and Writing

Some of the most investigated aspects of fine motor manual control are the techniques and processes involved in drawing and writing. These skills progress from primitive scribbling and coloring to the highly coordinated and dynamic fine motor movements used to draw figures and write in cursive. In general, the development of drawing and writing follows the *proximodistal* trend, with males lagging behind females at virtually all ages; this is due in large part to females' advanced neurological maturity (e.g., Blote & Van Haasteren, 1989). However, keep in mind that experience and sociocultural factors play an influencing role.

focus on change

Change in children's handwriting ability is closely associated with academic performance.

Around the age of 18 months, children can hold a writing or coloring implement (e.g., pencil or crayon) and by 6 years have acquired an array of holding grips. Although a number of grips are applicable depending on the implement (e.g., pencil or paintbrush) and the condition (e.g., on a desk or at an upright easel), two basic developmental styles appear to be most prominent: the power grip and the tripod (Fig. 9.23). From these two basic styles, several variations exist.

The palmar grasp, also referred to as the *power grip*, is usually the initial technique used among children below the age of 3 years. With this style, all four fingers and the thumb are wrapped around the implement and most movement is initiated and guided by the shoulder and arm. The more advanced holding style is the *tripod*, in which the implement is held by the thumb, index finger, and middle finger. During initial use of this style, the child will hold the implement with the proper tripod grip, but movement will still be controlled by the arm rather than hand.

The mature version of the basic tripod is the *dynamic tripod*. At this stage, development has reached the level of using the proper grip and skillfully manipulating the implement with the wrist, fingers, and thumb. The beginnings of dynamic manual control in this context are usually evident by age 4 years and progress to a relatively mature level by 7 years, with refinement continuing through early

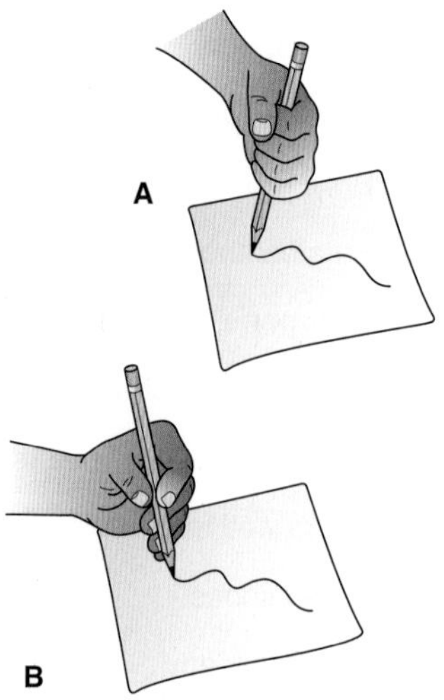

Figure 9.23 Basic holding grips: **(A)** the immature power grip and **(B)** the more advanced tripod.

think about it

What are the constraints to handwriting in an elderly person?

adolescence (Ziviani, 1983). From the ages of 2 to 6 years, children's writing ability increases dramatically as the hand moves closer to the tip of the implement. See Henderson and Pehoskil (2006) for detailed description and assessment techniques for the development of prehension skills, including writing and drawing grips.

The following discussion describes typical age-related drawing and writing characteristics noted in the literature.

By the age of 2 years, children can crudely draw circular, vertical, and horizontal lines that follow the appropriate direction. However, the quality of performance among children may vary considerably. The general progression and approximate age expectancies for common figure copying are circle (36 months); cross (48 months); square (54 months); triangle (60 months); and the more difficult, diamond (72 months). Tracing abilities for all forms are generally mature by 6 years.

The task of forming letters and numbers as required in handwriting tasks presents the child with additional manual challenges. By the age of 4 years, most children are capable of printing at least a few recognizable letters but frequently position them in a disorganized manner on the page. With adequate practice, most 6-year-olds are capable of printing their first names, the alphabet, and numbers up to 10. Younger children (ages 4 and 5 years) typically write in large letters and numbers. The ability to space letters remains a difficult task for many children until around 9 years of age.

For a more precise observation of the development of fine motor control associated with drawing and handwriting, Rueckriegel and colleagues (2008) collected kinematic data on individuals aged 6 to 18 years. The researchers noted a strong association between age and performance, speed, and automation increased with increasing age. As one might expect, age of completed maturation depended on task complexity and kinematic parameters. For example, handwriting movements finished maturing later than circle drawing. The average for drawing was 12 years, whereas for sentence writing was 15 years. The researchers hypothesized that the increase in handwriting speed was predominantly due to improved motor planning of complex stroke and loop sequences, which is faster and more efficiently processed simultaneously to execution. In summary, this study indicates that quality of movements associated with drawing and writing may not mature until the adolescent ages. This study also provides an excellent review of research on children's drawing and handwriting abilities.

Bimanual Control

Several manipulative activities require the controlled use of the two hands, or **bimanual control**, in a symmetrical or asymmetrical function. In *symmetrical function*, the two hands perform similar and simultaneous movements, such as those used in clapping and performing selected calisthenic exercises. The other form of bimanual control is more common to general manipulative behavior and is referred to as *asymmetrical function*. This term describes the function in which the two hands make different movements in a coordinated and complementary manner. This ability is evident in the performance of such tasks as cutting paper with scissors, tying shoelaces, and dealing cards (Fig. 9.24). In each of these conditions, one hand is the primary manipulator, whereas the other functions in a complementary manner to position and stabilize the object.

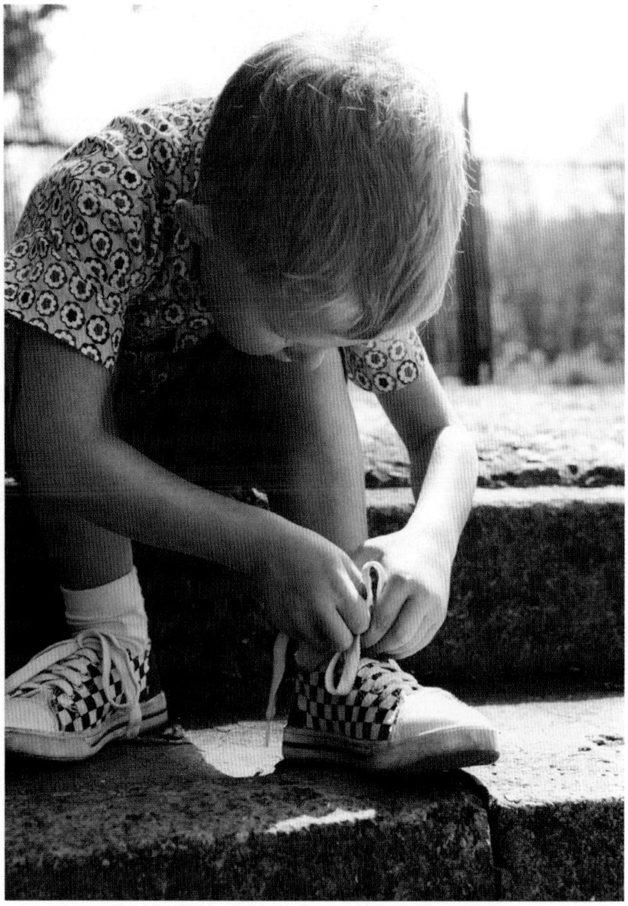

Figure 9.24 For a young child, tying shoes can be a difficult asymmetrical function.

Although they are not intentional (i.e., voluntary), symmetrical bilateral arm movements can be observed at birth in the form of primitive reflexes (e.g., the Moro reflex) and in the spontaneous behavior of newborns during the first month of life. The earliest patterns of bimanual activity (e.g., hand interplay and clasping) are primarily nonvisual and occur after 3 months of age. By 4 to 4½ months, when crude attempts at voluntary reaching are displayed, arm actions are still basically bilateral and symmetrical, although one hand contacts the object first. Although some form of asymmetrical behavior also has been noted around this age, it is generally not before the end of the first year that the complementary characteristics of bimanual asymmetrical coordination are unquestionably present. The variety and complexity of tasks that can be performed using bimanual control increase enormously during childhood, although they may be unrefined.

Closely associated with proficiency of asymmetrical bimanual control are hemispheric lateralization and the establishment of a consistent hand preference. Although specific age-related changes are difficult to establish, children display basic mastery of asymmetrical and symmetrical bimanual control by 6 years, just after hand preference has been established. From this basic foundation develops the motor control that ultimately manifests itself in the ability to perform complex bimanual skills.

Although age-related characteristics and the nature of developmental change have not been clearly established, a general trend has been noted. Apparently, children progress from an early stage of crude bimanual movements that tend to be symmetrical to the development of unilateral behavior, or establishment of a preferred limb. With the development of a preferred and nonpreferred hand evolves more refined bimanual control that culminates in the role differentiation of the hands that is observed in most forms of asymmetrical manipulative behavior. For a dynamic systems/constraints perspective of the development of bimanual coordination, refer to Mason et al. (2013) and Serrien et al. (2014).

FUNCTIONAL (MOTOR) ASYMMETRIES

Objective 9.7

Complementing the development of motor control, especially during early childhood, is establishment of limb (hand and foot) and eye preference. As noted in previous chapters (brain lateralization), although the human body (and brain hemispheres) is symmetrical in general appearance, the paired limbs (hands and feet) and sensory organs (eyes and ears) are used in an asymmetric manner. The behavioral manifestations of this phenomenon are referred to as **functional asymmetries.** For example, in tasks where only one limb can be used, such as throwing or kicking a ball, most individuals exhibit a consistent preference for the use of one limb over the other (also known as *handedness* and *footedness*).

Although lateral preference most often is identified as *right-sided* or *left-sided*, some individuals do not consistently favor the use of one limb or the other on a specific task; these individuals are identified as *mixed-sided. Ambidexterity* is a somewhat confusing term in a neurological context and one that has received little attention in the developmental psychology literature. This term describes the use of either limb with somewhat equal proficiency on the same task. This characteristic does not necessarily indicate dual dominance of hemispheric control. It is generally believed that individuals possessing this ability with a specific task have adapted or trained their nonpreferred side to be as, or perhaps more, skillful than their dominant side for a specific skill(s). This type of behavior is evident in skilled (practiced) activities such as soccer, handball, and boxing that require proficiency in both limbs.

Following are brief discussions of the developmental characteristics associated with handedness, footedness, and eye preference behavior, which, as noted earlier, are closely linked with the development of motor control during early childhood.

Handedness

Of the motor asymmetries, handedness has been investigated more than all others combined. Hand preference on tasks such as writing, throwing a ball, hammering, stacking cubes, and cutting with scissors is currently the most widely used method of determining degree of handedness. It is generally acknowledged that handedness (and footedness) is a trichotomous continuum ranging from left to mixed to right, rather than a dichotomy (right or left only). With a series of tasks, many individuals will not exhibit a totally consistent right- or left-hand preference.

As noted in Chapter 8, individuals generally become more right-handed with increasing age; in addition, it is widely known that approximately 90% of the population establishes this preference. By the middle of the first year, handedness becomes more evident, with most infants exhibiting a preference for the right hand for visually directed reaching. By 3 to 4 years of age, children generally show

think about it

Recent theory suggests that although we have a hand preference, environmental (attentional) stimuli tied to task demands can modify limb selection. What is an example?

differential hand preference (about 75% prefer the right limb at this time) and hand skill of a kind comparable to adult characteristics. At about 6 years, handedness (i.e., direction) is stable in most children, with about 90% preferring the right hand.

Is there a disadvantage to being left-handed? For many years, left-handedness was associated with cognitive and language dysfunctions and general motor clumsiness because left-handed individuals more often were found to have such deficits. However, these findings and assumptions were based more on clinical samples and have not been supported by more recent investigations of normal individuals.

More contemporary views on hand preference and selection suggest that to fully understand one's preference, the context of the action should be considered. For example, as a right-hander, would you cross your midline to the far left to pick up a water bottle or a cube and stack it on top of the others? Research indicates that many right-handers switch limbs, suggesting that hand selection is to some extent adaptable to task demand and environmental context (e.g., Sivagnanasunderam et al., 2014; Hill & Khanem, 2009).

Footedness

A myriad of data are available on hand preference, but research on foot laterality is relatively limited. By operational definition, the preferred foot is the one used to manipulate an object or to lead out, as in kicking or jumping, whereas the nonpreferred limb is used as the primary stabilizer. Recommended tests of footedness include kicking a ball, figure tracing with toes while standing, and foot stamping a target.

The developmental course of foot preference behavior follows a similar general developmental trend as handedness; that is, there is a significant shift toward greater right-sidedness with increasing age. In comparison to handedness, however, the genesis of foot preference exhibits a few unique characteristics. During early childhood, about twice as many individuals are mixed-footed, compared to persons who do not exhibit a preferred hand. During late childhood, a significant shift toward greater right-footedness with a corresponding decrease in mixed-footedness occurs, after which preferences remain relatively stable into adulthood with approximately 80% favoring the ride side (Gabbard & Ityea, 1996).

What accounts for the mixed-footed phenomenon? One explanation is that environmental factors such as culture (the right-sided world phenomenon) and experience may influence *direction and/or degree* of preference. For example, activities that require use of the feet (relative to those of the hands) are usually less complex and practiced. From these observations, it seems likely the environmental factor that may affect (e.g., strengthen) degree of hand preference during childhood may be less of an influence on foot laterality.

An interesting issue has emerged in contemporary literature associated with footedness: Which is the dominant limb, the one used to stabilize the body or the foot that is mobilized to lead out or manipulate? The consensus of research suggests that most humans are right-footed for actions of mobilization (operationally defined as the dominant limb) and left-sided for postural stabilization. However, in virtually all of these observations, the task of stabilizing was arguably easier than that required of the manipulating foot (e.g., kicking a stationary ball). There is evidence that when individuals are placed in a unilateral condition (e.g., one-leg static balance), they also prefer the right limb or have no preference (e.g., see review by Hart & Gabbard, 1997). That is, although most individuals stabilize on the left side in the bilateral condition, they switch to the right in the unilateral context of balance. Interestingly, with virtually all foot tasks used in behavioral inventories (because most are bilateral actions), stabilizing requirements such as postural support while kicking a ball and foot-tracing letters are relatively simple, compared to the demands of focused mobilization. What does this research suggest? Although these findings are not conclusive, they hint that in foot dominance, the preferred limb is reserved for the more difficult aspect of a behavioral activity. And, foot dominance should be defined operationally, in light of behavioral context (unilateral or bilateral) and demands (level of complexity) of the particular task performed.

Eye Preference

Eye preference can be observed when sighting a telescope or aiming a gun-like instrument. A review of research on eyedness suggests that, as with the other asymmetries described, most individuals prefer the right side, and degrees of right-eyedness increase between childhood and maturity. The levels of right-sidedness in adults, however, are not as high as with hand and foot preference. Approximately 70% of adults prefer the right eye (Bourassa et al., 1996), whereas values for the same preference in children range between 55% and 60% (Nachshon et al., 1983).

Summary

Early childhood is characterized by fundamental movement actions that can be categorized into locomotor, nonlocomotor, and manipulative (gross and manual) behaviors. The developmental characteristics of locomotor and gross motor manipulative skills can be described according to process-related movement pattern changes. Movement pattern status frequently is identified using terms that represent proficiency ranging from immature to sport skill form.

Two general approaches associated with describing and interpreting qualitative movement changes across time are the composite approach and component method. The composite approach describes the sequence of movement pattern changes through a series of total body (general pattern) stages. The component approach divides pattern changes into substages that depict specific body component changes.

A scientific and applied (e.g., teaching) body of information is available concerning the sequential progression and developmental characteristics of most fundamental locomotor and gross motor manipulative skills.

Manipulation refers to the skillful and refined use of the hands, such as that displayed in tasks of finger differentiation, construction and self-help skills, and drawing and writing. As one would expect, the development of manual control abilities generally proceeds in a proximodistal direction.

Bimanual control involves the use of two hands in a symmetrical or asymmetrical function. Bimanual coordination clearly improves during childhood, with the initial actions being more symmetrical before complete role differentiation of the hands can be observed. Mastery of asymmetrical bimanual control seems to be associated with the development of hand preference. A general developmental trend for all functional asymmetries is a shift toward greater right-sidedness with increasing age.

think about it

1. **Describe what a comprehensive study of walking skills could involve.**
2. **What is the role of biology/environment in the development of fundamental movement patterns during early childhood? Consider information from previous chapters to support biological change.**
3. **What are the individual *constraints* driving efficient running for speed?**
4. **What forms of jumping do we typically use in everyday life? What do young and older persons use?**
5. **How does Wild's stages (composite of throwing) and Table 9.3 (components for throwing) compare?**
6. **What task *constraints* could you provide to improve catching behavior?**
7. **Of the fundamental skills described in the "Movement Patterns" section, which are culturally gender-biased in children's play and youth sport activities?**
8. **Identify which prenatal factors could affect manipulation.**
9. **What do you think is the effect, both short- and long-term, of early use of electronic devices by this generation on finger differentiation?**
10. **What are the constraints to handwriting in an elderly person?**
11. **Recent theory suggests that although we have a hand preference, environmental (attentional) stimuli tied to task demands can modify limb selection. What is an example?**

LEARNING ACTIVITIES

Objective: To gain experience in observing and analyzing movement patterns of young children. First, review text material on the developmental stages of running, throwing, and jumping. Next, searching YouTube and similar sites depicting those movements, find at least one child 3 to 4 years of age and one child 5 to 7 years of age. For each child, analyze their movement pattern and provide recommendations for improvement.

Objective: To observe behavior and administer tests associated with manual manipulation. Obtain permission to study a 4- to 5-year-old child's fine motor manipulation behavior. Review the information and developmental milestones associated with this age range: Look at construction and self-help skills (e.g., buttons shirt, laces shoes), writing grips (e.g., power grip, tripod), and drawing or writing skills (e.g., ability to draw a circle, lines, square, and other figures). Develop a checklist of characteristic behaviors likely to be observed or elicited during visits. Most of the expected behaviors can be observed in either the school or home setting. However, an interview with the aid of a parent is recommended if more information is needed.

Chapter 10

Motor Behavior During Later Childhood and Adolescence

OBJECTIVES

Upon completion of this chapter, you should be able to

10.1 Provide an overview of the developmental milestones that occur during later childhood and adolescence.

10.2 Discuss quantitative (product) motor performance changes and describe gender trends during later childhood and adolescence.

10.3 List and briefly describe the quantitative changes that occur in motor performance.

10.4 Discuss the influence of physical activity and sport participation on motor skill refinement.

KEY TERMS

product performance
gender motor performance trends
youth sports
physical education
developmentally appropriate

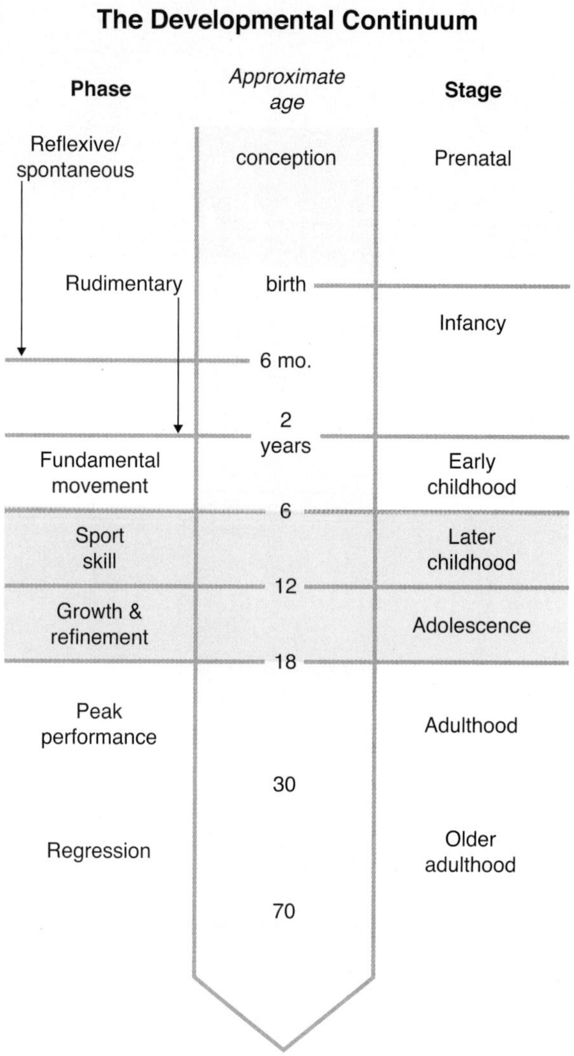

Objective 10.1

The period from later childhood through adolescence (approximately 7 to 18 years of age) is characterized by several growth and development milestones, many of which are manifested in significant improvements in motor skill performance. Around the beginning of later childhood, individuals begin to use with increasing frequency the fundamental movement abilities acquired during early childhood. At the same time, changes in physical growth, body structure, and physiological development combine to produce greater **product performance**—that is, performance (outcome) values—while continuing to refine "process" form characteristics (Chapter 9). This period is also distinguished by the emergence of sport skill behaviors. In essence, these behaviors are advanced versions of basic skills that are the primary vehicle by which the individual's increased level of motor behavior is displayed. Along with improvements in motor performance that appear in both sexes during this period, differences in **gender motor performance trends** also come increasingly into play. These trends are especially apparent during the adolescent growth spurt. In addition to biological changes, skill practice and sociocultural factors play a significant role in behavior.

This chapter focuses on the description and bases for quantitative changes in motor performance exhibited during preadolescence and the adolescent years.

It also addresses the related issue of gender trends in motor performance and the refinement of fundamental skills as displayed by sport skill behavior. An excellent model for studying this period, and other, is the bioecological model described in Chapter 1 and in more detail in Chapter 14. That model considers, for example, family, community, government, a national influence.

QUANTITATIVE (PRODUCT) MOTOR PERFORMANCE CHANGES

Objective 10.2

Quantitative changes in motor performance tend to parallel increasing levels of experience and changes in physical growth, physiological development, and neurological functioning. Previous chapters that described these changes have established that with advancing age, most individuals experience increases in such characteristics as body size, muscle mass, strength, cardiorespiratory capacity, and perceptual-motor ability (e.g., coincident timing and reaction time [RT]). As a result of these and other developmental changes, virtually all aspects of product-oriented motor performance show an upward trend beginning at the preschool level.

Differences between genders before puberty are minimal and if they do exist are driven in large part by sociocultural influences. Some reports suggest that young boys tend to outperform females on selected tasks of running, throwing, and jumping. Females, on the other hand, appear to excel in hopping, skipping, and tasks requiring fine motor control, balance, and flexibility. Some performance differences have been attributed to biological factors such as body fat, which favor males, and advanced neurological development, which favor females. But it also seems quite likely that at this age level, environmental agents are a primary determinant. Several studies confirm that, beginning at the preschool level, males are generally more active than females (e.g., Baranowski et al., 1993; Troiano et al., 2008). Complementing this is the fact that parents and teachers usually express specific gender role expectations, which dictate that males and females should behave differently at play and sport. Thomas et al. (1991) note that from a physiological perspective, young females' overall motor performance should be better due to the faster maturation rate prior to puberty. The fact that their overall motor performance generally is not better argues for a sociocultural explanation.

think about it

What are the implications of being an early or late mature regarding this discussion?

focus on change

Later childhood and adolescence presents significant *change* in motor performance—*change* that affects biological maturity and sociocultural experience.

think about it

Do you think the hypothetical gender trend for females has changed in the last 10 years?

If you will recall from Chapter 4 in reference to the National Youth Fitness Survey (NYFS) (2012), although results were limited to four health-related factors of strength, there was no significant differences between boys and girls aged 6 to 11 years; only after that (ages 12 to 15 years) did males perform better.

With the onset of the adolescent growth spurt (from ages 10 to 12 years), differences in motor performance product characteristics between the sexes become increasingly evident and generally favor the male. The literature reveals a consistent trend that shows males continue to improve in motor performance on a variety of skills through adolescence, but females have a tendency to peak around the age of 14 years and then level off (plateau) or decrease in performance (e.g., Malina et al., 2004). Given that females mature earlier, part of this trend maybe expected; however, the age of 14 years has stimulated considerable debate.

Figure 10.1 illustrates hypothetical gender age performance (quantitative) trends for the basic motor skills including running, jumping, and throwing. This information is described in subsequent sections of this chapter.

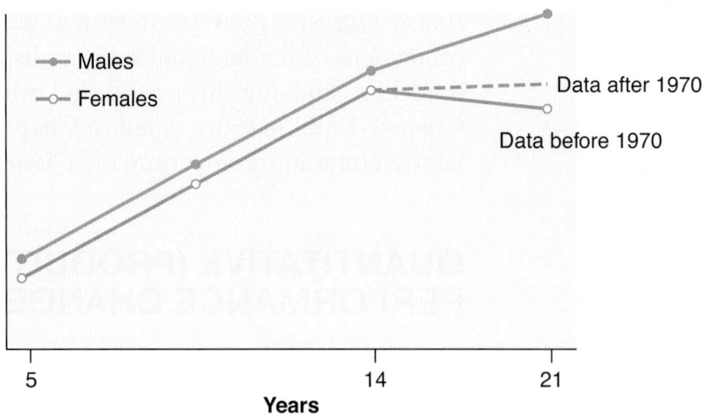

Figure 10.1 Hypothetical gender age performance (quantitative) trends.

Although cultural practices and participation levels may significantly influence the range of individual differences within and between genders during this period, numerous biological factors may provide an advantage to males in several motor skill activities. Earlier discussions have highlighted that the primary factors that provide males with a biological advantage over females in motor performance are sex chromosomes and hormones. Most of these factors become increasingly apparent after the age of 10 years. The earlier chapters on physical growth (Chapter 3) and physiological changes (Chapter 4) are useful for reviewing the discussion of the biological differences between genders.

In general, males tend to be larger and have more muscle mass, less body fat, and a greater oxygen transport capacity than their female counterparts. These characteristics give males the biological advantage in performing activities that require strength, power, and endurance. Because females possess more body fat and less muscle mass than males do, females are at a distinct disadvantage in performing motor tasks that require lifting the body (e.g., jumping) or moving their mass against gravity (e.g., running).

As noted earlier, several research studies that involve children and adults confirm a negative relationship between body fatness and performance on tasks that require the vertical and horizontal movement of the body weight. In essence, body fat adds to the mass of the body without contributing to force-producing capacity. Swimming is one activity for which a higher body fat value may be an advantage. Higher values of body fat have been shown to allow individuals to swim higher in the water with less body drag. Although this factor may decrease the difference between the sexes, males still tend to outperform females in swimming events simply because they are stronger.

Structural factors that provide a mechanical advantage also may favor males in sprinting, jumping, and throwing skills. Males have longer arms and wider shoulders, which produce the leverage and rotation torque needed to forcefully propel objects in throwing or striking activities. Longer legs and narrower hips also may tend to be advantageous in sprinting and jumping tasks. Greater proportionate hip width and angle of insertion of the femur in females has been suggested as a mechanical disadvantage in achieving maximal running speed for sprinting. On the other hand, because females generally have a lower center of gravity and wider hips, they may have the advantage in motor skills that require a high degree of balance. Although females tend to outperform males at virtually all ages on tests of flexibility, current evidence does not suggest that biological factors account for the difference.

think about it

What is your community's view of female participation in all types of sport?

Although biological factors can influence performance differences, social and cultural agents also may offer the explanation for some of the variation. This may be the case particularly when the motor task involves a high degree of skill (e.g., skipping and throwing) rather than higher levels of basic strength and cardiorespiratory endurance.

Performance of tasks that require a higher degree of skill (i.e., coordination and refinement) can be influenced significantly by practice. Although the trend certainly is changing, males and females in the United States tend to practice only those physical activities traditionally regarded as male- or female-oriented, respectively. Although females today participate in many more traditionally male-oriented activities (e.g., females play baseball, softball, soccer, and football) and vice versa (e.g., males dance and play volleyball), some segments of society still adhere to the more traditional gender roles. It can be speculated that this practice may discourage individuals from attaining their potential in specific motor skills.

Interestingly, in describing data collected during the 1950s, Eckert (1987) notes European females continue to improve their running, throwing, and jumping skills up to 16 to 18 years of age. Their American counterparts, in contrast, displayed a leveling off between age 13 and 15 years. It may be assumed from this data that cultural values have an effect on motor skill performance.

Although differences that favor males still exist for most tests of motor performance (especially on strength-related tasks), in recent years, females appear to be narrowing that differential. This trend seems to be related to increased participation in physical fitness and sports programs, effective school and university programs, an increase in athletic scholarships and participation opportunities (through Title IX), and a gradual change in society's view of female participation in sports.

In addition to this interesting developmental issue, Figure 10.2 shows life-span physical activity levels for the years 2003 to 2004 (Troiano et al., 2008). Over 20 years ago, it was reported (as noted earlier in Chapter 5) that after the age of about 12 years, activity levels decline to those exhibited by adults. Have the levels changed? As shown in the figure, levels after ages 6 to 11 years, "drop" to less than

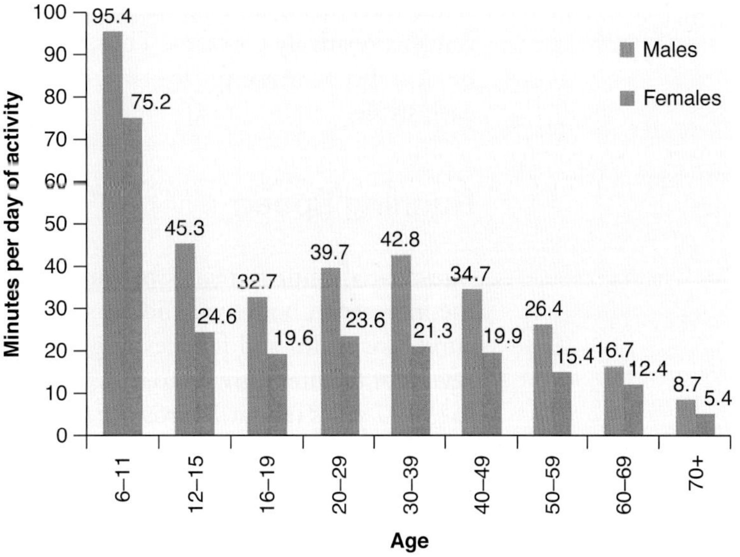

Figure 10.2 Minutes per day of moderate to vigorous physical education activity across the life span.

SOURCE: Modified from Troiano, R. P., Berrigan, D., Dodd, K. W., Mâsse, L. C., Tilert, T., & McDowell, M. (2008). Physical activity in the United States measured by accelerometer. *Medicine and Science in Sports and Exercise*, *40*(1), 181–188.

think about it

What ideas do you have to change these trends (obesity and being less active after childhood)?

WebLink

http://www.cdc.gov/; see NYFS (2012) report.

50 percent. Furthermore, these statistics confirm the observation that females (across all ages) are not as active as males. With all three of these observations—gender performance trends, the dramatic decline in activity after 11 years, and females being less active—important challenges and explanations await researchers and practitioners. Add to these observations, the continuing troublesome issue of overweight/obesity. Another fact of note is the latest data from the NYFS report (2012), only 42% of U.S. youth, aged 12 to 15 years had acceptable levels of cardiorespiratory fitness. That number was a decrease from a 1999 to 2000 study showing 52%. Another important finding was that fitness level decreased as body weight increased.

A word of caution should be given regarding the general interpretation of gender differences. Although clear-cut differences that generally favor males are evident sometimes very early in their development, comparisons normally are based on average performance data by group (males and females). In nearly all motor performance studies, large individual differences exist within the sexes at each age level. For example, although the mean performance of males may be significantly greater on a specific motor skill, the performance of some females certainly may equal or exceed that of some males. Therefore, mean data may be useful from a developmental perspective, but the true developmentalist is also sensitive to individual progress.

QUANTITATIVE (PRODUCT) CHANGES IN MOTOR PERFORMANCE

Objective 10.3

Running performance commonly is measured by requiring the individual to run as fast as possible (sprint) over a distance of 30 to 50 yards. Performance times usually are reported in tenths of a second and then, for comparative purposes, are converted to feet or yards covered per second. The speed with which an individual can run depends significantly on the length of the stride as well as the stride rate. Stride and leg length generally increase with age, whereas stride rate remains relatively constant. Thus, an increase in running velocity may not be due to an ability to move the legs more frequently but to propel the body farther with each stride.

Running Speed

Age-related improvements in running speed can be explained in large part by the increase in body size and muscular strength. Figure 10.3 shows performance curves for males and females originally composed by Espenschade (1960) after a review of the literature up to that period. Males continue to increase in velocity up to age 17 years (about 7 yards per second), but females begin to level off or regress slightly beginning around age 13 years. A review of studies since 1960 confirms this trend for males but reports slightly higher scores for females (Haubenstricker, Wisner, Seefeldt, & Branta, 1997). The review did not find a regression of performance in females after age 13 or 14 years but identified a plateauing trend up to age 17 years. Similar performance patterns have been reported for a test of *agility*, the ability to change the direction of the body rapidly. A popular test is the 30-feet shuttle run. Improvement occurs through childhood with males displaying an edge that increases after 13 years and females plateauing around age 15 years (Fig. 10.4).

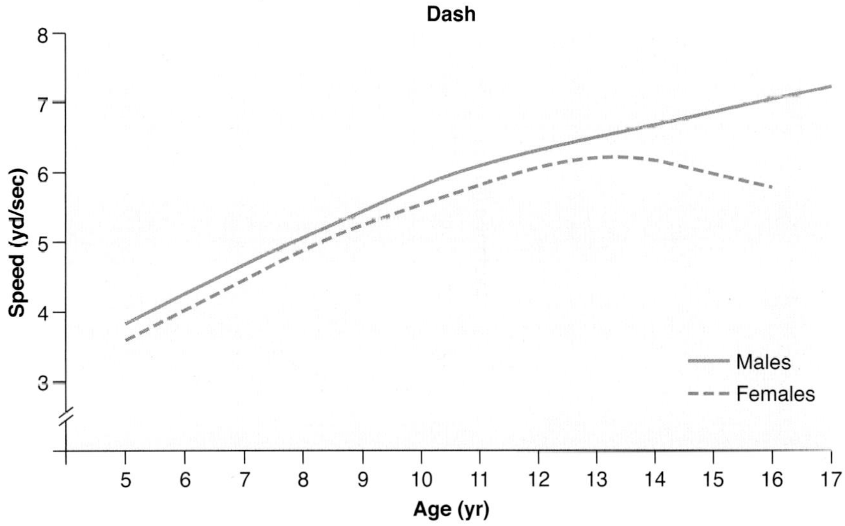

Figure 10.3 Running speed curves.

Throwing

The quantitative characteristics of throwing most often are determined by measuring the maximum distance thrown, throwing velocity, and accuracy. Both sexes improve dramatically from childhood to adolescence on all three abilities, but gender differences (that favor males) appear quite early and are relatively large in comparison to other fundamental skills. As noted earlier, it may be speculated that much of the difference that favors males is due to their greater strength and biomechanical

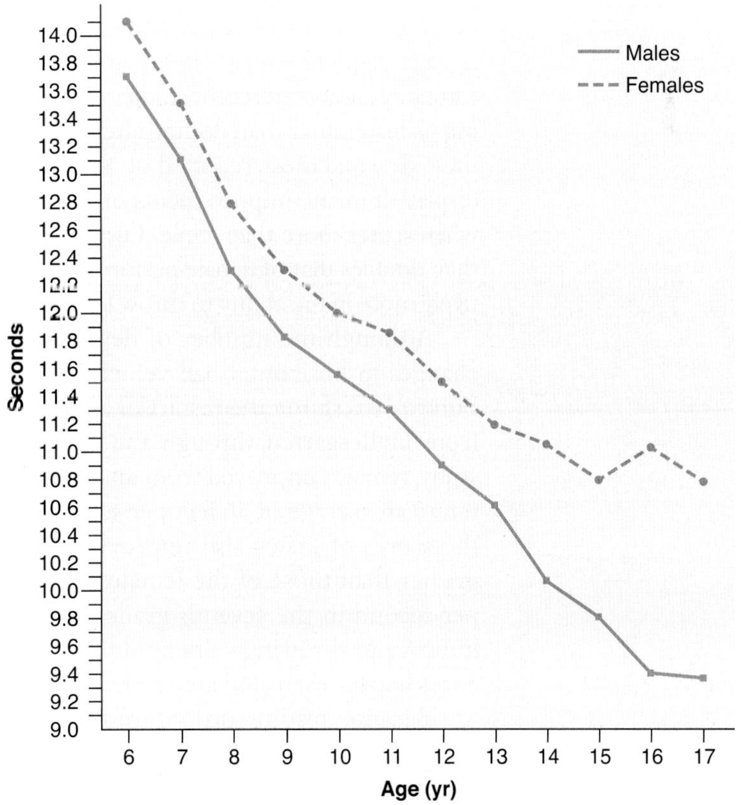

Figure 10.4 Agility run scores (30-foot shuttle).

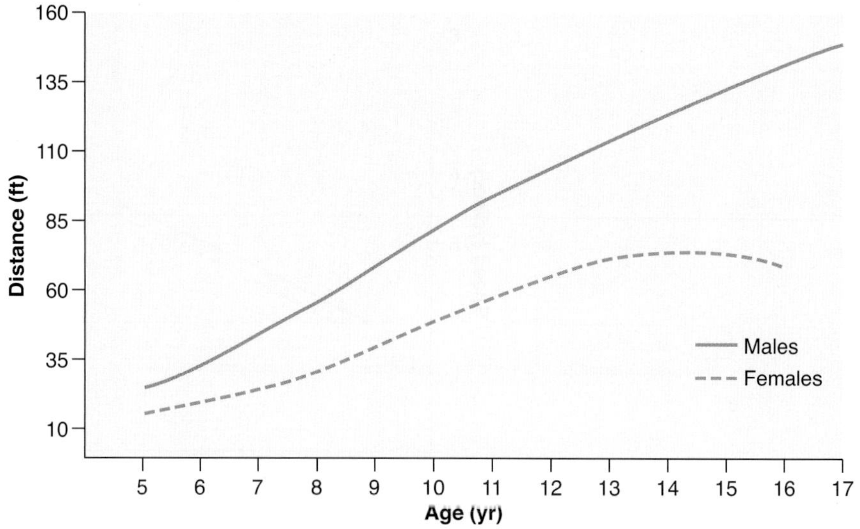

Figure 10.5 Throwing distance curves.

characteristics, and the fact that females generally exhibit less mature throwing patterns. Another consideration is the possibility that cultural and social factors provide a positive influence for the development of throwing among males.

Regardless of throwing task, balls projected by the overhand throw have been measured more frequently than those of any other movement pattern. The distance an individual can throw has received the most attention in the developmental literature. Although gender differences are more obvious at the younger ages and become greater over time, throwing distance performance curves show trends similar to those found with running speed performance (Fig. 10.5). That is, both genders improve up to puberty (12 to 14 years). After this, males continue to improve performance, and females begin to level off and then decline in performance. Unlike running speed performance, however, recent studies do not indicate that female performances in throwing plateau rather than decline after puberty (Haubenstricker & Seefeldt, 1986). From these data and those reported by Keogh and Sugden (1985), it is clear that both sexes display dramatic improvements in distance thrown during the preadolescent period, when scores more than triple. Furthermore, male performance by age 17 years more than doubles that of female performance. Females and males apparently increase relatively more in the ability to throw for distance than they do in other fundamental skills.

Although the number of developmental studies has been somewhat limited, changes in horizontal ball velocities (speed) at various ages have been reported. Figure 10.6 shows the results of a longitudinal study of throwing velocity changes from kindergarten through the seventh grade (Halverson et al., 1982). In this study, females improved from an average of 29 feet per second while in kindergarten to an average of 56 feet per second by the seventh grade. As one would expect, the scores of males also improved over the study period and were significantly greater than those of the females—39 feet per second in kindergarten to 78 feet per second in the seventh grade. Like distance thrown, both males and females improve in throwing velocity dramatically through childhood, and gender differences appear early and are relatively large.

Because testing procedures associated with throwing accuracy have varied considerably, an acceptable developmental description of throwing cannot be given. However, the general statement that individuals improve with age through childhood and that males are usually more accurate than females are is

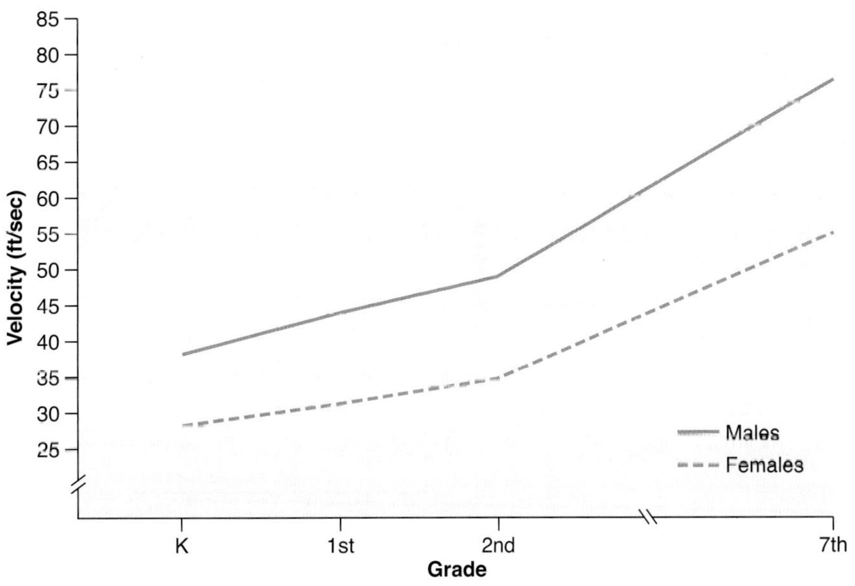

Figure 10.6 Longitudinal changes in ball throwing velocities.

well supported. Because distance and the target area usually are confined and the production of force is not as critical, that is, throwing for maximum distance and velocity, gender differences in throwing accuracy are not as marked.

Jumping

A considerable amount of developmental information has been gathered on jumping ability as measured by the standing (horizontal) long jump and vertical jump. Although data have been amassed from a multitude of studies, the general patterns of change are quite similar.

Figure 10.7 shows general performance curves for the standing long jump. Both sexes improve approximately 3 to 5 inches per year to around age 11 years;

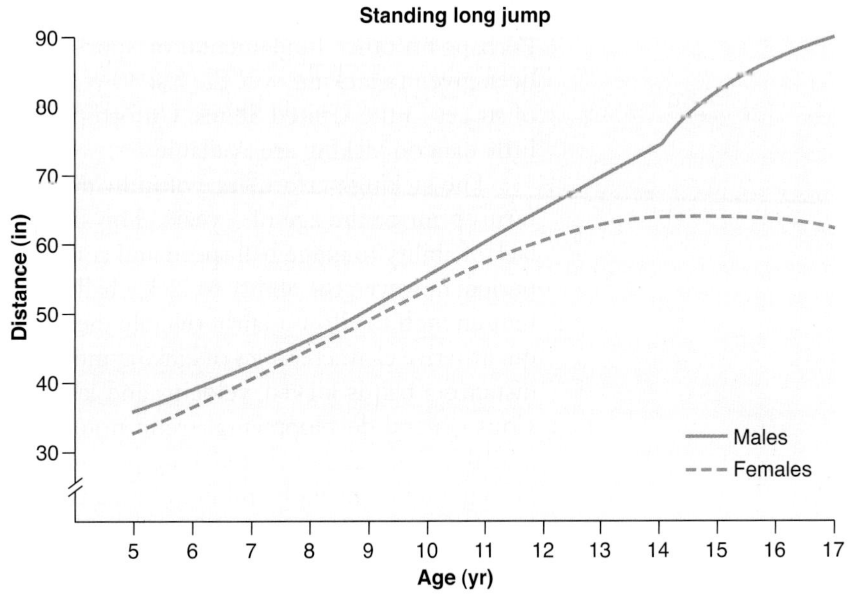

Figure 10.7 Standing long jump performance curves.

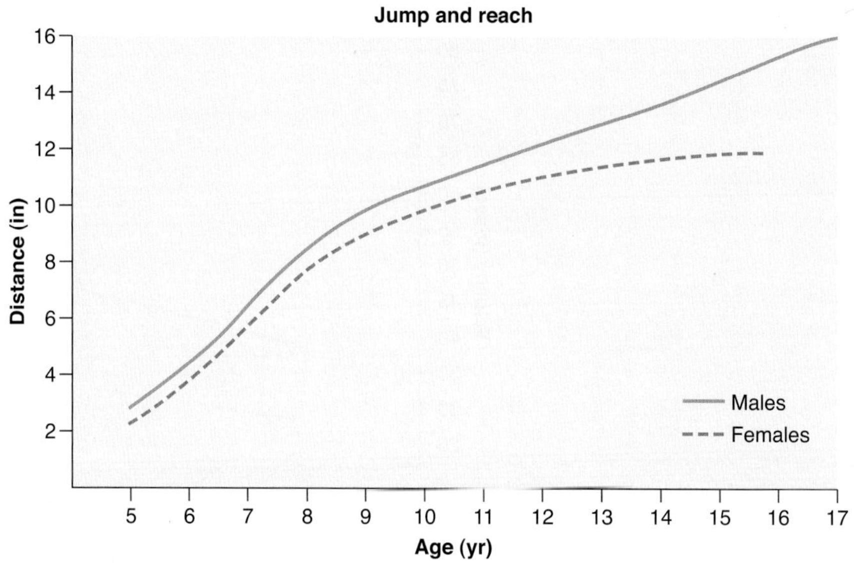

Figure 10.8 Vertical jump performance curves.

males jump 3 to 5 inches farther than females do at each age (Keogh & Sugden, 1985). After that period, males continue to improve to at least age 17 years, whereas the female scores begin to level off and reach a peak at around age 14 years. Haubenstricker and associates (1997) confirm the general trend across time but report somewhat higher scores for females.

Data for the vertical jump (jump-and-reach task) provide similar performance curves to those for horizontal jumping (Fig. 10.8). Males improve from approximately 2 inches at age 5 years to about 17 inches at age 17 years. Females also show significant improvement by starting out just below the males at age 5 years and reaching a peak of approximately 12 inches by age 16 years. A plateauing of female performance begins around the age of 11 years.

Kicking

Perhaps no other fundamental or sport skill has received the attention that has been given to kicking over the last 30 years or so, due to the increasing popularity of soccer in the United States. Unfortunately, even with such focus on this sport, little data on kicking are available.

The kicking performance of individuals is difficult to measure in quantitative terms prior to the age of 5 years. This is due primarily to lack of experience and lack of ability to judge ball speed and coordinate the movement pattern. After this period, however, the ability to kick a ball with force and accuracy becomes consistent enough to allow a fairly reliable measurement and assessment of ability. The quantitative characteristics of kicking most often are determined by measuring the distance a ball is kicked, velocity, and kicking accuracy. In keeping with the previous general developmental trend noted with running, throwing, and jumping, available data suggest that kicking performance improves with increasing age (for both genders) through childhood regardless of the test; males generally perform better than females do. In addition, the differences between male and female kicking performance tend to increase as children get older. However, as noted earlier, much of the available data predate 1970. As of this writing, little has been reported for ages beyond 12 years.

Catching

Catching is a coincident timing task that involves the complex interplay of coordinating visual information and motor behavior to a single point of interception (refer to Chapter 6). The information-processing literature suggests the ability of individuals to accurately time their movements to an interception point with a moving object improves through childhood before it reaches a relatively mature level in the early teens. In the review by Williams (1983), it was noted that several developmental trends in the ability to judge the speed, direction, and interception point of a moving object can be observed between the ages of 6 and 12 years. Older children (from ages 9 to 12 years) are generally much more accurate in judging the flight of a moving object than younger children are. Although these data provide useful information with which to understand the perceptual and motor mechanisms' prerequisite to the successful interception of objects, they do not provide specific product performance information. One should also keep in mind that experience has been shown to be a better indicator of coincident timing ability than age. Unfortunately, much of the literature concerning the quantitative characteristics of young children's catching ability is unclear because many research studies have used scoring systems that reflect the process by which the object is intercepted as well as the actual success of the catch. It also should be noted that although much of the literature describes 6- to 8-year-olds as relatively proficient catchers, much of this information was collected when a large ball was used and the thrower was positioned directly in front of a ball tossed slowly from about 6 feet away.

Studies that have focused primarily on the end product characteristics of catching (i.e., interception and control of the ball), under simple and complex conditions, suggest that males and females display yearly increases in performance through the elementary years and, in some cases, beyond (e.g., Fischman, Moore, & Steele, 1992). These data appear to parallel the information related to the development of perceptual-motor and coincident timing abilities. In the Fischman et al. (1992) investigation, one-hand catching was studied among a sample of 5- to 12-year-olds. Subjects were tossed tennis balls at four different locations (waist height, shoulder height, above the head, and out to the side) from 9 feet away and scored by the number caught. Results indicated that catching performance improved with age, with males outperforming females. One of the noted conclusions is that even 5-year-olds were able to integrate, to some degree, perception and motor response. The literature is mixed with regard to gender differences; therefore, a clear-cut statement cannot be made. Along with the general age-related trend of increased catching ability, the literature also suggests that improvement is characterized by the ability to catch increasingly smaller balls and display more sophisticated hand-catching techniques.

Striking with an Implement

Striking is a coincident timing skill that presents difficulty for those who would attempt to establish a precise developmental picture of product performance. This inherent problem is that striking skills are performed in a variety of planes (overhand, sidearm, and underhand) and under widely varying conditions. Along with a wide assortment of striking motions, other variables include the size and type of ball, and the striking implement. The diversity of popular sports that use striking skills includes softball, tennis, hockey, golf, and volleyball. Although a limited number of studies have assessed product characteristics across the broad spectrum of striking, a clear and persistent trend of yearly increases through childhood (and perhaps beyond) has been identified. In contrast to the interception skill of catching, however, most data indicate that males are better strikers than females.

Much of the data on the product characteristics of striking have been collected by measuring striking velocity, distance the ball travels, and number of hits (out of a set number of trials). Williams (1983) reported that velocity with the one- and two-arm sidearm motion (using a racquetball racquet) improved substantially for both sexes from 4 to 8 years. Interestingly, one-arm striking performances were slightly better than two-arm striking performances. It has been speculated that this is due to a young child's difficulty in effectively timing the motion with two hands. Unfortunately, little information is available in relation to the distance a ball travels after being struck. One generally would expect distance (force) performance trends to parallel those found in velocity scores (as in throwing and kicking); however, there has not been enough evidence gathered to make such a statement.

Perhaps the most commonly used measure of striking performance has been number of hits. Two studies cited most often were conducted by Seils (1951) and Johnson (1962). In both investigations, children were positioned with a bat in a typical batter's stance and asked to strike a ball attached at the end of a rope and swung over the plate. Similar results were found; both sexes increased in their striking ability at successive grade levels; at each grade, males performed better than females.

Although there appears to be a general trend toward improvement through the childhood years, the characteristics associated with change in general striking ability have not been identified clearly.

Hopping

We learned in Chapter 9 that hopping is the most difficult form of basic jumping and is an integral part of several advanced movement skills used in games, dance, and gymnastic activities. The movement presents difficulty because it requires leg strength, balance, and controlled rhythmical movement. During the childhood years, hopping is one of the fundamental skills in which gender differences favor the female. In terms of quantitative characteristics, hopping usually is measured by determining (a) the number of consecutive hops completed before balance is lost, (b) the ability to complete a specified distance (usually 25 or 50 ft) while in balance, and (c) the time required to hop a specified distance. Available data suggest that hopping abilities, regardless of the particular type of task, generally improve with age through childhood and that females perform better than males. Unfortunately, minimal data are available for individuals beyond the elementary years; thus, the developmental perspective is limited.

By 3½ years of age, most children have the ability to hop repeatedly for three steps (the definition of a true hop); by age 5 years, the ability to hop 10 consecutive times is normal. Keogh (1965) investigated the ability of children from ages 5 to 9 years to hop 50 feet without stopping or exchanging hopping legs. In his findings, he reported that with advancing age, an increasing percentage of children completed the distance and females were approximately 1 year ahead of the males in acquiring the ability. Hopping speed over a specified distance also improves with age during childhood. Cratty (1986) suggests that by age 5 years, most children can hop a distance of 50 feet in about 10 seconds and females are approximately 3.5 seconds faster than males are.

Ball Bouncing and Dribbling

Although ball bouncing and dribbling (i.e., three or four consecutive bounces) are two of the most widely practiced fundamental and sport skills, little data are available. In an unpublished study by Williams and Breihan (1979) as reported by Williams (1983), males and females aged 4, 6, and 8 years were asked to use one hand to bounce an 8-inch ball repeatedly within a 12-inch square. Results indicated that performances for both genders improved with advancing age. Although males performed better than the females at ages 4 and 6 years, females were substantially better at 8 years. As a group, the 4-year-olds averaged less than two successful bounces within the square before they lost control. In contrast, 6-year-olds averaged four controlled four bounces and the 8-year-olds slightly more than five good bounces.

This topic should be studied more extensively to develop a more complete picture of dribbling as a sport skill. Currently, no information is available that assesses dribbling performance in which the child uses the right and left hands while moving.

Balance

As noted in the discussion of vestibular awareness in Chapter 6, the successful performance of virtually all motor skills depends on the individual's ability to establish and maintain equilibrium, or balance. Refer to Chapter 6 for a review of the development of balancing abilities through adolescence.

MOTOR SKILL REFINEMENT

Objective 10.4

Sports and physical education are two of the most influential developmental factors in motor skill development and refinement during childhood and adolescence. Sport and other physical activity participation normally occur through school programs, spontaneous play activities, and organized youth sport programs. The dramatic increase in nonschool youth sport programs has received considerable attention from developmentalists in recent years.

focus on change

Youth sport and school physical education can have a dramatic effect on performance *change* and lifelong well-being.

Youth Sport Participation

An estimated 50 million children and youth ages 5 to 18 years participate in non-school-sponsored sport activities. These activities include team sports, club sports (e.g., swimming, running, and gymnastics), and recreational sport programs. Females account for approximately 45% of the total, which represents a continuing trend of increased female participation over the last decade. The term **youth sports** refers to any athletic program that provides a systematic sequence

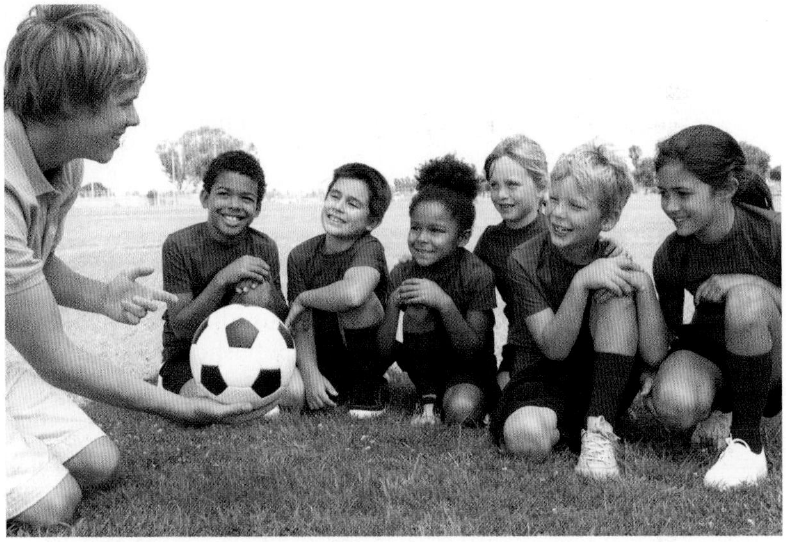

Figure 10.9 Soccer accounts for a large portion of youth sport participation.

of practices and contents for children and youth. Approximately 75 different individual and team sport activities are available for youth (Fig. 10.9).

Seefeldt and Branta (1984) suggested six explanations for the increased participation of children in youth sport programs. Although older than 30 years, mention is still given to these observations.

1. Passage of Title IX, which mandates equal opportunities in sport at all levels for females. This has had a great impact on overall participation. In 1971, the year before Title IX, less than 300,000 girls participated in high school sports, about 1 in 27. Today (2016), the number approaches 3 million, or approximately 1 in 1 million. The number of women participating in intercollegiate sports in that same span has gone from about 30,000 to more than 150,000. In the last 20 years alone, the number of women's college teams has nearly doubled.
2. Greater accessibility to programs due to the gradual movement of the population from rural to urban residences
3. Changing lifestyles of adults, including greater concern for health and physical fitness, may be influencing the decisions parents make about children's participation in physical activities that include sports.
4. An increase in the number of women in the workforce. It may be speculated that this has led to an increase in the enrollment of children in activity programs as a caretaking function. It also may be that some single-parent mothers view the coach as an additional role model for their child and want to encourage that interaction. Of course, this could be true for single-parent fathers as well.
5. Glorification of sport. The media's constant focus on the glory of sport undoubtedly leads some parents to involve their child in sport at an early age. Some parents perceive sport involvement as an avenue through which to increase their child's opportunities for social and financial success.
6. Declining role of public schools in providing sport programs below the high school level. This has stimulated increased involvement by municipal recreation and community agencies in providing activity programs.

Focus on Application
Head Collisions in Sport and Brain Function

An estimated 350,000 sports-related brain injuries, of mild to moderate severity, most of which can be classified as concussions, occur in the United States each year. Although the significance of that has drawn strong public attention in recent years (even a movie), scientists have been aware of the issue for close to two decades. For example, in 2001, the Society for Neuroscience conducted a review of the research concerning head collisions resulting from activity in contact sports such as football, hockey, boxing, and soccer. An interesting finding was the evidence for supposedly "minor" injuries. Evidence confirms that even minor head collisions can create changes in mental function. For example, most of the time, contacts are not hard enough to actually cause an open wound or large bump, but they can cause the brain to reverberate around in the skull. Typical effects include a brief loss of consciousness, lightheadedness, and dizziness—which many parents and coaches consider just part of the game and no big deal. However, the evidence indicates that such contact can cause problems with memory and attention. For example, in one study, researchers gave a series of written and verbal tests to college football players before their season started. Those who experienced a concussion during play were retested. The players' performance on tests of verbal learning, memory, and speed of information processing was noticeably worse for up to 1 week after the blow. Another study examined amateur soccer players who previously experienced concussions as part of the match. Similarly, their performance on tests of memory and information processing was impaired. Furthermore, the research indicated that those with the most concussions did the worst. This suggests that hits to the head, even supposedly minor ones, may lead to lasting, cumulative damage in the brain. Studies of brain activity complement those findings. That is, athletes who suffered several concussions had weaker activity in brain regions that play a role in certain memory functions. They also had problems conducting memory tasks.

For a debate on the issue of "Tackling in Youth Football," see the American Academy of Pediatrics policy statement (WebLink provided).

Source:

Society for Neuroscience. (2001). Knocking noggins, *Brain Briefings*. Retrieved from http://www.sfn.org/

WebLink

See "Concussions."
http://www.brainfacts.org
http://www.aap.org
http://www.pbs.org
(brain trauma)

think about it

From your experience, what are the positives and negatives in youth sport?

Another significant reason for the increase in youth sport participation is the fact that children are getting involved at an earlier age; programs for 5-year-olds are commonplace today. Modifications of popular sports, such as T-baseball and small fry soccer, make such programs more enticing to parents. Other explanations are the increased participation in what are considered nontraditional sport activities (e.g., roller hockey, in-line skating, and snowboarding) and the dramatic increase in the number of programs and events organized for handicapped individuals (e.g., wheelchair bowling, tennis, and softball, and the Special Olympics) are two other areas of increased involvement in sport activity.

With that said, concerning the overall total participation increase over the last 30 years, recent reports present somewhat troublesome decline (Sports and Fitness Industry Association, 2015). Among 6- to 17-year-olds, the average number of team sports per participant has declined 6% from 2009 to 2014. Why? Among the explanations is increased focus on "specialization and year-round play"—a situation that may lead to burnout. That speculation is supported in part by the observation that about 75% of participants drop out by age 15 years (Merkel, 2013). The issues of burnout, specialization, and sports injuries are discussed in a subsequent section of this chapter.

INTERSCHOLASTIC SPORTS

With regard to number of participants in interscholastic sports in high school, Table 10.1 shows figures from the 2014 to 2015 school year regarding the 10 most popular activities. The report noted that participation among females had increased significantly over the years, especially in soccer, volleyball, and softball (Fig. 10.10). It can be speculated that much of this interest is due to the growing popularity of female sport in general, as evidenced by the increase in programs (and scholarship opportunities) at the college and university levels. Overall, about 7 million students (4 million males and 3 million females) participated in high school athletics.

COLLEGE SPORTS

WebLink
http://www.ncaa.org/; see "Sport Participation Report."

According to the National Collegiate Athletic Association (2015), participation in college athletics continues to rise—more than 480,000 participated. That is more than 19,000 teams in 23 sports. A positive note is that the gap between male and females continues to narrow. Whereas more male athletes participated (57%), around 53% of teams were female. Female participation has increased every year since 1981 to 1982. To illustrate the impact of females, there were 80 soccer teams in 1981 to 1982; in 2014 to 2015, there were 1,030.

Although involvement in sport programs has been found to contribute significantly to the participant's physical, psychomotor, social, and emotional development, several issues have been raised in relation to potential psychological and physical harm. Frequently addressed issues include the related competitive stress and anxiety; dropout rate; the physical risks, especially in contact and collision sports; and the effects of intense early participation.

DEBATING PARTICIPATION

Are youth sports harmful? In addition to the debate of participation in contact sports such as youth football, noted earlier, in Chapter 5, we addressed this question with

TABLE 10.1 Ten Most Popular Interscholastic Sports[a]

Boys	Rank	Girls
Football	1	Outdoor track and field
Outdoor track and field	2	Volleyball
Basketball	3	Basketball
Baseball	4	Soccer
Soccer	5	Fast-pitch softball
Wrestling	6	Cross-country
Cross-country	7	Tennis
Tennis	8	Swimming/diving
Golf	9	Competitive spirit squad
Swimming/diving	10	Lacrosse

[a]Denoted number of participants.
SOURCE: National Federation of State High School Associations (2015).

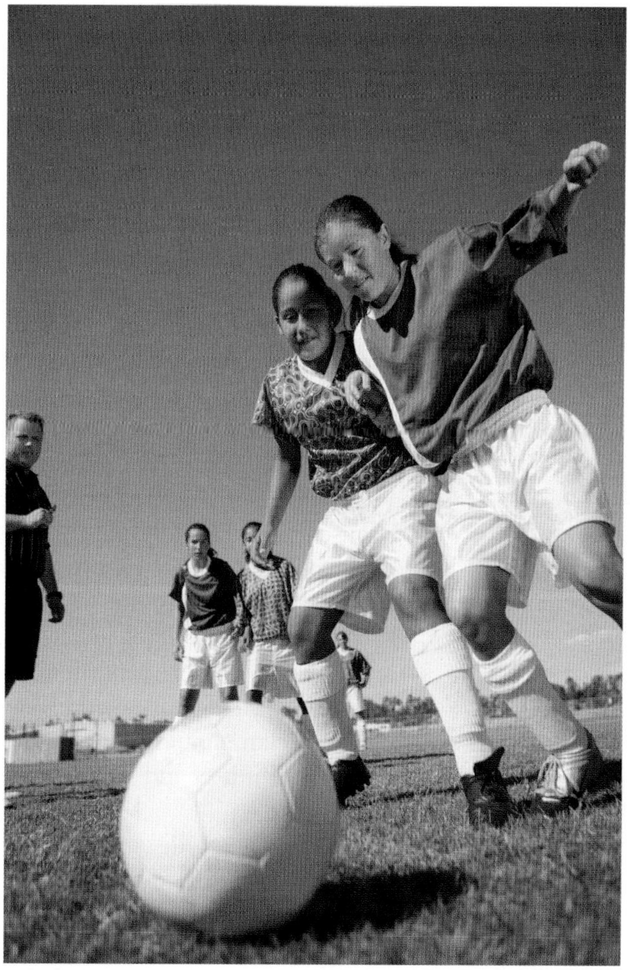

Figure 10.10 Title IX has helped considerably to increase female participation in sports.

regard to sport training effects and childhood growth—namely, pubertal growth. In general, the evidence suggests that growth is not affected adversely by typical sports training of less than 18 hours per week. Of course, both physical and psychological intensity with fewer or more hours could produce a different conclusion. For example, as noted in Chapter 5, a consistent body of evidence indicates that intense training in selected female athletes (e.g., gymnasts and ballet dancers) results in menarche later than that of the general population.

The importance of this issue prompted the American Academy of Pediatrics (2000) to form a statement regarding "intensive training and sports specialization in young athletes." The primary concern is young athletes who specialize in just one sport may be denied the benefits of varied activity while they face additional physical and psychological demands from intense training and competition. As noted earlier, there is speculation that specialization and year-round training may lead to burnout by early adolescence. Although supporting selected psychological (self-esteem) and physical benefits (cardiac and musculoskeletal growth) of sports training, the report states that little information is available on the possible short-term and long-term health consequences of intensive training in young athletes. One of the difficulties is lack of a clear definition of *specialized* and *intensively trained*. In addition, as a general human development principle, there is a wide variation in individual tolerance to specific conditions. The reports confirm that only a small minority of young athletes experience adverse effects. It appears, however, that those who participate in a variety of sports and specialize only after reaching puberty tend to be more consistent performers, have fewer injuries, and adhere to sports play longer than those who specialize early. In conclusion, the report recommended the following:

1. Children should be encouraged to participate in sports at a level consistent with their abilities and interests. Pushing children beyond these limits is discouraged as is specialization in a single sport before adolescence.
2. The child athlete should be coached by persons knowledgeable about proper training techniques, equipment, and the unique physical, physiological, and emotional characteristics of young competitors.
3. In the absence of prospective markers of excessive physical stress, physicians and coaches should strive for early recognition, prevention, and treatment of overuse injuries (tendinitis, apophysitis, stress fractures, and shin splints).
4. A pediatrician should regularly monitor the conditions of child athletes involved in intense training.
5. The intensely trained, specialized child athlete needs ongoing assessment of nutritional intake, with particular attention to total calories, a balanced diet, and intake of iron and calcium.
6. A pediatrician should educate the child athlete, family, and coach about the risks of heat injury and strategies for prevention.

For an excellent discussion of the positive and negative impact of youth sports, see Merkel (2013) and updates at the WebLinks noted earlier. Chapter 14 discusses selected psychological considerations (e.g., self-esteem, gender roles, sex-stereotyping).

Ironically, even with the large number of youth participating in sports and other community activities, a large portion of American youth 12 to 21 years of age are not active on a regular basis. In fact, as noted in Chapter 5, physical activity declines dramatically with age for both genders during adolescence.

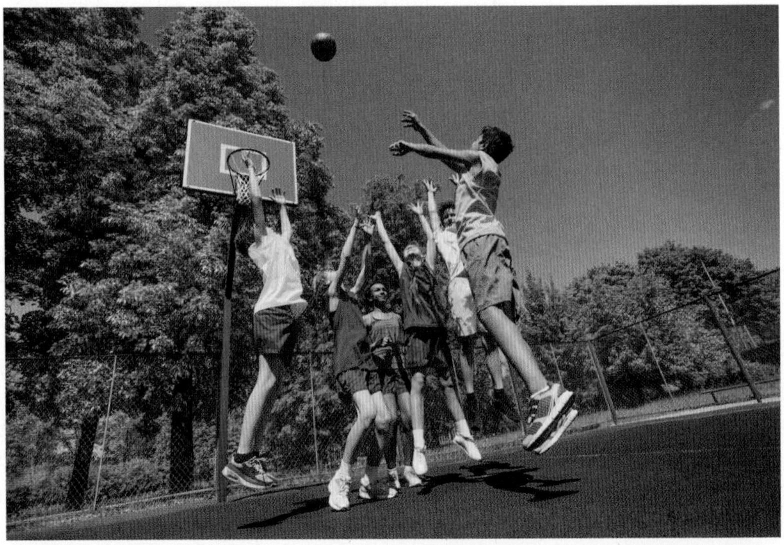

Figure 10.11 According to the CDC (2014), basketball is the most common activity for boys; for girls it is running.

Focus on Application
Drug Use and Young Athletes

Ergogenic drugs are substances used to enhance athletic performance. Such drugs have been used widely by professionals and elite athletes for several decades; however, research indicates that younger athletes are increasingly experimenting with these substances. Commonly used ergogenic drugs include anabolic–androgenic steroids, creatine, and ephedra alkaloids. Anabolic steroids and creatine have been shown to offer potential gains in body mass and strength, but use confers adverse effects to multiple organ systems.

Recent surveys report that children are exposed to these substances at younger ages than in years past and use starts as early as middle school. Estimates of high school steroid use range from 4% to 11% in boys and up to 3% in girls. Forty-two percent of college athlete users report that their first use occurred in high school, and 15% say that they started in junior high or before. Furthermore, up to one-third of high school students who use anabolic steroids are in the population of nonathletes who use steroids to improve their appearance.

Nearly 30% of steroid users experience mild subjective adverse effects. Adverse effects include premature balding, acne, precocious puberty, high blood pressure, and left ventricular hypertrophy. Psychologically, steroid users may experience severe mood swings from depression to mania and aggression that cannot be channeled properly outside the athletic arena. The bottom line is that athletes, parents, physicians, and coaches all need to be educated on the prevention and monitoring of ergogenic drug use.

Source:

Calfee, R., & Fadale, P. (2006). Popular ergogenic drugs and supplements in young athletes. *Pediatrics*, *117*(3), e577–e589.

School Physical Education

Another potentially powerful source for motor skill and physical fitness development is the school **physical education** program. As noted in Chapter 5, the problem of national health among children and adults is clear. For example, about 69% of the adults in the United States are overweight or obese, and 50% of adults are not active enough physically to reap any significant health benefits (Centers for Disease Control and Prevention [CDC], 2016). A sedentary lifestyle almost doubles one's risk for coronary heart disease, a condition that can begin to develop in childhood. With regard to children and youth, almost one-third of children are now overweight; overall, the percentage has tripled in the last 30 years. With this has emerged type 2 diabetes, which is strongly linked to obesity in adults.

WebLink

See "Physical Education and Fitness."
http://www.fitness.gov
http://www.shapeamerica.org
http://www.cdc.gov

Many children spend too much time viewing electronic devices (up to 6 hours a day) and are not active physically. Participation in all types of physical activity declines dramatically as age and grade in school increase. For example, nearly 50% of young people aged 12 to 21 years are not active on a regular basis. This trend results in about 50 percent of adults who do not achieve the recommended amount of physical activity (CDC, 2016).

Although awareness appears to have increased, according to a national survey, only six states in the United States require physical education in every grade (National Association for Sport and Physical Education & American Heart Association, 2012). Only 14 states (27%) require schools to perform fitness assessment. Declining activity levels typically mean declining physical fitness levels, which is associated with increased prevalence of a multitude of medical problems.

think about it

Reflect on your physical education experience in schools. Did it promote health-related activity?

Most researchers and educators agree that one of the solutions to the problem is *quality school physical education*, more specifically, school programs that are **developmentally appropriate**. This means a program of activities that meets the individual's level of physical and psychological development (see the latest information from the Society of Health and Physical Educators [SHAPE]). Activities may be age-related, but not age-determined, which thus supports the principle of individual differences. Such programs have high priority for the development of fundamental motor skills, health-related fitness, and healthy living education (Fig. 10.12).

SHAPE provides a variety of resources (e.g., national standards, appropriate practices, outcomes, and guidelines) to help parents, schools, and communities develop quality sport and physical education programs. Their position is that children and youth should learn how to be physically active in ways that increase physical competence, self-esteem, and enjoyment through physical activity. An example of a quality physical education program would include the following characteristics:

- Instruction by physical education specialists who have baccalaureate degrees
- Required physical education for all grade levels, preferably 150 minutes a week for elementary grades and 225 minutes for middle and high school students
- Instruction in a variety of developmentally appropriate physical activities
- Use of fitness assessment and education to help children understand, enjoy, improve, and/or maintain their physical health and well-being
- Opportunities through physical activity participation to develop social and cooperative skills and to gain a multicultural perspective
- Classes designed for ALL children to be involved in activities that provide maximum opportunity to be active continuously
- Instruction in healthy eating habits and good nutrition

One trend that has shown promise in recent years is "school-based physical education." These are more comprehensive programs that structure health-related activities into not only physical education classes but also the classroom, recess, and before/after school. Some of these programs provide intervention for those

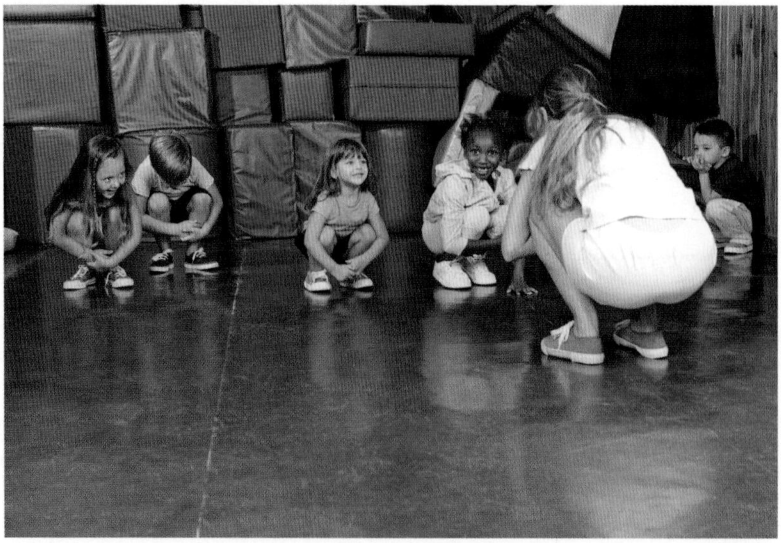

Figure 10.12 Quality physical education provides the foundation for lifelong fitness habits.

WebLink

http://www.shapeamerica.org; http://www.physicalactivityplan.org

students assessed at lower fitness levels. One of the driving goals is to increase education and level of daily physical activity. Obviously, due to time constraints, for most schools, it is not feasible to program 60 minutes of physical activity per day (the CDC recommendation for children) in physical education class.

The improvement of physical education programs is a priority goal of several major health agencies, including the CDC, American Heart Association, American Academy of Pediatrics, and the President's Council on Fitness, Sports & Nutrition. Also refer to the National Physical Activity Plan for a review of research and recommendations.

Summary

The period from later childhood through adolescence encompasses the sports skill and growth and refinement phases of motor behavior and is marked by rapid biological change, increases in product performance, gender-related differences, and the emergence of sport skill behavior. Many of the quantitative (product) changes in motor performance are based on increasing levels of experience, biological change associated with the adolescent growth spurt (e.g., increased body size, muscle mass, strength, and cardiorespiratory capacity), sociocultural practices, and participation levels. In general, females appear to be closing the gender gap that was quite wide in earlier years. This trend seems to be related to increased participation and a change in society's view of females in sporting activities. However, a general and rather consistent trend in product performance (e.g., run, jump, and throw) change is that both genders improve significantly from childhood to adolescence and that males continue to improve on a variety of skills through adolescence (to at least age 17 years), whereas females have a tendency to peak around early adolescence.

Organized youth sport programs and school physical education programs are two of the most influential factors in motor skill development and refinement. In recent years, there has been a dramatic increase in youth sport participation with a wide variety of activities offered for both genders. Although numerous developmental contributions have been linked to participation in organized youth sport programs, several issues have been raised in relation to their potential to result in psychological and physical harm.

School physical education, if presented in a developmentally appropriate manner, can do much to improve the state of physical fitness in the United States.

think about it

1. **What are the implications of being an early or late mature regarding this discussion?**
2. **Do you think the hypothetical gender trend for females has changed in the last 10 years?**
3. **What is your community's view of female participation in all types of sport?**

4. **What ideas do you have to change these trends (obesity and being less active after childhood)?**
5. **From your experience, what are the positives and negatives in youth sport?**
6. **Reflect on your physical education experience in schools. Did it promote health-related activity?**

LEARNING ACTIVITIES

Objective: To examine local school district (or your hometown) physical education (PE) policy. Select a school district. Ask for information about their PE program for grades K to 12 including basic curriculum by grade, time/days a week, and teacher requirements. Compare to national recommendations and create a report of your findings, including your suggestions.

Objective: To determine youth sport injuries that require follow-up therapy. Ask local physical therapists what are the most common youth sport injuries that they work with and, then via the Web or interview with therapists, what are the typical therapy applications for each injury. Create a two- to three-page report.

Suggested Reading

Siedentop, D., Hastie, P., & van Der Mars, H. (2011). *Complete guide to sport education* (2nd ed.). Champaign, IL: Human Kinetics.

Chapter 11

Motor Behavior in the Adult Years

OBJECTIVES

Upon completion of this chapter, you should be able to

11.1 Provide a brief overview of motor behavior in the adult years.

11.2 Describe the growth and physiological characteristics associated with peak maturity.

11.3 Identify the motor performance characteristics that parallel peak biological maturity.

11.4 Describe the various biological theories of advanced aging.

11.5 Explain the term *regression* and distinguish between chronological and physiological age.

11.6 Briefly introduce and outline the characteristics associated with biological regression and motor performance.

11.7 Describe the changes in movement patterns that occur with advancing age.

11.8 Discuss the relationship between physical activity and longevity.

KEY TERMS

peak motor performance
aging
gerontology
chronological age
physiological age
regression
psychomotor slowing
longevity
daily living skills (DLS)

The Developmental Continuum

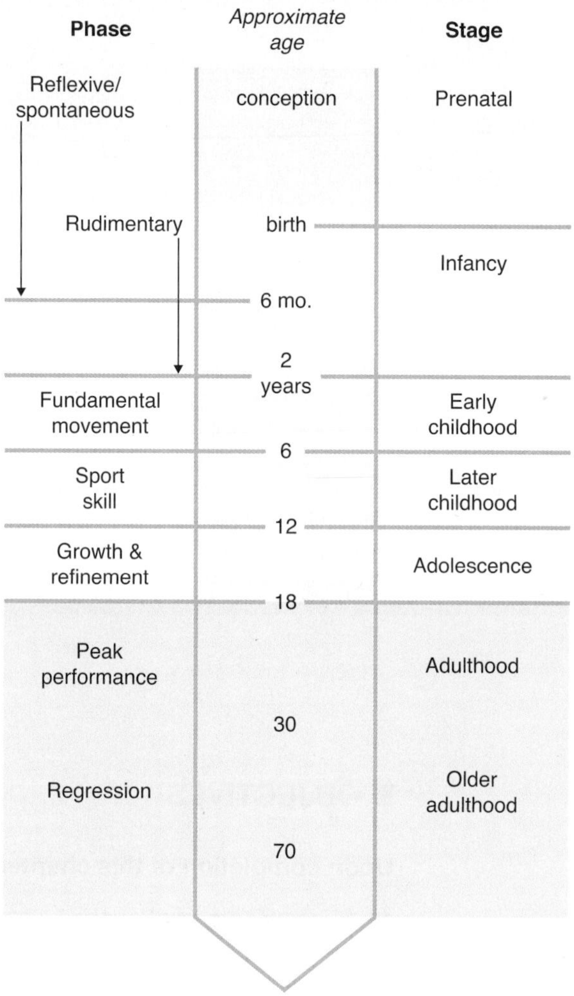

Objective 11.1

Much of the information to this point in the text has provided the basis for understanding lifelong motor development by describing the biological and information-processing characteristics associated with motor behavior across the life span. Part Four began with an introduction to the developmental approach to motor performance and identified each of the contributing phases of motor behavior. In keeping with this approach, Chapter 8 presented the initial phase of motor behavior by describing actions exhibited prior to birth. Subsequent chapters have traced the evolution of movement abilities and the acquisition of fundamental and basic sport skills through childhood and adolescence.

This chapter describes the final phases and associated "typical" behaviors in the lifelong process of motor development. The next chapter briefly describes "atypical" populations that are commonly observed in teaching and clinical settings. Motor behavior during the adult years is characterized by two distinguishing milestones—peak performance, which is associated with biological maturity during early adulthood, and the emergence of performance regression, which is linked with the latter stages of aging.

The information presented in this chapter constitutes a brief review of those biological distinctions and motor performance characteristics that distinguish adulthood from the other periods of the total life span. A timely discussion of the possible effects of physical activity on longevity also is presented.

PEAK MOTOR PERFORMANCE

Objective 11.2

Although adolescence generally is accepted as the most distinctive period of biological growth and motor skill development, most individuals reach their peak of physical performance, health, and sexual maturity in early adulthood. It is also during the early adult years that gender differences in motor performance are maximized. Wide variation among young adults is common. But it is during this period in the life span that individuals attain **peak motor performance** partly because the different physiological systems have become capable of working together so efficiently.

Growth and Physiological Function

focus on change

Change continues through the life span with advanced aging presenting new and exciting challenges.

Skeletal maturity is one example of continued growth into the adult years. Although most epiphyseal growth is completed in late adolescence (16 to 18 years), the long bones may continue to grow until approximately age 25 years, and the vertebral column may continue to grow until about age 30 years. This continued growth in the long bones may add up to one-fourth of an inch to an individual's height. In addition, certain areas of the braincase do not reach maturity until well into adulthood. This continued growth is evident when men (and women) who wear hats notice they have to purchase larger sizes as they age.

According to most sources, peak physiological function generally occurs between the approximate ages of 25 and 30 years of age (Kenney, Wilmore, & Costill, 2015; McArdle et al., 2015). As a general rule, females tend to mature at the lower end (22 to 25 years) and males at the upper end (28 to 30 years) of the range. This is especially evident in three of the most influential factors in motor performance: muscular strength, cardiorespiratory efficiency, and processing speed (reaction/movement time).

Maximum strength for both genders generally is achieved at a time when the muscular cross-sectional area is the largest, which is between the approximate ages of 20 and 30 years. Maximal strength for most muscle groups takes place between the ages of 25 and 29 years. Support for this assertion is shown in Figure 11.1, which illustrates that male grip strength values peak in the late 20s and early 30s and then decline steadily. These data represent both cross-sectional and a 9-year longitudinal study (Kallman, Plato, & Tobin, 1990); note the striking agreement between the two data sets.

Peak physiological function in maximum oxygen consumption and cardiorespiratory work for both genders typically occurs during the third decade. Several reviews and studies report peak values within the range of 25 to 29 years. Figure 11.2 shows maximal oxygen uptake as a function of age, with peak uptake occurring around age 25 years and declining steadily thereafter. Figure 11.3 is a frequently cited illustration that depicts maximum work at various ages based on a two-step climbing test. Based on this information, peak work performance for females is said to occur around the age of 25 years, and for males, approximately 3 years later. In the early 1960s, Shock (1962) conducted what is now referred to

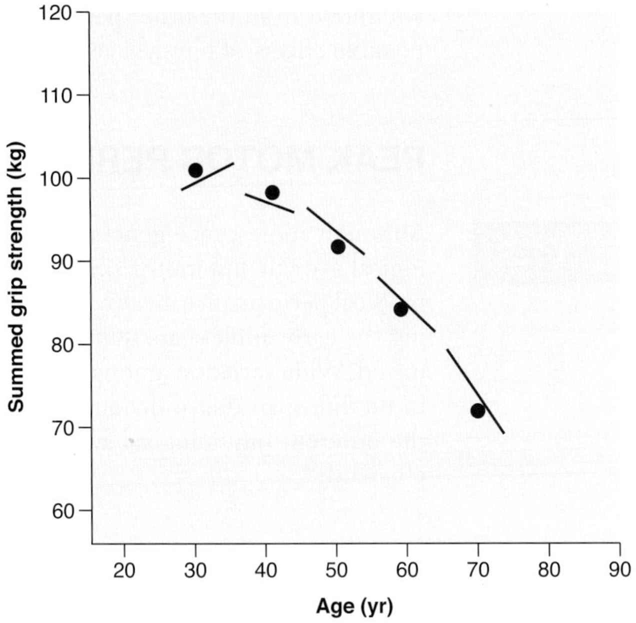

Figure 11.1 Changes in grip strength with age.

as a classic aging and physical performance study. Included in that series of experiments was a test to determine the amount of work that males could do using a crank ergometer. Among the physiological variables measured were oxygen consumption and cardiac output. The researchers found work rate peaked around the age of 28 years.

The importance of neurophysiological function and processing speed in the performance of a motor act is obvious. Assessments of successful motor performance frequently are based on the combination of perceptual recognition (attention), speed of memory, and neuromuscular response time (reaction/movement time). Processing speed, as determined by reaction time, improves with age up to the early adult years; peak performance occurs in the 20s (Salthouse, 2007) (Fig. 11.4).

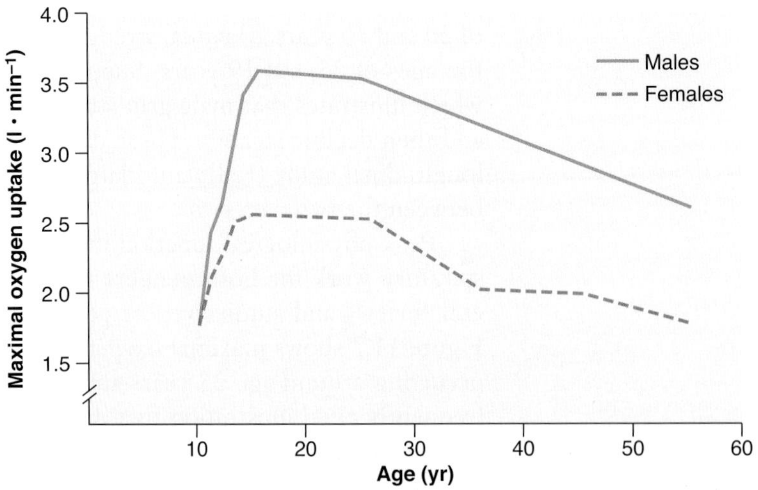

Figure 11.2 Changes in maximum oxygen consumption with age.

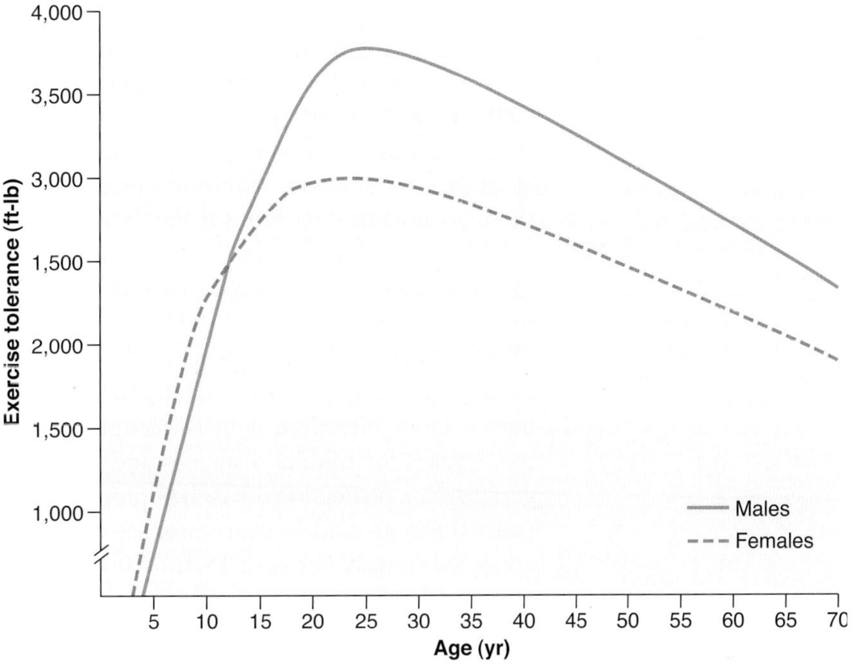

Figure 11.3 Relationship of age to exercise tolerance (in foot-pounds of work per minute).

SOURCE: Data from Master, A. M. (1935). The two-step test of myocardial function. *American Heart Journal*, *10*, 495–510.

Motor Performance Characteristics

Objective 11.3

Peak physiological function, which occurs in the approximate range of 25 to 30 years, closely parallels maximal motor performance. A general observation of the sporting world quickly leads to the speculation that college athletes are better than those of high school age, and few professional or Olympic-caliber athletes participate at these levels beyond their early 30s.

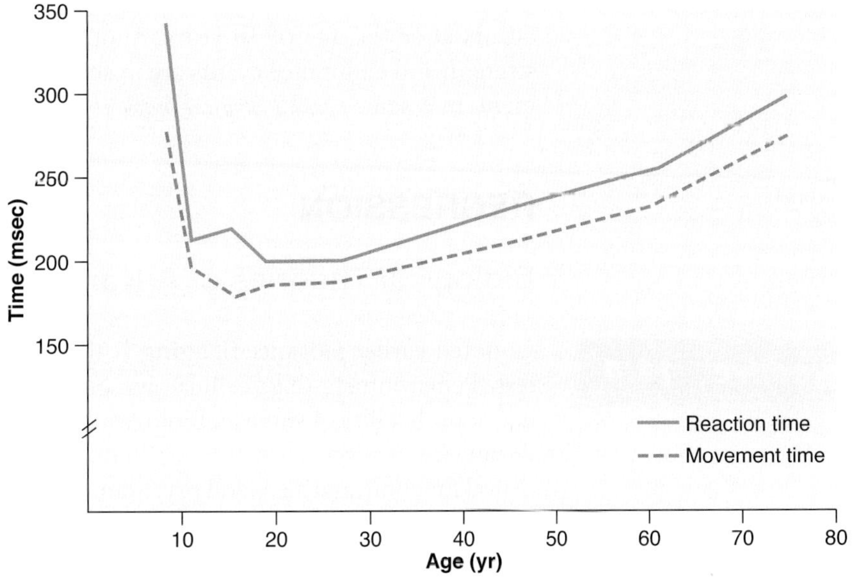

Figure 11.4 Reaction time and movement time as functions of age.

Because the majority of physical growth and development occurs during adolescence, the increases in motor performance during the adult years are due primarily to training, practice, experience, and motivation. Peak proficiency may be studied from the perspective of a highly trained population (i.e., athletes) that seeks maximum motor performance or from the perspective of a population of average or normal ability. Although considerable diversity and variability exist within these groups, and normal is difficult to define, certain trends can be identified.

With the intent of determining age at peak athletic performance, Schulz and Curnow (1988) analyzed records and national ranking from track and field, swimming, baseball, tennis, and golf. In track and field, for example, they examined Olympic results from 1896 to 1980. Overall, the mean age of winners in seven events was about 25 years. Comparing running events, the average age at peak performance increased with the length of the race: from 22 years in the sprints to 24 years for middle distances and 27 years for distances of 5,000 meters and greater. For professional baseball players, the mean age of peak performance was consistently around 27 years (also see Schulz et al., 1994). Swimming performance appeared to peak between 18 and 20 years, and record performances in golf were achieved between the ages of 30 and 31 years. An examination of world professional tennis rankings suggested that 24 to 25 years of age was best for optimal performance. Females generally achieved peak performance about 1 to 2 years before males did. A review of 1993 world record holders at the times the records were broken for open-class track and field and swimming reveals similar findings (Stone & Kozma, 1996). Track and field records (male and female ages combined) were broken at 24 to 29 years, whereas most swimming achievements were attained at ages 17 to 19 years; the backstroke was the exception at age 24 years. Interestingly, a more recent study of Olympic athletes in track and field and swimming, reported peak at 26 and 21 years, respectively (Berthelot et al., 2012).

think about it

Speculate on a secular trend for peak physiological function and performance 50 years from now. Relate your projections to specific types of activities.

The conclusion drawn from reviews of the data on this topic has been that younger athletes generally challenge performance records that require greater levels of strength, speed, and endurance. Furthermore, older athletes frequently obtain peak proficiency in activities that require a high skill level and experience but less vigorous physical demands (e.g., golf). Although research in this area is limited, it allow us to speculate that maximum proficiency in relatively less physically demanding motor skills such as shooting, bowling, golf, and billiards generally occurs after the age of 30 years. Another observation is that the data for more strength and endurance events are in accordance with peak physiological development. In essence, *peak biological maturity parallels peak performance.*

REGRESSION

Biological Theories of Advanced Aging

Objective 11.4

As noted earlier (advanced), **aging** is the diminished capacity to regulate the internal environment (e.g., cellular and organismic structures), which results in a reduced probability of survival. Biological aging commonly is equated with biological decline (regression), such as losses in muscle, bone mass, and cardiorespiratory and neural function, and a general psychomotor slowing of the body. Although the body is aging continuously from conception to death, after about age 30 years, regression in some form typically develops. There are numerous theories, subtheories, and lines of research on aging; no single hypothesis answers all of the questions proposed.

WebLink

http://www.nia.nih.gov/; see "Theories on Aging."

The study of older people and the aging process is known as **gerontology**. The following discussion briefly describes some of the general explanations of biological aging. For a more detailed discussion, refer to the "Suggested Reading" and the WebLink for the National Institute on Aging (NIA). As pointed out in previous chapters and noted in this unit, although advanced aging typically complements a decline in function, physical activity and health habits are significant factors in the rate of degradation. According to McArdle, Katch, and Katch (2010), "sedentary living produces losses in functional capacity at least as great as the effects of aging" (p. 853). Underscoring this observation is the fact that aging is an individual experience that has considerable variability. Two 70-year-olds may be so different that one swims a mile three times a week, whereas the other must be helped to bathe.

GENETIC THEORY

Also referred to as *cellular clock theory*, genetic theory suggests that aging is under the direction of the DNA in human genes. Evidently, there are proliferative and antiproliferative genes that, in theory, provide checks and balances of biological systems. Antiproliferative genes result in decreased cell division, which represents a weakening agent to the body. Once these genes become more active, regression develops. It seems clear, based on several lines of supportive research, that some sort of genetic program determines the aging process, but our understanding of the specifics remains unclear. This theory places the upper limit of the life span at 125 years.

WEAR-AND-TEAR THEORY

The relatively simple premise of this theory is that aging is a result of long-term, accumulated damage to various vital bodily systems. In the course of daily living, the body suffers some damage but repairs itself under relatively normal conditions. With advancing age, this ability gradually becomes less effective. Although some aspects of this notion appear reasonable, such as wear due to prolonged exposure to sunlight and other damaging elements, there is no evidence that hard work causes early death. To the contrary, vigorous exercise is a factor in predicting longer, not shorter, life. Similarly, in some aspects, the brain functions better with use.

think about it

Does exercise influence any of these theories? How? What does research tell us?

CELLULAR GARBAGE/MUTATION THEORIES

These theories suggest that with advancing age, the body accumulates cellular garbage (waste products) due to destructive mutation, which results in a decline in functioning. Two of the most noted views on this approach are the *free radical* and *cross-linking* theories. Free radicals are highly unstable molecules that react with other molecules in a way that may damage cells and diminish bodily functions. The normal process of cellular metabolism produces some free radicals; other free radicals are derived from the environment. Although the body can protect itself against some free radicals, with time the number builds up, resulting in signs of aging. Related to this view is the cross-linking theory, which focuses on the processes by which different types of molecules are joined together permanently (cross-linked). This results in deterioration such as wrinkling (due in part to collagen change) and atherosclerosis. Another substance connected with the wear-and-tear of the body over time is *lipofuscin*. As the body ages, this inert granulated pigment, which accumulates in nerve, cardiac, and skeletal cells, fills spaces and interferes with function. It has been suggested that lipofuscin may be created during metabolism, and it is probably an effect rather than a cause of aging.

IMMUNE SYSTEM THEORIES

With aging, the immune system's response decline, thus the body's ability to fight many infections diminishes. It is suggested that many symptoms of aging are a result of the accumulated effect of past and present disease that the system was or is unable to control. From another perspective, some researchers suggest that with aging, the body loses its ability to distinguish between its own specific materials and threatening foreign organisms (e.g., bacteria, viruses, and fungi). Thus, it attacks and annihilates its own tissues at a gradually progressing rate. Although these theories do not address aging of the immune system itself, it stands to reason that life expectancy would increase if the power of the system were sustained.

HORMONAL THEORIES

One possible cause for decline in the immune system's effectiveness and the subsequent aging effects has been atrophy of the thymus gland, which influences immune functioning via thymic hormone. Its progressive, age-related loss has been linked with declines in functioning of certain immune cells. Other examples of hormonal influence on characteristics associated with advanced aging are estrogen decline and bone loss in women, and loss of growth hormone (GH), which is related to a decline in muscle mass, bone density, and body fat and the occurrence of thin, wrinkled skin. Individuals who have been treated with GH (discussed in Chapter 5) have shown improvements in these areas.

With the advancement in scientific methodology, new theories of aging are emerging; see NIA website for updates.

focus on change

Physical activity and healthy living habits play a major role in influencing negative *change*.

Objective 11.5

The differences between **chronological age** and **physiological age** become increasingly evident with advancing age. In general physiological function, active individuals appear physiologically superior to their counterparts of the same chronological age (see Fig. 11.5). From a general observation of human performance and attitude, this phenomenon is also apparent. Although some people consider themselves old by the age of 30 years, others continue to pursue a highly

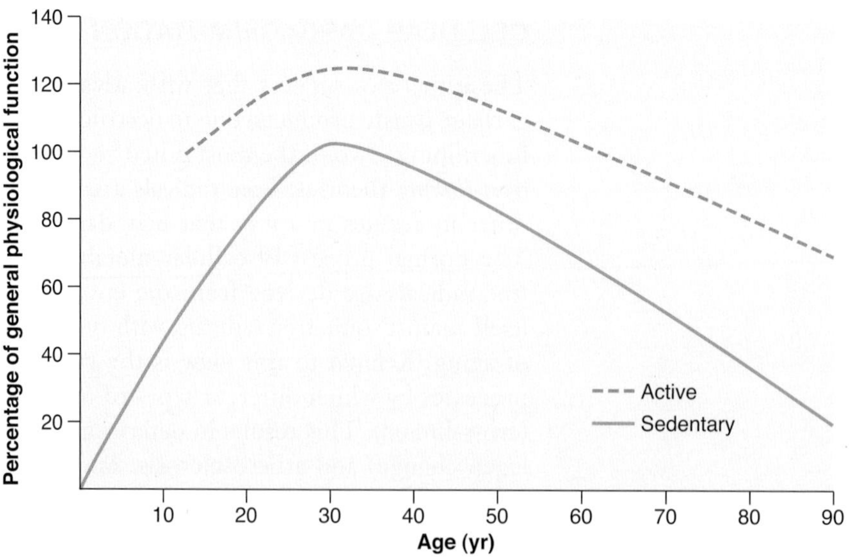

Figure 11.5 General physiological function across the life span for active and sedentary persons.

active lifestyle through old age. Several major championships and records in such sports as track and field, tennis, baseball pitching, and golf have been held by individuals in their 40s. One of the truly remarkable athletic feats by an older individual was accomplished by John Kelley. In the 1992 Boston Marathon at the age of 84 years, Kelley completed the course (26 miles, 365 yards) in close to 5 hours. It was the 61st time he had run this race, which he won in 1935 and 1945.

However, although there are numerous benefits from a healthy and active lifestyle during adulthood, it appears that no matter how well people take care of themselves, the effects of advancing age will result in **regression** of physiological processes and motor performance.

Biological Regression and Motor Performance

Objective 11.6

After an individual reaches peak maturity at approximately 30 years of age, most physiological factors begin to show decrements at a rate of about 0.75% to 1% a year. This is a general trend of decline; however, differences between individuals and the function of specific organs can vary considerably. There is some suggestion from the research community that up to 50% of the loss usually attributed to physiological aging may be due to inactivity and other poor health habits. The decline in biological capacity and associated motor performance generally is characterized by decrements in cardiorespiratory function, muscular strength, neural function, balance, and flexibility. Additional age-related factors that may affect one's motor performance are changes in the skeletal system (bone tissue) and increased body fat.

think about it

How much do genetics influence the regression of motor behavior?

For a summary of selected biological changes that occur with aging after peak maturity, refer back to Table 4.4 on page 120. The following is a summary of those changes and a description of associated decrements in motor performance.

CARDIORESPIRATORY FUNCTION

Cardiovascular capacity as measured by maximal oxygen consumption (maximal aerobic power) declines approximately 30% between the ages of 30 and 70 years (see Fig. 11.2 on page 314). Closely associated with this general physiological decrement is a decrease in cardiac output (stroke volume and maximal heart rate) and respiratory (pulmonary) function. Complementing Figure 11.6, research consistently shows that active individuals maintain a higher aerobic capacity than their sedentary counterparts. As noted in Chapter 4, *sedentary persons have nearly a twofold faster rate of decline* in VO_2max as they age (McArdle et al., 2015). In addition to diminished cardiac capacity, respiratory function decreases with advancing age, as evidenced by an estimated 40% loss in vital capacity between the ages of 30 and 70 years.

Parallel to the loss in aerobic capacity after peak maturity is a slightly greater decline in anaerobic power (about 40% by age 70 years). This loss is linked, in part, to the aging body's diminishing capacity to turn over lactic acid accumulation during short bouts of intense physical activity. Other significant cardiovascular changes include increased blood pressure and blood flow resistance. Thus, aging produces significant decreases in the body's oxygen transport and extraction capacities.

Motor performance decrements in physical work capacity tasks and high-level aerobic activities clearly follow the general aging trend. Figures 11.3 (on page 315), 11.6, and 11.7 show examples of this trend. Figure 11.3 depicts changes in work capacity (exercise tolerance) in a laboratory setting, and Figures 11.6 and 11.7 illustrate

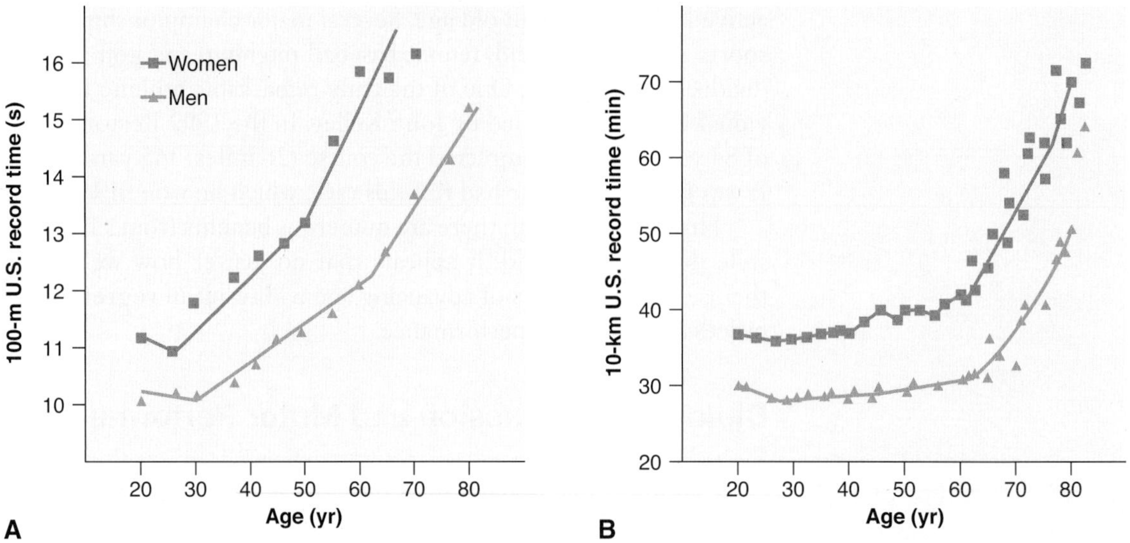

Figure 11.6 Change with age in male and female world records for **(A)** 100-meter and **(B)** 10-kilometer runs.

age-related changes in U.S. record 100-meter and 10-kilometer run times and master's level freestyle swimming events, respectively. It also may be suggested from the data shown on run and swim times that regardless of training experience, performance (aerobic capacity) diminishes with advancing age. Kenney and colleagues (2015), in reference to Figure 11.6, note that run performance decreases by about 1% per year from age 25 to 60 years. After that, the rate is approximately 2% decline per year.

MUSCULAR STRENGTH

The primary factor in the loss of muscular strength after peak performance is the decrease in muscle mass that occurs with advancing age. Although the average estimate is a 25% to 30% loss in muscle mass between ages 30 and 70 years, some

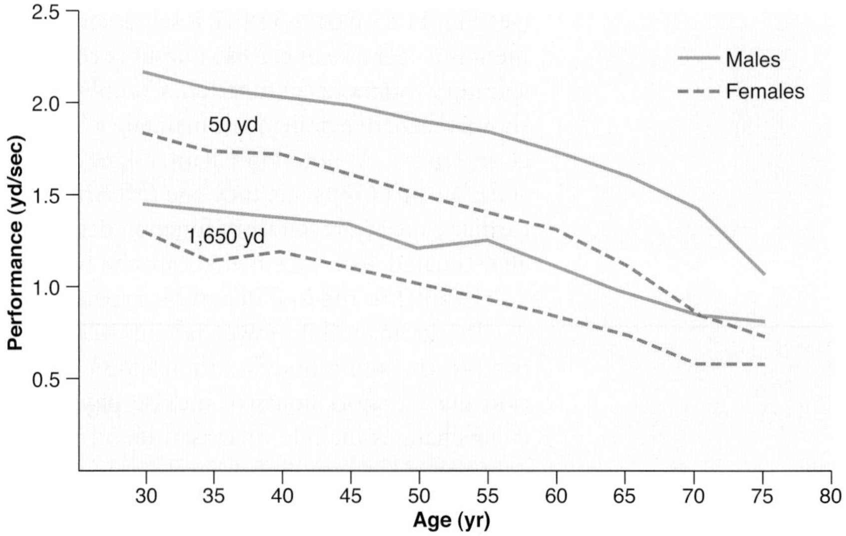

Figure 11.7 Mean performance for short- and long-distance master's level freestyle swimming events.

SOURCE: Data from Hartley, A. A., & Hartley, J. T. (1984). Performance changes in champion swimmers aged 30 to 84 years. *Experimental Aging Research*, *10*(3), 141–147.

reports show a loss of up to 50% by age 80 years. This general loss of body tissue is characterized by specific decreases in the size and number of muscle fibers, loss of biochemical capacity, increases in connective tissue and fat, and a general dehydration in body cells. Concerning fiber type, it appears that type II fast twitch may be lost at a faster rate (McArdle et al., 2015). In addition to affecting isometric and dynamic strength, these changes also hamper mobility and speed of movement, especially among the elderly.

The general decline with advancing age in maximal muscular strength seems to parallel the loss in muscle mass. That is, there is a 25% to 30% decline in strength between the ages of 30 and 70 years. It also has been suggested that the rate of decline in leg and trunk muscles in both sexes is greater than in arm and hand-grip muscles. As evidenced in Figure 11.1 on page 314, grip strength decreases slowly after peak performance and does not show a marked decline until after the approximate age of 40 years. For this aspect of muscular strength, the total loss from 30 to 60 years usually does not exceed 10% to 20% of maximum; the degree of decrement is somewhat greater in females than in males. The decrement in grip-strength endurance, usually measured by the amount of force that can be held for 1 minute, is not as great as the decline in grip strength; estimates suggest a decrease of about 30% from age 20 to 75 years.

Interestingly, a study of maximal grip strength and grip-strength endurance among males, all of whom performed similar work in a machine shop, revealed no change in strength or endurance from age 22 to 62 years (Petrofsky & Lind, 1975). These data suggest the changes found in a more typical population may be due largely to disuse rather than to aging. Although activity may slow the effects of aging, however, there is little question that sizable decrements occur in old age, regardless of activity level.

NEURAL FUNCTION

As noted in Chapter 7, with regard to information processing, one of the most consistently observed and significant changes with advancing age is the decline in processing (behavioral) speed, described as **psychomotor slowing.** Over the years, several theories have been proposed regarding this phenomenon; some focus on neuromuscular factors, others on a breakdown in the central nervous system (CNS). Perhaps the most compelling explanation is a *general biological degradation*. That is, with advanced aging, there is a deterioration of the neural network functioning that affects processing durations (e.g., Salthouse, 2007, 2009). Part of this degradation described earlier is the significant reduction in brain cells, increased synaptic delay, an approximate 15% decrease in nerve conduction velocity, and an estimated loss of 37% in the number of spinal cord axons. All of these structures and processes are a part of the links and nodes that form the neural network. Theoretically, with aging, links in the network are broken or disrupted, which causes the decline in processing.

Evidence of age-related psychomotor slowing has been reported with several laboratory motor tasks based on reaction time and speed of movement. In general, greater reductions in both reaction time and movement speed tend to occur in the lower parts of the body in contrast to the areas of most frequent use, such as the fingers. The rate of psychomotor slowing also is affected by the complexity of the motor task; tasks of greater complexity are associated with increased rates of decline. That is, as movement complexity increases, the effects of adult aging on reaction time increase (e.g., Ketcham & Stelmach, 2001). Refer back to Chapter 7, Figure 7.8, in reference to Hick's law and age.

Data reported by Williams (1990) clearly support this contention. The research showed that between the ages of 50 and 90 years, there was a 32% decrement in speed of simple discrete and repetitive arm/hand movements. In contrast, a 65% decrease in speed was found in the performance of complex sequential arm/hand/finger movements. The researcher also found substantial decrements of about 30% in timed bilateral and unilateral object manipulation tasks. Evidence also suggests that fine motor actions that require steadiness, such as writing digits and letters, undergo even greater decrements (68% to 78%) during the adult years. Complementing these findings are comparative reports of large decrements with greater age in the performance of a variety of rapid hand-aiming movements (e.g., Yan et al., 2000).

think about it

What are some implications for psychomotor slowing in the elderly?

In general, after performance peaks during the 20s, a gradual slowing of the body occurs in relation to reaction time and speed of movement (i.e., movement time), with more marked increases occurring after the age of 60 years (see Fig. 11.4 on page 315). Thus, the general trend is one of increasing proficiency, then peak performance, and finally the psychomotor slowing in finger, hand, and arm speed tasks with age.

Although it does appear that there is a general age-related decline in movement processing and speed of actions, Krampe (2002) contends that this general model does not represent the wide variability among individuals in fine motor control. For actions such as typing and playing the piano, for example, there are wide processing differences in timing, sequencing, and executive control. It appears that some older individuals selectively rely on processing mechanisms that are less sensitive to age-related decline. That is, these individuals learn (adapt) to internal and external *performance constraints*.

The suggestion that a healthy, physically active lifestyle may reduce the decrement in psychomotor slowing (i.e., CNS deterioration) has some support in research findings. In studies that have compared groups of physically active (i.e., aerobic-type activity) and nonactive young and old persons on reaction and movement time tasks, similar results have been reported (Rikli & Busch, 1986; see review by Spirduso et al., 2004). That is, reaction and movement time scores for the active groups (young or old) were considerably faster than the scores for the corresponding age group that was less active. As one would expect, when scores for the age groups were averaged across activity levels, the young groups were faster than their older counterparts were. Studies also found that scores for the nonactive older group were substantially slower than those of the other groups were. Figure 11.8 shows the movement time characteristics for simple and complex motor tasks.

think about it

How would you set up a study to test the influence of aerobic and weight-training exercises on psychomotor slowing?

What about the effects of training (practice) on reaction time and speed of movement among the elderly? One of the more common measurements of cognitive function with advanced aging is information-processing speed in the form of reaction time tasks and timed behavior with daily living tasks. Although studies confirm a general decline with increasing age, there are indications that training may reduce the long-term outcome. For example, Rebok and colleagues (2014) tested the effects of a cognitive and daily living skills training program over 10 years starting at age 65 years and older (average age at the end was 82 years). Results indicated training produced significant improvements in processing speed and better preserved functional status than in nontrained persons 10 years later.

As a general observation, both studies suggest that "activity" during older age may offset the negative effects of aging. Complementing those reports are findings that exercise, primarily aerobic-type, is linked to improved brain and cognitive

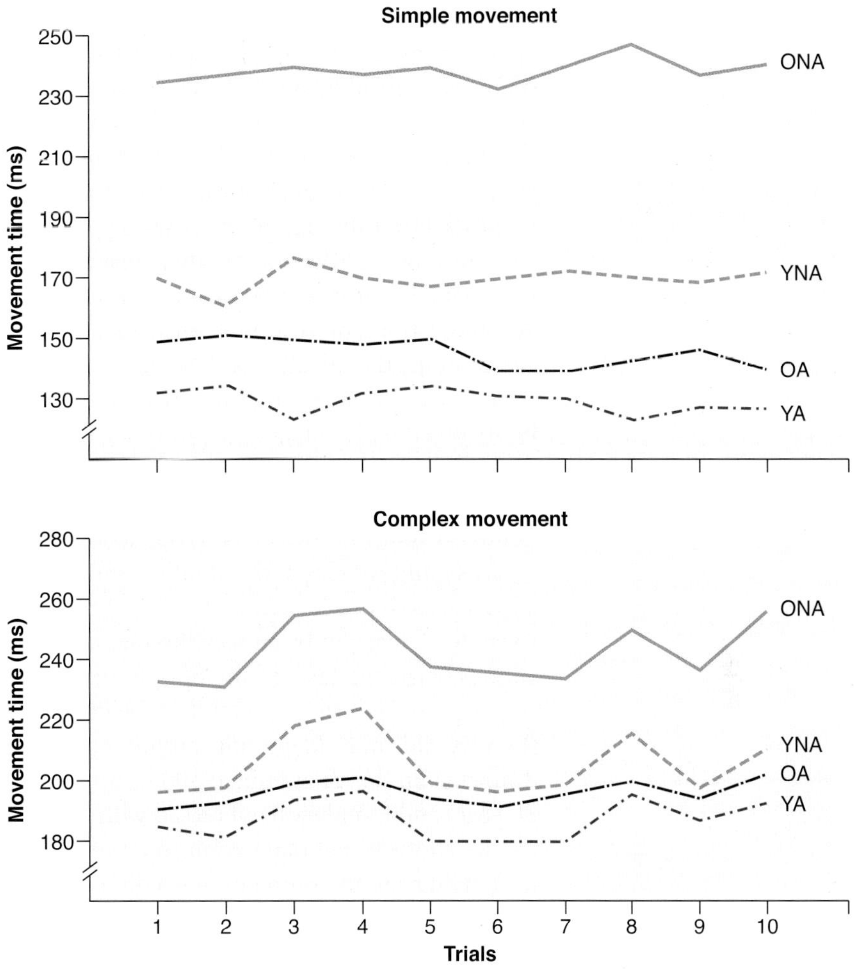

Figure 11.8 Movement time characteristics in young (Y), old (O), active (A), and nonactive (NA) subjects.

functioning in younger and older adults (see review by Colcombe & Kramer, 2003; Nagamatsu et al., 2014).

Evidence has also been documented that practice with videogame playing among elderly individuals who averaged 70 years of age improved response speed (i.e., reaction time) and, in essence, reversed the age-related decline in processing (Clark, Lanphear, & Riddick, 1987). This research suggested that central mechanisms (e.g., information-processing strategies), rather than neuromuscular factors, were most influenced by the practice.

BALANCE (POSTURAL STABILITY)

Associated with the age-related decline in neuromuscular capacity is the loss of balance (postural stability). Any movement that requires balance involves the successful integration of several anatomical, muscular, and neurological functions. The deterioration of any of these functions may impede the ability to maintain equilibrium. For example, loss of brain cells (primarily in the cerebellum and brain stem) with advancing age may hinder the capacity to use proprioceptive information. That is, the kinesthetic information received concerning the position of the body's various parts is less accurate and thus inhibits precise postural control. From approximately 40 years of age, there is a gradual deterioration of vestibular nerve cells. Sensory cell loss may begin as early as the fifth decade in the semicircular canals and may be quite marked in the saccule and utricle as well after the age of 70 years. In addition, with advancing age, there are deficits in the somatosensory system that involve tactile (touch) sensitivity.

Visual perception also plays a significant role in maintaining stability, especially when the body is moving. For most people, the decrement in visual acuity begins around the age of 40 years; by 60 years, the ability to focus on objects at close distance is affected greatly. A loss in the ability to judge depth is also particularly evident after age 60 years. Although performance (balance) and symptomatic indications of vestibular malfunction (vertigo and dizziness) in older adults are evident, the specific underlying mechanisms responsible for these responses have not been clearly defined. It is likely, however, that a number of causes may be involved with balance loss in older adults; they include disease, weak muscles, limited range of motion, abnormal reflexes, visual/vestibular deficits to central sensory integration, deficiencies in motor programming, and motor control difficulties (Shumway-Cook & Woollacott, 2012; Sullivan et al., 2009).

A significant loss in the ability to establish and maintain balance can affect virtually all gross motor activities. However, the research technique most frequently used to study changes in balance is the measurement of postural sway while performing various balancing tasks in the upright position. In general, research findings suggest the magnitude of the sway tends to be greater (i.e., less stable) in the very young and the very old, and older adults are less stable than younger adults are. For example, Toupet et al. (1992) examined 500 healthy (free of pathology) adults from ages 40 to 80 years and found sway increased with each decade of advancing age. More recent studies confirm that older adults tend to display both a shorter time to lose stability in standing and the problem of needing more time to reacquire stability (Slobounov et al., 2006; Tucker et al., 2009). The factor of stability is closely associated with falls in older persons (Fig. 11.9).

WebLink
http://www.cdc.gov; see "Falls."

According to 2016 CDC statistics, more than one-third of adults 65 years and older *fall* each year in the United States. Among older adults, falls are the leading cause of injury deaths. They are also the most common cause of nonfatal injuries

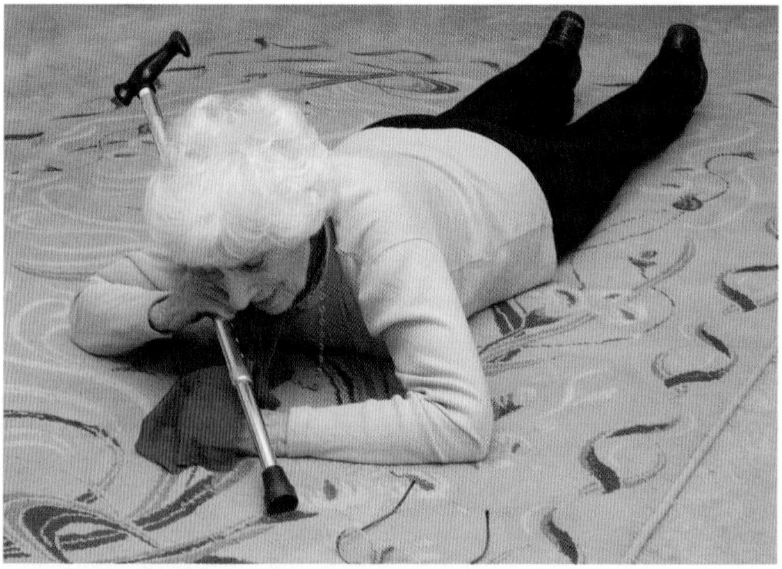

Figure 11.9 Loss of postural stability can be a critical safety factor in older persons (falling).

and hospital admissions for trauma. Factors other than lack of balance that have been mentioned as contributors to falling include decreased levels of physical activity, stroke, arthritis, low blood pressure, muscle weakness, poor eyesight, ineffective walking pattern (especially, reduced foot raise), and adverse effects of medication. Compared to males, females tend to inherit a much greater possibility of hip fracture as a result of falling due to structural and bone characteristics. The angle of insertion of the head of the femur into the hip socket creates a structural weakness more conducive to hip fracture. Females also lose considerably more bone mineral mass and have a much greater incidence of osteoporosis in late adulthood. About 76% of all hip fractures occur in women, with people 85 years and older being 10 to 15 times more likely to sustain hip fractures than are people ages 60 to 65 years.

A paradox exists with regard to the difference between males and females in the frequency of falls. Information presented earlier in this text suggested females have the structural advantage (lower center of gravity and wider base relative to height) in maintaining stability. An example of this advantage is evidenced by superior scores in balance beam walking. One could speculate that, at worst, females should be no more prone to falling than males are. The research literature provides little support for a significant gender difference in kinesthetic mechanisms (including vestibular functions) or visual processes. In fact, available information appears to favor females for balancing mechanisms. It seems plausible (although speculative) that although the female physique is more suited to balancing tasks, practice and environmental influences are also significant factors in optimal balance development. To illustrate, females generally perform better than males do on balancing tasks during childhood—a time when the female anatomical structure (a higher center of gravity and longer legs) should not provide an advantage. Based on this hypothesis, a possible explanation for the gender difference in frequency of falls in old age could be that higher participation levels by males in physical activities are conducive to maintaining bone density and efficient stability.

> **think about it**
>
> Based on the multiple factors underlying falls, what prevention strategies/practices would you recommend?

Included in the Rikli and Busch (1986) study of active and inactive young and old females was a difficult balancing task, the one-foot stand for time (60-sec limit). The active older group performed significantly better than the inactive older group, which indicates physical activity level may influence balancing ability. It also was noted that both young groups (active and inactive) performed the task equally well and did considerably better than the active older group, which suggests a healthy, active lifestyle does not prevent the age-related decrement in balancing performance but may change the rate of decline.

FLEXIBILITY

One of the most obvious changes associated with advancing age is the loss of joint mobility (range of motion). Closely linked to this general decline are changes in the joints and muscles and the presence of degenerative joint diseases. A smooth functioning of the joints is made possible by the strength and elasticity of the tendons and ligaments (forms of connective tissue that encompass the joint) and the synovial fluid. After the early adult years (or later adult years for some individuals), the joints become less stable and mobility diminishes. In addition, collagen fibers and synovial membranes degrade, and the viscosity of the synovial fluid decreases. As a result of these decrements, the joints become stiff, which may decrease the range of motion (flexibility). However, *there is no conclusive evidence that biological aging inherently causes decreased flexibility*. A considerable amount of research also links the decline in range of motion with degenerative joint diseases such as

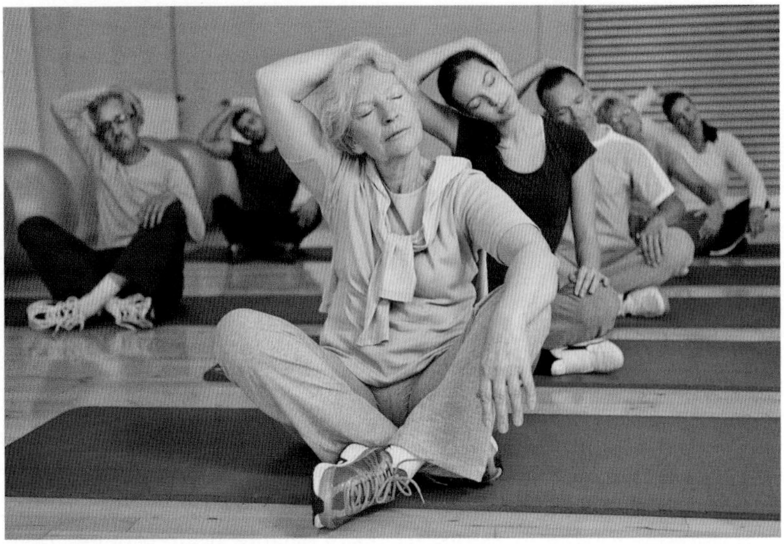

Figure 11.10 Activity level and not age is the best predictor of flexibility.

osteoarthritis and osteoarthrosis. There are indications that more than two-thirds of individuals 55 to 64 years of age have signs of osteoarthrosis in some joint.

The inherent difficulty with using a general performance curve to describe changes in flexibility across the life span is that activity level is a better indicator of flexibility than age (Fig. 11.10). With that said, research suggests that general range of motion increases steadily through childhood and flexibility starts to decline around 10 years of age in males and 12 years of age in females; once again, the likely factor is activity level.

The three factors that appear to have the greatest influence on flexibility during adulthood are physical activity level, the inherent effects of aging, and degenerative joint diseases. The effects of aging on joint and muscle tissue have been verified, as well as the presence of joint diseases in the majority of elderly persons. Results of the Rikli and Busch (1986) investigation of active and inactive young and old females demonstrated clearly that physical activity level was a strong factor in maintaining flexibility in old age. In this study, the old active females performed significantly better on a sit-and-reach (trunk flexibility) test than their inactive counterparts of the same age group. In fact, the older active group demonstrated slightly greater flexibility than the young inactive group.

CHANGES IN SKELETAL TISSUE AND BODY FAT

It is typical for aging humans to increase in body weight and fat and to show a decrease in height and bone mass. The average female loses a striking 30% of bone mass between the approximate ages of 35 and 70 years. Bone mass loss among males generally does not begin until about age 55 years and reaches a smaller total loss between 10% and 15% by age 70 years. With advancing age also comes a slight decrease in height, due primarily to bone mass loss, increased kyphosis (rounding of the back), compression of intravertebral disks, and deterioration of vertebrae.

For the average person, gains in body weight and fat begin gradually in the late 20s and continue to increase until approximately age of 55 or 60 years, when the gains show signs of decreasing. The typical increase in body weight and fat from age 20 to 60 years for both sexes is approximately 15%. This value is highly variable and may be considerably less among highly active, diet-conscious individuals. Lean body mass also tends to decrease with age. This overall effect is due primarily to bone mass loss and the reduction of muscle mass. As noted earlier, in most individuals, there is a marked deterioration in muscle mass with aging.

The effects of skeletal and body composition changes on motor performance are generic; that is, rather than affecting the performance of a specific type (group) of motor activities, these changes influence the overall ability to perform a wide scope of motor skills. For example, bone mass loss results in bone that has less density and tensile strength. Therefore, it is generally weaker and more prone to injury and fracture. Due to the increased likelihood of injury, many older persons limit their physical exertion levels and modify movement patterns for fear of physical harm. The presence of kyphosis (rounding of the back) also may significantly alter basic and advanced movement patterns (e.g., swimming, running, and throwing).

An increase in adult body fat of 10% to 15% may have implications for physiological functions and motor performance. In general, a significant increase in body fat impairs cardiac function by increasing the mechanical work the heart must perform and thus affects aerobic and muscular endurance activity. Numerous research studies that involve young and older adults have found the percentage of body fat to be related inversely (negatively) to the ability to move the total body weight. This is especially true for motor performance tasks that require horizontal acceleration (e.g., running) or vertical lifting of the total body (e.g., jumping). Theoretically, this relationship is based on the fact that body fat adds to the total mass of the body without contributing to the force-producing capability. Therefore, the additional body fat gained during adulthood becomes excess weight to be moved during locomotor activity.

think about it

In what way has research (science) helped curb the rate of regression?

Changing Movement Patterns

WALKING

Objective 11.7

Although the information on age-related changes in movement patterns during the adult years is limited, a number of studies have focused on walking—the most used movement pattern. In general, a deterioration in walking gait occurs with advancing age, beginning with late adulthood (more than 60 years). The stereotypic gait of an elderly person normally is characterized by slow, short, shuffling steps in which there is little range of motion and a slumping of the head, shoulders, and trunk. Differences in performance among individuals of similar age can be considerable, however.

Murray and associates (1970) have conducted several investigations on gait patterns in individuals 20 to 87 years of age. In summary, when males older than age 65 years were compared to males ages 20 to 25 years, the older males displayed *shorter steps* (i.e., linear distance traveled of alternate feet), *shorter stride lengths* (i.e., linear distance traveled of same foot), *increased out-toeing*, and *less pelvic rotation and ankle extension*. Out-toeing is a technique used to improve lateral stability. Similar results also were found among females. When only able-bodied older persons were compared with younger individuals, fewer differences were noted—namely, shorter steps, a shorter stride length, and increased out-toeing. Other significant changes noted with advancing age are less step height (foot raise), slower walking speed, and wider steps. Compared to young adults, the ability to raise each foot during walking (step height) decreases in individuals older than 70 years. As one might expect, after reviewing the information on falling frequency, older females in particular have difficulty with step height. Gait initiation, which refers to stance at the beginning of movement, has been linked to falls. After comparing active 65- to 79-year-olds to young adults, Henriksson and Hirschfeld (2004) reported that the older group stood more unequally and were considerably slower to react than the young adults were.

think about it

What are the similarities between an infant and an older adult in walking?

Focus on Application
Growth Hormone for Older Adults

Chapter 3 described the issue of using GH in prepubertal children diagnosed with severe delays in skeletal development (primarily short stature). In aging men, GH secretion declines by 50% every 7 years after age 25 years. The declines in GH production and the decrease in muscle mass and increase in adiposity (fat) that typically occur in healthy older adults have led to attempts to determine whether the administration of GH is beneficial. GH is available by prescription to treat adults who have GH deficiency, not the expected decline in GH due to aging. Although the evidence is limited, studies of adults who have GH deficiency show that injections can increase muscle mass and bone density, decrease body fat, and increase exercise capacity. Because of such results, some people believe that GH can help healthy older adults who have naturally occurring low levels of GH.

One interesting finding is that the increase in muscle doesn't directly translate to increased strength. One study compared older men who took GH with older men who went through strength-training programs. The study revealed that strength training can increase both muscle mass and strength, making it cheaper and more effective than taking GH. Overall, it isn't clear whether GH can provide benefits to healthy adults because most of the research has focused on the people who have deficiencies. How much does GH treatment cost? It costs $10,000 to $30,000 a year, depending on body weight, and it requires long-term treatment.

Sources:
Gentili, A., Adler, R. A., Talavera, F., Schalch, D. S., & Griffing, G. T. (2005). *Growth hormone replacement in older men*. Retrieved from http://emedicine.medscape.com/
Mayo Clinic. (2014). *Human growth hormone (HGH): Does it slow aging?* Retrieved from http://www.mayoclinic.org/healthy-lifestyle/healthy-aging/in-depth/growth-hormone/art-20045735

By what standard should normal walking speed be judged? One suggestion of particular relevance to older adults is that the minimum velocity needed to cross a traffic intersection should be used as one criterion for measuring normal speed. Based on this criterion, Aniansson and colleagues (1980) determined that the normal walking speed of the general adult population is about 1.4 meters per second. However, the average normal, functional walking speed of adults 70 years and older was found to be much slower than the criterion speed was; the average speed was 1.2 meters per second for males and 1.1 meters per second for females.

think about it

Summarize the constraints to efficient walking in the typical elderly person. What about driving a car at the age of 90 years?

Another consideration among older adults in relation to gait pattern is the psychological factor. It may be speculated that many elderly persons shuffle cautiously and use short steps in fear of falling. Evidence for this speculation is supported to some degree by the findings of a study reported by Willmott (1986). The researcher found that among elderly hospital patients, gait speed and step length were significantly greater on a carpeted surface compared to a vinyl surface. More confidence and little fear were expressed about walking on the carpeted surface in comparison to the vinyl surface.

Table 11.1 summarizes gait pattern changes in the elderly, as reported by Shumway-Cook and Woollacott (2012).

RUNNING AND JUMPING

There are some indications that basic running and jumping patterns also change with aging. With the growing senior population, increasing numbers of older persons participate in competitive sporting events (e.g., Senior Olympics, Senior Games, marathons, and triathlons) and engage in a regular routine of fitness-oriented

TABLE 11.1 Summary of Gait Changes in the Older Adult

Temporal/distance factors
Decreased velocity
Decreased step length
Decreased step rate
Decreased stride length
Increased stride width
Increased stance phase
Increased time in double support
Decreased swing phase
Kinematic changes
Decreased vertical movement of the center of gravity
Decreased arm swing
Decreased hip, knee, and ankle flexion
Flatter foot on heel strike
Decreased ability to couple hip/knee movements
Decreased dynamic stability during stance
Muscle activation patterns
Increased coactivation (increased stiffness)
Kinetic changes
Decreased power generation at push-off
Decreased power absorption at heel strike

SOURCE: From Shumway-Cook, A., & Woollacott, M. (2012). *Motor control* (4th ed.). Philadelphia, PA: Lippincott Williams & Wilkins.

activities, but most older individuals do not include running and jumping or other basic sport skills (e.g., throwing, catching, and kicking) in their lives. In an unpublished study by Adrian and Cooper (1995), the kinematics (movement pattern characteristics) of healthy, active females aged 60 to 80 years were identical to university track team females during a paced run. However, when the sprint patterns were compared, there was little similarity. More specifically, the younger females exhibited greater leg flexion and extension. Other information suggests that older runners do not tuck (flex) their recovery leg as completely; they display a shorter stride and take a greater number of strides to complete the distance.

Associated with the general age-related psychomotor slowing and decrements in anaerobic function and strength is the expected decline in running speed (Ko et al., 2010; Nelson, 1981). A fact that is also associated with elite senior runners. With regard to jumping, little has been studied among the adult population and, in particular, among the elderly. The kinematics of the vertical jump of college-aged females and females older than the age 60 years have been compared

(Klinger et al., 1980). Results suggested that, in general, the patterns of both groups were similar. However, the older persons displayed less knee flexion and could not extend their legs (at the knee joint) as quickly as the younger individuals could.

THROWING AND STRIKING

Also included in the Klinger et al. (1980) study was a comparison of several throwing and striking patterns (tennis backhand and batting). In each case, the extension velocities older individuals achieved were slower than those of the younger group were. It should be noted, however, that in many instances, the older individuals had no athletic background or had gone years without practicing any of the skills. Individuals identified as more active displayed a more sophisticated movement pattern (e.g., better coordination, faster movement, and greater range of motion) than those in their age group who were less active.

In a series of studies by Williams (1990) and Williams, Haywood, and Van Sant (1991), similar findings were reported for the overarm throw in the elderly (ages 63 to 78 years). That is, ball velocities approximated speeds usually generated by 8- to 9-year-olds; this was accompanied by a relatively shorter backswing (i.e., less range of motion). In addition, those individuals who participated in throwing-oriented sports in their past exhibited better movements. As one might expect, males generally had better form and threw faster than females did.

Some generalizations may be made concerning the changing of movement patterns in adulthood. In general, the average elderly person shows a definite *slowing of movements* and *less flexion* and *extension* compared to his or her younger counterpart. However, among active older persons, the decrement in speed is not as great and the characteristics of the movement pattern are generally well maintained from younger years.

Physical Activity and Longevity

Objective 11.8

This text has presented numerous assertions with regard to the potential benefits of physical activity to growth, development, and motor performance (Fig. 11.11). Discussions have affirmed that physical activity and exercise can have positive effects on bone and muscle tissue, body composition, and cardiorespiratory development. Performance characteristics in the form of strength, aerobic and anaerobic function, flexibility, coordination, balance, speed, and numerous motor skills all have been shown to progress through the psychomotor mode. Several assertions also were made in this chapter concerning the contribution of a healthy, physically active lifestyle toward delaying and modifying the effects of aging on various physiological functions and motor performance. In essence, physical activity was suggested as an important factor in the association between physiological age and chronological age (see Figure 11.5 on page 318).

The effects of physical activity on motor development are generally positive and, in some instances, dramatic. But what about the effects of physical activity on **longevity** (length of life)? Since the 1970s, a vast amount of research has been conducted and reported to the public concerning factors associated with human health and life expectancy (e.g., smoking, high cholesterol, coronary heart disease, high blood pressure, nutrition, and exercise). Several studies report convincing evidence that asserts that regular (habitual) physical activity and physical fitness of a *moderate level* is associated with increased longevity in comparison to sedentary and less active lifestyles. One of the most significant and common findings from this research is that physical activity is inversely associated with the rate of certain

Focus on Application

You Are Never Too Old to Learn

Jeanne Louise Calment, once listed as the world's longest living person, died at the age of 122 years. Heredity most likely contributed to her longevity: Her father lived to age 94 years and mother to 86 years. However, physical activity was a major factor in her lifestyle. As a young girl, she was active with tennis, bicycling, swimming, and roller skating. Perhaps most interesting, she took up fencing lessons at the age of 85 years and rode a bicycle until 100 years old! Although her longevity is certainly unique, she was also an excellent example of maintaining life satisfactory via activity, which is in reference to *activity theory* (Chapter 14).

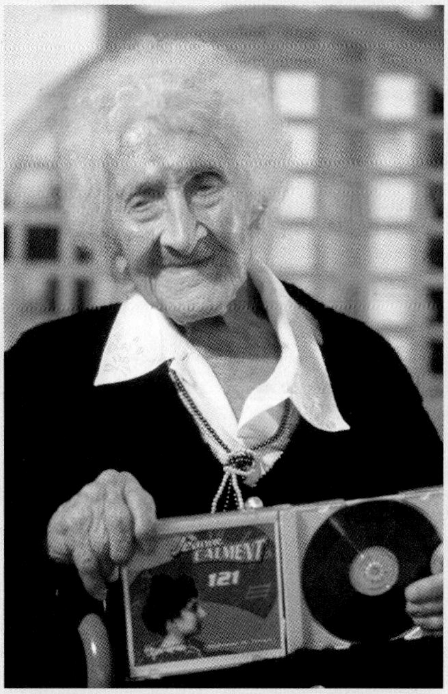

Source:
Robine, J. M., & Allard, M. (1999). Jeanne Calment: Validation of the duration of her life. In B. Jeune & J. W. Vaupel (Eds.), *Validation of exceptional longevity* (pp. 145–172). Odense, Denmark: Odense University Press.

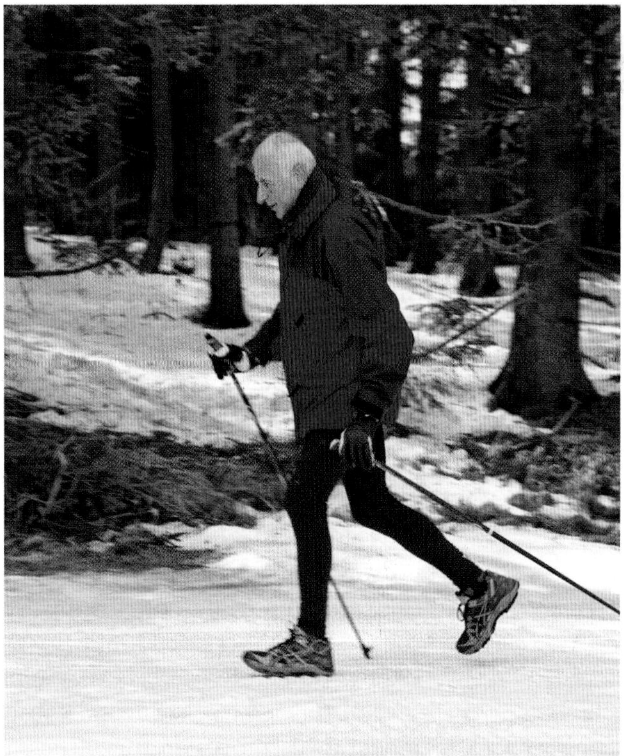

Figure 11.11 For the active older person, the decline in performance is not as great.

WebLink

See "Benefits of Exercise." http://www.acsm.org; http://www.ama.org

diseases and early mortality. Furthermore, many researchers and physicians promote the idea that "exercise is medicine."

One of the most comprehensive investigations collected data on 16,936 Harvard alumni, aged 35 to 74 years, with 12 to 16 years of follow-up (Paffenbarger et al., 1986). The physical activity level for each subject was measured as the total amount of energy expended (in kilocalories) at physical activity (e.g., sports, yard work, and walking) per week. Results indicated that physical activity level is related inversely to total mortality. That is, death rates declined steadily as physical activity (energy expenditure) increased. This trend continued with the increase in expenditure from less than 500 kilocalories to 3,500 kilocalories per week; beyond that amount, the rates increased slightly. In males, mortality rates were one-fourth to one-third lower among those individuals who expended at least 2,000 kilocalories per week, compared to less active males.

Perhaps most important, the researchers further concluded that regardless of whether the individual smoked, had high blood pressure, experienced extreme gains or losses in body weight, or had parents who died early, mortality rates were considerably lower among the more physically active. This general finding was confirmed in a report by Powell and Blair (1994). The researchers concluded that lack of regular physical activity contributes to heart disease in a cause-and-effect relationship, with sedentary individuals almost twice as likely to develop heart disease as the most active persons were. And inadequate physical activity is responsible for about 30% of all deaths due to heart disease, colon cancer, and diabetes. Numerous studies that used general adult populations also have reported an inverse relationship between coronary heart disease, death, and regular physical activity. In addition to the inverse trends (of heart disease and mortality) with leisure time habitual physical activity, similar results also have been associated with occupational activity.

think about it

How would you use the information on physical activity and longevity to have an impact on society; that is, what strategies would you recommend?

All of the aforementioned studies used physical activity as determined by various units of measurement (e.g., kilocalories expended and hours participated) as the factor with which to compare rates of disease and death. An alternative approach perhaps more specific and objective is the use of physical fitness level. Most studies identify the level and type of physical activity, but few investigations provide the additional insight of comparing the physiological (physical fitness) state of the body to rate of disease and death.

One of the landmark investigations using the latter approach was conducted by Blair and associates (1989) and reported in the *Journal of the American Medical Association*. The study consisted of more than 13,000 males and females, who ranged from 20 to older than 60 years of age. They were tested for aerobic fitness and then assigned to one of five physical fitness groups (low-fit to high-fit) based on age, sex, and fitness test results. Results indicated a strong, graded, and consistent inverse relationship between physical fitness and mortality due to all causes (i.e., smoking, cholesterol level, parent history, cardiovascular disease, and cancer). When comparing least-fit to most-fit groups, the chances of a low-fit individual experiencing an early death were 3.44 times greater for males and 4.65 times more likely among females. However, one of the most important conclusions of the study was that the fitness standard associated with increased longevity may be attained by individuals who engage in regular moderate exercise that approximates a brisk walk of about 30 minutes several times a week. Several subsequent studies show similar results. That is, moderate cardiorespiratory fitness provides some protection from cardiovascular disease mortality.

Focus on Application

Delayed Onset of Dementia via Exercise

Research clearly indicates that the elderly as well as younger persons are in need of moderate exercise for their physical health. However, the benefits are linked not only to the physical domain but also to the cognitive domain as well. An increasing body of evidence points to an association between lack of exercise and cognitive decline. Although research with exercising animals (mice) has shown a positive effect of exercise on cognition, only in recent years have data for humans been reported. One result of the animal research is the finding that exercise in the form of voluntary running reduces the cognitive decline and brain pathology that characterize Alzheimer's disease.

Larson and colleagues (2006) found that among adults 65 years of age and older, those who exercised had a lower incidence of dementia at the end of a 6-year tracking period. The incidence rate of dementia was 13.0 per 1,000 person-years for participants who exercised three or more times per week when compared with 19.7 per 1,000 person-years for people who exercised fewer than three times per week. These results suggest that regular exercise is associated with a delay in the onset of dementia and Alzheimer's disease, further supporting its value for elderly persons.

Other studies with humans have reported benefits to executive control, attention, and memory. Due in large part to research such as this, the NIA now offers a guide for suggested exercises (Exercise: A Guide from the National Institute on Aging) through their Website (https://www.nia.nih.gov/health).

Sources:

Adlard, P. A., Perreau, V. M., Pop, V., & Cotman, C. W. (2005). Voluntary exercise decreases amyloid load in a transgenic model of Alzheimer's disease. *Journal of Neuroscience, 25*(17), 4217–4221.

Larson, E. B., Wang, L., Bowen, J. D., McCormick, W. C., Teri, L., Crane, P., & Kukull, W. (2006). Exercise is associated with reduced risk for incident dementia among persons 65 years of age and older. *Annuals of Internal Medicine, 144*(2), 73–81.

National Institutes on Aging. (2006). *Exercise associated with reduced risk of dementia in older adults.* Retrieved from https://www.nia.nih.gov/newsroom/2006/01/exercise-associated-reduced-risk-dementia-older-adults

In summary, it appears from the data that regular physical activity of a moderate level of intensity can prolong life. Longevity, however, is more associated with the prevention of early mortality than with extending one's potential life span.

A term commonly associated with older persons as a form of motor behavior is **daily living skills (DLS)**; also known as *activities of daily living*. These are basic self-care tasks such as feeding, toileting, putting on clothes, tying shoes, getting in/out of bed, bathing, and walking. DLS are often a primary component in geriatric assessment (see Chapter 13) and therapeutic intervention in the elderly. Although cognitive impairment and DLS status are correlated, they are separate dimensions of functioning—not all persons with substantial cognitive impairment have DLS dysfunctions. Obviously, the ability to execute such activities typically declines with age; however, there are considerable individual differences depending on overall health, exercise, disease, and environmental conditions. For example, in a review of the research on this topic, Vermeulen and colleagues (2011) found that individual physical frailty indicators, such as weight loss, gait speed, grip strength, physical activity, balance, and lower extremity function were predictors of future DLS disability in community-dwelling elderly people. With that said, there is also evidence that exercise in these and other populations has helped. In 2012, a review by Chou, Hwang, and Wu found that exercise programs improved performance in DLS in frail older adults; most notably improved was quality of walking.

Summary

Motor behavior during the adult years is characterized by two distinguishing milestones: peak performance (associated with biological maturity) and regression. Peak physiological function, for the most part, occurs between the approximate ages of 25 and 30 years. Closely associated with peak physiological function is maximal motor performance in several activities.

A basic fact of development during the adult years is the difference between chronological and physiological age. However, it appears that no matter how well people take care of themselves, some degree of regression in physiological processes and associated motor performance is inevitable. After peak maturity, most physiological functions begin to show decrements at a general rate of 0.75% to 1% per year. The decline is characterized by decrements in cardiorespiratory function, muscular strength, neural function, balance, and flexibility. There is some suggestion that much of the loss in physiological aging may be attributed to inactivity and poor health habits.

During late adulthood, a deterioration in specific movement patterns (e.g., walk, run, and jump) also may occur. Although wide differences in performance exist, in general, elderly persons exhibit a definite slowing of movements with less flexion and extension compared to younger persons. Physical activity, especially habitual participation, has been shown to have positive effects on several aspects of growth, development, and motor performance.

think about it

1. **Speculate on a secular trend for peak physiological function and performance 50 years from now. Relate your projections to specific types of activities.**
2. **Does exercise influence any of these theories? How? What does research tell us?**
3. **How much do genetics influence the regression of motor behavior?**
4. **What are some implications for psychomotor slowing in the elderly?**
5. **How would you set up a study to test the influence of aerobic and weight-training exercises on psychomotor slowing?**
6. **Based on the multiple factors underlying falls, what prevention strategies/practices would you recommend?**
7. **In what way has research (science) helped curb the rate of regression?**
8. **What are the similarities between an infant and an older adult in walking?**
9. **Summarize the constraints to efficient walking in the typical elderly person. What about driving a car at the age of 90 years?**
10. **How would you use the information on physical activity and longevity to have an impact on society; that is, what strategies would you recommend?**

LEARNING ACTIVITIES

Objective: To test older person for DLS. First, create a checklist of DLS (found in this text and additional on the Web). Then, observe if possible, or ask the individual or his or her assistant if applicable. Write a brief one- to two-page summary with recommendations for improvement.

Objective: To design a fall prevention program for an elderly person. Look on the Web for ideas and create a comprehensive prevention (not remedial) program. Provide a general outline that includes the major components and two to three activities.

Suggested Reading

Taylor, A. W., & Johnson, M. J. (2008). *Physiology of exercise and healthy aging*. Champaign, IL: Human Kinetics.

Chapter 12

Atypical Motor Behavior

OBJECTIVES

Upon completion of this chapter, you should be able to

12.1 Describe the relevance of studying populations that display atypical behaviors.

12.2 Briefly describe the various atypical populations and the most frequently observed motor deficits.

KEY TERMS

attention deficit hyperactivity disorder (ADHD)

autism spectrum disorder (ASD)

cerebral palsy (CP)

developmental coordination disorder (DCD)

Down syndrome (DS)

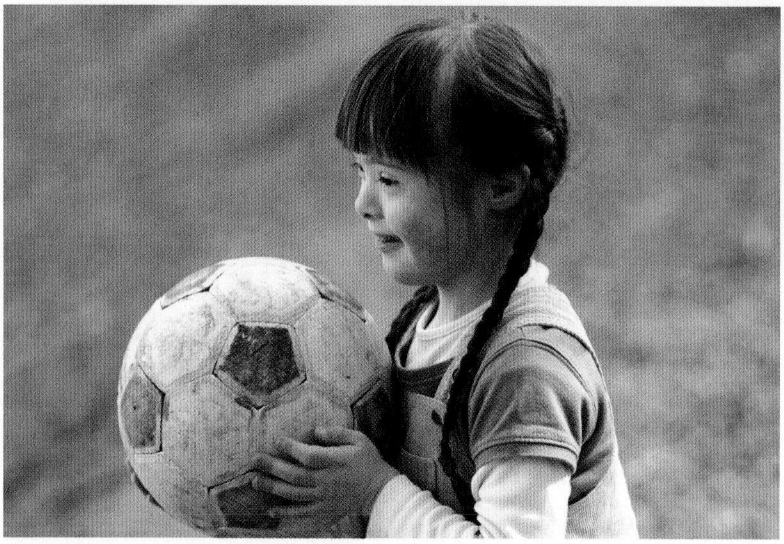

Figure 12.1 Motor skills typically develop at a slower rate for special populations.

Objective 12.1

Up to this point in the textbook, information has predominately focused on lifelong growth and motor development of typically developing humans. However, most of you at some point in your career, some of you more so (e.g., rehabilitation, physical therapy), will encounter individuals with special needs that display atypical motor behavior. That is, individuals who have conditions that are commonly associated with motor impairments. In fact, a significant portion of motor development research today involves special populations (Fig. 12.1). Obviously, a detailed discussion of this topic is beyond the scope of this text. Going back to Chapter 1 and the question of why study motor development?—a few items have relevance here:

1. To interact effectively with other individuals, we need to be aware of what they can and cannot do.
2. If we understand what constitutes the normal range of motor development, we can better understand and guide individuals who may be developing atypically.
3. We can use our understanding of motor development to improve health and optimize motor performance.

WebLink
http://www.cdc.gov

The following is a brief description of the more common conditions that are associated with motor impairment in infants, children, and adolescents. For more information on motor control and clinical applications with atypical populations, refer to Shumway-Cook and Woollacott (2012) and note WebLinks for national organizations, including the Centers for Disease Control and Prevention (CDC).

ATTENTION DEFICIT HYPERACTIVITY DISORDER

Objective 12.2

Attention deficit hyperactivity disorder (ADHD) is one of the most common neurobehavioral disorders of childhood. It is usually first diagnosed in childhood, is more prevalent in boys, and often lasts into adulthood. Individuals with ADHD are easily distracted, have trouble focusing on any one thing, show impulsive behaviors, and in some cases, are overly active. All of which may affect motor behavior. The cause(s) and risk factors for ADHD are unknown, but current research shows that genetics plays an important role. Other causes are brain injury, environmental

WebLink

http://www.chadd.org (National Resource Center for Attention Deficit Hyperactivity Disorder); http://www.help4adhd.org

exposure to teratogens (lead, alcohol, tobacco prenatally), premature birth, and low birth weight. Although the specific neurological deficits associated with ADHD and motor control are still unsolved, one point of focus has been on deficits in executive functions (the ability to organize and act on information). According to the CDC, approximately 3% to 7% of school-aged children suffer from ADHD.

In regard to motor difficulties, several studies indicate that individuals with this condition also have a comorbidity of developmental coordination disorder (discussed later). In general, these individuals display motor difficulties with the following (see review by Kaiser et al., 2014; also, Cheng, Ji, Zhang, & Feng, 2012; Klotz et al., 2012):

think about it

What instructional strategies would you use to help this population?

- Fine and gross motor development
- Balance being a major problem
- Slower and more variable reaction times
- Timing perception
- Kinesthetic acuity
- Visual-spatial organization

AUTISM SPECTRUM DISORDER

Autism spectrum disorder (ASD) refers to a group of complex neurodevelopment disorders characterized by repetitive and characteristic patterns of behavior and difficulties with social communication and interaction. The symptoms are present from early childhood and affect daily functioning, including motor behavior. According to the CDC, 1 in 68 children have ASD. Studies suggest that ASD could be a result of disruptions in normal brain growth very early in development. These disruptions may be the result of defects in genes that control brain development and regulate how brain cells communicate with each other (e.g., Doll & Broadie, 2014; Verly et al., 2014). Autism is more common in children born prematurely. Characteristic motor behaviors include repetitive movements or unusual behaviors such as arm flapping and rocking from side to side, and atypical responses to sensory information. Common motor difficulties include the following (Johnson et al., 2013; Liu & Breslin, 2013):

WebLink

http://nationalautism association.org (National Autism Association); http://www.ninds.nih.gov/; see Autism Spectrum Disorder.

- Fine motor: manual dexterity, especially handwriting
- Gross motor: balls skills, static/dynamic balance

For additional information on motor behavior and assessment of this special population see the chapter by Liu et al. (2016).

CEREBRAL PALSY

Cerebral palsy (CP) is a disorder that primarily affects a person's ability to move and to maintain balance and posture. It is due to a nonprogressive brain abnormality that affects the reflexes and control of muscle tone, which underscores the ability to maintain stability and move efficiently. CP is the most common cause of physical disability in childhood, occurring in 1 in 500 children. Reported causes include premature birth, lack of enough blood and oxygen before or during birth, brain injury, and serious brain infection. CP can extend into adulthood (Usuba et al., 2014).

WebLink

http://www.ninds.nih.gov/; see Cerebral Palsy. http://yourcpf.org (Cerebral Palsy Foundation)

think about it

What are the major individual constraints for persons with CP?

Severity level for CP varies considerably but is generally classified by motor impairment as mild, moderate, and severe. In some cases, only a single limb may be affected and in other cases, all four limbs are impaired. And, as one might expect, movement ability varies from walking with little aid at an age of normally developing children, to severe delays with a multitude of motor skills. Common motor difficulties include the following (e.g., Gofer-Levi et al., 2013; Janssen & Steenbergen, 2011):

- Controlling postural stability (balance); less capability of adaptation
- Gross motor function; movements are typically slower with a higher energy cost, compared to typically developing persons.
- Motor planning
- Performing bimanual tasks
- Learning motor sequencing

DEVELOPMENTAL COORDINATION DISORDER

WebLink

http://www.canchild.ca; see Developmental Coordination Disorder.

Developmental coordination disorder (DCD) is a condition marked by poor coordination and clumsiness. Formally, it describes motor impairment in the absence of neurological disease, any known physical disorder, mental retardation, and low IQ. Individuals with this condition often have ADHD. Studies indicate that DCD interferes with a wide variety of behaviors and skills, including academic achievement, daily living skills (e.g., dressing, tying shoelaces, and brushing teeth), and engaging in sporting activities.

The prevalence of DCD has been estimated to be as high as 6% for children in the age range of 5 to 11 years; with about 2% being affected severely. It is now acknowledged that the signs and symptoms of DCD persist into adolescence and adulthood (e.g., Kirby et al., 2013; Purcell et al., 2015). The literature indicates quite clearly that children with DCD display deficits with the following:

- An array of perceptual-motor skills including handwriting (which may persist into adulthood) (Fig. 12.2)
- Generating and monitoring internal models of action; that is, an inability to mentally represent and efficiently plan actions
- Gross motor skills and fundamental movement skills (Yu et al., 2016)
- Driving a car (adults)

A popular assessment for identifying DCD is the Movement Assessment Battery for Children-2 (MABC-2; Henderson, Sugden, & Barnett, 2007), described in Chapter 13. A common criterion is children with motor performance in the lower 15th percentile. For more information, see *Developmental Coordination Disorder and its Consequences* by Cairney (2015).

DOWN SYNDROME

Down syndrome (DS), the most commonly identified cause of mental retardation, occurs in about 1 in 800 births. Despite many years of research to identify

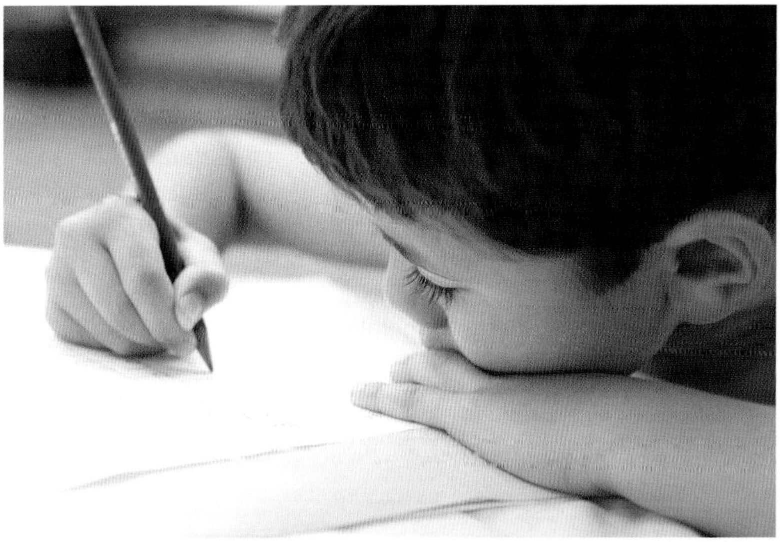

Figure 12.2 Handwriting problems may persist into adulthood for those with DCD.

risk factors associated with DS, only one factor, advanced maternal age, has been well established. As noted in Chapter 5, older mothers (>35 years) are at an increased risk of having children with DS. It occurs as a result of an extra chromosome, that is, individuals with DS have 47 rather than 46. DS children are identified by characteristic facial and body features—almond-shaped eyes and a flatness of the nose.

Although some DS children may have motor difficulties due to their mental delay, research shows that others have delays that are more of a motor nature (keep in mind that all voluntary motor actions have some link to mental processes). Specific problem areas include the following (e.g., Cardoso et al., 2015; Pereira et al., 2013):

- Gross motor skills including fundamental rudimentary behaviors such as sitting, standing, and walking. In fact, a considerable amount of research with DS has focused on walking. Due to problems with, for example, joint laxity and decreased muscle tone, DS children typically exhibit delayed walking onset.
- Postural control, which is closely associated with the deficits mentioned with gross motor skills
- Fine motors such as drawing
- In general, children with DS require more time to learn movements.

WebLink

http://www.nads.org (National Association for Down Syndrome); http://www.ndss.org (National Down Syndrome Society)

Infants with DS learn to walk about 1 year later than typically developing infants. Ulrich et al. (2008) and Ulrich et al. (2001) conducted experiments to determine if practice stepping on a motorized treadmill could help reduce the delay in walking onset. Interestingly, the experimental group learned to walk with help and to walk independently significantly faster than the group of DS infants that did not receive the practice. In essence, results provided evidence that, with training and support, parents can use these treadmills in their homes to help their infants with DS learn to walk earlier than they normally would.

think about it

Considering all of the special populations described, many are not physically active as typically developing persons. Why?

Summary

Although the focus on this course is no typically developing behavior, most of you at some point in your career will encounter individuals that display atypical motor behaviors. For some of you that will be in the clinical professionals (e.g., rehabilitation, physical therapy, occupational therapy), these special populations and circumstances will be your primary responsibility.

Populations that exhibit frequently atypical motor behaviors are ADHD, ASD, CP, DCD, and DS. As with typically developing populations, keep in mind that individual behavior may vary depending on severity of the condition and environmental influence.

think about it

1. **What instructional strategies would you use to help this population?**
2. **What are the major individual constraints for persons with CP?**
3. **Considering all of the special populations described, many are not physically active as typically developing persons. Why?**

LEARNING ACTIVITIES

Objective: To create a motor program for a special population. Select one of the special populations described in this chapter. Pick an age group (infancy, early childhood, etc.) and design a program to improve two fine motor and two or gross motor skills.

Objective: To discover new information about a special population. After selecting one of the special populations, search the Web for two up-to-date (no more than 2 years old) articles on instructional or intervention techniques. Write a brief one- to two-page summary of each article. Option: Present your findings to the class.

Suggested Readings

Behrmann, M., & Minshew, N. J. (2015). Sensory processing in autism. In M. Leboyer & P. Chaste (Eds.), *Autism spectrum disorders: Phenotypes, mechanisms and treatments.* Basel, Switzerland: Karger.

Piek, J. P. (2006). *Infant motor development*. Champaign, IL: Human Kinetics.

part five

Assessing Change

Chapter 13: Assessment

part five consists of a single chapter that provides information on assessing change in growth, development, and motor performance. Along with a discussion of the purposes and considerations for selecting and implementing a wide variety of instruments, this chapter features examples of the most widely used and contemporary instruments available.

Chapter 13

Assessment

OBJECTIVES

Upon completion of this chapter, you should be able to

13.1 Discuss the general scope of motor assessment.

13.2 List and define the basic terms associated with motor assessment.

13.3 Describe the purposes of motor assessment.

13.4 Identify the considerations for selecting an assessment instrument.

13.5 Provide examples of product-oriented assessment instruments.

13.6 Provide examples of process-oriented assessment instruments.

13.7 Identify assessment instruments appropriate for older persons.

KEY TERMS

assessment
measurement
evaluation
norm-referenced standards
criterion-referenced standards
product-oriented assessment
process-oriented assessment

Objective 13.1

The operational definition of motor development in this text is the study of the process of change in growth, development, and motor behavior (performance) across the life span. Assessment, in general, provides the opportunity to observe, document, and interpret this process of change as well as the ability to determine the growth and developmental status of the individual at that particular time in the life span. Motor assessment can be as diverse as the field of motor development itself. Table 13.1 presents items that may be used in a comprehensive physical-motor assessment. They are grouped according to each of the different perspectives of growth, development, and performance from which motor development may be observed and assessed. An aspect that could be added to the assessment of performance is the evaluation of either the process (qualitative) or product (quantitative) characteristics of the movement action. Chapter 9 described these perspectives under the discussion of fundamental movement skills.

think about it

Describe how you could use Table 13.1 to assess lifelong motor development (developmental continuum).

An example of the dynamic nature and potential for assessment through motor performance may be illustrated using the skill of running. From a development, or level of functioning, perspective, running may be used as an indicator of cardiorespiratory function, speed, agility, general coordination, and reaction time. From the viewpoint of motor performance, running may be judged by its process characteristics (movement pattern) or by the product produced (e.g., performance times in the 50-yard dash or the marathon).

Numerous component- and task-specific tests are available for assessing the physical and motor behavior characteristics of individuals at virtually all ages. Unfortunately, no assessment batteries include norms that reflect the lifelong perspective. Most batteries were developed to assess a diversity of age-span

TABLE 13.1 Comprehensive Physical-Motor Assessment

Biological Growth	Development (Level of Functioning)	Motor Behavior (Performance)
Body mass	Cardiorespiratory	Reflex behavior
Height	Muscular strength/ endurance	Spontaneous movement behavior
Body weight	Flexibility	Rudimentary behavior
Physique (body build)	Coordination	Fundamental movement behavior
Posture	Speed	Sport skill behavior
Anthropometric measures	Agility	Daily living skills (DLS)
Circumference	Power	
Breadth/length	Visual	
Skeletal maturity (age)	Balance	
Body composition	Reaction time	
Body fat	Kinesthetic	
Lean body mass	Temporal (rhythm) timing	
Secondary sex characteristics	Menarche	

characteristics (e.g., motor, mental, and social) displayed during the primary growth and development years of infancy through childhood.

This chapter provides an understanding of the basic terms, purposes, and considerations for motor assessment. Also presented are a description and review of selected popular and contemporary assessment instruments. For additional information, refer to the "Suggested Readings" at the end of this chapter.

BASIC TERMINOLOGY OF ASSESSMENT

Objective 13.2

Before the student of motor development can grasp a functional understanding of motor assessment with regard to the purpose, selection, and administration of assessment instruments, a review of basic terminology is warranted.

focus on change

Quality assessment of growth, development, and motor performance is vital to identifying and understanding *change*.

Assessment is a process that involves both measurement and evaluation. **Measurement** refers to the collection of information on which a decision is based. In measurement, various instruments and techniques are used to collect data. **Evaluation** is the process of decision making with regard to the value or worth of collected information. Support for such judgments commonly is based on norm- or criterion-referenced standards. For cases in which such standards are not available or an overall judgment is needed for several measurements that represent a diverse spectrum of traits, evaluation is frequently thought of as the process that qualitatively (subjectively) appraises the quantitative data. For example, the results of three groups of tests (e.g., physical growth, fundamental motor skill process characteristics, and motor performance product results) may be combined to produce a single assessment score.

Criterion- and norm-referenced standards are the two most widely used types of standards. **Norm-referenced standards** involve the hierarchical ordering of individuals. Assessment instruments that use this form of evaluation are basically quantitative evaluations designed to compare an individual's characteristics with those of other persons of similar sex, age, and socioeconomic group. Quality norm-referenced tests are based on statistical samplings of hundreds or, ideally, thousands of individuals.

The most common descriptors used to communicate norm-referenced standards are *percentile norms*. This type of norm describes the percentage of a given group that can be expected to score above or below a given value. For example, 40 modified sit-ups in a 1-minute period for a boy 10 years of age is at the 75th percentile. This means that only 25% of the boys in this age group did more sit-ups and about 75% did less. For purposes of practical interpretation, the 50th percentile mark (and above) often is used as the level of acceptability. Norm-referenced standards are particularly useful for making comparisons among individuals when the situation requires a degree of selectivity, such as in identifying excellence or extremely low status values.

Criterion-referenced standards are concerned with the degree to which an individual achieves a specified level of development, motor performance, or physical status. This type of standard has received considerable attention in recent years, as evidenced by its use with most national physical fitness assessment batteries. In this case, the value of the criterion standard represents the acceptable level of performance, which is usually based on normative data and expert judgment. For example, the criterion standard for the acceptable level of flexibility on the sit-and-reach test is 25 centimeters, or 2 centimeters beyond the toes. In contrast to norm-referenced standards, individuals are compared to the criterion value and not to others of the same sex and age. Criterion-referenced standards are useful for setting performance standards for all individuals. However, a limitation of its use is that the tester knows only when an individual has met an acceptable performance level, not to what degree the person actually performed.

Some assessments are specific to motor behavior, such as fundamental movement skill performance; these are referred to as product- or process-oriented instruments. With the **product-oriented assessment**, the examiner is primarily interested in the performance outcome, or the product of the behavior. Product values are described as *quantitative data*, such as the yards a ball is thrown, running velocity in seconds, and feet and inches jumped.

In contrast, **process-oriented assessment** involves the measurement and evaluation of the characteristics of the process, or form, such as those used in rudimentary actions and fundamental movement patterns. These types of data are most often *qualitative* rather than quantitative. Although product-oriented data can be used with either norm- or criterion-referenced standards, they commonly are associated with population norms. On the other hand, process-oriented assessment instruments are most often criterion-referenced, that is, individuals are compared to themselves in relation to established criteria. This chapter highlights such examples based on contemporary motor development theory.

PURPOSES OF ASSESSMENT

Objective 13.3

Assessment instruments are employed for many reasons, and the applications of the information obtained are varied. Whether the setting is in schools, child care centers, university laboratories, or at home, assessment provides vital services in the areas of teaching, learning, and science. Although most people associate measurement and evaluation with grading as is practiced in the schools, this is perhaps one of the least useful reasons to assess. Regardless of the setting and type of program, the most important factor is to conduct assessment with a specific purpose. The following discussion explains some of the more widely accepted purposes for assessment.

Diagnosis/Screening. Some of the frequently used assessment instruments are known as *diagnostic/screening tools* (e.g., Apgar scale and Bayley III Screening Test). Assessments such as these provide a means of differentiating normal-functioning individuals (usually newborns to middle childhood) from those who may not be developing normally. If weaknesses are detected, this information is then used to determine whether the individual should be referred for additional testing or remedial work. Basic screening procedures at the beginning of any physical education or motor development program are an excellent means of identifying individuals who may have special needs.

Determine Status. Perhaps the most commonly stated purpose of assessment is to determine individuals' status, progress, or achievement. This information may be used for a multitude of reasons related to more specific purposes. One indispensable practice of any instructional program is to determine whether objectives have been reached. Assessment is also essential for providing feedback on the individual's physical status or level of performance.

Placement. The results of assessment instruments are frequently used to place individuals in classes or groups according to their motor abilities. A common practice within instructional programs is to arrange individuals into homogeneous groups. In several cases, this practice enhances the teaching or learning process (e.g., swimming, gymnastics, and fitness classes).

Program Content. After student behaviors and characteristics have been assessed, results can be used to plan program content and guide individual progress. Assessment information is a considerable aid in writing student and program objectives that are reasonable and challenging.

Program Evaluation. Program directors and administrators frequently use assessment results to evaluate the program and thereby determine the possible need for change. A common change that occurs is a modification of program standards.

Construction of Norms and Performance Standards. Measurement, especially among large populations, provides data that can be used in establishing norms and performance standards. Group norms enable comparisons with other groups, such as those based on a nationwide sample. When criterion standards for specific performance tasks are not available, local norms (or a combination of local and national) can be used to establish criterion standards. Norms and performance standards are instrumental in providing motivation and interest within a program.

think about it

Explain how you could apply the purposes of assessment if you were a director of an early childhood learning center that has a motor development program.

Research. Measurement and evaluation conducted scientifically can add significantly to the body of motor development research and provide information on which educational programs can improve. Research is an important responsibility of any outstanding program.

Prediction. Theoretically, some aspects of assessment may be used to a limited degree to predict future performance. That is, specific information may be useful to directors in selecting activities that individuals are most likely to master. For example, an individual who has a high maximal oxygen consumption may decide to participate in triathlons or other endurance events.

Motivation of Individuals. Assessment instruments can be used as motivational tools. Individuals who know how well they are performing and how they can improve are likely to be better motivated than those who receive no feedback.

CONSIDERATIONS FOR PROPER ASSESSMENT

Objective 13.4

After the purposes for assessment have been established, additional considerations are warranted, especially with regard to instrument selection. Along with deciding what physical and motor characteristics are to be measured (which usually accommodate program objectives), a review of available instruments should be conducted. In addition to including the desired assessment items, only instruments that have an acceptable level of validity, reliability, and objectivity should be selected.

Validity refers to the degree to which an assessment item measures that which it is intended to measure. For example, if the purpose of the assessment is to measure aerobic capacity, experts have determined that a 1-mile run or 12-minute run is a valid indicator of this characteristic, whereas a half mile run is not a valid indicator.

Reliability is a measurement of the repeatability of assessment results. An individual's scores should not differ markedly on repeated administrations of the same assessment. Factors related to repeatability are consistency (dependability) of the instrument used to measure the individual's status (e.g., skinfold calipers and grip dynamometers), the examiner's instructions, and the subject's effort. One also should be aware that a test can be reliable without being valid, whereas a valid test must also be reliable.

The *objectivity* of a test refers to the degree of agreement among examiners. That is, a test that is completely objective will be scored identically by different examiners. The level of acceptability of these basic test characteristics can vary widely, even among the most popular assessment instruments. The statistical term related to the comparison of test characteristics and repeated occurrences is a *correlation*; a correlation coefficient of .80 or above generally is deemed quite acceptable.

Additional considerations for the selection of an assessment instrument include the following:

1. Is the instrument norm- or criterion-referenced? Care should be taken to determine if the sampled population is representative of the population of individuals in the program.
2. Is the instrument feasible to administer? This consideration may involve several things, including time, cost, equipment, space requirements, and personnel needed. Because time is often a perpetual problem facing program administrators who have large and small numbers of participants, instruments should be evaluated in terms of time economy.
3. Are the funds available? Some assessment instruments cost hundreds of dollars and require expensive equipment, whereas others may accomplish the basic objectives with only minor compromises at a much lower price. For example, the best measurement of aerobic capacity is maximal oxygen consumption. However, thousands of dollars' worth of equipment are needed to carry it out, and each test requires about 45 minutes to administer. Less accurate but acceptable and more feasible measures (field tests) are the 1-mile walk/run and 12-minute walk/run (using norm- or criterion-referenced standards). In general, however, the cost factor should consider accuracy, durability, and long-term use.
4. What levels of training and expertise are required to administer the items and interpret the data? Additional training and practice may be needed. In the interest of time economy, more than one examiner is usually imperative. This may call for considerable planning in order to provide reliable and objective assessment.

For a more thorough treatment of measurement and test evaluation, refer to the Suggested Readings.

ASSESSMENT INSTRUMENTS

The possibilities of assessing the various aspects of physical growth, development, and motor behavior are numerous (see Table 13.1 on page 346). In the areas of physical growth and physiological assessment alone, there are hundreds of instruments. Many of these have been mentioned or described throughout the text (e.g., skinfolds, anthropometric measures, and various physiological tests). This discussion focuses on some of the more widely used and readily available product-oriented motor assessment batteries and process-oriented instruments.

Motor behavior assessment items have been included in general child development batteries since the 1920s (Gesell, 1925). Since that time, numerous instruments have been developed. However, although the quantity of instruments seems sufficient, the quality has been suspected. Many motor behavior items have minimal, if any, rationale for development and are based on generalized product (quantitative) characteristics (e.g., how far, how fast, or how many). Other global assessment items merely ask if the child can throw a ball, kick a ball forward, stack cubes, or balance on one foot—all of which, to a great extent, underscore neuromaturational theory. Although some of these types of assessments may have an acceptable level of validity and reliability, they are limited from a motor development perspective, especially in describing the process of change. In recent years, greater focus has centered on the qualitative characteristics of motor behavior as evidenced by the development of process-oriented assessment instruments based on contemporary motor development theory. From this perspective, there may be large variability in scores within, among, and across developmental domains.

The following pages describe only a selected number of assessment instruments. The intent of this discussion is to provide the student of motor development with a glimpse into the diversity of assessment items and formats available. For additional information on specific instruments, the latter part of this chapter provides a list of recommended sources. Refer to the "Suggested Readings" at the end of this chapter for resources that provide in-depth descriptions of these and other physical and motor assessment tests.

The following examples represent standardized and accessible instruments that have received considerable recognition for the assessment of newborns, infants, school-age populations, and older persons.

Newborn Assessment

Objective 13.5

THE APGAR SCALE

The Apgar scale (Apgar, 1953) is used in delivery rooms all over the world to test the physical health of newborns. The scale typically is administered to newborns 1 minute and 5 minutes after delivery and measures the appearance (skin color), pulse, grimace (reflex irritability), activity (muscle tone), and respiratory effort (APGAR) of the infant. Each characteristic is rated on a scale of 0 to 2, in which 2 denotes normal function, 1 denotes reduced function, and 0 denotes seriously impaired function (Table 13.2). Thus, a total score of 10 is perfect.

Approximately 90% of all newborns score 7 or higher. A score of 4 or less is generally an indication that immediate medical assistance is needed. The Apgar scale is an important tool for assessing the state of the infant at birth, but it has limited predictive value given that 75% of children who have a low score develop normally (Piek, 2006).

THE NEONATAL BEHAVIORAL ASSESSMENT SCALE

Among the unique characteristics of the *Neonatal Behavioral Assessment Scale* (NBAS) (Brazelton & Nugent, 2011) is that it provides an assessment 2 or 3 days

TABLE 13.2 The Apgar Scale

	0	1	2
Appearance (skin color)	White or blue	Limbs blue, body pink	Pink
Pulse (rate)	No pulse	100 beats/min	More than 100 beats/min
Grimace (reflexive grimace initiated by stimulating the plantar surface of the foot)	No response	Facial grimaces, slight body movement	Facial grimaces, extensive body movement
Activity (muscle tone)	No movement, muscles flaccid	Limbs partially flexed, little movement, poor muscle tone	Active movement, good muscle tone
Respiratory effort (amount of respiratory activity)	No respiration	Slow, irregular respiration	Good, regular respiration, strong cry

SOURCE: From Apgar, V. A. (1953). A proposal for a new method of evaluation of a newborn infant. *Current Researches in Anesthesia and Analgesia*, *32*, 260–267. Copyright © 1953 Williams & Wilkins, Baltimore, MD. Reprinted by permission.

after the baby is born, then another assessment on day 9 or 10 after the baby is home from the hospital and has had the opportunity to relax from the stress of delivery. The NBAS was designed to examine individual differences in newborn behavior and is appropriate for infants up to 2 months of age. Typically, the scale is administered to at-risk babies or those for whom there is a concern about development.

The instrument generates results in three areas. One consists of *reflex* items designed to screen for neurological soundness. The second is the neonate's *interactive behavioral repertoire*. The third area of assessment, which is not as closely linked to motor behavior, is a rating of *attractiveness behavior* (i.e., the baby's contribution to and readiness for interaction) and need for stimulation (i.e., the need for and use of stimulation as it relates to organizing responses).

In the reflex assessment, each reflex is scored on a 4-point scale. Babies with 3 or more low scores typically are referred for additional neurological assessment. The 28 behavioral items are considered the most important assessment area. Each item is scored on a continuum of 1 to 9. A score of 1 represents the lowest state, whereas the ideal state varies from item to item and lies somewhere between 1 and 9. The baby's performance also may be rated on each item with a more simplistic good, adequate, or deficient.

Although evidence of the NBAS's validity has been verified, its test-retest reliability and standardization have been questioned. The reliability problem is due primarily to the fact that the instrument assesses the neonate's current status, which can change rapidly. One problem plaguing standardization is that newborns from different cultures tend to behave differently. However, the NBAS remains a popular tool for identifying high-risk infants.

INFANT ASSESSMENT

THE BAYLEY SCALES OF INFANT DEVELOPMENT

The *Bayley-III Motor Scale* (Bayley, 2006), is a norm-referenced instrument designed to measure the developmental functioning of infants and toddlers aged 1 to 42 months (Table 13.3). The motor scale (four other scales are available, e.g., cognitive, adaptive) consists *of fine motor* and *gross motor* subtests. The fine motor subtest contains 66 items and is purported to measure skills associated with eye movements, perceptual-motor integration, motor planning, and motor speed (e.g., grasping, drawing, writing). The gross motor subtest contains 72 items and is designed to measure movements of the limbs and torso (e.g., postural control, sitting, walking, jumping, throwing). The highest possible score on a subtest is 19, and the lowest possible score is 1. Administration of the motor scale takes 20 to 30 minutes. The author reports good reliability (test-retest) ranging from .86 to .91 and moderate correlations (validity) between the Bayley-III motor composite and other well-known motor assessments. Reports of the ability of the instrument to predict (predictive validity) motor outcome have not been strongly supportive

TABLE 13.3 Bayley-III Motor Scale Items

Group	Motor Area (Number of Items)
Gross motor	Head control
	Hands posture
	Turning
	Imitative behavior
	Preambulatory skills
	Body positioning
	Sitting
	Stairs
	Balance
	Walking
	Jumping
	Throwing
Fine motor	Grasping
	Drawing
	Pencil grasp/writing
Ungrouped (e.g., retains ring, buttons one button, tactile discrimination)	
Motor quality (behavioral rating scale)	

SOURCE: Bayley, N. (1993). *Bayley scales of infant development* (2nd ed.). San Antonio, TX: The Psychological Corporation.

think about it

As you review the tests, how does each relate to the behaviors noted in the "phases" of motor behavior?

WebLink

http://www.albertainfantmotorscale.com; also, see YouTube for demos.

(Anderson et al., 2010). Nonetheless, the Bayley-III is currently one of the most commonly applied measurement tools for assessing early development both in clinical practice and research settings.

A *Bayley-III Screening Test* is also available. It is composed of select items from three of the subtests: cognitive, language, and motor and takes roughly 15 to 25 minutes to administer. It is a normative-referenced assessment instrument.

THE ALBERTA INFANT MOTOR SCALE

The *Alberta Infant Motor Scale* (AIMS) (Piper & Darrah, 1994) is an observational assessment designed to evaluate the motor development of infants from 2 weeks through independent walking (18 months). The authors identify two purposes of the AIMS: (a) to identify infants delayed or impaired in their motor development and (b) to evaluate motor development over time. This uniquely qualitative test consists of 58 developmentally sequenced pictorial items that describe the infant's posture, weight bearing, and spontaneous antigravity movements while in four postural positions: prone, supine, sitting, and standing (Fig. 13.1 provides an example). To score the items (observed/not observed), the infant is observed in an unobtrusive environment with minimal handling. The total test easily is completed in 20 to 30 minutes. Normative data are available, and the raw scores can be converted to percentile ranks from monthly age levels.

The AIMS has demonstrated excellent psychometric properties with high test-retest and interrater reliability and concurrent validity with the Bayley III and Peabody Scales. There is evidence suggesting that the AIMS measures infant ability best from 3 to 9 months (Liao & Campbell, 2004). Complementing the qualitative nature of the assessment, it also has been reported that the descriptive indicators are consistent with functional movement. For example, the infant's skill level is represented by a developmental window (range of skills), which hypothetically depicts the dynamic nature of movement in transition (Case-Smith, 1996). Darrah and colleagues (2014) asked the question, "Are the AIMS norms collected over 20 years ago, still valid?" The answer was yes.

The AIMS is a popular and widely used instrument for the assessment of infant motor development.

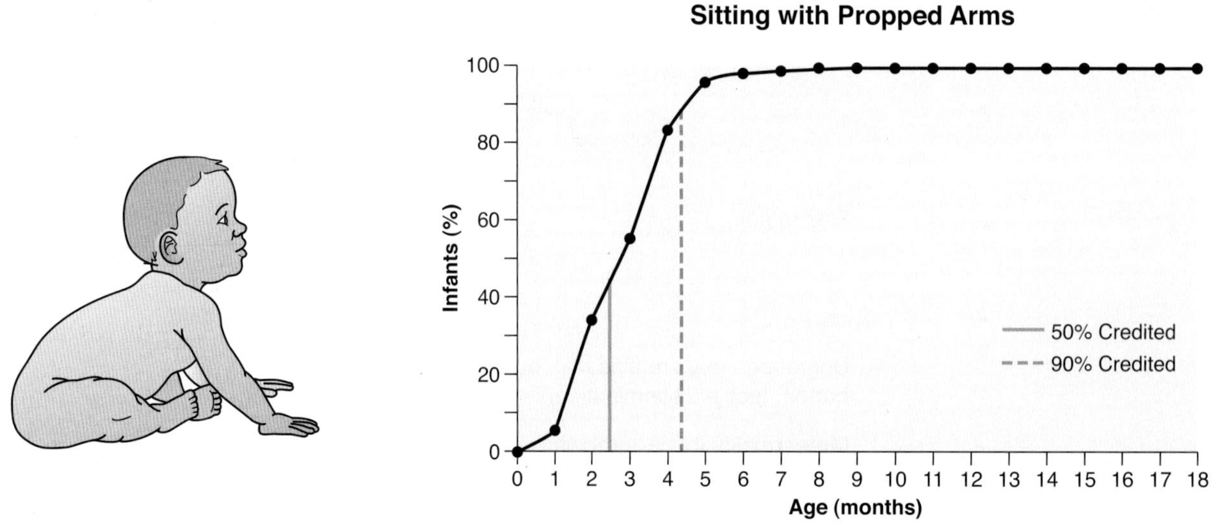

Figure 13.1 Example of an AIMS item.

Posture in Prone

Observe the infant in a prone position with a toy placed in front of him or her.

1. Stability of posture
1. Lies flat on the supporting surface
2. Assumes an upright posture momentarily
3. Maintains an upright posture for less than 10 seconds
4. Maintains an upright posture for more than 10 seconds

2. Movement against gravity
1. Lies flat on the supporting surface
2. Infrequently and momentarily moves against gravity
3. Lifts head and chest from surface in the vertical plane
4. Moves side to side

3. Trunk stability and extension
1. Does not lift head or demonstrates neck extension only
2. Trunk extension through the scapular region
3. Trunk extension to the lumbar spine
4. Trunk extension to pelvis

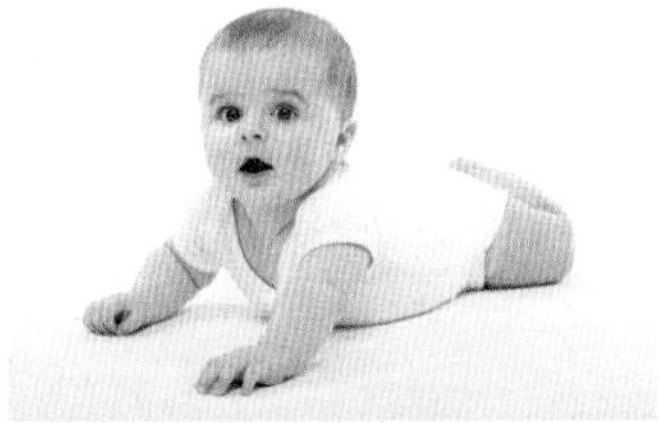

Figure 13.2 Example of a PFMAI assessment item (posture: ages 2 to 6 months).

POSTURE AND FINE MOTOR ASSESSMENT OF INFANTS

Based on contemporary dynamic systems theory, the *Posture and Fine Motor Assessment of Infants* (PFMAI) (Case-Smith & Bigsby, 2000) measures qualitative aspects of motor skill development by using systems that rate the dynamic quality of postural control and grasping/manipulation (fine motor) patterns in infants in the first year of postnatal life (2 to 12 months). The PFMAI is sensitive to small increments of change in individual infants. A 4-point criterion-referenced scale is used to rate the specific aspects of movement believed to be important in attaining functional mobility and manipulation. An additional purpose of the PFMAI is to measure progress or developmental change. Figure 13.2 presents an example of a PFMAI assessment item.

The Fine Motor section has 41 items that measure accuracy and quality of reach and grasping patterns, precision of release, and control of arm and hand movements when specific objects are presented. In addition to its qualitative merits, the PFMAI Fine Motor section is unique because it provides a method for assessing the influence of object affordances in eliciting a range of manipulative movements. This is accomplished by presenting the infant with objects of different size and action potential, which thereby facilitates different movement patterns.

The Posture Scale consists of 31 items designed to measure postural control and proximal stability/mobility, and the infant's ability to move within and between postures. According to the authors, psychometric properties include high interrater reliability (.86 to .99), moderate test-retest reliability (.58 to .96), and a high correlation with chronologic age (r = .94).

TODDLER AND INFANT MOTOR EVALUATION

The stated purposes of the *Toddler and Infant Motor Evaluation* (TIME) are (a) to diagnose motor delays, (b) to plan intervention, and (c) to evaluate change due to intervention and/or maturation (Miller & Roid, 1994). The TIME was designed to assess the quality of movement in children 4 to 42 months of age. The qualitative assessment includes standard scores on eight subtests, five of which have been standardized: Mobility, Stability, Motor Organization, Social/Emotional Abilities, and Functional Performance.

Holding to the dynamic systems perspective, the TIME identifies the components of specific actions and assesses the infant's ability to organize those components. For example, the Mobility subtest assesses the infant's ability to move within and from five starting positions (supine, prone, sitting, quadruped, and standing) that complement his or her developmental age. The scale analyzes the maturity and number of variations within and between positions and the highest developmental level obtained. The test provides a measurement of the patterns of transitional movements observed over a 20-second time.

Standardized with a sample of 144 children who have motor delays and 173 children who are developing normally, the TIME has good test-retest and inter-rater reliability (.89 to .99). The authors report excellent sensitivity in identifying infants with motor dysfunction.

TEST OF INFANT MOTOR PERFORMANCE

The *Test of Infant Motor Performance* (TIMP) (Campbell et al., 1994) is an assessment of motor function in infants at risk for developmental disabilities. The test was designed for use by physical therapists (PTs) and occupational therapists (OTs) who assess and treat infants from 32 weeks' gestational age through 4 to 5 months postterm equivalent age. The concepts underlying the test include the notion that movement assessment must be based contextually, must reveal the development of postural control synergies that lead to functional movement in daily life, and must reflect the hypothesis that development of postural control may be a rate-limiting factor in motor development and motor learning. The TIMP assesses the infant's ability to sustain postures in a variety of spatial orientations; regain postural stability following perturbations; and make transitions between postures for orienting to interesting events and people, changing positions, and self-comforting. The test consists of two scales. The infant's ability to make coordinated postural responses when positioned in a variety of spatial orientations is rated with the *Elicited Scale* (e.g., "Head turn in prone position to sound"). The *Observed Scale* assesses the infant's attempt to change positions, orient head and trunk, and selectively initiate individual body segments into action (e.g., "Reaches for person or object" and "Reciprocal kicking").

WebLink
http://www.timp.com

think about it
What do the tests for infants (birth to 2 years) have in common?

Recent studies indicate the test discriminates among children with varying degrees of risk for motor dysfunction in the first year of life, is reliable in the hands of experienced clinicians, and has test-retest stability (Campbell & Eaton, 1999; Campbell & Kolobe, 2000). An independent review of the test by Case-Smith (1996) concludes that the TIMP is a "sensitive measure of motor development in the first 4 months of life" (p. 36).

Assessment of (Up to) School-Age Populations

AGES AND STAGES QUESTIONNAIRE

The *Ages and Stages Questionnaire* (ASQ-3) (Squires & Bricker, 2009) is a standardized parent-friendly questionnaire used to *screen* children from 1 month to 5½ years. Among the areas screened are parent observations of fine and gross motor responses. For example, "Does your baby pick up a crumb or Cheerio with the tips of his or her thumb and a finger?" and "Does your child stack a small block or toy on top of another one?"

The ASQ-3 is based on a sample of 15,000 children with excellent validity and reliability (all above .82, reported by the authors). Rosenbaum and colleagues (2009), in their review and recommendations for epidemiological studies in children, note that the ASQ-3 is a well-validated and highly recommended instrument. The questionnaire takes 10 to 15 minutes to complete and typically 1 to 3 minutes to score. For more information, see the website http://www.agesandstages.com.

MOVEMENT ASSESSMENT BATTERY FOR CHILDREN

The *Movement Assessment Battery for Children* (ABC-2) (Henderson et al., 2007) is designed for children and adolescents aged 3 to 16 years. The instrument is well known as a research tool for identifying children with developmental coordination disorder (DCD) and as a general screening instrument for motor problems in typically developing children. It also has uses in planning and evaluating an intervention program in either a school or clinical setting. The test consists of eight tasks for each of three age bands (3 to 6, 7 to 10, and 11 to 16 years) involving *manual dexterity*, *ball skills*, and *static and dynamic balance*. Each item is rated on a 6-point rating scale, where 5 equates to the weakest performance and 0 equals the best performance. Total standard scores and percentiles are provided. Although the Movement ABC-2 is a product-oriented test with norms, qualitative observations are available.

Several reports of the psychometric properties of the instrument suggest that it is a valid and reliable tool (e.g., Gard & Rösblad, 2009; Smits-Engelsman et al., 2011). The Movement ABC-2 has universal appeal and has been validated in several countries. The test is relatively simple to administration in approximately 20 to 40 minutes.

The *Movement ABC-2 Checklist*, for ages 5 to 12 years, focuses on how a child manages everyday tasks encountered in school and at home. The checklist has a motor and a nonmotor component that provides information on direct and indirect factors that might affect movement. Supplemental to the evaluation is an excellent "ecological intervention" guide based in large part of the constraints model (Child–Task–Environment). Figure 13.3 shows an example of process and product assessment for manual dexterity.

Manual Dexterity 1: PLACING PEGS

Record: Preferred hand: R/L (should be same as for Drawing Trial); Time taken (secs); F for failure; R for refusal; I if inappropriate (note reasons below)

Preferred hand		Only administer a second trial if the first trial takes longer than the time stated below:					Non-preferred hand		Only administer a second trial if the first trial takes longer than the time stated below:				
Trial 1			7:0-7:11	8:0-8:11	9:0-9:11	10:0-10:11	Trial 1			7:0-7:11	8:0-8:11	9:0-9:11	10:0-10:11
Trial 2			37 secs	33 secs	32 secs	29 secs	Trial 2			47 secs	41 secs	36 secs	34 secs

Qualitative observations

Posture/body control

- Sitting posture is poor ☐
- Holds head too close to task ☐
- Holds head at an odd angle ☐
- Does not look at board while inserting pegs ☐
- Does not use pincer grip to pick up pegs ☐
- Exaggerates finger movement in releasing pegs ☐
- Does not use the supporting hand to hold board steady ☐
- Does extremely poorly with one hand (asymmetry striking) ☐
- Changes hands or used both hands during a trial ☐
- Hand movements are jerky ☐
- Moves constantly/fidgets ☐

Adjustment to task requirements

- Misaligns pegs with respect to holes ☐
- Uses excessive force when inserting pegs ☐
- Is exceptionally slow/does not change speed from trial ☐
- Goes too fast for accuracy ☐
- **Other** ______ ☐

Comments: ______

Figure 13.3 Sample of the Movement ABC-2; qualitative and quantitative assessment.

WebLink
http://www.dcdq.ca

For screening of probable DCD, the Developmental Coordination Disorder Questionnaire (DCDQ) (Wilson et al., 2007) is a brief parent questionnaire designed for children aged 5 to 15 years. It has wide acceptance internationally with cross-cultural adaptations in several countries—see WebLink.

PEABODY DEVELOPMENTAL MOTOR SCALES II

WebLink
See YouTube for demos.

The *Peabody Developmental Motor Scales II* (PDMS-2) (Folio & Fewell, 2000) assesses the quantitative and qualitative aspects of gross and fine motor ability of children from birth through 5 years of age. The Fine Motor section consists of test items that measure (a) controlled use of the fingers and hands under the general heading of grasping and (b) visual-motor integration, using such test items as reaching and grasping an object, building with blocks, and copying designs.

The normative sample for the PDMS-2 consisted of 2,003 persons who resided in 46 states and were considered to be representative of the current U.S. population. The manufacturer claims that with regard to psychometrics, this version is an improvement over the original. For example, it has good reliability and validity within a variety of subgroups as well as with the general population. According to the manual for the 1983 version, the test has acceptable test-retest reliability (.95 and .80, for the Gross and Fine Motor scales) and outside reviews of the test's psychometric properties are generally supportive (e.g., van Hartingsveldt et al., 2005; Wang et al., 2006).

BRUININKS-OSERETSKY TEST OF MOTOR PROFICIENCY

The *Bruininks-Oseretsky Test of Motor Proficiency* (BOT-2) (Bruininks & Bruininks, 2005) is a clinical and research tool used to assess fine and gross movement skill development in individuals aged 4 to 21 years. The complete BOT-2 features 53 items and is divided into 8 subtests: *fine motor precision*, *fine motor integration*, *manual dexterity*, *bilateral coordination*, *balance*, *running speed and agility*, *upper limb coordination*, and *strength*. The items in every subtest become progressively more difficult. The scoring system varies according to the individual items; it ranges from a 2-point scale to a 13-point scale. Results are available in composite scores for fine manual control, manual coordination, body coordination, and a strength and agility composite. The sum of scores results in a total motor composite. The time required to assess one individual varies between 45 and 60 minutes.

think about it
Have you noticed any commonalities among the product-oriented tests? Describe some of them.

A short form of the BOT-2 is available to be used as a screening tool. The BOT-2 Short Form comprises a subset of 14 items of the BOT-2 Complete Form. The Short Form features items from all subtests. The authors report a high correlation (r = .80s) between the Short and Complete Form. Administration of this version takes between 15 and 20 minutes.

Internal (authors) and external reports of the psychometric properties (reliability, validity) of the BOT-2 and Short Form have been reported as acceptable to quite good (e.g., Venetsanou et al., 2009; Wuang & Su, 2009). More recently, Hands et al. (2015), after a review of five popular tests to identify motor coordination difficulties in adults, ranked the BOT-2 as the best.

AFFORDANCES IN THE HOME FOR MOTOR DEVELOPMENT

The *Affordances in the Home for Motor Development* (AHEMD) (Caçola et al., 2015; Rodrigues et al., 2005) are an innovative parental self-report instruments for assessing the quality and quantity of factors (affordances and events) at home that are conducive to enhancing motor development in children ages 3 to 18 months (Infant Scale [IS] version) and 18 to 42 months old. The instruments were designed based on a contemporary view of early childhood motor development, which considers environmental influences as critical factors in optimal growth and behavior and in which the home is the primary agent. Each instrument consists of one section on child and family characteristics, and three sections on home environment characteristics and affordances: physical space, daily activities, and play materials. Assessment items, which are grouped according to common content in 20/35 (IS) variables, "representing expected markers of the meaningful characteristics of the home environment" (Rodrigues et al., 2005, p. 143). The variables are further grouped according to inside space, outside space, variety of stimulation, fine motor, and gross motor. In addition to simple dichotomic and Likert-type questions, the instrument uses description-based questions that provide pictorial examples to give the responder an idea of material category (group) (Fig.13.4). For both versions, parent self-report reliability and reliability against actual home visits by trained observers were acceptable. Overall, the AHEMD is a valid and reliable tool for assessing the home environment for motor affordances. In addition to being used as a research tool, the instruments are popular with PTs and OTs for assessing and providing intervention at home. As of the date of this writing, the AHEMD has been translated from English into eight languages. Tests are available free via contact with authors.

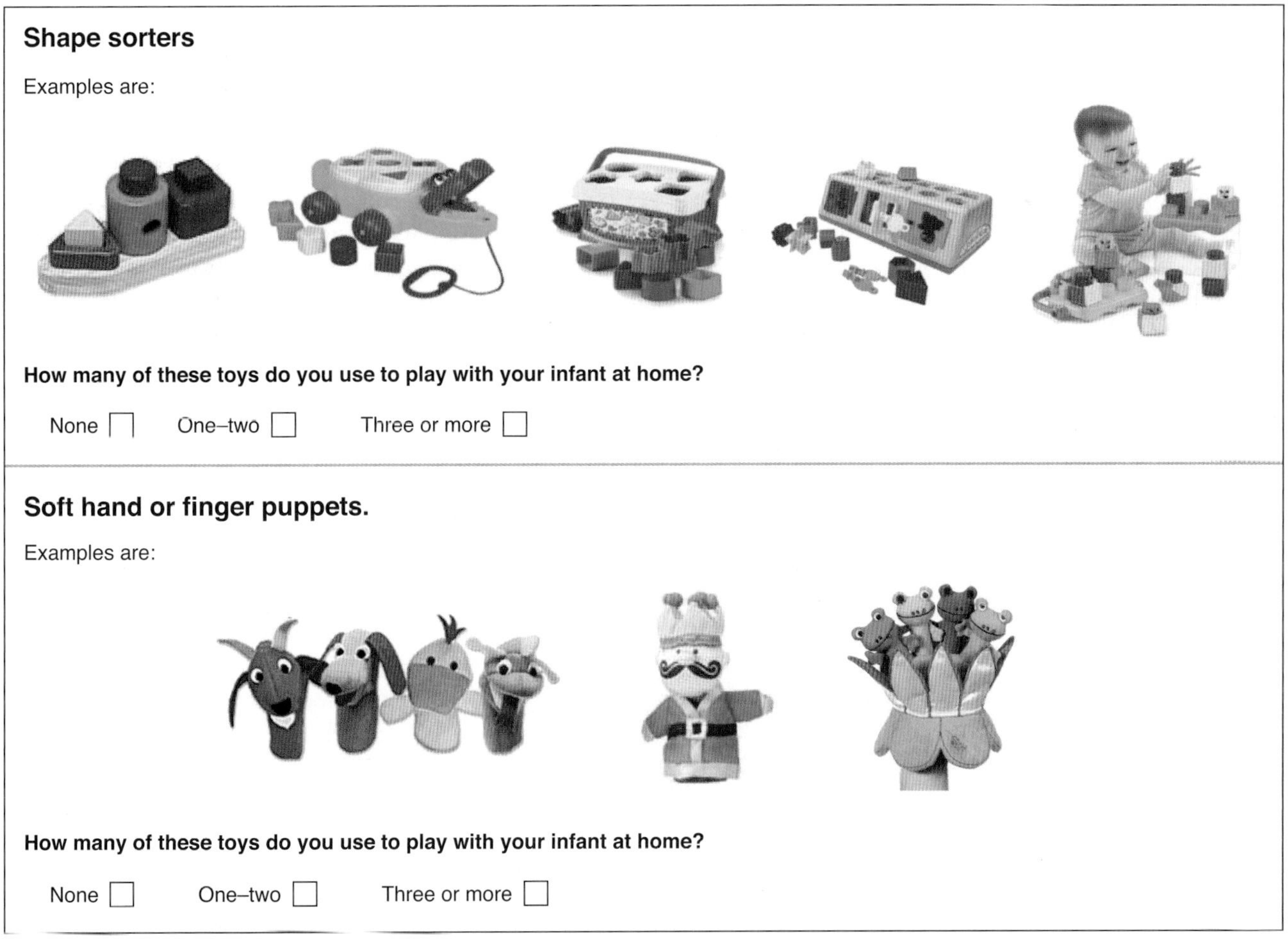
Shape sorters

Examples are:

How many of these toys do you use to play with your infant at home?

None ☐ One–two ☐ Three or more ☐

Soft hand or finger puppets.

Examples are:

How many of these toys do you use to play with your infant at home?

None ☐ One–two ☐ Three or more ☐

Figure 13.4 Examples of fine motor toy items with AHEMD-IS.

BEERY-BUKTENICA DEVELOPMENTAL TEST OF VISUAL-MOTOR INTEGRATION

The *Beery-Buktenica Developmental Test of Visual-Motor Integration* (Beery VMI) (Beery et al., 2010) was designed to assess the extent to which individuals (ages 2 years to adult) can integrate their visual and motor abilities. The Short Format and Full Format tests present drawings of geometric forms arranged in order of increasing difficulty that the individual is asked to copy. The Short Format is often used with children ages 2 to 7 years. The VMI also provides supplemental *Visual Perception* and *Motor Coordination* tests, which use the same stimulus forms as the Short Format and Full Format tests. These optional assessments were designed to be administered after results from the Short Format or Full Format test show the need for further testing. The instrument also provides age-specific norms from birth through age 6 years for basic gross, fine, visual, and visual fine motor developmental "stepping stones."

WebLink
See YouTube for demos.

According to the authors, the instrument has high test-retest reliability (.90 to .92) and acceptable concurrent and predictive validity. A more recent study using children 4 to 12 years of age, supports this claim (Wuang & Su, 2009). Both formats (Short and Full) take approximately 15 minutes to complete and the supplemental tests about 5 minutes each. The instrument has an international reputation as an excellent clinical and research tool to screen for visual-motor deficits. The authors state that the VMI is useful with individuals of diverse environmental, educational, and linguistic backgrounds.

DEVELOPMENTAL TEST OF VISUAL PERCEPTION (DTVP-3)

The *Developmental Test of Visual Perception* (DTVP-3) (Hammill et al., 2013), frequently used by OTs, assesses visual perception and visual-motor integration in individuals ages 4 to 12 years. The DTVP-3 comprises five subtests: Eye-Hand Coordination, Copying, Figure-Ground, Visual Closure, and Form Constancy. Results of the subtests are combined to form three composites: motor-reduced visual perception, visual-motor integration, and general visual perception (combination of motor-reduced and motor-enhanced subtests). The authors report the instrument as highly reliable at the .80 level or above for all subtests and .90 or above for the composites for all age groups. Outside review supports those claims (Brown & Hockey, 2013).

Process-Oriented (Fundamental Movement) Assessment Instruments

Objective 13.6

A variety of assessment instruments are designed to examine the process (i.e., qualitative) characteristics of movement. Inherent in these instruments is the intent to identify an individual's current movement qualities and compare the actions to an established developmental sequence. (Chapter 9 discussed the research and applied information concerning developmental sequence with regard to specific fundamental movement skills. It may be helpful to review that information. Particularly relevant are the discussions related to stage theory and Roberton's intratask component theory of identifying change in motor behavior.) Generally, accompanying process-oriented instruments are criterion-referenced standards that compare individuals to themselves and to the criterion standard rather than to other people as with norm-referenced standards.

Keep in mind that the instruments described in the following pages represent practical attempts to observe, measure, and assess the process characteristics of movement. Research endeavors in this field are relatively recent; not a great deal has been established concerning the validity of several developmental movement pattern sequences. To more accurately assess the developmental change of an individual's movement pattern characteristics, film analysis over time is desirable (although it is generally not practical).

Because the use of sophisticated instrumentation and film analysis is needed to detect precise changes, most process-oriented instruments use a global analysis. That is, the developmental sequence of a specific skill is identified using three to five total body stages (e.g., immature, elementary, and mature) rather than making a developmental-level analysis of specific body segments. There are also instruments that use identifiers considered to be relatively subjective; these are useful primarily as global screening and diagnostic devices.

WebLink

See thePoint FMS collection, YouTube, and other sites for fundamental movement skill videos.

As noted in Chapter 9, several excellent videos are available. In addition to the detailed written movement descriptions provided in that chapter, videos offer dynamic visual depictions of skill in action.

TEST OF GROSS MOTOR DEVELOPMENT-3

The *Test of Gross Motor Development-3* (TGMD-3) (Ulrich, 2016) is the latest update of one of the best examples, to date, of a practical, easily administered instrument developed to assess the sequence and qualitative aspects of motor skill behavior. Designed for use with children 3 to 11 years of age, the TGMD-3 provides assessment of 13 of the most commonly practiced locomotor and manipulative motor skills. The locomotor skill assessment includes running, horizontal jumping, hopping, galloping, skipping, and sliding. The Ball Skills section includes one- and two-handed striking, stationary ball dribbling, catching, kicking, and overhand/underhand throwing. Table 13.4 presents a sample of the qualitative assessment format.

The TGMD-3 is considered quite comprehensive in the number and diversity of the motor skills that it assesses; it also can be administered with a minimum amount of special training and takes only about 15 minutes to complete per child. Another attractive characteristic is that it provides both norm-referenced and criterion-referenced interpretations. The instrument has well-established validity and reliability characteristics and, for an instrument of this type, is standardized on a diverse and relatively large normative sample.

WebLink

See YouTube for TGMD-3 demos.

For additional information on developmental sequences and instructional strategies, see Cleland Donnely et al. (2016).

In addition to the resources described, recall that Chapters 8 and 9 provide useful information of assessing rudimentary behaviors and fundamental movement patterns. For example, in Chapter 9, the information related to the mature characteristics and developmental sequence of each skill may be used to create a useful observation instrument.

Tests for Older Persons

Objective 13.7

Because physical function can differ considerably in the elderly, a wide range of tests is needed. Test categories correspond to general capability level and range from physically elite and fit, to the physically independent (low-level function), to the physically frail and dependent. Tests for the frail and dependent typically

TABLE 13.4 Samples of TGMD-3 Items

Locomotor Subtest

Skill	Materials	Directions	Performance Criteria	Trial 1	Trial 2	Score
1. Run	60 feet (18.3 meters) of clear space to run, and two cones or markers	Place two cones 50 feet (15.2 meters) apart. Make sure there is at least 8–10 feet (2.4–3.1 meters) of space beyond the cone for a safe stopping distance.	1. Arms move in opposition to legs with elbows bent			
			2. Brief period where both feet are off the surface			
		Tell the child to run fast from one cone to the other cone when you say, “Go.”	3. Narrow foot placement landing on heel or toes (not flat-footed)			
		Repeat a second trial.	4. Nonsupport leg bent about 90 degrees so foot is close to buttocks			
				Skill Score		
2. Horizontal jump	A minimum of 10 feet (3.1 meters) of clear space, and tape or markers	Mark off a starting line on the floor, mat, or carpet. Position the child behind the line. Tell the child to jump far. Repeat a second trial.	1. Prior to take off both knees are flexed and arms are extended behind the back.			
			2. Arms extend forcefully forward and upward reaching above the head.			
			3. Both feet come off the floor together and land together.			
			4. Both arms are forced downward during landing.			
				Skill Score		

Ball Skills Subtest

Skill	Materials	Directions	Performance Criteria	Trial 1	Trial 2	Score
3. Two-hand catch	A 4-inch (10.2-centimeter) plastic ball, 15 feet (4.6 meters) of clear space, and tape or a marker	Mark off two lines 15 feet apart. The child stands on one line and the tosser stands on the other line. Toss the ball underhand to the child aiming at the child’s chest area. Tell the child to catch the ball with two hands. Only count a trial in which toss is near child’s chest. Repeat a second trial.	1. Child’s hands are positioned in front of the body with the elbows flexed.			
			2. Arms extend reaching for the ball as it arrives.			
			3. Ball is caught by hands only.			
				Skill Score		

4. Overhand throw	A tennis ball, a wall, and 20 feet (6.1 meters) of clear space	Attach a piece of tape on the floor 20 feet from the wall. Have the child stand behind the tape line facing the wall. Tell the child to throw the ball hard at the wall. Repeat a second trial.	1. Windup is initiated with a downward movement of hand and arm.			
			2. Rotates hip and shoulder to a point where the nonthrowing side faces the wall			
			3. Steps with the foot opposite the throwing hand toward the wall			
			4. Throwing hand follows through after the ball release, across the body toward the hip of the nonthrowing side.			
				Skill Score		

Ball Skills Subtest Total Score ____________

Total Gross Motor Score ____________

SOURCE: From Ulrich, D. A. (2016). *Test of gross motor developments* (3rd ed.). Reprinted with permission of the author and Pro-Ed, Inc., Austin, TX.

Focus on Application
Assessment of Cross-Cultural Samples

Cross-cultural research examines different cultural groups to determine in what ways development is universal and in what ways it is culturally different. For example, do children in Africa sit, crawl, and walk at the same approximate time that U.S. infants do? One of the ways researchers compare cultural groups is to use a well-known assessment instrument. This method helps if the objective is to compare a study with previous research. Common "universal" (motor) tests for children include the Bayley Scales of Infant Development, the Peabody Developmental Motor Scales, and the Test of Gross Motor Development (all three are described in this chapter).

These tests and several others provide norms established using U.S. samples. Is it appropriate to use these norms to compare children from other countries? It depends on the intent of the research. If the intent is to compare how a set of children compares to the U.S. standard, the tests may be appropriate. For example, if the children as a group are below the norm, is there a cultural explanation, such as a specific child-rearing practice? On the other hand, is it meaningful to compare the norm of U.S. children for placekicking ability with that of Brazilian children, a culture that has a strong cultural bias for soccer? What about throwing ability, which very likely would favor U.S. children? Perhaps a better question for Brazil would be, "What is the norm for Brazilian children?" And, from an intervention perspective, what is the lower 25th percentile? One solution is to use the standard scores rather than norms. Another is to create a specific set of norms for the population (country or segment of it) using the same test items.

Getting back to the example stated earlier, how do African infants compare to U.S. infants? One difference is that African (more specifically, Ugandan) babies tend to be more advanced in sitting, walking, and running than U.S. infants (Gardiner & Kosmitzki, 2005). Once again, researchers suggest that child rearing is a major factor; some cultures encourage and some discourage early motor development.

Source:
Gardiner, H. W., & Kosmitzki, C. (2005). *Lives across cultures: Cross-cultural human development*. Boston, MA: Allyn & Bacon.

think about it

In contrast to being physically elite as an older person, a minimal level of physical function is essential to daily living. Provide some specific examples of the latter.

WebLink

http://www.humankinetics.com/; see demos.

include items that assess function of basic daily living skills (DLS) (e.g., feeding, tying shoelaces, and basic mobility). Physically fit individuals can be tested using routine laboratory items with some or no modification (e.g., treadmill, bicycle ergometer, and dynamometer). (For a description of testing the elderly at this level, see "Suggested Readings.") The highlights of three attractive test batteries follow; each is appropriate for the physically independent.

SENIOR FITNESS TEST

Although tests and components of physical fitness are beyond the scope of this text, the Senior Fitness Test (Rikli & Jones, 2013) provides assessment items to test actions used by older persons in ordinary, everyday tasks. For example, older adults require adequate strength, flexibility, balance, and endurance to accomplish even ordinary, everyday tasks. Here is a list of the test items.

Chair stand—testing lower body strength
Arm curl—testing upper body strength
Chair sit and reach—lower body flexibility test
Back scratch—upper body flexibility test
8-Foot up and go—agility test

Walk or step in place—the walk test is used to assess aerobic fitness unless the person uses orthopedic devices when walking or has difficulty balancing, in which case they do the step in place test. The test is safe and enjoyable for older adults and the authors report acceptable reliability and validity. The test has performance norms based on actual performance scores of over 7,000 men and women between the ages of 60 and 94 years. One of the merits of the test is that it provides information on ways to modify test protocols for those with limiting conditions (e.g., diabetes, recover from stroke, heart conditions, and joint replacement).

BRUININKS MOTOR ABILITY TEST

The *Bruininks Motor Ability Test* (BMAT) (Bruininks & Bruininks, 2012) is one of the newest to attract attention for use with adults 40 years and older. The BMAT, ideal for clinical and research settings, is designed to determine functional status and, if needed, set intervention goals and monitor progress. The test provides three composite scores for fine motor, gross motor, and total motor. There are five subtests consisting of 32 items to determine: fine motor integration, manual dexterity, coordination, balance and mobility, and strength and flexibility. Each subtest can be administered in about 15 minutes. There is also a short form that offers a quick assessment of motor ability in about 20 minutes. The BMAT provides standard scores and percentile rank. In regard to its psychometrics properties, the authors report content validity was well established with the BOT-2 and the Beery VMI. Test-retest values ranged from .77 to .92 and interrater reliability was .95 to .99.

WebLink
See YouTube for demos.

PHYSICAL PERFORMANCE TEST

As noted earlier, with older persons, the assessment of functional status in the form of DLS is important in determining level of independent living; *Physical Performance Test* (*PPT*) provides a good example of such a test. Developed by Reuben and Siu (1990), the PPT is an objective measure of physical function in the elderly. Test items were designed to simulate daily living activities that vary in level of difficulty and measure a variety of fitness components (Table 13.5). The test discriminates well among older adults from a variety of clinical settings. The values shown in the table represent individuals from hospital primary care units, assisted living homes,

TABLE 13.5 Physical Performance Test Items

Timed Physical Performance Test Item	Percentage Able to Complete	Average Time to Complete (s)
Writing a sentence	94	16.7
Simulated eating	100	15.4
Lifting a book and putting it on a shelf	94	4.0
Putting on and removing a jacket	97	15.6
Picking up a penny	98	3.5
Walking 50 feet	98	25.0
Climbing a flight of stairs	91	10.6

SOURCE: Modified from Reuben, D. B., & Siu, A. L. (1990). An objective measure of physical function of elderly outpatients. The physical performance test. *Journal of the American Geriatrics Society*, *38*, 1105–1112.

TABLE 13.6 Summary Information on Selection Instruments

Instrument	Age Range	Type of Items	Source
AIMS	2 wk–18 mo	Process (rudimentary motor skills)	Elsevier http://www.elsevier.com
Bayley-III	1–42 mo	Product (fine and gross motor)	Pearson http://www.pearsonassessment.com
BOT-2	4–21 y	Product (fine and gross motor)	Pearson
Movement ABC-2	3–16 y	Product/process (fine and gross motor)	Pearson
PFMAI	2–12 mo	Process (posture/manipulative)	Pearson
TGMD-3	3–11 y	Process (fundamental motor skills)	PRO-ED http://www.proedinc.com
Beery VMI	2–adult	Process (visual-motor)	Pearson
Senior Fitness Test	>60 y	Product (fitness)	Human Kinetics http://www.humankinetics.com
BMAT	>40 y	Product (fine and gross motor)	Pearson

AIMS, Alberta Infant Motor Scale; BOT-2, Bruininks-Oseretsky Test of Motor Proficiency-2. ABC-2, Assessment Battery for Children-2. PFMAI, Posture and Fine Motor Assessment of Infants. TGMD-3, Test of Gross Motor Development-3. VMI, visual-motor integration. BMAT, Bruininks Motor Ability Test.

and senior citizen housing. Reports of use with diverse samples indicate that the PPT is a valid and reliable instrument (Paschal et al., 2006; Wilkins et al., 2010).

Table 13.6 provides some information about a few of the more recommended and available motor assessment instruments. Refer to the "Suggested Readings" (Physical and Motor Assessment) for single-test and laboratory-oriented recommendations.

Summary

Assessment provides the opportunity to observe, document, and interpret change across the life span as well as to determine the growth and developmental status of an individual at a particular time. The possibilities for physical and motor assessment as associated with growth, development, and motor performance are vast.

Assessment involves both measurement (collection of information) and evaluation (process of judgment). The two most widely used types of standards by which performance is judged are norm- and criterion-referenced standards. The assessment of movement skill performance usually is conducted with process-oriented (form characteristics) or product-oriented (performance outcome) assessment instruments.

After the purpose for conducting the assessment has been established, additional considerations are warranted with regard to instrument selection. Considerations should include a review of the instrument with regard to its psychometric properties (e.g., validity, reliability, and norm sample), feasibility (e.g., cost, equipment, space, personnel needed, and time), and level of training and expertise needed.

Most instruments are based on generalized product (quantitative) characteristics and provide little insight into the process of developmental change. These shortcomings have been addressed to some degree in recent years, as evidenced by the introduction of several process-oriented instruments and motor-specific, product-oriented assessment batteries.

think about it

1. **Describe how you could use Table 13.1 to assess lifelong motor development (developmental continuum).**
2. **Explain how you could apply the purposes of assessment if you were a director of an early childhood learning center that has a motor development program.**
3. **As you review the tests, how does each relate to the behaviors noted in the "phases" of motor behavior?**
4. **What do the tests for infants (birth to 2 years) have in common?**
5. **Have you noticed any commonalities among the product-oriented tests? Describe some of them.**
6. **In contrast to being physically elite as an older person, a minimal level of physical function is essential to daily living. Provide some specific examples of the latter.**

LEARNING ACTIVITIES

Objective: To test older person for DLS. First, create a checklist of DLS (use textbook information and Web). Then, observe if possible, or ask the individual or his or her assistant if applicable. Write a brief one- to two-page summary with recommendations for improvement.

Objective: To explore the Web for widely used assessment tools used in the chosen career. Search the Web for assessment tools that you might be using, especially those not mentioned in this text. Provide a two- to three-page summary of the tests (purpose, ages, etc.) and your personal evaluation of each instrument.

Suggested Readings

General Assessment

Baumgartner, T. A., Jackson, A. S., Mahar, M., & Rowe, D. (2015). *Measurement for evaluation in kinesiology* (9th ed.). Burlington, MA: Jones & Bartlett Learning.

Physical and Motor Assessment

Kaplan, R. M., & Saccuzzo, D. P. (2013). *Psychological testing* (8th ed.). Belmont, CA: Cengage Learning.

Salvia, J., Ysseldyke, J. E., & Witmer, S. (2017). *Assessment in special and inclusive education* (13th ed.). Boston, MA: Cengage Learning.

part six

Sociocultural Influences on Motor Development

Chapter 14: Sociocultural Influences on Motor Development

part six **The final chapter** of this text describes the role of sociocultural factors in motor development. This information addresses the primary sociocultural factors from infancy to old age that may influence the individual's participation in sport and physical activity.

Chapter 14

Sociocultural Influences on Motor Development

OBJECTIVES

Upon completion of this chapter, you should be able to

14.1 List and identify the basic terminology associated with socialization.

14.2 Describe the processes involved in socialization.

14.3 Define *socializing agent* and provide primary examples of those agents.

14.4 Explain Bronfenbrenner's bioecological systems model.

14.5 Briefly discuss the importance of socialization to motor development.

14.6 Identify and elaborate on the primary sociocultural influences that may affect motor development during childhood and adolescence.

14.7 Describe Parten's four categories of play.

14.8 Define *gender roles* and *gender-role stereotyping* and discuss their influence on motor development.

14.9 Explain the role of self-esteem in motor development.

14.10 Explain the possible influences of race on socialization into physical activity and sport.

14.11 Identify the primary sociocultural influences that can affect physical activity involvement during adulthood.

14.12 Describe the social views of aging that have implications for socialization into physical activity.

KEY TERMS

- socialization
- socializing agent
- Bronfenbrenner's bioecological systems model
- Parten's play model
- peers
- gender roles
- gender-role stereotyping
- self-esteem
- self-concept
- age-related stereotyping
- activity theory

At birth, newborns are very much alike in that they have similar needs for nurturing, progress through the same general sequence in developing locomotion and speech, and must learn appropriate social behavior. However, children become different due to sociocultural influences, experience, and their biological uniqueness. Chapter 5 addressed factors that affect growth and development: maternal and external influences on prenatal development, nutrition, hormones, and the effects of physical activity (and exercise) on lifelong human development. This chapter focuses specifically on the influences and importance of sociocultural factors on lifelong motor development.

BASIC TERMINOLOGY OF SOCIALIZATION

Objective 14.1

focus on change

An individual's sociocultural setting has a profound effect on *change* in growth and motor development.

think about it

How would you describe your particular context (home/community/state) in regard to being *socialized* into sport and physical activity?

Although socialization commonly is linked with child and adolescent development, it is a lifelong process. As individuals vary their social environment, they must learn to adapt to new situations. **Socialization** refers to a set of events and processes by which individuals acquire the beliefs and behaviors of the particular society and subgroup in which they live and, in most cases, are born into. Many goals of socialization are common to all societies, but each society and subgroup develops its own unique practices and goals to maintain itself in its particular ecological context.

Culture, which is generally thought of as a subset of society, is the collection of specific attitudes, behaviors, and products that characterize an identifiable group of people. Because societies and cultures frequently differ, it is reasonable to assume that expectations would vary from culture to culture. Although differences exist between our society and those of other countries, differences exist within our society between cultural groups. Some cultures place a higher priority on leisure, recreation, and sports than do others; this will have an effect on the motor development of its members.

Four general concepts frequently used to describe the structure of socialization are status, class, role, and norm. *Status* refers to an individual's position in society. One individual can hold many positions—father, brother, coach, mentor, friend, athlete, and so on. Some positions are conferred on individuals due to their experience or expertise, whereas others are simply a function of sex (e.g., mother, wife) or age (e.g., family leader and grandparent). Individuals learn to assume the role associated with the established position of status.

A complementary term to one's status in society is social class. *Social class*, also called *socioeconomic status*, refers to a grouping of people who have similar economic, educational, and occupational characteristics. Cross-cultural studies often use terms such as *lower*, *middle*, and *upper socioeconomic class* as a factor for making comparisons.

Accordingly, a *social role* is the particular behavior an individual uses to fulfill a position of status. One may describe a role as the set of dynamics and expectations that complements the status; in essence, it is the job description that goes with a position. For example, a quarterback holds the status of team leader on the field. With that status, the individual is expected to do such things as organize the group and carry out the game plan. As role expectations for a specific position of status are developed and a relatively predictable set of characteristics is formed, norms are established.

A *norm* refers to a standard of behavior that would be expected from members of a similar group of society. For instance, common and expected behaviors are associated with specific groups of teachers and coaches in addition to their individual personalities.

Cultural socialization should be viewed as an interactive process between society and the individual, with one intricately influencing the other. Socialization is a lifelong dynamic process that allows people to use their individual differences to make unique contributions.

SOCIALIZING PROCESSES AND AGENTS

Objective 14.2

Socialization involves acquiring knowledge and various types of skills, including those related to the motor domain. There are three principal modes of socialization: direct instruction, shaping, and modeling. All three modes are used to teach individuals about social roles they and others can play in the culture. Each also is mediated by the individual's social cognition or understanding of the social world.

Direct instruction deals primarily with concepts and ideas conveyed through language. This mode of socialization includes specific or general information about how to act and what to say and when to act and speak. *Shaping* refers to the social learning processes that allow an individual to benefit from experience. The concept that individuals can learn social behaviors by observing other people who serve as models is known as *modeling*. Frequently associated with cognitive-social learning theory and the works of Bandura (2009) (refer to Chapter 1), it is suggested that individuals cognitively represent the behavior of others through observational learning and then possibly adopt, or model, this behavior themselves. Modeling can have a profound effect on the development of motor skills, especially during childhood and adolescence when individuals frequently attempt to model the behavior of famous athletes.

Objective 14.3

Socialization depends on the contexts and settings in which it occurs. Individuals may be influenced by the overlapping factors of society at large, one or more subcultures, socioeconomic class, institutions, and individuals. Each can play a significant role in the socialization process. Complementary to the processes of socialization are the various agents influential in affecting social behavior and motor development.

A **socializing agent** is an individual, group, or institution that interprets culture to the individual. Although there are numerous subagents, the major socializing influences are family, school, peer group, church, and community. Of this group, it is generally acknowledged that the family is the primary socializing agent that transmits cultural content during the early developmental years. The family not only passes on its attitudes, prejudices, and health habits but also determines social class, ethnic origin, race, and religious beliefs. As individuals grow older, the school and peer group characteristically become stronger influences in socialization. More specific to motor development, teachers and coaches are in positions of powerful influence in the school and community. Other potentially strong agents (medium) through which individuals may be socialized are play and sports involvement. Subsequent discussions of the primary factors that influence development during childhood, adolescence, and adulthood will incorporate these primary agents.

Objective 14.4

One of the few comprehensive frameworks for understanding sociocultural influences on socialization was developed by Bronfenbrenner (2005) (Fig. 14.1). **Bronfenbrenner's bioecological systems model** places the individual at a theoretical center surrounded by five environmental systems: microsystem, mesosystem, exosystem, macrosystem, and chronosystem. The most direct interactions are with the *microsystem*, the environment in which the person lives. Influential agents include the family, school, peers, church, and neighborhood play area. Within these contexts, the individual is viewed as one who helps construct the environment.

Influences that occur as a result of relationships between different microsystems are part of the *mesosystem*. For example, the relation of family experiences to school experiences, or church training to family experiences, falls within the mesosystem. Developmentalists suggest that it is important to observe the

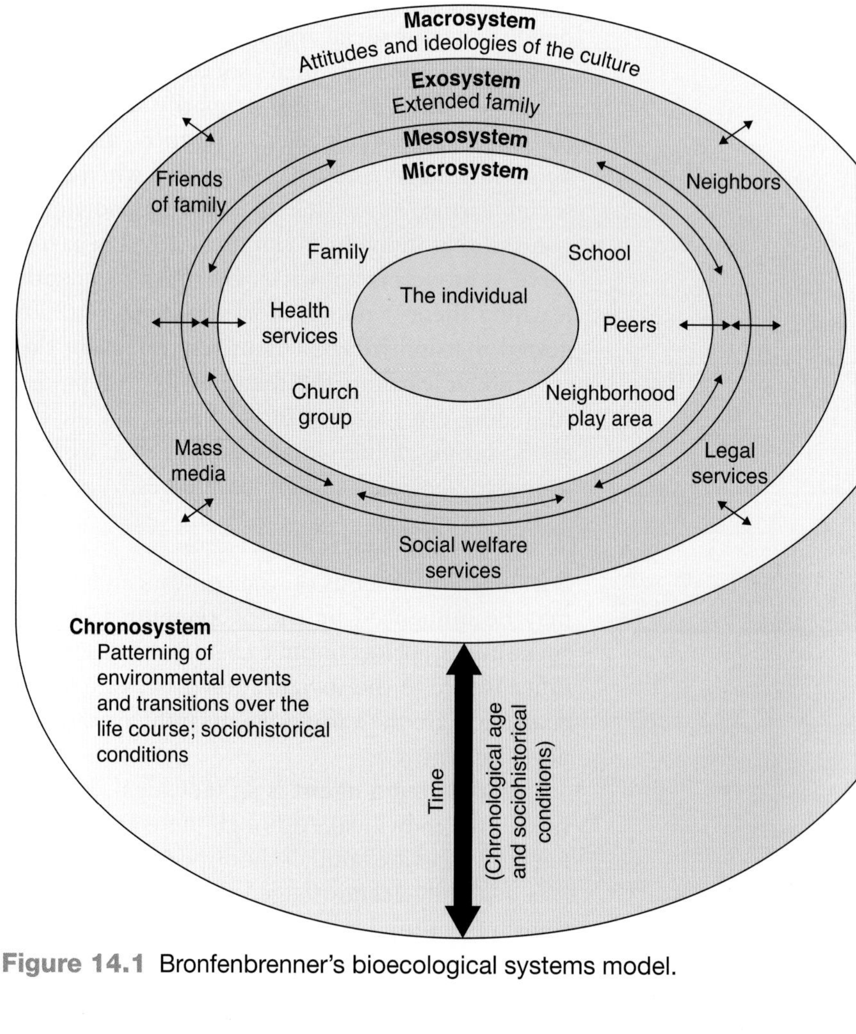

Figure 14.1 Bronfenbrenner's bioecological systems model.

think about it

How could you use Bronfenbrenner's bioecological systems framework and Process–Person–Context–Time (PPCT) model to study environmental effects on motor behavior?

individual's behavior in multiple contexts to provide a more complete picture of social development.

The *exosystem* involves indirect influences from another social context that affect what the person experiences in an immediate setting. This would include, for instance, the school board and city government, both of which have control over the quality of physical education and recreational facilities available to individuals.

The *macrosystem* incorporates the broad-based attitudes and ideologies of the society and specific culture in which the individual lives. It is suggested that these influences may permeate virtually all of the other systems within the individual's ecological world. As mentioned earlier, different societies and cultures place varying levels of importance on influential factors such as education, leisure time, sports, and health promotion, all of which may have a powerful impact on motor development across the life span.

The final influence is the *chronosystem*, which involves the patterning of environmental events and transitions over the life span, that is, the sociohistorical contexts. For example, females today are much more likely to participate in athletic activities than they were in the 1950s and 1960s.

THE PROCESS–PERSON–CONTEXT–TIME MODEL

Although the systems model (see Fig. 14.1) theoretically represents broad-based influences on and options for studying human development, the likelihood of undertaking such a venture in its entirety is arguably not feasible for most researchers (we view the model as a general framework for variable selection). With the idea of providing a more applicable model with focus on the individual, Bronfenbrenner (1995) introduced the PPCT model—a model that in recent years has gathered the attention of the research community interested in the environment influence on human (biological) development. More specific, this construct encompasses particular forms of interaction between organism and environment, called *proximal processes*, which operate over time and are posited as the primary mechanism producing human development. The power of such processes to influence development is a function of the characteristics of the developing person, and the immediate and more remote environmental context and the time, in which the proximal processes take place. The model allows for examination of the following:

Process: what is happening to the person, for example, physical education, sport, recess
Person: biological, cognitive, and emotional characteristics
Context: nested levels or systems of the ecology
Time: multiple dimensions of temporality

Bronfenbrenner referred to time as the historical period through which the person lives and the timing of biological and social transitions as they relate to the culturally defined age, role expectations, and opportunities occurring throughout the life course.

Objective 14.5

Socialization affects behaviors that include values, knowledge, social skills, and traits and is vital for optimal physical and motor development. Societies, cultures, or families that do not expose their members or their children to physical activities, sports, and proper health practices are limiting the human potential for optimal development.

focus on change

Ecological systems have an interactive and cumulative effect on *change*.

The following discussion focuses on the primary sociocultural influences that can affect motor development through involvement in sports and other physical activity across the life span. Although it has been shown that sociocultural factors begin to show their influence on growth and development in the prenatal stages (when the mother's health practices may be affected by socioeconomic status) and become more direct after birth, this discussion focuses on the primary factors associated with early childhood through adulthood.

PRIMARY INFLUENCES DURING CHILDHOOD AND ADOLESCENCE

Objective 14.6

The primary sociocultural influences on sports involvement and physical activity during childhood and adolescence are the family, peer relations in play and sport participation, and the relationship to coaches and teachers in the school and community. Additional factors to be discussed are gender-role expectations, self-esteem, and race.

The Family

The family is the socializing agent most directly responsible for the communication of cultural content to the growing child. This observation is relevant not only to socialization in general but also with regard to the child's movement endeavors. Significant changes in the family unit have taken place in recent decades, brought about by an increase in the number of working mothers and single-parent homes. In fact, several surveys indicate that the majority of mothers of children and youth now work outside of the home. According to Pew Research Center report (Cohen et al., 2012), only 29% of families had a stay-at-home mother. That report also notes that 34% of American children spend some time in a single-parent family, usually with their mother. Despite all of these changes and their ramifications, the family is still the primary caregiver and socializing agent during infancy and childhood.

Of the many influences associated with the family, perhaps the most dominant are parental beliefs and attitudes. Parents who believe in the importance of an active, healthy lifestyle usually share it with their children. Many parents take their children along to such settings as tennis courts, swimming pools, health clubs, and other recreational areas. With this positive attitude and the knowledge that physical activity is beneficial, it is usually the parent's wish that their children adopt these characteristics. Consequently, these parents usually provide their children with early experiences (Fig. 14.2).

The first contact young children have with motor activities and sports normally takes place with the family. Along with taking their children to fitness and sporting activities, parents may give sport equipment and clothing as presents and introduce the basic skills and concepts of selected activities. All of this may begin at a very young age. As children grow older, they are encouraged to participate in more formal settings (e.g., youth sports) and to maximize their abilities. Sports involvement for the vast majority of eventual participants normally begins by the age of 8 years; if parental interest is high, the likelihood of participation is much greater.

focus on change

The family is a strong agent for *change*.

As a result of early experiences and watching their parents participate in physical activity regularly over the years, children also may develop a positive

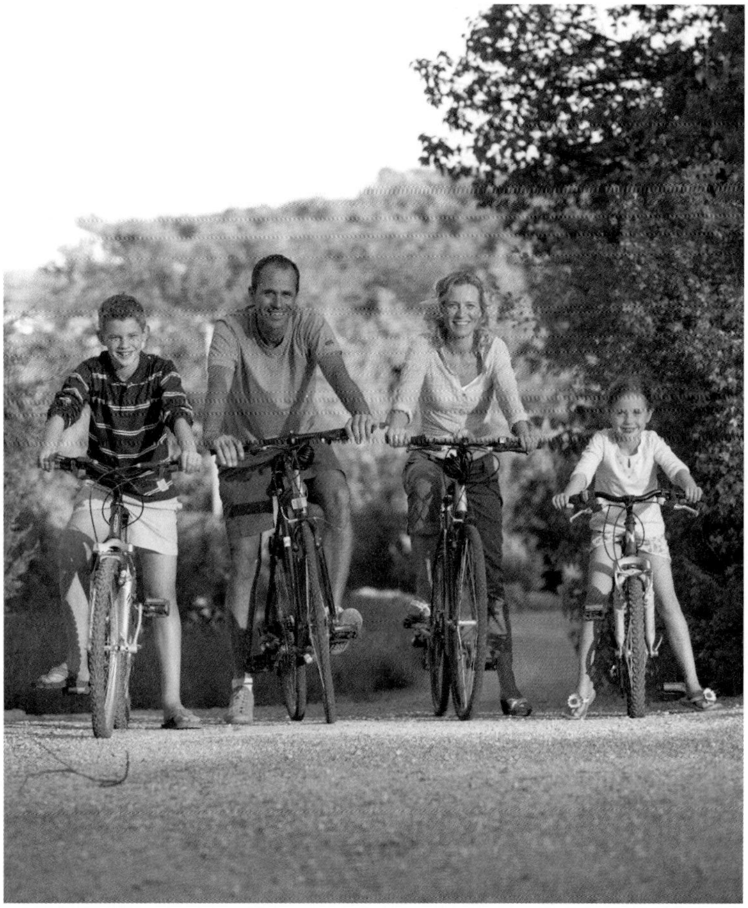

Figure 14.2 Parental beliefs and attitudes toward a healthy lifestyle are important in socializing the child.

attitude about physical activity and thus become socialized into an active physical lifestyle. Participation in sport activities in later years (i.e., older childhood through adulthood) reflects, at least to some degree, their parent's beliefs, attitudes, and encouragement during earlier years. Although other influences are likely to be present, research findings indicate that the best predictor of participation in physical activities and sports by adults is activity and skill proficiency during childhood and adolescent involvement (e.g., Barnett et al., 2009; Jaakkola et al., 2015).

The research is clear that parental approval and active involvement are important in youth sport participation, especially so at the more elite athlete level. Research findings with regard to individual *family member influence*, although somewhat inconsistent, indicate that specific members of the unit likely play differential roles in play and sport socialization. One body of literature suggests that the same-gender parent has the most influence on the extent of the child's involvement (DiLorenzo et al., 1998). Although the more traditional view that males are more "sport-oriented" and therefore should be more encouraged (than females) to participate still exists, as noted in Chapter 10, views are changing, as evidenced by the significant increase in female sport participation over the last 30 years.

There is also evidence that the opposite-gender parent influences involvement, but that fathers are the primary influencing agent for both girls and boys

(Moore et al., 1991). Evidence from this investigation also found the mother's role in influencing sport participation of either gender child was minimal, which supports the more traditional view that the father is responsible for initiating sport involvement of the offspring, especially the male child.

The literature concerning sibling influence seems to be inconsistent. However, it appears that older brothers and sisters may be important agents in the sport socialization of younger siblings. Overall, it is clear that the family, especially the father, is the significant agent in the socialization of its children to physical activity and sport.

Along with determining religious beliefs, race, and ethnic origin, the family also serves as the economic unit. Economic factors can affect nutritional practices and corresponding physical growth and development. There are also indications that socioeconomic status may be an influential factor in motor development. Although research on this topic is gravely lacking, it appears as though children from low-income families (especially single-parent homes) may be limited in motor development experiences due at least in part to lack of financial resources, parental involvement time, and the parents' experience. Living on a tightly budgeted low income may present a shortage of funds for such items as toys, sport equipment, and activity program enrollment fees.

There are also indications that children in low-income or single-parent homes may have limited exposure to different kinds of play activities and sports in comparison to children of higher income families. For instance, Greenspan (1983) found that age-group skiers, gymnasts, and swimmers come primarily from homes of upper-middle-class socioeconomic status, whereas young boxers, wrestlers, and baseball players derive from less economically endowed families. Empirical evidence also would suggest that activities such as golf and tennis are associated with higher income families.

Another consideration is socioeconomic status as it relates to education and knowledge of the importance of motor activities in child and adolescent development. Low-income families, which generally lack higher education, may be less knowledgeable about the importance of physical activity to health and thus may be less apt to consider motor activities important to their children's development. On the other hand, some highly educated people may view the time spent on motor activities as detrimental to optimal cognitive development.

Peer Relations

The influence of peers and participation in play and sport activities become increasingly powerful socializing influences through the childhood years. As the effects of these factors increase through later childhood and adolescence, family dominance tends to decrease on several socialization issues. From a motor development perspective, the influence of both of these agents are intertwined. Although research has not shown that participation in play and sport activities systematically produces positive social characteristics, it does suggest that when good consequences occur, they are tied to the social relationships found in these settings (Coakley, 2015).

Play, as it relates to socialization and other aspects of human behavior, has been one of the most extensively studied areas of child development. In addition to stimulating peer relations, play also has been shown to advance cognitive development, increase exploration, release tension, enhance self-esteem, influence attitude formation, and stimulate moral growth. In fact, a report of the American Academy

Focus on Application

Child-Rearing Practices and Cross-Cultural Difference in Motor Development

A frequently asked question about motor development is "At what age should children master a particular motor skill, such as walking?" As our textbook notes, the environment and child-rearing practices are an important factor. With this in mind, using U.S. norms as the worldwide standard presents a problem for some countries. For example, in some cultures, early movement is discouraged as practiced when infants are held longer by the mother and not allowed to explore by the typical means of crawling and creeping. This may be due to hazards in and around the home (e.g., cooking fires, potentially harmful animals, or rough terrain), or the simple fact that the flooring (e.g., dirt, stones) is not suitable, such as in very rural areas. In addition, there are cultural practices that do not allow the freedom of mobility that is typical in our nation. For example, babies from the Yucatan (in Mexico) are traditionally bound (swaddled) during the period that most babies in the United States are learning locomotion. The inserted photo shows an example of swaddling.

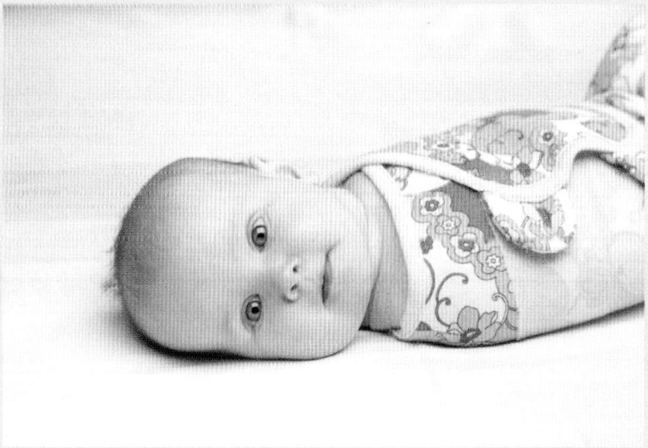

Alternatively, in some countries, such as parts of Africa and the West Indians of Jamaica, early development of motor skills as a general practice is encouraged by using bouncing and stepping practice to strengthen the legs: a practice selectively done in many cultures as a bonding or play time activity but not as a traditional practice. Keep in mind that even though many of those babies that were "held back" fall below the "typical" norm for early movement behavior, many are able to catch-up if they are allowed to explore and play.

of Pediatrics (Ginsburg, 2007) stated that play was an essential component in a child's learning (also see updated report by Milteer & Ginsburg, 2012). As mentioned earlier, Piaget (1952) viewed play as a medium that advances the child's cognitive development. Several traditional and contemporary theorists share the general notion that play is a positive influence in child development. Play and sport activities take up a sizable amount of time during childhood and adolescence and provide many opportunities for enhancing physical and motor development. Although numerous research papers have been written on the topic, the term *play* remains an elusive concept. Descriptions of play range from an infant's simple display of a newly discovered perceptual-motor talent, to a parent and child catching a ball, to an older child's involvement in organized youth sports. In general, play can be described as a pleasurable activity engaged in for its own sake (Fig. 14.3).

Objective 14.7

Many years ago, Parten (1932) identified categories of play (**Parten's play model**) still recognized by developmentalists today as relevant forms of social development. These include the categories of solitary, parallel, associative, and cooperative play. In *solitary play*, the child plays alone or independently of those around him or her. Solitary play is characteristic of 2- and 3-year-olds. *Parallel play* is similar to

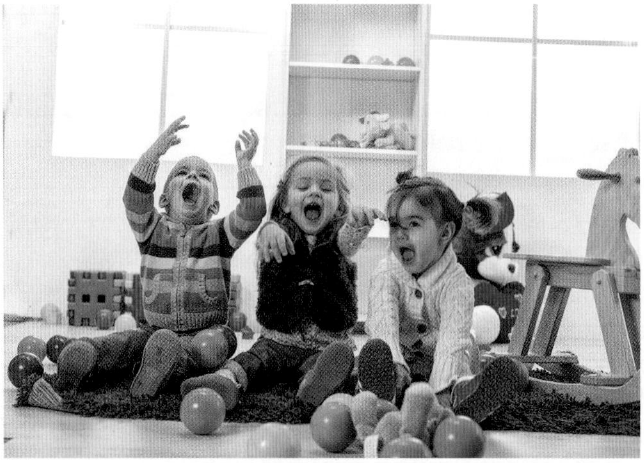

Figure 14.3 Play is considered a primary mode of social development during childhood.

solitary play in that the child still plays independently but plays with toys like those other children are using. Thus, parallel play mimics the behavior of children who are playing alongside. Although this type of play decreases in frequency with age, older preschool children can be observed in this behavior often.

focus on change

Play has a significant role in physical, social, and cognitive *change*.

WebLink

http://www.a4pt.org/ (Association for Play Therapy)

Social interaction in the form of play with little or no organization is described as *associative play*. At this time in social development, children seem to be more interested in associating with each other than in the tasks around them. Specific characteristic behaviors include follow-the-leader and invitation-type activities, along with borrowing and sharing toys. This type of play often is observed between the ages of 3½ to 5 years.

Around the age of 5 years marks the beginning of purposeful, cooperative play, which represents social interaction in a group with a sense of group identity and organization. This category is characterized by formal games, competitive group activities, and activities in which children must work together to achieve a common goal. *Cooperative play* at this level is the precursor to forms of movement activities and sport observed during older childhood and adolescence. Observation also suggests that as children grow older, they tend to form more complex and larger social structures when at play. Table 14.1 presents a summary of Parten's categories of play.

There are indications that play behavior, as described by these categories, has changed over the last half century. Some of this change has implications for motor development. It appears that children do not engage in as much associative and cooperative play as they did in the past. In addition to being less physically active in general, it has been suggested that children may be expressing more passive solitary and parallel play behavior as a reflection of the extended time they spend watching television, operating computers, and playing video games. Beginning at approximately age 5 years, individuals engage in physical activities that are more cooperative and complex (i.e., group-oriented). The need for this type of play appears to increase with age (and peak during adolescence) due in part to the individual's strong social desire to be a part of a peer group. Cooperative play may take the form of informal or formal games (and sports). In informal activities, children usually get together on their own to play with equipment at hand and use makeshift or flexible rules.

Focus on Application

Is Recess Important?

This chapter and previous chapters (Chapters 1 [Piaget, 1985] and 5) underscore the importance of play in child development. Given that more and more formal instruction is placed in the school day for children, some schools have considered either shortening or ending recess, especially if physical education is provided. Is recess important? According to the American Academy of Pediatrics and several national education agencies, such as the National Association of Elementary School Principals and the National Association for the Education of Young Children, recess is an important component of a child's physical, social, and cognitive development. In addition, Article 31 of the United Nations Convention on Children's Rights states "that every child has the right to leisure time. Taking away recess, whether as a disciplinary measure or abolishing it in the name of work, infringes on that right."

Recess is not a physical education and should not substitute for or be excluded in favor of physical education. In addition to the physical benefits, recess provides children with discretionary time and opportunities to practice life skills such as conflict resolution, cooperation, respect for rules, taking turns, sharing, using language to communicate, and problem solving in real situations.

Organized activities such as youth sport and school athletic programs often demand significant time commitments by the participant and family. It is not uncommon for parents to adjust meal and work schedules and weekend plans to get their children to practices and games. Along with probable financial requirements, these considerations, when compared to other family commitments and priorities, can be important factors in the degree of organized sport socialization.

TABLE 14.1 **Parten's Categories of Play**

Play Category	Description
Solitary independent play	The child plays alone with toys that are different from the toys used by nearby children, and the child makes no effort to get close to the other children and toys.
Parallel play	The child plays independently among other children with toys like those used by the other children. The child is not necessarily playing with the toys in the same way as the other children are. The parallel player plays beside rather than with other children and does not try to influence the other children's play.
Associative play	The child plays with other children. The children play similarly, if not identically, and there is no division of labor and no organization around a goal. Each child acts as he or she wishes, and each child is more interested in being with the other children than in the activity.
Cooperative or organized play	The child plays in a group that is organized for a goal, such as making something or playing a formal game. By dividing the labor, the children take on different roles and supplement their mutual efforts.

SOURCE: Adapted from Parten, M. (1932). Social participation among pre-school children. *Journal of Abnormal and Social Psychology*, *27*, 243–269.

In addition to being influential in developing social behaviors and stimulating peer relations, sport settings also provide excellent opportunities for advancing motor development and physical fitness (refer to Chapter 10).

One of the most frequently cited reasons for involvement in play and sport activities is the desire to interact with peers. **Peers** are individuals of about the same age or maturity level and, in some instances, social class. A common characteristic of the peer group during childhood and adolescence is that its members are usually of the same sex. This provides an extremely powerful socialization environment. Most peer relations arise from associations made in the school, particularly if the schools are attended by individuals from the same neighborhood. The desire to fit in and the need to belong and be identified as part of a group, team, or club can be compelling socialization forces. Adolescent peer groups are often organized around *cliques*—small groups of people that have similar interests. As individuals enter later childhood and adolescence, influence from the peer group becomes increasingly important, whereas that of the family and other social agents may diminish.

Some research has also examined the influence of friends, more specific "best friends," on sport and physical activity. For example, Lopes and colleagues (2016) report significant similarity patterns among adolescent best friends. Interestingly, it was also noted that regardless of the sex of the individual, having a male best friend was a factor in being more active.

Coakley (2015) notes that children's involvement in informal or organized sports is influenced by (a) the availability of opportunities; (b) support from the family, peers, role models, and the general community; and (c) the child's self-perception as a participant. Of these influences, there are strong indications that the peer group is a dominant factor with respect to socialization into physical activity and sport from childhood through early adulthood. Peers have the potential to reinforce family influence concerning socialization into physical activity and sport and to provide new considerations not stressed at home. There also may be situations when peer influence challenges those values set by other social agents (e.g., family, school, and church).

Throughout childhood and adolescence, this influence seems to be stronger with regard to involvement in team (group) activities rather than individual sport endeavors. However, regardless of the type of activity into which the individual is drawn by peer influence to participate, peer relations can be a powerful social agent in enhancing motor development.

Coaches and Teachers

Usually associated with the school and community social structures, teachers and coaches have the potential for being influential agents with regard to sport involvement. In fact, in some situations in which few other influential adults are available, these agents may become significant others for the child. Although some suspicion has been cast regarding the primary motives of coaches (e.g., too much emphasis on winning), in most cases, these agents are genuinely concerned with helping members of the team to experience positive socialization outcomes. Unfortunately, little evidence can be found on the extent to which coaches affect behaviors that transcend sport situations and influence individuals in later life. There is an evidence, however, that adolescent athletes are more likely to be influenced in regard to self-concept by coaches, compared to parents (Jowett & Cramer, 2010).

think about it

Using your experience, describe how the various socializing agents (family members, peers, coaches, and teachers) have influenced your participation in physical activity.

In general, coaches and teachers appear to influence males more than females with regard to involvement in sport and physical activity. This statement, although quite true even today, was much more profound just a few decades ago (Ennis, 1996). With the increase in high school sport programs for females, we could assume stronger overall support for female participation and success.

Gender-Role Expectations and Stereotyping

Objective 14.8

Gender roles are social expectations of how individuals should act and think as males and females. Along with being influenced by biological factors (primarily sex hormones), socializing agents such as family members, schools, peers, and the media can have a significant effect on this aspect of human behavior. In general, parents tend to encourage boys and girls to engage in different types of play and activities (e.g., Campbell & Eaton, 1999; McBride-Chang & Jacklin, 1993).

Related to this aspect of sociocultural influence is **gender-role stereotyping**, the use of different methods to introduce boys and girls to physical activities and sports. Even as infants, girls tend to be handled more gently and protectively than boys (Fig. 14.4). Infant boys, on the other hand, are perceived as tougher, stronger, and more athletic and are more often given toys that require active play and the use of motor skills.

Toy selection and marketing traditionally are based on gender-role stereotyping and tied to socialization into physical activity and sport. For example, when a parent gives a basketball to a young boy, the gesture usually promotes physical activity in the form of shooting and dribbling and introduces the child to the sport. Although basketball also is considered a female sport, there seem to be few promotional products that use females as gender-role models. By about 3 years of age, most children have a firmly established preference for gender-appropriate play items. Although biological disposition cannot be completely ruled out, early preferences for play items probably are influenced strongly by parents and significant others. Social learning theory (Chapter 1) provides some insight into this phenomenon by suggesting that gender development occurs

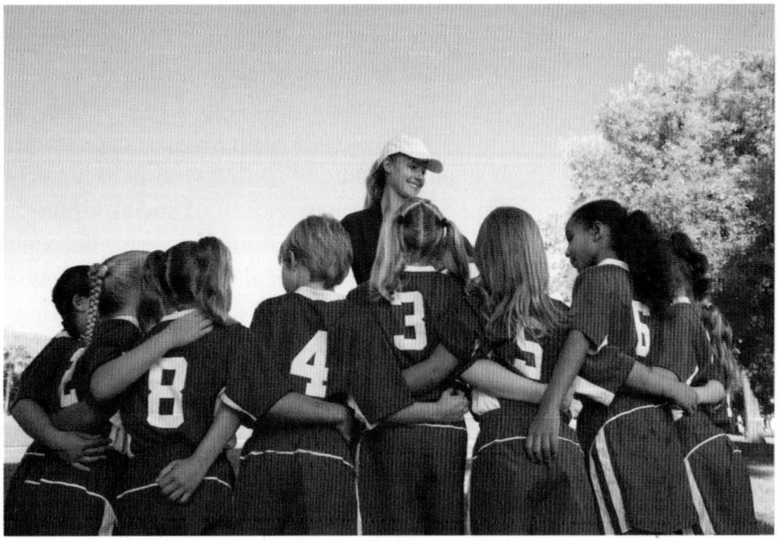

Figure 14.4 Encouragement with young girls can narrow the sports gender gap and encourage lifelong play.

WebLink

http://www.womenssports foundation.org

think about it

Explain your view of gender-role behavior.

think about it

Today, females participate more openly in what traditionally has been called "male-oriented" sports such boxing, body building, and wrestling. What are some of the issues and considerations?

primarily through observation and imitation of behavior and through reward and punishment with experience.

As children enter school, they also tend to be treated differently. For instance, males are more likely to receive strong support from family, relatives, peers, teachers, and coaches to begin and continue in sports. For boys, sport involvement is viewed as part of the young man's path to manhood, whereas such endeavors are traditionally not linked to becoming a woman. Because many girls are not encouraged to participate in skilled, vigorous motor activities, many never develop their skills to full potential. These attitudes also have an effect on the motivation to get involved seriously in sports and to train to achieve maximum performance.

During adolescence, gender-role expectations can be of primary influence in the individual's decision to get involved in sport activities. *Gender-role conflict* may be created when adolescents decide to participate in certain sport activities. Although it still appears today, in the past, this was a greater issue for female participation in sport—which form a traditional (outdated) perspective viewed as more of a masculine endeavor. A survey of high school graduates of the 1980s reported indications of less traditionalism (Suitor & Reavis, 1995). That is, compared to younger cohorts, those who graduated in the late 1980s noted an increase in gaining prestige through sports and a decrease in gaining prestige through cheerleading. For an excellent book on the rise of females in sport see Cahn (2015).

For males, however, involvement in sport seems to cause little gender-role conflict and is viewed as stereotypic of ideal male characteristics. Related research findings also suggest males are more easily socialized into sports than females are (Coakley, 2015).

However, society's view that females are the weaker gender appears to be changing. In more recent years, female participation in sports has increased not only at the youth sport level but also in school, university, and professional programs.

Self-esteem

Objective 14.9

Also referred to as self-image, **self-esteem** is the evaluative and *personal judgment of one's self*. The judgment does not necessitate accuracy so much as one's belief that it is correct. The term is often used interchangeably with **self-concept**. However, this term correctly refers to *domain-specific evaluations of the self* rather than a global (overall) evaluation. For example, you may have a low self-concept about math ability but a high self-concept regarding ability with a specific sport. Self-esteem is included in this section as a sociocultural factor because it is considered, in large part, a reflection of social support in the form of parents, peers, teachers, and coaches, and so on. For example, a child who is highly praised by a teacher for his or her physical ability and is preferred by peers as a teammate for games generally has a good sense of worth for this particular endeavor. Self-esteem is considered by some to be a critical index of mental health; a high sense of worth during childhood is linked to satisfaction in later life. However, global self-esteem judgments should be viewed with caution, for an individual's sense of worth may vary according to different skill domains and areas of competence. Variation within skill domains is not uncommon. Some individuals may have a strong sense of self-worth in, for example, basketball but not in baseball or track. Indications are that feelings about self-esteem are relatively well established by middle childhood (Harter, 2013).

Within the context of physical activity and youth sports involvement, researchers have found that such participation generally is associated with higher self-esteem (e.g., Raustorp & Lindwall, 2015; Schmidt et al., 2015). It would seem reasonable to expect a person who has good self-esteem regarding physical ability to be more likely to engage in complementary activities such as youth sports. On the other hand, research confirms that a person who has a low sense of physical competence is more likely to avoid these opportunities (see discussion on perceived motor competence in Chapter 9). Along with the internal factors associated with personality type and emotions, social interactions play a vital role in the development of self-esteem.

Although children younger than the age of about 10 years depend primarily on parents and the outcomes of contests for appraisals, those who are older tend to rely more on comparison to and appraisals provided by their peers (Horn & Weiss, 1991). In addition, feedback from teachers and coaches also may be influencing factors. For example, young athletes tend to exhibit higher self-esteem while playing for coaches who give frequent encouragement and corrective feedback, especially if the individual begins the sport with a relatively low sense of worth. Obviously, mental maturity, emotional state, manner of delivery, and rapport between athlete and coach are critical factors in effectiveness of communication and development of self-esteem.

Individuals with high self-esteem in their physical abilities may be more apt to join in sport programs. Nevertheless, a large portion of children and youth, especially females, drop out. Why is there a dropout (for both gender but more so for females)? According to a Women's Sports Foundation (2008) report, boys and girls between the ages of 6 and 9 years are equally interested in sport participation. *However, by age 14 years, girls drop out at a rate that is six times greater than boys.* One suggestion is that during adolescence, interest in sports conflicts with other opportunities more than it did in childhood. That is, adolescents have a greater number of desirable options during leisure time and more demands on how they use their time. This dropout dilemma may reflect a normal trial-and-error sampling done in research of an enjoyable activity or achievement domain. A second (general) perspective emphasizes the negative aspects of youth sports and disenchantment with participation. Such experiences as loss of interest, not having fun, lack of playing time, dislike for the coach, pressure to perform (or win), and lack of success have been suggested as factors in dropping out (e.g., Coakley, 2015; Craike et al., 2009).

Although different age groups may state different reasons for participating and continuing in youth sport programs, the most commonly stated reasons include to have fun, to improve skills, to demonstrate competency, the desire to compete, to please family and friends, to affiliate with or make new friends, and to be part of a team. There have been critics who suggest that much of youth sport is emotionally stressful due to, for example, an overemphasis on winning and maximum performance. However, in a thorough review of studies of state anxiety and associated symptoms in young athletes, Gould and Eklund (1996) estimated that only a small percentage (5% to 10%) was experiencing high levels of stress (e.g., loss of sleep and appetite).

Possible Influences of Race

Objective 14.10

One should be cautious when trying to discuss gender and race socialization in sport and physical activity due to the wonderful diversity in our culture and individual families. Earlier reports (1980s) provided indications that African American and

Caucasian children are socialized into sports differently. A generalization was that possible success in sports took on more importance for black youths compared to their white counterparts, especially for males from lower socioeconomic homes.

Encouragement from family members, same-sex peers, coaches, teachers, and the community may be more influential for blacks than for whites. It was suggested that some of this encouragement originates from the somewhat misleading perception that sports offer blacks more opportunities than other careers in society and therefore provide a more readily conceivable means for increasing social status; obviously, much of that has changed for many but not all. Harris and Hunt (1984) found that encouragement for involvement in sports among black youth gets stronger as they move through adolescence and begin to perceive major obstacles to success in careers outside of sports and entertainment. Adding to this view is the fact that although professional black athletes are strong role models for young blacks and whites, blacks have had fewer role models from other occupations to emulate. Certainly, this has changed in recent years with more minority role models in government, business, and education.

PRIMARY INFLUENCES DURING ADULTHOOD

Objective 14.11

Just as society and various cultures have expectations for individual behavior from infancy through adolescence, numerous sociocultural influences and expectations are also present through adulthood. Although home and school settings were dominant socializing factors prior to adulthood, these agents become less of a primary influence in establishing or changing behavior characteristics as individuals attain independence from the family and complete formal schooling. For the remainder of life, the primary agents are usually the media, peers, spouses, and other individuals in the community (e.g., doctors and class instructors). In addition to these influences, seasonal, personal, and situational factors that are continuous and dynamic over the life cycle (e.g., marriage, children, and employment situation) play an important role in adult sport socialization. Just as there are varying sociocultural views and expectations for behavior concerning health practices and physical activity in earlier years, a variety of views and trends are evident during adulthood. Society in general, as expressed through various media, places a premium on youth and good looks. The idea of living a zestful, active lifestyle while at the same time eating and drinking things that allow one to remain slim has been one of the central themes in advertising. In today's world, advertising is a powerful socializing agent.

WebLink

http://www.ncoa.com/ (National Council on Aging); http://www.nia.nih.gov/ (National Institute on Aging, see "Health and Aging")

During early adulthood, individuals can still be quite impressionable; the need for self-esteem and peer acceptance has led many to take up or continue physical activity in some form. This is also the period in the life span when most individuals are at their healthiest and reach peak physical performance (around age 30 years). For many individuals, the notion that they are at their best and not slowing down physically needs to be tested on a regular basis. However, many young adults have not been influenced by or do not have the desire to engage in physical activities as part of their lifestyle. In fact, empirical evidence suggests that due at least in part to their relatively healthy status during this period in their lives, many individuals do not think about how their lifestyles will affect their health in later years. College students specifically seem to have unrealistic and overly optimistic views about their future health and longevity. Unfortunately, many of the college students who are not healthy (e.g., overweight and unfit) have established attitudes concerning physical activity that are difficult to overcome.

As individuals approach middle age (ages 35 to 40 years), concern for health and physical appearance becomes more evident. For most individuals, this is a time when the regression of physical skills and signs of physical aging begin, which causes more attention to be drawn to these characteristics. Part of the stimulus for personal concern is likely related to two sociocultural influences. As mentioned earlier, our society places a premium on a healthy, youthful physical appearance. This factor alone is responsible for millions of dollars spent nationally each year on health and beauty items and on products to help preserve youthfulness. Many individuals begin dyeing gray hair, undergoing cosmetic surgery, and enrolling in weight reduction and conditioning classes, all in effort to maintain a healthy, youthful appearance.

Another major influence that has drawn attention and concern to health status and promoted physical activity is the flood of educational information that comes by way of the media. This information also is conveyed by physicians, peers, spouses, and various community agents (e.g., class instructors and pharmacists). For several years, there has been a national effort to make the general public aware of such health concerns as obesity, cardiovascular disease, high blood pressure, too much salt, high cholesterol, and lack of exercise.

Although recent trends seem to suggest that attitudes have changed with regard to involvement in physical activity and active sports among the middle-aged and elderly, as noted in previous chapters, many adults still decrease their level of involvement as they age. These views, by the individual and from others, may be described as a form of **age-related stereotyping**. Although such activities as swimming, jogging, and tennis currently are encouraged as lifelong pursuits, there are sociocultural forces that reinforce the idea that aging adults (especially the elderly) should be more sedentary with age. It is not uncommon to hear teenagers and adult children say, "You need to slow down, you are going to get hurt . . . ."

Objective 14.12

Although several social views of aging have been proposed, few have received more support than **activity theory**. Most research studies have found that when individuals continue to live active (including physically) and productive lives as older adults, their satisfaction with life, in general, does not decline and may even go up (Oerlemans et al., 2011; Phillips et al., 2013). In a large-scale study of Canadian older adults, Azagba and Sharaf (2014) observed that *those who were more physically active had greater life satisfaction and social interaction*. In essence, the more active older people are, the less likely they are to age atypically and show discontent with life (Fig. 14.5).

think about it

If you were presenting a speech on physical activity to senior adults, what would you say? Consider other chapter topics also.

In addition to this general view of aging, several theories related to exercise motivation in older adults have been proposed. One of the more interesting perspectives proposes that Bandura's social cognitive theory may be an appropriate framework to study this behavior (Dzewaltowski, 1989; Resnick, 2004). Using the triadic causation concept (the person, behavior, and context) as the basis for affecting change across the life span, three mechanisms are suggested as important mediators in influencing exercise motivation. Foremost is *self-efficacy*, defined as the individual's judgment of his or her capabilities to complete courses of action. Older adults who lack this characteristic usually drop out of or do not participate in exercise programs. As with younger populations, a strong influence in self-efficacy is interaction with various social agents. Mental and physical health directly influence this factor. A second factor is the value older persons place on the outcome and the provision of incentives, which is associated with *outcome expectations*.

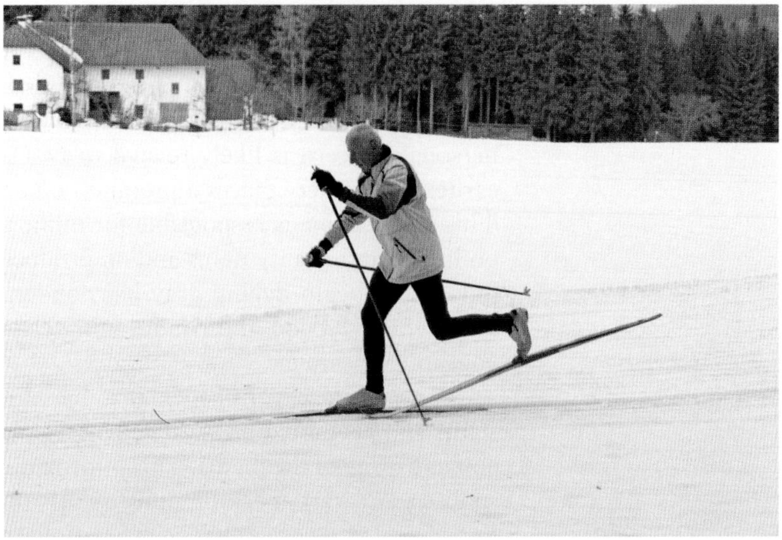

Figure 14.5 An active lifestyle during later adulthood increases the likelihood of life satisfaction.

The third mechanism, *self-evaluated dissatisfaction*, is illustrated by individuals who are motivated to exercise because they are not satisfied with their current level of performance (e.g., muscular strength and flexibility). Many older persons will continue exercising to avoid becoming dissatisfied if they quit. This perspective in general recognizes that in addition to psychological factors, social contexts and biological constraints are strong influences in exercise motivation in the elderly.

Summary

Sociocultural influences have been shown to have a lifelong effect on involvement in physical activity and motor development. Socialization is a lifelong process that refers to a set of events and processes by which individuals acquire the beliefs and behaviors of a particular society and subgroup (culture). Socialization is strongly influenced by various sociocultural agents that interpret culture to the individual. The major socializing agents are the family, school (teachers and coaches), peers, church, and the community. Within these agents are the influences of play and sport participation.

Gender-role stereotyping is practiced by several social agents. As a result of these influences, young males and females develop a preference for gender-appropriate play items and physical activities.

Self-esteem is a more global view of one's self, whereas self-concept reflects one's domain specific view. Both characteristics influence participation in play and sports involvement. Children praised by others generally have good self-esteem and are more likely to participate in organized activities.

Beginning with early adulthood, the primary social agents are the media (education), peers, spouses, and individuals in the community. Society in general, as expressed predominantly through the media, places a premium on youth and physical appearance. This influence, along with the positive habits formed in earlier years, causes many young adults to continue, improve on, or take up a physically active lifestyle.

As individuals approach middle age and enter later adulthood, concern for health status and physical appearance normally receives more attention. Society's emphasis on good health and youthfulness stimulates many to become involved in physical activity. Another strong agent is the extensive media promotion of information concerning the need for good health practices. Similar information may also be transmitted through peers, spouses, and members of the community.

Although recent trends seem to suggest that attitudes have changed with regard to involvement in physical activity among older adults, many still decrease their level of involvement as they age. However, of the various social views of aging, activity theory seems to have the most support. According to this view, an active lifestyle during later adulthood increases the likelihood for life satisfaction.

think about it

1. **How would you describe your particular context (home/community/state) in regard to being *socialized* into sport and physical activity?**
2. **How could you use Bronfenbrenner's bioecological systems framework and Process–Person–Context–Time (PPCT) model to study environmental effects on motor behavior?**
3. **Using your experience, describe how the various socializing agents (family members, peers, coaches, and teachers) have influenced your participation in physical activity.**
4. **Explain your view of gender-role behavior.**
5. **Today, females participate more openly in what traditionally has been called "male-oriented" sports such boxing, body building, and wrestling. What are some of the issues and considerations?**
6. **If you were presenting a speech on physical activity to senior adults, what would you say? Consider other chapter topics also.**

LEARNING ACTIVITIES

Objective: To observe and evaluate children engaged in various forms of play. Arrange permission to visit an early childhood or day-care facility where there are children 2 to 5 years of age. Select two children, observe and record play behavior using Parten's four categories over a period of 2 or 3 days.

Objective: To evaluate exercise program advertisements for adults. Search the Web or local newspaper for at least two exercise program advertisements. Using the causation mechanisms of self-efficacy, outcome expectations, and self-evaluated dissatisfaction, how would you describe their approach?

Adolph, K. E. (2008). Learning to move. *Current Directions in Psychological Science, 17*, 213–218.

Adolph, K. E., & Berger, S. E. (2015). Physical and motor development. In M. H. Bornstein & M. E. Lamb (Eds.), *Developmental science: An advanced textbook* (7th ed., pp. 261–333). New York, NY: Psychology Press.

Adolph, K. E., Cole, W. G., Komati, M., Garciaguirre, J. S., Badaly, D., Lingeman, J. M., . . . Sotsky, R. B. (2012). How do you learn to walk? Thousands of steps and dozens of falls per day. *Psychological Science, 23*, 1387–1394.

Adolph, K. E., Eppler, M. A., & Gibson, E. J. (1993). Crawling versus walking infants' perception of affordances for locomotion over sloping surfaces. *Child Development, 64*, 1158–1174.

Adolph, K. E., & Robinson, S. R. (2013). The road to walking: What learning to walk tells us about development. In P. Zelazo (Ed.), *Oxford handbook of developmental psychology* (pp. 403–443). New York, NY: Oxford University Press.

Adolph, K. E., & Robinson, S. R. (2015). Motor development. In L. Liben & U. Müller (Eds.), *Handbook of child psychology and developmental science: Cognitive processes* (7th ed., Vol. 2, pp. 114–157). Hoboken, NJ: Wiley.

Adolph, K. E., Vereijken, B., & Denny, M. A. (1998). Learning to crawl. *Child Development, 69*(5), 1299–1312.

Adrian, M., & Cooper, J. M. (1995). *Biomechanics of human movement* (2nd ed.). Madison, WI: Brown & Benchmark.

American Academy of Pediatrics. (2000). Intensive training and sports participation in young athletes. *Pediatrics, 106*, 154–157.

American Academy of Pediatrics. (2016). *Breastfeeding Initiatives*. Retrieved from https://www2.aap.org/breastfeeding/

Anderson, P. J., De Luca, C. R., Hutchinson, E., Roberts, G., & Doyle, L. W. (2010). Underestimation of developmental delay by the new Bayley-III Scale. *Archives of Pediatrics & Adolescent Medicine, 164*(4), 352–356.

Aniansson, A., Rundgren, A., & Sperling, L. (1980). Evaluation of functional capacity in activities of daily living in 70-year-old men and women. *Scandinavian Journal of Rehabilitation Medicine, 12*(4), 145–154.

Annett, M. (1970). The growth of manual preference and speed. *British Journal of Psychology 61*, 545–558.

Annett, M. (1985). *Left, right, hand, and brain: The right shift theory*. London, United Kingdom: Lawrence Erlbaum Associates.

Annett, M. (1996). In defence of the right shift theory. *Perceptual and Motor Skills, 82*, 115–137.

Apgar, V. A. (1953). A proposal for a new method of evaluation of the newborn infant. *Current Research in Anesthesia & Analgesia, 32*, 260–267.

Aslin, R. N. (2007). What's in a look? *Developmental Science, 10*(1), 48–53.

Astle, D. E., & Scerif, G. (2008). Using developmental cognitive neuroscience to study behavioral and attentional control. *Developmental Psychobiology, 51*(2), 107–118.

Azagba, S., & Sharaf, M. F. (2014). Physical inactivity among older Canadian adults. *Journal of Physical Activity & Health, 11*(1), 99–108.

Baddeley, A. D. (2012). Working memory: Theories, models, and controversies. *Annual Review of Psychology, 63*, 1–29.

Bandura, A. (1986). *Social foundations of thought and action: A social cognitive theory*. Englewood Cliffs, NJ: Prentice Hall.

Bandura, A. (2009). Social and policy impact of social cognitive theory. In M. Mark, S. Donaldson, & B. Campbell (Eds.), *Social psychology and evaluation* (pp. 33–70). New York, NY: Guilford Press.

Baranowski, T., Thompson, W. O., DuRant, R. H., Baranowski, J., & Puhl, J. (1993). Observations on physical activity in physical locations: Age, gender, ethnicity, and month effects. *Research Quarterly for Exercise and Sport, 64*(2), 127–133.

Barela, J. A., Godoi, D., Freitas Júnior, P. B., & Polastri, P. F. (2000). Visual information and body sway coupling in infants during sitting acquisition. *Infant Behavior and Development, 23*, 285–297.

Barnett, L. M., Ridgers, N. D., & Salmon, J. (2015). Associations between young children's perceived and actual ball skill competence and physical activity. *Journal of Science and Medicine in Sport, 18*(2), 167–171.

Barnett, L. M., van Beurden, E., Morgan, P. J., Brooks, L. O., & Beard, J. R. (2009). Childhood motor skill proficiency as a predictor of adolescent physical activity. *Journal of Adolescent Health, 44*, 252–259.

Barr, H. M., & Streissguth, A. P. (2001). Identifying maternal self-reported alcohol use associated with fetal alcohol spectrum disorders. *Alcoholism, Clinical and Experimental Research, 25*, 283–287.

Barsalou, L. W. (2008). Grounded cognition. *Annual Review of Psychology, 59*, 617–645.

Barto, A. G. (2002). Reinforcement learning in motor control. In M. Arbib (Ed.), *The handbook of brain theory and neural networks* (pp. 968–972). Cambridge, United Kingdom: MIT Press.

Bauer, P. J. (2009). Learning and memory: Like a horse and carriage. In A. Woodward & A. Needham (Eds.), *Learning and the infant mind* (pp. 3–28). New York, NY: Oxford University Press.

Bayley, N. (2006). *Bayley Scales of Infant and Toddler Development—Third Edition*. San Antonio, TX: Harcourt Assessment.

Beery, K. E., Buktenica N. A., & Beery N. A. (2010). *The Beery-Buktenica Developmental Test of Visual-Motor Integration: Administration, scoring, and teaching manual* (6th ed.). Minneapolis, MN Pearson.

Bennell, K., Khan, K., Matthews, B., Cook, E., Holzer, K., McKay, H., & Wark, J. (2000). Activity-associated differences in bone mineral are evident before puberty: A cross-sectional study of 130 female novice dancers and controls. *Pediatric Exercise Science*, *12*, 371–381.

Berardi, N., Sale, A., & Maffei, L. (2015). Brain structural and functional development: Genetics and experience. *Developmental Medicine and Child Neurology*, *57*, 4–9. http://dx.doi.10.1111/dmcn.12691

Berkey, C. S., Rockett, H. R., Field, A. E., Gillman, M. W., Frazier, A. L., Camargo, C. A., Jr., & Colditz, G. A. (2000). Activity, dietary intake, and weight changes in a longitudinal study of preadolescent and adolescent boys and girls. *Pediatrics*, *105*(4), E56.

Bernstein, N. (1967). *The coordination and regulation of movements*. London, United Kingdom: Pergamon Press.

Bertenthal, B. I., Boker, S. M., & Xu, M. (2000). Analysis of the perception-action cycle for visually induced postural sway in 9-month-old sitting infants. *Infant Behavior and Development*, *23*, 299–315.

Bertenthal, B. I., Rose, J. L., & Bai, D. L. (1997). Perception-action coupling inthe development of visual control of posture. *Journal of Experimental Psychology: Human Perception and Performance*, *23*, 1631–1643.

Berthelot, G., Len, S., Hellard, P., Tafflet, M., Guillaume, M., Vollmer, J. C., . . . Toussaint, J. F. (2012). Exponential growth combined with exponential decline explains lifetime performance evolution in individual and human species. *Age*, *34*(4), 1001–1009.

Berthier, N. E., & Carrico, R. L. (2010). Visual information and object size in infant reaching. *Infant Behavior & Development*, *33*(4), 555–566.

Berthier, N. E., Rosenstein, M. T., & Barto, A. G. (2005). Approximate optimal control as a model for motor learning. *Psychological Review*, *112*, 329–346.

Biddle, S. J. H., Whitehead, S. H., O'Donovan, T. M., & Nevill, M. E. (2005).Correlates of participation in physical activity for adolescent girls: A systematic review of recent literature. *Journal of Physical Activity & Health*, *2*, 423–434.

Bjorklund, D. F. (2004). *Children's thinking: Developmental function and individual differences* (4th ed.). Belmont, CA: Wadsworth.

Blair, S. N., Kohl, H. W., III, Paffenbarger, R. S., Jr., Clark, D. G., Cooper, K. H., & Gibbons, L. W. (1989). Physical fitness and all-cause mortality. A prospective study of healthy men and women. *JAMA*, *262*, 2395–2401.

Blake, R., & Sekuler, R. (2005). *Perception* (5th ed.). New York, NY: McGraw-Hill.

Blanchette, N., Smith, M. L., Fernandes-Penney, A., King, S., & Read, S. (2001). Cognitive and motor development in children with vertically transmitted HIV infection. *Brain and Cognition*, *46*, 50–53.

Blote, A. W., & Van Haasteren, R. (1989). Developmental dimensions in the drawing behavior of pre-school children. *Journal of Human Movement Studies*, *17*, 187–205.

Bornstein, M. H., Hahn, C. S., & Suwalsky, J. T. (2013). Physically developed and exploratory young infants contribute to their own long-term academic achievement. *Psychological Science*, *24*, 1906–1917.

Botwinick, J., & Storandt, M. (1974). *Memory, related functions and age*. Springfield, IL: Charles C. Thomas.

Bourassa, D. C., McManus, I. C., & Bryden, M. P. (1996). Handedness and eye-dominance: A meta-analysis of their relationship. *Laterality*, *1*(1), 5–34.

Bower, T. G. R. (1976). Repetitive processes in child development. *Scientific American*, *235*(5), 38–47.

Bower, T. G. R. (1989). *The rational infant: Learning in infancy (A series of books of psychology)*. New York, NY: Freeman.

Boyce, B. A., Coker, C. A., & Bunker, L. K. (2006). Implications for variability of practice from pedagogy and motor learning perspectives: Finding a common ground. *Quest*, *58*, 330–343.

Brazelton, T., & Nugent, J. (2011). *The neonatal behavioral assessment scale* (4th ed.). London, United Kingdom: MacKeith Press.

Broca, P. (1865). Sur le siège de la faculté du langage articulé. *Bulletins de la Société d'anthropologie de Paris*, *6*, 377–393.

Broekhoff, J. (1986). The effect of physical activity on physical growth and development. In G. A. Stull & H. M. Eckert (Eds.), *Effects of physical activity on children* (pp. 75–87). Champaign, IL: Human Kinetics.

Bronfenbrenner, U. (1986). Ecology of the family as a context for human development: Research perspectives. *Developmental Psychology*, *22*, 723–742.

Bronfenbrenner, U. (1995). Developmental ecology through space and time: A future perspective. In P. Moen, G. H. Elder, & K. Luscher (Eds.), *Examining lives in context: Perspectives on the ecology of human development* (pp. 599–618). Washington, DC: American Psychological Association.

Bronfenbrenner, U. (2005). The bioecological theory of human development. In U. Brofenbrenner (Ed.), *Making human being human: Bioecological perspectives on human development* (pp. 3–15). Thousand Oaks, CA.

Brown, T., & Hockey, S. C. (2013). The validity and reliability of developmental test of visual perception-2nd edition (DTVP-2). *Physical & Occupational Therapy in Pediatrics*, *33*(4), 426–439.

Brown-Séquard, C. E. (1877). *Dual character of the brain, etc. (The toner lectures. Lecture II)*. Washington, DC: Smithsonian Institute.

Bruininks, B. D., & Bruininks, R. H. (2012). *Bruininks Motor Ability Test (BMAT)*. Minneapolis, MN: Pearson.

Bruininks, R. H., & Bruininks, B. D. (2005). *Bruininks-Oseretsky Test of Motor Proficiency, second edition (BOT-2)*. Minneapolis, MN: Pearson.

Caçola, P. M., Gabbard, C., Montebelo, M. I., & Santos, D. C. (2015). Further development and validation of the Affordances in the Home Environment for Motor Development-Infant Scale (AHEMD-IS). *Physical Therapy*, *95*(6), 901–923.

Campbell, D., & Eaton, W. (1999). Sex differences in the activity levels of infants. *Infant and Child Development*, *8*, 1–17.

Campbell, J. M., Marcinowski, E. C., Babik, I., & Michel, G. F. (2015). The influence of a hand preference for acquiring objects on the development of a hand preference for unimanual manipulation from 6 to 14 months. *Infant Behavior & Development*, *39*, 107–117.

Campbell, S. K., & Kolobe, T. H. A. (2000). Concurrent validity of the test of infant motor performance with the Alberta Infant Motor Scale. *Pediatric Physical Therapy*, *12*, 1–8.

Campbell, S. K., & Kolobe, T. H. A., Osten, E., Girolami, G. L., & Lenski, M. (1994). *Test of Infant Motor Performance*. Chicago, IL: Department of Physical Therapy, University of Illinois.

Cao, X., Laplante, D. P., Brunet, A., Ciampi, A., & King, S. (2014). Prenatal maternal stress affects motor function in

5½-year-old children: Project ice storm. *Developmental Psychobiology*, *56*(1), 117–125.

Cardoso, A. C., Campos, A. C., Santos, M. M., Santos, D. C., & Rocha, N. A. (2015). Motor performance of children with Down syndrome and typical development at 2 to 4 and 26 months. *Pediatric Physical Therapy*, *27*(2), 135–141.

Carlson, J. L. (2015). The menstrual cycle. In C. Gordon & LeBoff, M. (Eds.), *The female athlete triad: A clinical guide* (pp. 29–38). New York, NY: Springer Publishing.

Carter, J. E. L. (2002). *The Heath-Carter anthropometric somatotype instruction manual*. San Diego, CA: San Diego State University.

Carter, J. E. L., & Heath, B. H. (1990). *Somatotyping—Development and applications*. Cambridge, United Kingdom: Cambridge University Press.

Carter, R. C., Jacobson, J. L., Sokol, R. J., Avison, M. J., & Jacobson, S. W. (2013). Fetal alcohol related growth restriction from birth through young adulthood and moderating effects of maternal prepregnancy weight. *Alcoholism, Clinical and Experimental Research*, *37*(3), 452–462.

Case-Smith, J. (1996). Analysis of current motor development theory and recently published infant motor assessments. *Infants & Young Children*, *9*(1), 29–41.

Case-Smith, J., & Bigsby, R. (2000). *Posture and fine-motor assessment of infants*. San Antonio, TX: Psychological Corporation.

Centers for Disease Control and Prevention. (2015). *Childhood overweight and obesity*. Atlanta, GA: U.S. Department of Health and Human Services.

Centers for Disease Control and Prevention. (2016). *Overweight & obesity*. Atlanta, GA: U.S. Department of Health and Human Services.

Chase, C., Ware, J., Hittelman, J., Blasini, I., Smith, R., Llorente, A., . . . Kaligh, L. I. (2000). Early cognitive and motor development among infants born to women infected with human immunodeficiency virus. *Pediatrics*, *106*(2), E25.

Cheng, W., Ji, X., Zhang, J., & Feng, J. (2012). Individual classification of ADHD patients by integrating multiscale neuroimaging markers and advanced pattern recognition techniques. *Frontiers in Systems Neuroscience*, *6*, 58.

Cherry, E. C. (1953). Some experiments on the recognition of speech, with one and with two ears. *Journal of the Acoustical Society of America*, *25*, 975–979.

Chi, M. (1978). Knowledge structures and memory development. In R. Siegler (Ed.), *Children's thinking: What develops?* (pp. 73–95). Hillsdale, NJ: Lawrence Erlbaum Associates.

Chou, C. H., Hwang, C. L., & Wu, Y. T. (2012). Effect of exercise on physical function, daily living activities, and quality of life in the frail older adults: A meta-analysis. *Archives of Physical Medicine and Rehabilitation*, *93*(2), 237–244.

Chugani, H. T. (1998). A critical period of brain development: Studies of cerebral glucose utilization with PET. *Preventive Medicine*, *27*, 184–188.

Clark, J. E., & Phillips, S. J. (1993). A longitudinal study of intralimb coordination in the first year of independent walking: A dynamical systems analysis. *Child Development*, *64*, 1143–1157.

Clark, J. E., Lanphear, A. K., & Riddick, C. C. (1987). The effects of videogame playing on the response selection processing of elderly adults. *Journal of Gerontology*, *42*(1), 82–85.

Clarke, H. H. (Ed.). (1975). Joint and body range of movement. *Physical Fitness Research Digest*, *5*, 16–18.

Cliff, D. P., Okely, A. D., Morgan, P. J., Jones, R. A., Steele, J. R., & Baur, L. A. (2012). Proficiency deficiency: Mastery of fundamental movement skills and skill components in overweight and obese children. *Obesity*, *20*(5), 1024–1033.

Clifton, R. K., Muir, D. W., Ashmead, D. H., & Clarkson, M. G. (1993). Is visually guided reaching in early infancy a myth? *Child Development*, *64*(4), 1099–1110.

Coakley, J. J. (2015). *Sport in society: Issues and controversies*. (11th ed.). New York, NY: McGraw-Hill.

Cohn, D., Livingston, G., & Wang, W. (2012). *After decades of decline, a rise in stay-at-home mothers*. Retrieved from http://www.pewsocialtrends.org/2014/04/08/after-decades-of-decline-a-rise-in-stay-at-home-mothers/

Colcombe, S., & Kramer, A. F. (2003). Fitness effects on the cognitive function of older adults: A meta-analytic study. *Psychological Science*, *14*(2), 125–130.

Corballis, M. C. (1983). *Human laterality*. New York, NY: Academic Press.

Corballis, M. C., & Morgan, M. J. (1978). On the biological basis of human laterality: I. Evidence for a maturational left–right gradient. *Behavioral and Brain Sciences*, *1*(2), 261–269.

Corbetta, D., Thelen, E., & Johnson, K. (2000). Motor constraints on the development of perception-action matching in infant reaching. *Infant Behavior and Development*, *23*(3–4), 351–374.

Coveney, P., & Highfield, R. (1995). *Frontiers of complexity: The search for order in a chaotic world*. New York, NY: Ballantine Books.

Cowan, N., Saults, J. S., & Clark, K. M. (2015). Exploring age differences in visual working memory capacity: Is there a contribution of memory for configuration? *Journal of Experimental Child Psychology*, *135*, 72–85.

Craike, M. J., Symons, C., & Zimmermann, J. A. M. (2009). Why do young women drop out of sport and physical activity? A social ecological approach. *Annals of Leisure Research*, *12*(2), 148–172.

Cratty, B. (1986). *Perceptual and motor development in infants and children* (3rd ed.). Englewood Cliffs, NJ: Prentice Hall.

Cummings, M. F., van Hof-van Duin, J., Mayer, D. L., Hansen, R. M., & Fulton, A. B. (1988). Visual fields of young children. *Behavioral Brain Research*, *29*, 7–16.

Currie, C., Ahluwalia, N., Godeau, E., Nic Gabhainn, S., Due, P., & Currie, D. B. (2012). Is obesity at individual and national level associated with lower age at menarche? Evidence from 34 countries in the Health Behaviour in School-Aged Children study. *Journal of Adolescent Health*, *50*, 621–626.

Czajkowska, M., Drosdzol-Cop, A., Gałązka, I., Naworska, B., & Skrzypulec-Plinta, V. (2015). Menstrual cycle and the prevalence of premenstrual syndrome/premenstrual dysphoric disorder in adolescent athletes. *Journal of Pediatric and Adolescent Gynecology*, *28*, 492–498.

Daly, R. M., Bass, S., Caine, D., & Howe, W. (2002). Does training affect growth? Answers to common questions. *The Physician and Sportsmedicine*, *30*(10), 21–29.

Damsgaard, R., Bencke, J., Matthiesen, G., Petersen, J. H., & Müller, J. (2000). Is prepubertal growth adversely affected by sport? *Medicine and Science in Sports and Exercise*, *32*(10), 1698–1703.

Dargent-Paré, C., De Agostini, M., Mesbah, M., & Dellatolas, G. (1992). Foot and eye preferences in adults: Relationship with handedness, sex and age. *Cortex*, *28*, 343–351.

Darrah, J., Bartlett, D., Maguire, T. O., Avison, W. R., & Lacaze-Masmonteil, T. (2014). Have infant gross motor abilities changed in 20 years? A re-evaluation of the Alberta Infant Motor Scale normative values. *Developmental Medicine and Child Neurology*, *56*(9), 877–881.

Datar, A., & Jacknowitz, A. (2009). Birth weight effects on children's mental, motor, and physical development: Evidence from twins data. *Maternal and Child Health Journal*, *13*(6), 780–794.

Davids, K., Bennett, S., Kingsbury, D., Jolley, L., & Brain, T. (2000). Effects of postural constraints on children's catching behavior. *Research Quarterly for Exercise and Sport*, *71*(1), 69–73.

Davis, W. E., & Broadhead, G. D. (Eds.). (2007). *Ecological task analysis and movement*. Champaign, IL: Human Kinetics.

Davison, K. K., Werder, J. L., Trost, S. G., Baker, B. L., & Birch, L. L. (2007). Why are early maturing girls less active? Links between pubertal development, psychological well-being, and physical activity among girls at ages 11 and 13. *Social Science & Medicine*, *64*(12), 2391–2404.

Deach, D. (1950). *Genetic development of motor skills in children two through six years of age* (Unpublished doctoral dissertation). University of Michigan, Ann Arbor.

de Jong, M., Verhoeven, M., Lasham, C. A., Meijssen, C. B., & van Baar, A. L. (2015). Behaviour and development in 24-month-old moderately preterm toddlers. *Archives of Disease in Childhood*, *100*(6), 548–553.

Delacato, C. H. (1966). *Neurological organization and reading*. Springfield, IL: Charles C. Thomas.

Deli, E., Bakle, I., & Zachopoulou, E. (2006). Implementing intervention movement programs for kindergarten children. *Journal of Early Childhood Research*, *4*(1), 5–18.

D'Hondt, E., Deforche, B., Gentier, I., De Bourdeaudhuij, I., Vaeyens, R., Philippaerts, R., & Lenoir, M. (2013). A longitudinal analysis of gross motor coordination in overweight and obese children versus normal-weight peers. *International Journal of Obesity*, *37*(1), 61–67.

D'Hondt, E., Deforche, B., Gentier, I., Verstuyf, J., Vaeyens, R., De Bourdeaudhuij, I., . . . Lenoir, M. (2014). A longitudinal study of gross motor coordination and weight status in children. *Obesity*, *22*, 1505–1511. http://dx.doi.org/10.1002/oby.20723

Diamond, A. (2016). *Developmental cognitive neuroscience*. Retrieved from http://www.devcogneuro.com

Dietz, W. (1997). Periods of risk in childhood for the development of adult obesity—What do we need to learn? *Journal of Nutrition*, *127*, 1884S–1886S.

DiLorenzo, T. M., Stucky-Ropp, R. C., Vander Wal, J. S., & Gotham, H. J. (1998). Determinants of exercise among children. II. A longitudinal analysis. *Preventive Medicine*, *27*(3), 470–477.

DiPietro, J. A., Novak, M. F., Costigan, K. A., Atella, L. D., & Reusing, S. P. (2006). Maternal psychological distress during pregnancy in relation to child development at age two. *Child Development*, *77*(3), 573–587.

Doll, C. A., & Broadie, K. (2014). Impaired activity-dependent neural circuit assembly and refinement in autism spectrum disorder genetic models. *Frontiers in Cellular Neuroscience*, *8*, 30.

Domellöf, E., Barbu-Roth, M., Rönnqvist, L., Jacquet, A. Y., & Fagard, J. (2015). Infant manual performance during reaching and grasping for objects moving in depth. *Frontiers in Psychology*, *6*, 1142.

Dominici, N., Ivanenko, Y. P., Cappellini, G., d'Avella, A., Mondì, V., Cicchese, M., . . . Lacquaniti, F. (2011). Locomotor primitives in newborn babies and their development. *Science*, *334*(6058), 997–999.

Doney, R., Lucas, B. R., Jones, T., Howat, P., Sauer, K., & Elliott, E. J. (2014). Fine motor skills in children with prenatal alcohol exposure or fetal alcohol spectrum disorder. *Journal of Developmental and Behavioral Pediatrics*, *35*(9), 598–609.

Dzewaltowski, D. A. (1989). A social cognitive theory of older adult exercise motivation. In A. C. Ostrow (Ed.), *Aging and motor behavior* (pp. 257–281). Indianapolis, IN: Benchmark Press.

Eckert, H. M. (1987). *Motor development* (3rd ed.). Indianapolis, IN: Benchmark Press.

Edelman, G. M. (1989). *The remembered present*. New York, NY: Basic Books.

Edelman, G. M. (1992). *Bright air, brilliant fire*. New York, NY: Basic Books.

Einkauf, D. K., Gohdes, M. L., Jensen, G. M., & Jewell, M. J. (1987). Changes in spinal mobility with increasing age in women. *Physical Therapy*, *67*, 370–375.

Einspieler, C., Prechtl, H. R. F., Bos, A., Ferrari, F., & Cioni, G. (2008). *Prechtl's method on the qualitative assessment of general movements in preterm, term and young infants*. Hoboken, NJ: Wiley.

Ennis, C. D. (1996). Student's experiences in sport-based physical education: More than apologies are necessary. *Quest*, *48*, 453–456.

Espenschade, A. (1960). Motor development. In W. R. Johnson (Ed.), *Science and medicine of exercise and sport*. New York, NY: Harper.

Eveleth, P. B., & Tanner, J. M. (1990). *Worldwide variation in human growth* (2nd ed.). Cambridge, United Kingdom: Cambridge University Press.

Fagard, J., & Jacquet, A. Y. (1996). Changes in reaching and grasping objects of different sizes between 7 and 13 months of age. *British Journal of Developmental Psychology*, *14*, 65–78.

Fagard, J., Spelke, E., & von Hofsten, C. (2009). Reaching and grasping a moving object in 6-, 8-, and 10-month-old infants: Laterality and performance. *Infant Behavior & Development*, *32*, 137–146.

Fakhouri, T. H., Hughes, J. P., Burt, V. L., Song, M., Fulton, J. E., & Ogden, C. L. (2014). Physical activity in U.S. youth aged 12–15 years, 2012. *NCHS Data Brief*, 141, 1–8.

Fenercioglu, A. K., Tamer, I., Karatekin, G., & Nuhoglu, A. (2009). Impaired postnatal growth of infants prenatally exposed to cigarette smoking. *The Tohoku Journal of Experimental Medicine*, *218*(3), 221–228.

Fiorentino, M. R. (1981). *A basis for sensorimotor development—Normal and abnormal: The influence of the primitive, postural reflexes on the development and distribution of tone*. Springfield, IL: Charles C. Thomas.

Fischman, M. G., Moore, J. B., & Steele, K. H. (1992). Children's one-hand catching as a function of age, gender, and ball location. *Research Quarterly for Exercise and Sport*, *63*(4), 349–355.

Fitts, P. M. (1954). The information capacity of the human motor system in controlling the amplitude of movement. *Journal of Experimental Psychology*, *47*, 381–391.

Flavell, J. H., Miller, P. H., & Miller, S. A. (1993). *Cognitive development* (3rd ed.). Englewood Cliffs, NJ: Prentice Hall.

Flegal, K. M., Carroll, M. D., Ogden, C. L., & Curtin, L. R. (2010). Prevalence and trends in obesity among US adults, 1999-2008. *JAMA*, *303*(3), 235–241.

Folio, R., & Fewell, R. (2000). *Peabody Developmental Motor Scales* (2nd ed.). Austin, TX: Pro ed.

Fox, N. A., & Rutter, M. (2010). Introduction to the special section on the effects of early experience on development. *Child Development*, *81*(1), 23–27.

Frankenburg, W. K., Dodds, J., Archer, P., Bresnick, B., Maschka, P., Edelman, N., & Shapiro, H. (1990). *Denver II screening manual*. Denver, CO: Denver Developmental Materials.

Freedland, R. L., & Bertenthal, B. I. (1994). Developmental changes in interlimb coordination: Transition to hands-and-knees crawling. *Psychological Science*, *5*(1), 26–32.

Friedman, D. (2013). The cognitive aging of episodic memory: A view based on the event-related brain potential. *Frontiers in Behavioral Neuroscience*, 7, 111.

Frisch, R. E. (1991). Puberty and body fat. In R. M. Lerner, A. C. Petersen, & J. Brooks-Gunn (Eds.), *Encyclopedia of adolescence* (pp. 884–892). New York, NY: Garland.

Gabbard, C., Gonçalves, V., & Santos, D. (2001). Visual-motor integration problems in low birth weight infants. *Journal of Clinical Psychology in Medical Settings*, *8*(3), 199–204.

Gabbard, C., & Hart, S. (1996). Probing Previc's theory of postural control. *Brain and Cognition*, *30*(3), 351–353.

Gabbard, C., & Iteya, M. (1996). Foot laterality in children, adolescents, and adults. *Laterality*, *1*(3), 199–205.

Galloway, J. C., & Thelen, E. (2004). Feet first: Object exploration in young infants. *Infant Behavior & Development*, *27*(1), 107–112.

Gard, L., & Rösblad, B. (2009). The qualitative motor observations in Movement ABC: Aspects of reliability and validity. *Advances in Physiotherapy*, *11*(2), 51–57.

Gesell, A. (1925). *The mental growth of the pre-school child: A psychological outline of normal development from birth to the sixth year, including a system of developmental diagnosis*. New York, NY: Macmillan.

Gibson, E. J. (2001). *Perceiving the affordances: A portrait of two psychologists*. Mahwah, NJ: Lawrence Erlbaum Associates.

Gibson, E. J., & Walk, R. D. (1960). The "visual cliff." *Scientific American*, *202*, 64–71.

Gibson, E. J., & Walker, A. S. (1984). Development of knowledge of visual-tactual affordances of substance. *Child Development*, *55*, 453–460.

Gibson, J. J. (1979). *The ecological approach to visual perception*. Boston, MA: Houghton Mifflin.

Gibson, J. J. (2014). *The ecological approach to visual perception: Classic edition*. New York, NY: Psychology Press.

Gilsanz, V., & Ratib, O. (2012). *Hand bone age: A digital atlas of skeletal maturity* (2nd ed.). Berlin, Germany: Springer.

Ginsburg, K. R. (2007). The importance of play in promoting healthy child development and maintaining strong parent-child bonds. *Pediatrics*, *119*(1), 182–191.

Glassy, D., & Romano, J. (2003). Selecting appropriate toys for young children: The pediatrician's role. *Pediatrics*, *111*(4), 911–913. Retrieved from http://pediatrics.aappublications.org/content/111/4/911

Glenberg, A. M. (2015). Few believe the world is flat: How embodiment is changing the scientific understanding of cognition. *Canadian Journal of Experimental Psychology*, *69*(2), 165–171.

Gofer-Levi, M., Silberg, T., Brezner, A., & Vakil, E. (2013). Deficit in implicit motor sequence learning among children and adolescents with spastic cerebral palsy. *Research in Developmental Disabilities*, *34*(11), 3672–3678.

Goldfield, E. (1995). *Emergent forms: Origins and early development of human action and perception*. New York, NY: Oxford University Press.

Goolsby, M. (2014). Female athlete triad. In M. L. Mountjoy (Ed.), *Handbook of sports medicine and science: The female athlete*. Hoboken, NJ: Wiley.

Gottlieb, G. (2007). Probabilistic epigenesis: A review. *Developmental Science*, *10*, 1–11.

Gould, D., & Eklund, R. C. (1996). Emotional stress and anxiety in the child and adolescent athlete. In O. Bar-Or (Ed.), *The child and adolescent athlete* (pp. 383–398). Oxford, United Kingdom: Blackwell.

Gracia-Bafalluy, M., & Noël, M. (2008). Does finger training increase young children's numerical performance? *Cortex*, *44*(4), 368–375.

Graham, G., Shirley, A., & Melissa, P. (2013). *Children moving: A reflective approach to teaching physical education with movement analysis* (9th ed.). New York, NY: McGraw-Hill.

Grattan, M. P., De Vos, E., Levy, J., & McClintock, M. K. (1992). Asymmetric action in the human newborn: Sex differences in patterns of organization. *Child Development*, *63*, 273–289.

Green, J. S., Stanforth, P. R., Rankinen, T., Leon, A. S., Rao, D. C., Skinner, J. S., . . . Wilmore, J. H. (2004). The effects of exercise training on abdominal visceral fat, body composition, and indicators of the metabolic syndrome in postmenopausal women with and without estrogen replacement therapy: The HERITAGE family study. *Metabolism*, *53*, 1192–1196.

Greenspan, E. (1983). *Little winners: Inside the world of the child sports star*. Boston, MA: Little Brown.

Hadders-Algra, M. (2010). Variation and variability: Key words in human motor development. *Physical Therapy*, *90*(12), 1823–1837.

Haehl, V., Vardaxis, V., & Ulrich, B. (2000). Learning to cruise: Bernstein's theory applied to skill acquisition during infancy. *Human Movement Science*, *19*, 685–715.

Hall, S. (2014). *Basic biomechanics* (7th ed.). New York, NY: McGraw-Hill.

Halford, G. S., & Andrews, G. (2011). Information-processing models of cognitive development. In U. Goswami (Ed.), *The Wiley-Blackwell handbook of childhood cognitive development* (2nd ed., pp. 697–722). Oxford, United Kingdom: Blackwell.

Halverson, L. E., Roberton, M. A., & Langendorfer, S. (1982). Development of the overarm throw: Movement and ball velocity changes by seventh grade. *Research Quarterly for Exercise and Sport*, *53*, 198–205.

Halverson, L. E., & Williams, K. (1985). Developmental sequences for hopping distance: A pre-longitudinal screening. *Research Quarterly for Exercise and Sport*, *56*, 37–44.

Hammill, D. D., Pearson, N. A., & Voress, J. K. (2013). *Developmental Test of Visual Perception-Second edition: DTVP-2*. Minneapolis, MN: Pearson.

Hands, B., Licari, M., & Piek, J. (2015). A review of five tests to identify motor coordination difficulties in young adults. *Research in Developmental Disabilities*, *41–42*, 40–51.

Harris, O., & Hunt, L. (1984).Race and sports involvement: Some implications of sports for black and white youth. Paper present at the meeting of the American Alliance for Health, Physical Education, Recreation, and Dance, Anaheim, CA.

Harter, S. (2013). The development of self-esteem. In M. H. Kernis (Ed.), *Self-esteem issues and answers: A sourcebook of current perspectives* (pp. 144–150). New York, NY: Psychology Press.

Hart, S., & Gabbard, C. (1997). Examining the stabilizing characteristics of footedness. *Laterality: Asymmetries of Body, Brain and Cognition, 2*(1), 17–26.

Haubenstricker, J., Branta, C., Seefeldt, V., Forsblom, L., & Kiger, J. (1990, June). *Prelongitudinal screening of a developmental sequence of skipping*. Paper presented at the annual meeting of the North American Society for the Psychology of Sport and Physical Activity, Houston, TX.

Haubenstricker, J., & Seefeldt, V. (1986). Acquisition of motor skills during childhood. In V. Seefeldt (Ed.), *Physical activity and well-being* (pp. 41–102). Reston, VA: American Alliance for Health, Physical Education, Recreation and Dance.

Haubenstricker, J. L., Wisner, D., Seefeldt, V., & Branta, C. (1997). Gender differences and mixed-longitudinal norms on selected motor skills for children and youth. *Journal of Sport & Exercise Psychology, 19*, S63.

Henderson, A., & Pehoski, C. (2006). *Hand function in the child: Foundations for remediation* (2nd ed.). St. Louis, MO: Mosby.

Henderson, S. E., Sugden, D. A., & Barnett, A. L. (2007). *Movement assessment battery for children, 2nd edition (MABC-2)*. London, United Kingdom: The Psychological Corporation.

Henriksson, M., & Hirschfeld, H. (2004). Physically active older adults display alterations in gait initiation. *Gait & Posture, 21*(3), 289–296.

Hepper, P. G. (2003). Prenatal psychological and behavioral development. In J. Valsiner & K. J. Connolly (Eds.), *Handbook of developmental psychology* (pp. 91–113). London, United Kingdom: Sage.

Hepper, P. G., McCartney, G. R., & Shannon, E. A. (1998). Lateralised behaviour in first trimester human foetuses. *Neuropsychologia, 36*(6), 531–534.

Hepper, P. G., Shahidullah, S., & White, R. (1991). Handedness in the human fetus. *Neuropsychologia, 29*(11), 1107–1111.

Heyward, V., & Wagner, D. (2004). *Applied body composition assessment* (2nd ed.). Champaign, IL: Human Kinetics.

Hill, E. L., & Khanem, F. (2009). The development of hand preference in children: The effect of task demands and links with manual dexterity. *Brain and Cognition, 71*(2), 99–107.

Holfelder, B., & Schott, N. (2014). Relationship of fundamental movement skills and physical activity in children and adolescents: A systematic review. *Psychology of Sport and Exercise, 15*(4), 382–391.

Horn, T. S., & Weiss, M. R. (1991). A developmental analysis of children's self-ability judgments in the physical domain. *Pediatric Exercise Science, 3*, 310–326.

Howley, E. T., & Thompson, D. L. (2012). *Fitness professional's handbook* (6th ed.). Champaign, IL: Human Kinetics.

Hubel, D. H., & Wiesel, T. N. (1970). The period of susceptibility to the physiological effects of unilateral eye closure in kittens. *The Journal of Physiology, 206*(2), 419–436.

Hughes, F. P., & Noppe, L. D. (1991). *Human development across the life span*. New York, NY: Macmillan.

Hume, C., Okely, A., Bagley, S., Telford, A., Booth, M., Crawford, D., & Salmon, J. (2008). Does weight status influence associations between children's fundamental movement skills and physical activity? *Research Quarterly for Exercise and Sport, 79*(2), 158–165.

Husby, I. M., Skranes, J., Olsen, A., Brubakk, A. M., & Evensen, K. A. (2013). Motor skills at 23 years of age in young adults born preterm with very low birth weight. *Early Human Development, 89*(9), 747–754.

Huttenlocher, P. R., & Dabholkar, A. S. (1997). Regional differences in synaptogenesis in human cerebral cortex. *The Journal of Comparative Neurology, 387*, 167–178.

Hyde, K. L., Lerch, J., Norton, A., Forgeard, M., Winner, E., Evans, A. C., & Schlaug, G. (2009). The effects of musical training on structural brain development: A longitudinal study. *Annals of New York Academy of Sciences, 1169*, 182–186.

Ishak, S., Franchak, J. M., & Adolph, K. E. (2014). Perception-action development from infants to adults: Perceiving affordances for reaching through openings. *Journal of Experimental Child Psychology, 117*, 92–105.

Jaakkola, T., Yli-Piipari, S., Huotari, P., Watt, A., & Liukkonen, J. (2015). Fundamental movement skills and physical fitness as predictors of physical activity: A 6-year follow-up study. *Scandinavian Journal of Medicine & Science in Sports, 26*, 74–81.

Jackson, A. S., Beard, E. F., Wier, L. T., Ross, R. M., Stuteville, J. E., & Blair, S. N. (1995). Changes in aerobic power of men, ages 25-70 yr. *Medical and Science in Sports Exercise, 27*, 113–120.

James, W. (1950). *The principles of psychology*. New York, NY: Dover.

Janssen, L., & Steenbergen, B. (2011). Typical and atypical (cerebral palsy) development of unimanual and bimanual grasp planning. *Research in Developmental Disabilities, 32*, 963–971.

Jersild, A. T., & Bienstock, S. F. (1935). Development of rhythm in young children. *Monographs of the Society for Research in Child Development, 22*.

Johnson, B. P., Phillips, J. G., Papadopoulos, N., Fielding, J., Tonge, B., & Rinehart, N. J. (2013). Understanding macrographia in children with autism spectrum disorder. *Research in Developmental Disabilities, 34*, 2917–2926.

Johnson, M. H., & de Haan, M. (2015). *Developmental cognitive neuroscience: An introduction* (4th ed.). Chichester, United Kingdom: Wiley.

Johnson, R. (1962). Measurements of achievement in fundamental skills of elementary school children. *Research Quarterly, 33*, 94–103.

Jowett, S., & Cramer, D. (2010). The prediction of young athletes' physical self from perceptions of relationships with parents and coaches. *Psychology of Sport and Exercise, 11*(2), 140–147.

Jwa, S. C., Fujiwara, T., & Kondo, N. (2014). Latent protective effects of breastfeeding on late childhood overweight and obesity: a nationwide prospective study. *Obesity, 22*(6), 1527–1537.

Kaiser, M. L., Schoemaker, M. M., Albaret, J. M., & Geuze, R. H. (2014). What is the evidence of impaired motor skills and motor control among children with attention deficit hyperactivity disorder (ADHD)? Systematic review of the literature. *Research in Developmental Disabilities, 36*, 338–357.

Kallman, D. A., Plato, C. C., & Tobin, J. D. (1990). The role of muscle loss in the age-related decline of grip strength: Cross-sectional and longitudinal perspectives. *Journal of Gerontology, 45*(3), M82–M88.

Karch, D., Kang, K. S., Wochner, K., Philippi, H., Hadders-Algra, M., Pietz, J., & Dickhaus, H. (2012). Kinematic assessment of stereotypy in spontaneous movements in infants. *Gait & Posture, 36*(2), 307–311.

Karpati, F. J., Giacosa, C., Foster, N. E., Penhune, V. B., & Hyde, K. L. (2015). Dance and the brain: A review. *Annals of the New York Academy of Sciences, 1337*, 140–146.

Kasch, F. W., Boyer, J. L., Van Camp, S. P., Verity, L. S., & Wallace, J. P. (1990). The effect of physical activity and inactivity on aerobic power in older men (a longitudinal study). *The Physician and Sportsmedicine, 18*, 73–83.

Katzmarzyk, P. T., Barreira, T. V., Broyles, S. T., Champagne, C. M., Chaput, J. P., Fogelholm, M., . . . Church, T. S. (2015). Relationship between lifestyle behaviors and obesity in children ages 9-11: Result from a 12-country study. *Obesity, 23*(8), 1696–1702.

Kavale, K., & Mattson, P. D. (1983). "One jumped off the balance beam": Meta-analysis of perceptual-motor training. *Journal of Learning Disabilities, 16*, 165–173.

Kenney, W. L., Wilmore, J., & Costill, D. L. (2015). *Physiology of sport and exercise* (6th ed.). Champaign, IL: Human Kinetics.

Keogh, J. F. (1965). *Motor performance of elementary school children.* Eugene, OR: University of Oregon, School of Health, Physical Education and Recreation.

Keogh, J. F., & Sugden, D. A. (1985). *Movement skill development.* New York, NY: Macmillan.

Kephart, N. C. (1971). *The slow learner in the classroom* (2nd ed.). Columbus, OH: Charles E. Merrill.

Ketcham, C. J., & Stelmach, G. E. (2001). Age-related declines in motor control. In J. E. Birren & K. W. Schaie (Eds.), *Handbook of the psychology of aging* (5th ed.). San Diego, CA: Academic Press.

King, S., Dancause, K., Turcotte-Tremblay, A. M., Veru, F., & Laplante, D. P. (2012). Using natural disasters to study the effects of prenatal maternal stress on child health and development. *Birth Defects Research Part C: Embryo Today: Reviews, 96*(4), 273–288.

Kirby, A., Williams, N., Thomas, M., & Hill, E. L. (2013). Self-reported mood, general health, wellbeing and employment status in adults with suspected DCD. *Research in Developmental Disabilities, 34*(4), 1357–1364.

Kliegman, R. M., Stanton, B., St. Geme, J., & Schor, N. (2015). *Nelson textbook of pediatrics* (20th ed.). Philadelphia, PA: Elsevier.

Klinger, A., Masataka, T., Adrian, M., & Smith, E. (1980, April). *Temporal and spatial characteristics of movement patterns of women over 60.* Paper presented at the National Conference of the American Alliance for Health, Physical Education, Recreation and Dance, Detroit, MI.

Klotz, J. M., Johnson, M. D., Wu, S. W., Isaacs, K. M., & Gilbert, D. L. (2012). Relationship between reaction time variability and motor skill development in ADHD. *Child Neuropsychology, 18*(6), 576–585.

Ko, S. U., Hausdorff, J. M., & Ferrucci, L. (2010). Age-associated differences in the gait pattern changes of older adults during fast-speed and fatigue conditions: Results from the Baltimore longitudinal study of ageing. *Age and Ageing, 39*, 688–694.

Konczak, J., Borutta, M., & Dichgans, J. (1997). The development of goal-directed reaching in infants. II. Learning to produce task-adequate patterns of joint torque. *Experimental Brain Research, 113*, 465–474.

Krampe, R. T. (2002). Aging, expertise and fine motor movement. *Neuroscience and Biobehavioral Reviews, 26*, 769–776.

Kuhlman, J. S., & Beitel, P. A. (1997). Developmental/learning of coincidence anticipation. *Journal of Sport & Exercise Psychology, 19*, S76.

Kugler, P. N., Kelso, J. S., & Turvey, M. T. (1980). On the concept of coordinative structures as dissipative structures: I. Theoretical lines of convergence. *Tutorials in Motor Behavior, 3*, 3–47.

Kugler, P. N., Kelso, J., & Turvey, M. (1982). On the control and coordination of naturally developing systems. In J. A. S. Kelso & J. E. Clark (Eds.), *The development of movement control and coordination* (pp. 5–78). New York, NY: Wiley.

Lai, S. K., Costigan, S. A., Morgan, P. J., Lubans, D. R., Stodden, D. F., Salmon, J., & Barnett, L. M. (2014). Do school-based interventions focusing on physical activity, fitness, or fundamental movement skill competency produce a sustained impact in these outcomes in children and adolescents? A systematic review of follow-up studies. *Sports Medicine, 44*(1), 67–79.

Lambert, J., & Bard, C. (2005). Acquisition of visuomanual skills and improvement of information processing capacities in 6- to 10-year-old children performing a 2D pointing task. *Neuroscience Letters, 377*, 1–6.

Langendorfer, S. J., & Roberton, M. A. (2002). Developmental profiles in overarm throwing: Searching for "attractors," "stages," and "constraints." In J. Clark & J. Humphrey (Eds.), *Motor development: Research and reviews* (Vol. 2, pp. 1–25). Reston, VA: National Association for Sport and Physical Education.

Latash, M. L. (2008). *Neurophysiological basis of movement* (2nd ed.). Champaign, IL: Human Kinetics.

Ledebt, A. (2000). Changes in arm posture during early acquisition of walking. *Infant Behavior and Development, 23*(1), 79–89.

LeGear, M., Greyling, L., Sloan, E., Bell, R. I., Williams, B. L., Naylor, P. J., & Temple, V. A. (2012). A window of opportunity? Motor skills and perceptions of competence of children in kindergarten. *The International Journal of Behavioral Nutrition and Physical Activity, 9*, 29.

Lerner, R. M. (2002). *Concepts and theories of human development* (3rd ed.). Mahwah, NJ: Lawrence Erlbaum Associates.

Lerner, R. M. (2012). Developmental science: Past, present, and future. *International Journal of Developmental Science, 6*, 29–36.

Leversen, J. S., Haga, M., & Sigmundsson, H. (2012). From children to adults: Motor performance across the life-span. *PloS One, 7*(6), e38830.

Liao, P. J., & Campbell, S. K. (2004). Examination of the item structure of the Alberta Infant Motor Scale. *Pediatric Physical Therapy, 16*(1), 31–38.

Lindemann, O., & Fischer, M. H. (2015). Cognitive foundations of human number representations and mental arithmetic. In R. Cohen Kadosh & A. Dowker (Eds.), *The Oxford handbook of numerical cognition* (pp. 35–44). Oxford, United Kingdom: Oxford University Press.

Liu, T., & Breslin, C. M. (2013). Fine and gross motor performance of the MABC-2 by children with autism spectrum disorder and typically developing children. *Research in Autism Spectrum Disorders*, 7(10), 1244–1249.

Liu, T., Breslin, C. M., & ElGarhy, S. (2016). Methods and procedures for measuring comorbid disorders: Motor movement and activity. In J. L. Matson (Ed.), *Comorbid conditions among children with autism spectrum disorders* (pp. 91–134). Baton Rouge, LA: Springer.

Londeree, B. R., & Moeschberger, M. L. (1982). Effect of age and other factors on maximal heart rate. *Research Quarterly for Exercise and Sport*, *53*, 297–304.

Lopes, V. P., Gabbard, C., & Rodrigues, L. P. (2016). Effects of psychosocial variables in the similarity and interdependence of physical activity levels among adolescent best friend dyads. *Journal of Sports Sciences*, *34*, 821–828.

Lopes, V. P., Stodden, D. F., Bianchi, M. M., Maia, J. A., & Rodrigues, L. P. (2012). Correlation between BMI and motor coordination in children. *Journal of Science and Medicine in Sport*, *15*, 38–43.

Lorton, E. L., & Lorton, J. H. (1984). *Human development through the lifespan*. Pacific Grove, CA: Brooks/Cole.

Luciana, M. (2007). Special issue: Developmental cognitive neuroscience. *Developmental Review*, *27*(3), 277–282.

Luciana, M. (2010). Adolescent brain development: Current themes and future directions. Introduction to the special issue. *Brain and Cognition*, *72*(1), 1–5.

Lund, R. D. (1978). *Development and plasticity of the brain*. New York, NY: Oxford University Press.

Magill, R. A., & Anderson, D. (2013). *Motor learning and control: Concepts and applications* (10th ed). New York, NY: McGraw-Hill.

Malina, R. M., Bouchard, C., & Bar-Or, O. (2004). *Growth, maturation, and physical activity*. (2nd ed.). Champaign, IL: Human Kinetics.

Marcovitch, S., Clearfield, M. W., Swingler, M., Calkins, S. D., & Bell, M. A. (2015). Attentional predictors of 5-month-olds' performance on a looking a-not-b task. *Infant and Child Development*. Advance online publication. http://dx.doi.org/10.1002/icd.1931

Mason, A. H., Bruyn, J. L., & Lazarus, J. A. (2013). Bimanual coordination in children: Manipulation of object distance. *Experimental Brain Research*, *231*(2), 153–164.

Matzkin, E., Curry, E. J., & Whitlock, K. (2015). Female athlete triad: Past, present, and future. *Journal of the American Academy of Orthopaedic Surgeons*, *23*(7), 424–432.

Mavilidi, M. F., Okely, A. D., Chandler, P., Cliff, D. P., & Paas, F. (2015). Effects of integrated physical exercises and gestures on preschool children's foreign language vocabulary learning. *Educational Psychology Review*, *27*(3), 413–426.

McArdle, W. D., Katch, F. I., & Katch, V. L. (2010). *Exercise physiology* (7th ed.). Philadelphia, PA: Lippincott Williams & Wilkins.

McBride-Chang, C., & Jacklin, C. (1993). Early play arousal, sex-typed play, and activity level as precursors to later rough-and-tumble play. *Early Education and Development*, *4*, 99–108.

McClelland, E., Pitt, A., & Stein, J. (2015). Enhanced academic performance using a novel classroom physical activity intervention to increase awareness, attention and self-control: Putting embodied cognition into practice. *Improving Schools*, *18*(1), 83–100.

McManus, I. C., Sik, G., Cole, D. R., Mellon, A. F., Wong, J., & Kloss, J. (1988). The development of handedness in children. *British Journal of Developmental Psychology*, *6*, 257–273.

Meeuwsen, H. J., Tesi, J. M., & Goggin, N. L. (1992). Psychophysics of arm movements and human aging. *Research Quarterly for Exercise and Sport*, *63*(1), 19–24.

Merkel, D. L. (2013). Youth sport: Positive and negative impact on young athletes. *Open Access Journal of Sports Medicine*, *4*, 151–160.

Miller, L. J., & Roid, R. G. (1994). *The T.I.M.E. Toddler and infant motor evaluation: A standardized assessment*. Tucson, AZ: Therapy Skill Builders.

Milteer, R. M., & Ginsburg, K. R. (2012). The importance of play in promoting healthy child development and maintaining strong parent-child bond: Focus on children in poverty. *Pediatrics*, *129*(1), e204–e213.

Moore, L. L., Gao, D., Bradlee, M. L., Cupples, L. A., Sundarajan-Ramamurti, A., Proctor, M. H., . . . Ellison, R. C. (2003). Does early physical activity predict body fat change throughout childhood? *Preventive Medicine*, *37*(1), 10–17.

Moore, L. L., Lombardi, D. A., White, M. J., Campbell, J. L., Oliveria, S. A., & Ellison, R. C. (1991). Influence of parents' physical activity levels on activity levels of young children. *Journal of Pediatrics*, *118*, 215–219.

Murray, M. P., Kory, R. C., & Sepic, S. B. (1970). Walking patterns of normal women. *Archives of Physical Medicine and Rehabilitation*, *51*, 637–650.

Nachshon, I., Denno, D., & Aurand, S. (1983). Lateral preferences of hand, eye and foot: Relation to cerebral dominance. *International Journal of Neuroscience*, *18*, 1–9.

Nagamatsu, L. S., Flicker, L., Kramer, A. F., Voss, M. W., Erickson, K. I., Hsu, C. L., & Liu-Ambrose, T. (2014). Exercise is medicine, for the body and the brain. *British Journal of Sports Medicine*, *48*, 943–944.

Nash, M. (1997). Fertile minds. *Time International*, *149*, 49–56.

National Center for Health Statistics. (2012). *National Youth Fitness Study*. Retrieved from http://www.cdc.gov/nchs/nnyfs/index.htm

National Association for Sport and Physical Education & American Heart Association. (2012). *2012 Shape of the nation report: Status of physical education in the USA*. Reston VA: American Alliance for Health, Physical Education, Recreation and Dance.

National Collegiate Athletic Association. (2015). *Student-athlete participation: 1981-82–2014-15*. Indianapolis, IN: Author.

National Institute of Diabetes and Digestive and Kidney Diseases. (2016). *National Diabetes Education Program*. Retrieved from http://www.niddk.nih.gov/health-information/health-communication-programs/ndep/Pages/index.aspx

Needham, A., Barrett, T., & Peterman, K. (2002). A pick-me-up for infants' exploratory skills: Early simulated experiences reaching for objects using 'sticky mittens' enhances young infants' object exploration skills. *Infant Behavior and Development*, *25*(3), 279–295.

Nelson, C. J. (1981). *Locomotor patterns of women over 57 (Unpublished master's thesis)*. Washington State University, Pullman.

Newell, K. M. (1986). Constraints on the development of coordination. In M. G. Wade & H. T. A. Whiting (Eds.), *Motor development in children: Aspects of coordination and control, 341–361*. Amsterdam, The Netherlands: Martinus Nijhoff.

Nickols-Richardson, S. M., Modlesky, C. M., O'Connor, P. J., & Lewis, R. D. (2000). Premenarcheal gymnasts possess higher bone mineral density than controls. *Medicine and Science in Sports and Exercise, 32*, 63–69.

Nilsson, M., Ohlsson, C., Odén, A., Mellström, D., & Lorentzon, M. (2012). Increased physical activity is associated with enhance development of peak bone mass in men: A five-year longitudinal study. *Journal of Bone and Mineral Research, 27*(5), 1206–1214.

Noël, M. (2005). Finger gnosia: A predictor of numerical abilities in children? *Child Neuropsychology, 11*, 413–430.

Oh, C. M., Oh, I. H., Choi, K. S., Choe, B. K., Yoon, T. Y., & Choi, J. M. (2012). Relationship between body mass index and early menarche of adolescent girls in Seoul. *Journal of Preventive Medicine and Public Health, 45*(4), 227–234.

Okely, A. D., Booth, M. L., & Chey, T. (2004). Relationships between body composition and fundamental movement skills among children and adolescents. *Research Quarterly for Exercise and Sport, 75*(3), 238–247.

Okely, A. D., & Janssen, X. (2015). Early physical activity and sedentary behaviours. In L. Stewart & J. Thompson (Eds.), *Early Years Nutrition and Healthy Weight* (pp. 46–58). Chichester, United Kingdom: Wiley.

Onushko, T., Kim, C., & Christou, E. (2014). Reducing task difficulty during practice improves motor learning in older adults. *Experimental Gerontology, 57*, 168–174.

Paffenbarger, R. S., Jr., Hyde, R. T., Wing, A. L., & Hsieh, C. C. (1986). Physical activity, all-cause mortality, and longevity of college alumni. *New England Journal of Medicine, 314*, 605–613.

Painter, M. A. (1994). Developmental sequences for hopping as assessment instruments: A generalizability analysis. *Research Quarterly for Exercise and Sport, 65*(1), 1–10.

Palmer, C. F. (1989). The discriminating nature of infant's exploratory actions. *Developmental Psychology, 25*, 885–893.

Parizkova, J., & Carter, J. E. (1976). Influence of physical activity on stability of somatotypes in boys. *American Journal of Physiology and Anthropology, 44*, 327–339.

Parten, M. (1932). Social participation among pre-school children. *Journal of Abnormal and Social Psychology, 27*, 243–269.

Paschal, K. A., Oswald, A., Siegmund, R., Siegmund, S., & Threlkeld, A. J. (2006). Test-retest reliability of the physical performance test for persons with Parkinson disease. *Journal of Geriatric Physical Therapy, 29*(3), 82–86.

Pennington, B. F., Snyder, K. A., & Roberts, R. J., Jr. (2007). Developmental cognitive neuroscience: Origins, issues, and prospects. *Developmental Review, 27*(3), 428–441.

Pereira, K., Basso, R. P., Lindquist, A. R., da Silva, L. G., & Tudella, E. (2013). Infants with Down syndrome: Percentage and age for acquisition of gross motor skills. *Research in Developmental Disabilities, 34*(3), 894–901.

Perry, B. (1997, February 3). Fertile minds. *Time, 149*(5), 49–56.

Peterson, M. L., Christou, E., & Rosengren, K. S. (2006). Children achieve adult-like sensory integration during stance at 12-years-old. *Gait & Posture, 23*(4), 455–463.

Petrofsky, J. S., & Lind, A. R. (1975). Aging, isometric strength and endurance, and cardiovascular responses to static effort. *Journal of Applied Physiology, 38*, 91–95.

Phillips, S. M., Wójcicki, T. R., & McAuley, E. (2013). Physical activity and quality of life in older adults: An 18-month panel analysis. *Quality of Life Research, 22*, 1647–1654.

Piaget, J. (1952). *The origins of intelligence in children* (M. Cook, Trans. 2nd ed.). New York, NY: International Universities Press.

Piaget, J. (1963). *The origins of intelligence in children* (M. Cook, Trans. 3rd ed.). New York, NY: Norton.

Piaget, J. (1985). *The equilibration of cognitive structures: The central problem of intellectual development* (T. Brown & K. J. Thampy, Trans.). Chicago, IL: University of Chicago Press.

Piek, J. P. (2006). *Infant motor development*. Champaign, IL: Human Kinetics.

Piek, J. P., & Carman, R. (1994). Developmental profiles of spontaneous movements in infants. *Early Human Development, 39*, 109–126.

Piper, M. C., & Darrah, J. (1994). *Motor assessment of the developing infant*. Philadelphia, PA: W. B. Saunders.

Poole, K. L., Schmidt, L. A., Missiuna, C., Saigal, S., Boyle, M. H., & Van Lieshout, R. J. (2015). Motor coordination difficulties in extremely low birth weight survivors across four decades. *Journal of Developmental and Behavioral Pediatrics, 36*(7), 521–528.

Poole, K. L., Schmidt, L. A., Missiuna, C., Saigal, S., Boyle, M. H., & Van Lieshout, R. J. (2016). Childhood motor coordination and adult psychopathology in extremely low birth weight survivors. *Journal of Affective Disorders, 190*, 294–299.

Powell, K. E., & Blair, S. N. (1994). The public health burdens of sedentary living habits: Theoretical but realistic estimates. *Medical and Science in Sports and Exercise, 26*, 851–856.

Prechtl, H., & Hopkins, B. (1986). Developmental transformations of spontaneous movements in early infancy. *Early Human Development, 14*, 233–238.

Provins, K. A. (1992). Early infant motor asymmetries and handedness: A critical evaluation of the evidence. *Developmental Neuropsychology, 8*(4), 325–365.

Purcell, C., Scott-Roberts, S., & Kirby, A. (2015). Implications of DSM-5 for recognising adults with developmental coordination disorder (DCD). *British Journal of Occupational Therapy, 78*(5), 295–302.

Raustorp, A., & Lindwall, M. (2015). Physical self-esteem—A ten-year follow-up study from early adolescence to early adulthood. *International Journal of Adolescent Medicine and Health, 27*(1), 31–39.

Rebok, G. W., Ball, K., Guey, L. T., Jones, R. N., Kim, H. Y., King, J. W., . . . Willis, S. L. (2014). Ten-year effects of the advanced cognitive training for independent and vital elderly cognitive training trial on cognition and everyday functioning in older adults. *Journal of the American Geriatrics Society, 62*(1), 16–24.

Reeb, B. C., Fox, N. A., Nelson, C. A., & Zeanah, C. H. (2009). The effects of early institutionalization on social behavior and underlying neural correlates. In M. de Haan & M. Gunnar (Eds.), *Handbook of developmental social neuroscience* (pp. 477–496). New York, NY: Guilford Press.

Reed, E. S. (1989). Chaining theories of postural development. In M. H. Woollacott & A. Shumway-Cook (Eds.),

Development of posture and gait: Across the life span (pp. 3–24). Columbia, SC: University of South Carolina Press.

Resnick, B. (2004). A longitudinal analysis of efficacy expectations and exercise in older adults. *Research and Theory for Nursing Practice*, *18*(4), 331–344.

Reuben, D. B., & Siu, A. L. (1990). An objective measure of physical function of elderly outpatients. The physical performance test. *Journal of the American Geriatrics Society*, *38*, 1105–1112.

Richter, C. P. (1934). The grasp reflex of the new-born infant. *American Journal of Developmental Children*, *48*, 327–332.

Rikli, R., & Busch, S. (1986). Motor performance of women as a function of age and physical activity level. *Journal of Gerontology*, *41*, 645–649.

Rikli, R. E., & Jones, C. J. (2013). *Senior fitness test manual*. Champaign, IL: Human Kinetics.

Rivera, J. A., Sotres-Alvarez, D., Habicht, J. P., Shamah, T., & Villalpando, S. (2004). Impact of the Mexican Program for Education, Health, and Nutrition (Progresa) on rates of growth and anemia in infants and young children: a randomized effectiveness study. *JAMA*, *291*, 2563–2570.

Roberton, M. A. (1990, June). *Interlimb timing changes in the development of hopping*. Paper presented at the annual meeting of the North American Society for Psychology of Sport and Physical Activity, Houston, TX.

Roberton, M. A., & Halverson, L. E. (1984). *Developing children—Their changing movement*. Philadelphia, PA: Lea & Febiger.

Robin, D. J., Berthier, N. E., & Clifton, R. K. (1996). Infant's predictive reaching for moving objects in the dark. *Developmental Psychology*, *32*(5), 824–835.

Robinson, L. E. (2011). The relationship between perceived physical competence and fundamental motor skills in preschool children. *Child: Care, Health and Development*, *37*(4), 589–596.

Rodrigues, L. P., Saraiva, L., & Gabbard, C. (2005). Development and construct validation of an inventory for assessing the home environment for motor development. *Research Quarterly for Exercise and Sport*, *76*, 140–148.

Rose, D., & Christina, R. (2006). *A multilevel approach to the study of motor control and learning* (2nd ed.). San Francisco, CA: Benjamin Cummings.

Rosenbaum, P. L., Missiuna, C., Echeverria, D., & Knox, S. S. (2009). Proposed motor development assessment protocol for epidemiological studies in children. *Journal of Epidemiology and Community Health*, *63*, i27–i36.

Rosenthal, T. L., & Zimmerman, B. J. (1978). *Social learning and cognition*. New York, NY: Academic Press.

Ross, E. J., Graham, D. L., Money, K. M., & Stanwood, G. D. (2015). Developmental consequences of fetal exposure to drugs: what we know and what we still must learn. *Neuropsychopharmacology*, *40*(1), 61–87.

Ross, J. [James] G., & Gilbert, G. G. (1985). The National Children and Youth Fitness Study: A summary of findings. *Journal of Physical Education, Recreation, & Dance*, *56*(1), 45–50.

Ross, J. [James] G., & Pate, R. R. (1987). The National Children and Youth Fitness Study II: A summary of findings. *Journal of Physical Education, Recreation, & Dance*, *5*(9), 51–56.

Ross, J. [Judith], Czernichow, P., Biller, B. M., Colao, A., Reiter, E., & Kiess, W. (2010). Growth hormone: Health considerations beyond height gain. *Pediatrics*, *125*(4), e906–e918.

Rovee-Collier, C., & Barr, R. (2001). Infant learning and memory. In A. Fogel & G. Bremner (Eds.), *Blackwell handbook of infant development* (pp. 99–138). Oxford, United Kingdom: Blackwell.

Rueckriegel, S. M., Blankenburg, F., Burghardt, R., Ehrlich, S., Henze, G., Mergl, R., & Hernáiz Driever, P. (2008). Influence of age and movement complexity on kinematic hand movement parameters in childhood and adolescence. *International Journal of Developmental Neuroscience*, *26*, 655–663.

Ruffman, T., Slade, L., Sandino, J. C., & Fletcher, A. (2005). Are A-not-B errors caused by a belief about object location? *Child Development*, *76*, 122–136.

Sadeghipour, A., & Kopp, S. (2012). Gesture processing as grounded motor cognition: Towards a computational model. *Procedia—Social and Behavioral Sciences*, *32*, 213–223.

Sallis, J. F., Prochaska, J. J., & Taylor, W. C. (2000). A review of correlates of physical activity of children and adolescents. *Medicine and Science Sports and Exercise*, *32*(5), 963–975.

Salthouse, T. A. (2007). Reaction time. In J. E. Birren (Ed.), *Encyclopedia of gerontology* (2nd ed., pp. 407–410). Boston, MA: Elsevier Academic Press.

Salthouse, T. A. (2009). When does age-related cognitive decline begin? *Neurobiology of Aging*, *30*, 507–514.

Salvia, J. Z., & Ysseldyke, J. E. (1991). *Assessment* (5th ed.). Boston, MA: Houghton Mifflin.

Schmidt, M., Blum, M., Valkanover, S., & Conzelmann, A. (2015). Motor ability and self-esteem: The mediating role of physical self-concept and perceived social acceptance. *Psychology of Sport and Exercise*, *17*, 15–23.

Schmidt, R. A. (1975). A schema theory of discrete motor skill learning. *Psychological Review*, *82*, 225–260.

Schmidt, R. A., & Lee, T. D. (2014). *Motor control and learning: A behavioral emphasis* (5th ed.). Champaign, IL: Human Kinetics.

Scholz, J., Allemang-Grand, R., Dazai, J., & Lerch, J. P. (2015). Environmental enrichment is associated with rapid volumetric brain changes in adult mice. *NeuroImage*, *109*, 190–198.

Schulz, R., & Curnow, C. (1988). Peak performance and age among superathletes: Track and field, swimming, baseball, tennis, and golf. *Journal of Gerontology*, *43*, 113–120.

Schulz, R., Musa, D., Staszewski, J., & Siegler, R. S. (1994). The relationship between age and major league baseball performance: Implications for development. *Psychology and Aging*, *9*(2), 274–286.

Seefeldt, V., & Branta, C. F. (1984). Patterns of participation in children's sport. In J. Thomas (Ed.), *Motor development during childhood and adolescence*. Minneapolis, MN: Burgess.

Seidler, R. D. (2007). Aging affects motor learning but not savings at transfer of learning. *Learning & Memory*, *14*(1–2), 17–21.

Seils, L. (1951). The relationship between measures of physical growth and gross motor performance of primary-grade children. *Research Quarterly for Exercise and Sport*, *22*, 244–260.

Serrien, D. J., Sovijärvi-Spapé, M. M., & Rana, G. (2014). Developmental changes in motor control: Insights from bimanual coordination. *Developmental Psychology*, *50*(1), 316–323.

Sheldon, W. H., Dupertuis, C. W., & McDermott, E. (1954). *Atlas of men: A guide for somatotyping the adult male of all ages*. New York, NY: Harper.

Shock, N. W. (1962). The physiology of aging. *Scientific American, 206*(1), 100–110.

Shonkoff, J. P., & Phillips, D. A. (2000). *From Neurons to neighborhoods: The science of early childhood development.* Washington, DC: National Academies Press.

Shors, T. J. (2014). The adult brain makes new neurons, and effortful learning keeps them alive. *Current Directions in Psychological Science, 23*(5), 311–318.

Shumway-Cook, A., & Woollacott, M. H. (2012). *Motor control: Translating research into clinical practice* (4th ed.). Philadelphia, PA: Lippincott Williams & Wilkins.

Siegler, R. S. (2006). Microgenetic analyses of learning. In D. Kuhn, R. S. Siegler, W. Damon, & R. M. Lerner (Eds.), *Handbook of child psychology: Cognition, perception, and language* (6th ed., Vol. 2., pp. 464–510). Hoboken, NJ: Wiley.

Sivagnanasunderam, M., Gonzalez, D. A., Bryden, P. J., Young, G., Forsyth, A., & Roy, E. A. (2014). Handedness throughout the lifespan: cross-sectional view on sex differences as asymmetries change. *Frontiers in Psychology, 5*, 1556.

Slater, A., Mattock, A., & Brown, E. (1990). Size constancy at birth: Newborn infants' responses to retinal and real size. *Journal of Experimental Child Psychology, 49*, 314–322.

Slobounov, S. M., Haibach, P. S., & Newell, K. M. (2006). Aging-related temporal constraints to stability and instability in postural control. *European Review of Aging and Physical Activity, 3*(2), 55–62.

Smits-Engelsman, B. C., Niemeijer, A. S., & van Waelvelde, H. (2011). Is the Movement Assessment Battery for Children-2nd edition a reliable instrument to measure motor performance in 3 year old children? *Research in Developmental Disabilities, 32*(4), 1370–1377.

Sorkin, J. D., Miller, D. C., & Andres, R. (1999). Longitudinal change in the heights of men and women: Consequential effects on body mass index. *Epidemiologic Reviews, 21*, 247–260.

Spelke, E. S. (1987). The development of intermodal perception. In P. Salapatek & L. Cohen (Eds.), *Handbook of infant perception: From perception to cognition* (Vol. 2, pp. 233–273). Orlando, FL: Academic Press.

Spencer, J. P., Samuelson, L. K., Blumberg, M. S., McMurray, B., Robinson, S. R., & Tomblin, J. B. (2009). Seeing the world through a third eye: Developmental systems theory looks beyond the nativist-empiricist debate. *Child Development Perspectives, 3*(2), 103–105.

Sporns, O., & Edelman, G. M. (1993). Solving Bernstein's problem: A proposal for the development of coordinated movement by selection. *Child Development, 64*(4), 960–981.

Sports and Fitness Industry Association. (2015). *2015 U.S. trends in team sports.* Silver Spring, MD: Author.

Squires, J., & Bricker, D. (2009). *Ages & Stages Questionnaires® (ASQ-3™): A parent-completed child monitoring system* (3rd ed.). Baltimore, MD: Brookes Publishing.

Staszewski, J. (Ed.). (2013). *Expertise and skill acquisition: The impact of William G. Chase.* New York, NY: Psychology Press.

Stice, E., & Martinez, E. E. (2005). Cigarette smoking prospectively predicts retarded physical growth among female adolescents. *Journal of Adolescent Health, 37*(5), 363–370.

Stodden, D., Langendorfer, S., & Roberton, M. A. (2009). The association between motor skill competence and physical fitness in young adults. *Research Quarterly for Exercise and Sport, 80*(2), 223–229.

Stone, M. J., & Kozma, A. (1996). Activity, exercise, and behavior. In J. E. Birren & K. W. Schaie (Eds.), *Handbook of the psychology of aging* (4th ed., pp. 338–352). San Diego, CA: Academic Press.

Strohmeyer, H. S., Williams, K., & Schaub-George, D. (1991). Developmental sequences for catching a small ball: A prelongitudinal screening. *Research Quarterly for Exercise and Sport, 62*(3), 257–266.

Suitor, J. J., & Reavis, R. (1995). Football, fast cars, and cheerleading: Adolescent gender norms, 1978-1989. *Adolescence, 30*, 265–272.

Sullivan, E. V., Rose, J., Rohlfing, T., & Pfefferbaum, A. (2009). Postural sway reduction in aging men and women: Relation to brain structure, cognitive status, and stabilizing factors. *Neurobiology of Aging, 30*, 793–807.

Summers, J. J., & Anson, J. G. (2009). Current status of the motor program: Revisited. *Human Movement Science, 28*(5), 566–577.

Sutherland, D. H. (1984). *Gait disorders in childhood and adolescence.* Baltimore, MD: Wolters Kluwer.

Svejme, O., Ahlborg, H. G., & Karlsson, M. K. (2012). Physical activity reduces bone loss in the distal forearm in post-menopausal women—A 25-year prospective study. *Scandinavian Journal of Medicine & Science in Sports, 24*, 159–165.

Swanson, M. W., Streissguth, A. P., Sampson, P. D., & Olson, H. C. (1999). Prenatal cocaine and neuromotor outcome at four months: Effect of duration of exposure. *Journal of Developmental and Behavioral Pediatrics, 20*(5), 325–334.

Tabibi, Z., & Pfeffer, K. (2007). Finding a safe place to cross the road: The effect of distractors and the role of attention in children's identification of safe and dangerous road-crossing sites. *Infant and Child Development, 16*, 193–206.

Tanner, J. M. (1990). *Fetus into man: Physical growth from conception to maturity.* Cambridge, MA: Harvard University Press.

Tanner, J. M., Healy, M. J. R., Goldstein, H., & Cameron, N. (2001). *Assessment of skeletal maturity and prediction of adult height (TW3 Method)* (3rd ed.). London, United Kingdom: W. B. Saunders.

Taylor, A. W., & Johnson, M. J. (2008). *Physiology of exercise and healthy aging.* Champaign, IL: Human Kinetics.

Thelen, E. (1979). Rhythmical stereotypies in normal human infants. *Animal Behaviour, 27*, 699–715.

Thelen, E. (2005). Dynamic systems theory and the complexity of change. *Psychoanalytic Dialogues, 15*, 255–283.

Thelen, E., & Fisher, D. M. (1982). Newborn stepping: An explanation for a "disappearing" reflex. *Developmental Psychology, 18*, 760–775.

Thelen, E., Fisher, D. M., & Ridley-Johnson, R. (2002). The relationship between physical growth and a newborn reflex. *Infant Behavior and Development, 25*(1), 72–85.

Thelen, E., & Smith, L. B. (1994). *A dynamic systems approach to the development of cognition and action.* Cambridge, MA: MIT Press.

Thelen, E., & Smith, L. B. (1998). Dynamic systems theories. In W. Damon & R. M. Lerner (Eds.), *Handbook of child psychology: Theoretical models and human development* (5th ed., Vol. 1, pp. 563–634). New York, NY: Wiley.

Thelen, E., Ulrich, B. D., & Wolff, P. H. (1991). Hidden skills: A dynamic systems analysis of treadmill stepping during the first year. *Monographs of the Society for Research in Child Development, 56*(1), 1–103.

Thomas, J. R., Thomas, K. T., Lee, A. M., Testerman, E., & Ashy, M. (1983). Age differences in use of strategy for recall of movement in a large scale environment. *Research Quarterly for Exercise and Sport, 54*(3), 264–272.

Thomas, R. J., Nelson, J. K., & Church, G. (1991). A developmental analysis of gender differences in health related physical fitness. *Pediatric Exercise Science, 3*, 28–42.

Tolonen, S., Sievänen, H., Mikkilä, V., Telama, R., Oikonen, M., Laaksonen, M., . . . Raitakari, O. T. (2015). Adolescence physical activity is associated with higher tibial pQCT bone values in adulthood after 28-years of follow-up—The Cardiovascular Risk in Young Finns Study. *Bone, 75*, 77–83.

Toumpaniari, K., Loyens, S., Mavilidi, M. F., & Paas, F. (2015). Preschool children's foreign language vocabulary learning by embodying words through physical activity and gesturing. *Educational Psychology Review, 27*(3), 445–456.

Toupet, M., Gagey, P. M., & Heuschen, S. (1992). Vestibular patients and aging subjects lose use of visual input and expend more energy in static postural control. In B. Vellas, M. Toupet, L. Rubenstein, J. L. Albarède, & Y. Christen (Eds.), *Falls, balance and gait disorders in the elderly* (pp. 183–198). Paris, France: Elsevier.

Troiano, R. P., Berrigan, D., Dodd, K. W., Mâsse, L. C., Tilert, T., & McDowell, M. (2008). Physical activity in the United States measured by accelerometer. *Medicine and Science in Sports and Exercise, 40*(1), 181–188.

Tucker, M. G., Kavanagh, J. J., Morrison, S., & Barrett, R. S. (2009). Voluntary sway and rapid orthogonal transitions of voluntary sway in young adults, and low and high fall-risk older adults. *Clinical Biomechanics, 24*(8), 597–605.

Tulving, E. (1985). How many memory systems are there? *American Psychologist, 40*, 385–398.

Ulrich, D. A. (2000). *Test of gross motor developments* (2nd ed.). Austin, TX: Pro-Ed.

Ulrich, D. A., Lloyd, M. C., Tiernan, C. W., Looper, J. E., & Angulo-Barroso, R. M. (2008). Effects of intensity of treadmill training on developmental outcomes and stepping in infants with Down syndrome: A randomized trial. *Physical Therapy, 88*(1), 114–122.

Ulrich, D. A., Ulrich, B. D., Angulo-Kinzler, R. M., & Yun, J. (2001). Treadmill training of infants with Down syndrome: Evidence-based developmental outcomes. *Pediatrics, 108*(5), E84.

Usuba, K., Oddson, B., Gauthier, A., & Young, N. (2014). Changes in gross motor function and health-related quality of life in adults with cerebral palsy: An 8-year follow-up study. *Archives of Physical Medicine and Rehabilitation, 95*, 2071.e1–2077.e1.

van der Fits, I. B. M., Klip, A. W. J., van Eykern, L. A., & Hadders-Algra, M. (1999). Postural adjustments during spontaneous and goal-directed arm movements in the first half year of life. *Behavioural Brain Research, 106*, 75–90.

van Hartingsveldt, M. J., Cup, E. H., & Oostendorp, R. A. (2005). Reliability and validity of the fine motor scale of the Peabody Developmental Motor Scales-2. *Occupational Therapy International, 12*(1), 1–13.

van Strien, J. (2000). Genetic, intrauterine, and cultural origins of human handedness. In M. Mandal, B. Bulman-Fleming, & G. Tiwari (Eds.). *Side bias: A neuropsychological perspective* (pp. 41–62). Dordrecht, The Netherlands: Kluwer Academic.

Venetsanou, F., Kambas, A., Aggeloussis, N., Fatouros, I., & Taxildaris, K. (2009). Motor assessment of preschool aged children: A preliminary investigation of the validity of the Bruininks-Oseretsky test of motor proficiency—Short form. *Human Movement Science, 28*(4), 543–550.

Verly, M., Verhoeven, J., Zink, I., Mantini, D., Van Oudenhove, L., Lagae, L., . . . Rommel, N. (2014). Structural and functional underconnectivity as a negative predictor for language in autism. *Human Brain Mapping, 35*(8), 3602–3615.

Vermeulen, J., Neyens, J. C., van Rossum, E., Spreeuwenberg, M. D., & de Witte, L. P. (2011). Predicting ADL disability in community-dwelling elderly people using physical frailty indicators: A systematic review. *BMC Geriatrics, 11*(1), 33.

von Hofsten, C., & Rönnqvist, L. (1993). The structuring of neonatal arm movements. *Child Development, 64*(4), 1046–1057.

Wagner, S., Winner, E., Cicchetti, D., & Gardner, H. (1981). "Metaphorical" mapping in human infants. *Child Development, 52*, 728–731.

Wang, H. H., Liao, H., & Hsieh, C. (2006). Reliability, sensitivity to change, and responsiveness of the peabody developmental motor scales-second edition for children with cerebral palsy. *Physical Therapy, 86*(10), 1351–1359.

Wang, L., & Pinkerton, K. E. (2008). Detrimental effects of tobacco smoke exposure during development on postnatal lung function and asthma. *Birth Defects Research. Part C: Embryo Today, 84*(1), 54–60.

Wang, Q. J., Suominen, H., Nicholson, P. H., Zou, L. C., Alen, M., Koistinen, A., & Cheng, S. (2005). Influence of physical activity and maturation status on bone mass and geometry in early pubertal girls. *Scandinavian Journal of Medicine & Science in Sports, 15*, 100–106.

Ward, E. V., Berry, C. J., & Shanks, D. R. (2013). Age effects on explicit and implicit memory. *Frontiers in Psychology, 4*, 639.

Whitall, J. (2009). Research on children: New approaches to answer old questions, but is this sufficient? *Quest, 61*, 93–107.

Wickstrom, R. L. (1983). *Fundamental motor patterns* (3rd ed.). Philadelphia, PA: Lea & Febiger.

Wild, M. (1938). The behavior pattern of throwing and some observations concerning its course of development in children. *Research Quarterly of the American Association for Health, Physical Education, & Recreation, 9*, 20–24.

Wilkins, C. H., Roe, C. M., & Morris, J. C. (2010). A brief clinical tool to assess physical function: The mini-physical performance test. *Archives of Gerontology and Geriatrics, 50*(1), 96–100.

Williams, H. G. (1983). *Perceptual and motor development.* Englewood Cliffs, NJ: Prentice Hall.

Williams, H. G. (1990). Aging and eye-hand coordination. In C. Bard, M. Fleury, & L. Hay (Eds.), *Development of eye-hand coordination across the life span* (pp. 326–357). Columbia, SC: University of South Carolina Press.

Williams, H. G., & Breihan, S. K. (1979). *Motor control tasks for young children.* Unpublished manuscript, University of Toledo, Toledo, Ohio.

Williams, J. L., Corbetta, D., & Cobb, L. (2015). How perception, action, functional value, and context can shape the development of infant reaching. *Movement & Sport Sciences-Science & Motricité, 89*, 5–15.

Williams, J. L., Corbetta, D., & Guan, Y. (2015). Learning to reach with "sticky" or "non-sticky" mittens: A tale of developmental trajectories. *Infant Behavior & Development*, *38*, 82–96.

Williams, J., Thomas, P. R., Maruff, P., & Wilson, P. H. (2008). The link between motor impairment level and motor imagery ability in children with developmental coordination disorder. *Human Movement Science*, *27*(2), 270–285.

Williams, K., Haywood, K., & Van Sant, A. (1991). Throwing patterns of older adults: A follow-up investigation. *International Journal of Aging & Human Development*, *33*, 279–294.

Willmott, M. (1986). The effect of vinyl floor surface and carpeted floor surface upon walking in elderly hospital in-patients. *Age and Ageing*, *15*, 119–120.

Wilson, B. N., Kaplan, B. J., Crawford, S. G., & Roberts, G. (2007). *The Developmental Coordination Questionnaire 2007 (DCDQ'07)*. Alberta, Canada: Alberta Children Hospital.

Wilson, M. R. (2009). *The endocrine system: Hormones, growth, and development*. New York, NY: Rosen Publishing Group.

Withagen, R., & van der Kamp, J. (2010). Towards a new ecological conception of perceptual information: Lessons from a developmental systems perspective. *Human Movement Science*, *29*(1), 149–163.

Wocadlo, C., & Rieger, I. (2008). Motor impairment and low achievement in very preterm children at eight years of age. *Early Human Development*, *84*(11), 769–776.

Women's Sports Foundation. (2008). *Go out and play—Youth sports in America*. East Meadow, NY: Author.

Wuang, Y., & Su, C. (2009). Rasch analysis of the developmental test of visual-motor integration in children with intellectual disabilities. *Research in Developmental Disabilities*, *30*(5), 1044–1053.

Yan, J. H., Thomas, J. R., Stelmach, G. E., & Thomas, K. T. (2000). Developmental features of rapid aiming arm movements across the lifespan. *Journal of Motor Behavior*, *32*(2), 121–140.

Yu, J., Sit, C. H., Capio, C. M., Burnett, A., Ha, A. S., & Huang, W. Y. (2016). Fundamental movement skills proficiency in children with developmental coordination disorder: Does physical self-concept matter? *Disability and Rehabilitation*, *38*(1), 45–51.

Zauner, C. W., Maksud, M. G., & Melichna, J. (1989). Physiological considerations in training young athletes. *Sports Medicine*, *8*(1), 15–31.

Zelazo, N. A., Zelazo, P. R., Cohen, K. M., & Zelazo, P. D. (1993). Specificity of practice effects on elementary neuromotor patterns. *Developmental Psychology*, *29*(4), 686–691.

Ziviani, J. (1983). Qualitative changes in dynamic tripod grip between seven and 14 years of age. *Developmental Medicine and Child Neurology*, *25*, 778–782.

Zmyj, N., Prinz, W., & Daum, M. M. (2015). Eighteen-month-olds' memory interference and distraction in a modified A-not-B task is not associated with their anticipatory looking in a false-belief task. *Frontiers in Psychology*, *6*, 857.

Credits

CHAPTER 1

Figure 1.3: Courtesy of Dr. Daniela Corbetta, Infant Motor Development Laboratory, University of Tennessee. **Figure 1.5 (A):** Courtesy of Dr. Elena Kushnerenko, UEL Babylab Leader, University of East London, London, United Kingdom. **Figure 1.5 (B):** Courtesy of Baby Research Center, Nijmegen, Netherlands. **Figure 1.7:** Courtesy of Claudia Paulussen/Shutterstock. **Figure 1.8:** Courtesy of Photographee.eu/Shutterstock.

CHAPTER 2

Figure 2.2: From Hole, J. W. (1984). *Human anatomy and physiology* (3rd ed.). Dubuque, IA: Wm. C. Brown Communications. Copyright © 1984 Wm. C. Brown Communications, Inc. All Rights Reserved. Reprinted by permission. **Figure 2.3:** From Sage, G. H. (1984). *Motor learning and control*. Dubuque, IA: Wm. C. Brown Communications. Copyright © 1984 Wm. C. Brown Communications, Inc. All rights reserved. Reprinted by permission. **Figure 2.4:** Courtesy of LifeART image. Copyright © 2016 Lippincott Williams & Wilkins. All rights reserved. **Figure 2.5:** From Conel, J. L. (1939–1963). *Postnatal development of the human cerebral cortex* (Vol. I–VI). Cambridge, MA: Harvard University Press. Copyright © Harvard University Press. Reprinted by permission. **Focus on Application, p. 49:** Courtesy of Dr. Henrietta Van Pragg. **Focus on Application, p. 50:** Courtesy of Laurel Trainor. **Figure 2.7:** Adapted from Rorke, L. B., & Riggs, H. E. (1969). *Myelination of the brain in the newborn*. Philadelphia, PA: Lippincott Williams & Wilkins; Dekaban, A. S. (1970). *Neurology of early childhood*. Baltimore, MD: Lippincott Williams & Wilkins; Yakovlev, P. I., Lecours, A. R. (1967). The myelogenetic cycles of regional maturation of the brain. In A. Minkowski (Ed.), *Regional development of the brain in early life* (pp. 3–70). Oxford, United Kingdom: Blackwell Scientific.

CHAPTER 3

Figure 3.1: Redrawn from Tanner, J. M. (1978). *Fetus into man: Physical growth from conception to maturity*. Cambridge, MA: Harvard University Press. **Figure 3.2:** Redrawn from Malina, R. M. (1975). *Growth and development: The first twenty years*. Minneapolis, MN: Burgess. **Figure 3.3:** Courtesy of Monkey Business Images/Shutterstock. **Figure 3.16:** Redrawn from Tanner, J. M. (1978). *Fetus into man: Physical growth from conception to maturity*. Cambridge, MA: Harvard University Press. **Figure 3.18:** Courtesy of Carolina Biological Supply Company. **Figure 3.19:** Modified from Tanner, J. M. (1990). *Fetus into man: Physical growth from conception to maturity*. Cambridge, MA: Harvard University Press. **Figure 3.20:** Adapted from Sorkin, J. D., Miller, D. C., & Andres, R. (1999). Longitudinal change in the heights of men and women: Consequential effects on body mass index. *Epidemiologic Reviews, 21*, 247–260. **Figure 3.22:** From Poss, R. (1992). *Natural factors that affect the shape and strength of the aging human femur*. Philadelphia, PA: J. B. Lippincott Co. Reprinted by permission. **Figure 3.24:** Courtesy of Body Comp, Inc. **Figure 3.25:** Adapted from Brooks, G. A., & Fahey, T. D. (1984). *Exercise physiology: Human bioenergetics and its applications*. New York, NY: Wiley. **Figure 3.26:** Adapted from Malina, R. M., & Bouchard, C. (1991). *Growth, maturation, and physical activity*. Champaign, IL: Human Kinetics. **Figure 3.27:** Adapted from Malina, R. M., & Bouchard, C. (1991). *Growth, maturation, and physical activity*. Champaign, IL: Human Kinetics. **Figure 3.28:** From Tanner, J. M. (1990). *Fetus into man: Physical growth from conception to maturity*. Cambridge, MA: Harvard University Press. **Figure 3.29:** Tanner, J. M. (1990). *Fetus into man: Physical growth from conception to maturity*. Cambridge, MA: Harvard University Press. **Figure 3.30:** Courtesy of University of California, Los Angeles Radnet. **Figure 3.31:** Adapted from Roche, A. F. (1979). Secular trends in stature, weight, and maturation. *Monographs of the Society for Research in Child Development*, 44(3–4), 3–27.

CHAPTER 4

Table 4.1: From Pollock, M. L., Wilmore, J. H., & Fox, S. M. (1978). *Health and fitness through physical activity*. New York, NY: Wiley. Copyright © 1978 John Wiley & Sons, Inc., New York. **Table 4.2:** Data recalculated from Lowrey, G. H. (1986). *Growth and development of children* (8th ed.). Chicago, IL: Year Book Medical; and Pollock, M. L., Wilmore, J. H., & Fox, S. M. (1978). *Health and fitness through physical activity*. New York, NY: Wiley. **Figure 4.5:** From Ferris, B. G., Jr., Whittenberger, J. L., & Gallagher, J. R. (1952). Maximum breathing capacity and vital capacity of male children and adolescents. *Pediatrics, 9*, 659–670. Copyright © 1952 and Ferris, B. G., Jr., & Smith, C. W. (1953). Maximum breathing capacity and vital capacity in female children and adolescents. *Pediatrics, 12*, 341–352. Copyright © 1953. Reproduced by permission of the American Academy of Pediatrics, Elk Grove Village, IL. **Figure 4.6:** Copyright: Mikkel Bigandt/Shutterstock. **Figure 4.9:** Adapted from Eckert, H. M. (1987). *Motor development* (3rd ed.). Indianapolis, IN: Benchmark Press. **Figure 4.10:** Adapted from Eckert, H. M. (1987). *Motor development* (3rd ed.). Indianapolis, IN: Benchmark Press. **Figure 4.11:** As reported by Ross, J. G., & Gilbert, G. G. (1985). The National Children and Youth Fitness Study: A summary of findings. *Journal of Physical Education, Recreation, & Dance, 56*(1), 45–50; and Ross, J. G., & Pate, R. R. (1987). The National Children and Youth Fitness Study II: A summary of findings. *Journal of Physical Education, Recreation, & Dance, 5*(9), 51–56. **Figure 4.14:** Adapted from Metter, E. J., Conwit, R., Tobin, J., & Fozard, J. L. (1997). Age-associated loss of power and strength in the upper extremities in women and men. *The Journals of Gerontology Series A. Biological Sciences and Medical Sciences, 52*(5), B267–B276.

CHAPTER 5

Figure 5.1: From Tecklin, J. S. (1998). *Pediatric physical therapy* (3rd ed.). Philadelphia, PA: Lippincott Williams & Wilkins. Copyright © Wolters Kluwer. **Focus on Application, p. 131:** Copyright: Flashon Studio/Shutterstock. **Figure 5.3:** Courtesy of Kjetil Kolbjornsrud/Shutterstock. **Focus on Application, p. 143:** Courtesy of bikeriderlondon/Shutterstock.

CHAPTER 6

Figure 6.3: Courtesy of Rubberball/Jupiter Images. **Figure 6.4:** George Zimbel. **Figure 6.6:** Courtesy of William Vandivert. **Figure 6.7:** Courtesy of blessings/Shutterstock. **Figure 6.8:** Courtesy of Karen E. Adolph. **Figure 6.9:** Courtesy of mike mols/Shutterstock.

CHAPTER 7

Figure 7.3: Courtesy of Carolyn Rovee-Collier, Rutgers University. **Figure 7.4:** From Hodgkins, J. (1962). Influence of age on the speed of reaction and movement in females. *Journal of Gerontology, 17*, 385–389. Copyright 1962 Gerontology Society of America. Reprinted by permission. **Figure 7.5:** Courtesy of Revenant/Shutterstock. **Figure 7.7:** Mark H. Johnson/ Department of Psychology, Birkbeck College, London, United Kingdom. **Figure 7.8:** Courtesy of Steve Wewerka/Impact Visuals. **Figure 7.10:** From Welford, T. A. (1977). Causes of slowing of performance with age. *Interdisciplinary Topics in Gerontology, 11, 46*. Copyright 1977 by S. Karger AG, Basel. Reprinted by permission.

CHAPTER 8

Table 8.1: Data from Forfar, J. O., & Arneil, G. C. (Eds.). (2003). *Textbook of pediatrics* (6th ed.). London, United Kingdom: Churchill Livingstone. **Figure 8.1:** From MacDonald, M. G., & Seshia, M. M. K. (2015). *Avery's neonatology* (7th ed.). Philadelphia, PA: Wolters Kluwer. Copyright © Wolters Kluwer. **Figure 8.2:** From Ricci, S. S., Kyle, T., & Carman, S. (2012). *Maternity and pediatric nursing* (2nd ed.). Philadelphia, PA: Wolters Kluwer. Copyright © Wolters Kluwer. **Figure 8.4:** Ricci, S. S. (2012). *Essentials of maternity, newborn, and women's health nursing* (3rd ed.). Philadelphia, PA: Wolters Kluwer. Copyright © Wolters Kluwer. **Figure 8.9:** From Pillitteri, A. (2013). *Maternal and child health nursing* (7th ed.). Philadelphia, PA: Wolters Kluwer. Copyright © Wolters Kluwer. **Figure 8.10:** AnikaNes/Shutterstock. **Focus on Application, p. 231:** Courtesy of wong sze yuen/Shutterstock. **Figure 8.14:** Courtesy of NatalieJean/Shutterstock. **Figure 8.17:** From *Experiment* by Thelen and Ulrich. Reprinted by permission of Esther Thelen. **Figure 8.19:** Courtesy of Amy Needham, Peabody College, Vanderbilt University.

CHAPTER 9

Figure 9.21: Courtesy of CroMary/Shutterstock. **Figure 9.24:** Courtesy of Soloviova Liudmyla/Shutterstock.

CHAPTER 10

Figure 10.6: From Thomas, J. R. (1984). *Motor development during childhood & adolescence*. Minneapolis, MN: Burgess Publishing. Data from Halverson, L., Roberton, M. A., & Langendorfer, S. (1982). Development of the overarm throw movement and ball velocity changes by 7th grade. *Research Quarterly for Exercise & Sport, 53*(3), 198–205. Reprinted by permission of Jerry R. Thomas. **Figure 10.9:** Courtesy of Monkey Business Images/Shutterstock. **Figure 10.10:** Courtesy of bikeriderlondon/Shutterstock. **Figure 10.11:** Courtesy of Sergey Novikov/Shutterstock. **Figure 10.12:** Courtesy of Robert Kneschke/Shutterstock.

CHAPTER 11

Figure 11.4: From Hodgkins, J. (1962). Influence of age on the speed of reaction and movement in females. *Journal of Gerontology, 17*, 385–389. Copyright © 1962 Gerontology Society of America. Reprinted by permission. **Figure 11.5:** From Smith, E. L., & Serfass, R. C. (Eds.), *Exercise and aging: The scientific basis*. Hillside, NJ: Enslow Publisher. Copyright © 1981 Enslow Publishers. Reprinted by permission. **Figure 11.9:** Courtesy of Stephen Rudolph/ Shutterstock. **Figure 11.10:** Courtesy of Robert Kneschke/ Shutterstock. **Focus on Application, p. 331:** Courtesy of Pascal Parrot/Corbis. **Figure 11.11:** Courtesy of Lisa S./ Shutterstock.

CHAPTER 12

Figure 12.1: Courtesy of Denis Kuvaev/Shutterstock. **Figure 12.2:** Courtesy of Juriah Mosin/Shutterstock.

CHAPTER 13

Figure 13.2: Courtesy of TRAIMAK/Shutterstock.

CHAPTER 14

Figure 14.2: From Williamson, P. (2011). *Exercise for special populations*. Philadelphia, PA: Wolters Kluwer. Copyright © Wolters Kluwer. **Focus on Application, p. 377:** Courtesy of Dmitry Naumov/Shutterstock. **Figure 14.3:** From Escott-Stump, S. (2016). *Nutrition and diagnosis-related care* (8th ed.). Philadelphia, PA: Wolters Kluwer. Copyright © Wolters Kluwer. **Figure 14.4:** Courtesy of bikeriderlondon/Shutterstock. **Figure 14.5:** Courtesy of Lisa S./Shutterstock.

Page references followed by *fig* indicate illustrated *fig*ures; followed by "t" indicate tables.

D

H

N